Nursing the Infant, Child & Adolescent

INTERACTIONS AND CARE

Volume 1

PART 1
Growth and Development: Body, Mind, Relationships and Emotions
PART 2
Alterations to Health in Infancy, Childhood and Adolescence

Anne Adams

RN BA MA DNE Cert Paed N FRCNA FCN(NSW)

Senior Lecturer, Faculty of Nursing
University of Technology, Sydney

Carmel Mcllin

RN Dip Teach (Nurs) BHS(Nurs) Cardio-Thoracic Nurs
Cert Acute Care Nurs CN(NSW)
Co-ordinator, Graduate Certifica atric Nursing Course
Woden Valley ACT

Sue y

RN PhD F N(NSW)

Professor ic Nursing
University rn Sydney
and Royal Alexandra Hospital for Children, Sydney

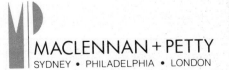

MACLENNAN+PETTY
SYDNEY • PHILADELPHIA • LONDON

First published 1996

MacLennan & Petty Pty Limited
809–821 Botany Road, Rosebery, Sydney NSW 2018 Australia

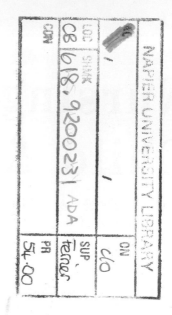

National Library of Australia
Cataloguing-in-Publication data:

Nursing the infant, child & adolescent: interactions and care.

Bibliography.

Includes index.

ISBN 0 86433 126 6.
ISBN 0 86433 105 3 (v. 1).
ISBN 0 86433 124 X (v. 2).

1. Teenagers — Medical care.   2. Pediatric nursing.
I. McQuellin, Carmel.   II. Adams, Anne, 1940– .   III. Nagy, Sue.
610.7362

Printed and bound in Australia

The authors, editors and publisher have done everything possible to make this book accurate, up to
date and in accord with accepted standards at the time of publication. They, however, are not
responsible for errors or omissions or for consequences arising from the use of the book. Information
in this book should be applied by the reader in accordance with professional standards of care
relevant to individual circumstances.

NOTE FROM THE PUBLISHER

In consideration of the range of readership and for ease of handling,
Nursing the Infant, Child & Adolescent is published in two volumes.

Volume 1 consists of PART ONE *Growth and Development: Body, Mind,
Relationships and Emotions* and PART TWO *Alterations to Health in Infancy,
Childhood and Adolescence* (ISBN 0–86433–105–3).

Volume 2 consists of PART THREE *Alterations to Health in Infancy,
Childhood and Adolescence: Special Problems* (ISBN 0–86433–124–X).

Page, table and figure numbers run continuously through the two volumes
and both contain the complete Contents, Appendices and Index.

Dedication

To

the many children and their families who have given our
endeavours purpose and meaning

and

to paediatric nurses everywhere who through their
commitment, sensitivity, optimism and capacity for joy
continue to make differences in the lives of others

Editors and Contributors

Anne Adams RN BA MA DNE Cert Paed N FRCNA FCN(NSW)
Senior lecturer, Faculty of Nursing
The University of Technology, Sydney

Gail Anderson RN CM BN Grad Dip Child Health Nursing, Adolescent Mental Health Certificate, MCN(NSW)
Clinical Nurse Consultant,
Adolescent Health
Westmead Hospital NSW

Jennifer Backhouse RN CM Grad Dip Child Health Nursing
Children's ward
Hills Private Hospital, Sydney

Julie Bleasdale RN
formerly Clinical Nurse Specialist
Royal Alexandra Hospital for Children,
Sydney

Katrina Brereton RN MRN ND
Pain Management Nurse Consultant
Royal Children's Hospital, Melbourne

Lynne Brodie RN BA Cert Paed N MRN
Nursing Unit Manager
Royal Alexandra Hospital for Children,
Sydney

Kim Burke RN LLB
Barrister-at-Law, formerly Clinical
Nurse Consultant, Oncology
Royal Alexandra Hospital for Children,
Sydney

Sue Casanelia RN BN Grad Dip Adv Nsg(Comm Hlth) Cert in Genetic Counselling
Genetics Department
Royal Children's Hospital, Melbourne

Kuei Meei Chen RN
Clinical Nurse Specialist
Royal Children's Hospital, Melbourne

Patricia Comerford RN BN Cert Paed N
formerly Nurse Unit Manager
Department of Paediatrics
John Hunter Hospital, Newcastle NSW

Marilyn Cruickshank RN BA(Hons) Neuro Cert PICU Cert FCN(NSW) FRCNA
Clinical Nurse Consultant
The Prince of Wales Children's
Hospital, Sydney

Victoria Cullins RN BN Cert NIC
Clinical Nurse Educator
Christchurch Women's Hospital,
New Zealand

Helen Dickinson RN
Clinical Nurse Specialist
Royal Children's Hospital, Melbourne

Laurence Dubourg RN Grad Dip Neuro Cert
Neuro Unit Manager — Nursing
Royal Children's Hospital, Melbourne

Jill Farquhar RN BHS(Nurs) Renal Certificate
Clinical Nurse Consultant
Renal Treatment Centre
Royal Alexandra Hospital for Children, Sydney

Glenys Goodwin RN CM PICU Cert Occ Health Management Cert IBCLC
formerly Clinical Nurse Consultant
Home Ventilation/Oxygen Support Program
Royal Alexandra Hospital for Children, Sydney

Maurice Hennessy RN RSCN B AppSci Ad Nsg(Ed)
Nurse Educator
Royal Children's Hospital, Melbourne

Angela Jones RN BEd Grad Dip Neurosciences CNRN
Case Manager — Neurosciences
The George Washington University Medical Center, Washington DC

Tina Kendrick RN BN MN PICU Cert FCN(NSW)
formerly Nurse Educator, Intensive Care
Royal Alexandra Hospital for Children, Sydney

John Leach RN Grad Dip Nurs Mgt Cert Paed N
formerly Nurse Unit Manager
Isolation ward/infectious diseases
Royal Alexandra Hospital for Children, Sydney

Paul Longridge RN Dip N
Clinical Nurse Specialist
Royal Children's Hospital, Melbourne

Jane Lush RN
Registered Nurse
Royal Children's Hospital, Melbourne

Carmel McQuellin RN BHS(Nurs) Dip Teach(Nurs) Cert Paed Cardio-thoracic N Cert Acute Care N MRCNA MCN(NSW)
Co-ordinator, Graduate Certificate in Paediatric Nursing Course
Woden Valley Hospital, Canberra ACT

Irene Mitchelhill RN, RMN, BHS(Nurs), Cert Paed & Child & Family Health
Clinical Nurse Consultant — Paediatric Endocrinology
Prince of Wales Children's Hospital, Sydney

Jill Molan RN BA Dip Ed(Nurs) Cert Opth N
formerly Course Co-ordinator
NSW College of Nursing

Sue Nagy RN PhD FRCNA FCN(NSW)
Professor of Paediatric Nursing
University of Western Sydney
and Royal Alexandra Hospital
for Children, Sydney

Gill Patterson RN MN Cert Paed N
Nurse Unit Manager
Royal Alexandra Hospital for Children, Sydney

Robyn Pedersen RN RM BA(Hons)
Certified Genetic Counsellor (HGSA)
Clinical Nurse Consultant (Genetics)
Prince of Wales Children's Hospital, Sydney

Mary Perisanidis-Douros RN Dip N
Clinical Nurse Specialist
Royal Children's Hospital, Melbourne

Helen Sharp RN BN Cert Paed N
Clinical Nurse Specialist
Royal Alexandra Hospital for Children, Sydney

Kaye Spence RN CM BEd(N) Cert NIC Cert Paed N MRCNA
Clinical Nurse Consultant, Neonatology
Royal Alexandra Hospital for Children, Sydney

David Sutton RN BHS(Nurs)
Associate Charge Nurse
Royal Children's Hospital, Melbourne

Lean Muar Tan RN BN MN
Registered Nurse
Royal Alexandra Hospital for Children, Sydney

Isobel Taylor RN Dip Teach(Nurs) Orth Cert
Lecturer, Faculty of Nursing
University of Sydney

Sandy Wales RN Cert Paed N
Clinical Nurse Specialist (Asthma Resource Nurse)
Prince of Wales Children's Hospital, Sydney

Margaret Yates RN Dip Teach(Nurs)
formerly Paediatric Nurse Educator
John Hunter Hospital, Newcastle NSW

Contents

PART ONE   Growth and Development: Body, Mind, Relationships and Emotions

**PART TWO   Alterations to Health in Infancy, Childhood and
Adolescence**

Forewords

I

The care of the sick child has seen many changes since the inception of the first hospitals for the care of sick children in Australia between 1870 and 1880. The evolution and development of nursing knowledge that is distinctly paediatric nursing is readily seen within the collective writings of this book.

Paediatric nursing is a discipline which builds upon the knowledge of the normal child as a basis for care and caring. It is therefore a tribute to the writers that the foundation of the text is that of growth and development, body and mind, relationships and emotions.

Keeping children healthy is more than nursing practice within the hospital. The writers of this book have given us to understand a function of wellness through health management, which includes the avoidance of infectious diseases through adequate and timely immunisation programs. The concept of health promotion extends the role of the paediatric nurse beyond the early aspirations of a nurse to care for sick children to that of a nurse caring for a child in illness and in health.

Care of the paediatric patient today requires a nurse who is a skilled professional member of a health team, able to keep pace with technical and scientific changes. The challenge is to acquire not only the technical skills of caring but a highly developed power of accurate observation which together with the knowledge of growth and development makes the nurse who cares for the child a specialist within the broader category of nursing.

Paediatric nursing practice, in keeping pace with changes in health service delivery, has recognised that while the majority of paediatric nurses continue to practise within a hospital there is an increasing need to support the child and family within their home. Every nurse must become familiar with teaching of patient, parents and the community at large to keep the continuity of care.

The challenge to paediatric nursing today is not the limitation of a nurse practising within a specialty, it is the opportunity for a nurse who has a responsibility of providing care for the infant, child and adolescent to influence the health of successive generations.

A defined paediatric nursing text written and edited by Australian nurses which, drawing on the knowledge of the nurse in clinical paediatric practice, embraces this challenge, is to be commended.

Jan Y. Minnis
Director of Nursing
Royal Alexandra Hospital for Children
Sydney

II

The paediatric nurse of the 1990s is a sophisticated clinician working as part of the health care team. The changing patterns of childhood disease and the focus of health promotion and maintenance are altering the way that nurses practise. The specialist paediatric nurse functions as clinical expert, educator of other staff and the family, role model, resource person and change agent. There has also been a change in community expectations of care and an explosion of knowledge and technology which contribute to a rapidly changing and increasingly complex health environment. Owing to the rapidity of change in the health sector, we need paediatric nurses who are well informed, open to change, capable of moving freely between practice settings and able to meet the needs of diverse cultural populations.

The changes in the focus and delivery of nursing care are also reflected in a broader educational preparation for nurses. However, in a bid to cover the breadth of clinical practice, nursing practice is often represented in a fragmented fashion to students of nursing. This may impede the development of an holistic understanding of, and approach to, the child and family with multiple needs for care. The demand for nurses with advanced clinical knowledge and skills imposes an imperative for quality educational activities and resources to foster and support competency in the nursing work force.

An effort has been made over the last decade to return care and caring to their essential places in nursing practice and education. Benner[1], who has written widely on the subject of practice, believed in the transformation of nursing practice through the exploration of the meaning of nursing. She also believed that nursing is a practice-based discipline with a knowledge base which should derive from and be explored through practice.

The editors are to be congratulated on their efforts in bringing together the clinical expertise of nurses caring for children in the Australian context. **Nursing the Infant, Child & Adolescent** aims to present a view of paediatric nursing which is practice-based. It is designed to meet the needs of all general and specialist nurses in the paediatric area. The book is a significant development in the history of nursing in Australia and encourages each learner to look beyond the immediate appearances in a nursing situation to consider medical, social, personal and other relationships.

Sandra Willis
Principal Nurse Educator
Mackinnon School of Nursing
Royal Children's Hospital
Melbourne

1. Benner, P. *From Novice to Expert: Excellence and Power in Clinical Nursing Practice*, Menlo Park: Addison Wesley, 1984.

Preface

The thinking in producing a text about the nursing care of infants, children, adolescents and their families began with the idea that a text written by nurses who could draw on their expert knowledge and experience in the Australian context would be a valuable resource and make a contribution to the practice of nurses who care for infants, children and adolescents in a range of settings. The editors were convinced that such a text was timely and have been encouraged throughout its production by the many expressions of affirmation for this work. Since that first idea was formed, the text has taken on a momentum of its own, reminiscent of the processes of growth and development. In content, there has been a steady growth in the scope and number of contributions and the detail within each section.

The content of the text has been arranged in three main parts in order to achieve a logical sequence. The first part is concerned with healthy growth and development and the management of health needs from birth to adolescence. Those alterations to health which nurses can expect to encounter in their care of infants, children and adolescents and the nursing management of such alterations are the concern of the second section. The third section is concerned with special problems which require highly specialised nursing. The content of the text is designed to meet the range of needs and interests of readers.

We are conscious that while the contributions in the text cover many topics there are some we have not been able to include. There is, however, a commitment to nursing throughout the text. Knowledge is presented as the basis for care and nursing management is the focus within each topic.

It is our belief that the text will be a useful source of information and a contribution to good practice in paediatric nursing.

The editors have been helped in their task in bringing this text to fruition. We are deeply grateful for the support, encouragement and direction we have received from Jenny Curtis. Her patience and constancy have sustained us. Jeremy Fisher has been a friend to the project and his positive approach is appreciated. We have been impressed by the efforts and perseverance of the many contributors and applaud their determination through numerous drafts and requests. We record our thanks for their efforts and commitment.

Anne Adams

Carmel McQuellin

Sue Nagy

GROWTH AND DEVELOPMENT: BODY, MIND, RELATIONSHIPS AND EMOTIONS

The growth and development of the child, from birth to maturity, is complex and dynamic. Growth is defined as the observable physical increase and change in the child's body; development refers to the continued and orderly increase in the child's functions and abilities. While, for convenience, growth and development are discussed separately in some parts of this section, it is emphasised that the progressive changes in body and mind, social and emotional experience are closely intertwined. It is their interrelatedness and their orderly progress which, over time, results in the ultimate maturity of the individual.

Part One concerns the healthy and anticipated growth and development of young individuals as newborns, infants, toddlers, pre-schoolers, school-age children and adolescents. The chapters in Part One are organised in sequence according to these stages with the aim of presenting the necessary information for nursing assessment of the healthy growth and development of the child.

Each chapter in Part One is organised according to physical growth and development, cognitive, social and emotional development. A section on the health management of the growing and developing child is included. It is hoped that such organisation makes for a logical flow of material and the easy location of content.

Chapter 1

Growth and Development: Birth to 18 Months

Physical Growth and Development

Anne Adams

ASSESSMENT OF NEWBORNS AND INFANTS

Growth and development before birth

Assessment of the newborn and young infant relies in part on knowledge of growth and development before birth. Development begins at conception and continues over the following 40 weeks. Stages within the 40 weeks of pregnancy have been defined according to age and development. In the 1st week or so, the zygote undergoes a series of cell divisions and then implants in the endometrium. The embryonic and fetal periods follow. During the embryonic period (until the end of the 8th week) the embryo undergoes rapid cell division, multiplication and differentiation. Tissues differentiate into organs and the body systems are organised. By 4 weeks the heart is beating and at 6 weeks the circulation is formed. At the end of the embryonic period the beginnings of all the main structures and systems exist. During the fetal period, from the 9th week to birth, these structures and systems undergo further growth and development. The rate of growth is rapid, particularly between the 3rd and 4th months, while the gain in weight is most marked in the final weeks before birth.[1,2]

Factors which influence the development of the embryo and fetus include the calibre of the ovum and sperm and the subsequent genetic inheritance, intrauterine conditions, maternal nutrition and exposure to harmful agents. Critical periods when the organism is particularly sensitive to the effects of harmful agents or teratogens, such as chemicals or viral organisms, are during the embryonic period when cellular differentiation leading to organ formation occurs. For example, 3 weeks after conception there is a potential for limb malformation, at 4 to 5 weeks oomphalocele and tracheoesophageal fistula may be precipitated, at 6 weeks cleft lip may occur while cleft palate and ventricular septal defects may form at 7 weeks.[2]

Physical assessment of the newborn

Early physical assessment of the newborn is carried out according to the Apgar scoring system. The newborn is scored at 1 minute after birth and again at 5 minutes. Scores of 0, 1 or 2 are made on 5 dimensions. These dimensions are heart rate, respiratory effort,

3

Table 1.1 Assessment of the newborn: the Apgar scoring system

	0	1	2
Heart rate	absent	slow (below 100)	over 100
Respiratory effort	absent	slow, irregular	good cry
Muscle tone	limp	some flexion of extremities	well flexed
Reflex response	no response	grimace	angry cry
Colour	blue, pale	body pink, extremities blue	completely pink

Modified from V Apgar, 1966[4]

muscle tone, reflex irritability and colour (**Table 1.1**). A total score of 10 across the 5 dimensions is optimal; between 7 and 10, satisfactory; between 4 and 6, a moderate difficulty in adjusting to extrauterine life; and below 4, the newborn is in severe distress. The score at 1 minute is usually lower than the score at 5 minutes, reflecting the physiological depression which is present immediately after birth.[3]

The heart rate is taken with a stethoscope at the apex and is correlated with the activity of the newborn. The respiratory rate is assessed by auscultation over a full minute. Muscle tone is determined by attempting to straighten the limbs. Reflex response is tested by flicking the sole of the foot or by briskly rubbing the back. Colour is observed over the whole body, extremities and within the mouth.[2,3,5]

During a physical examination the newborn and infant will be handled and coverings and clothing removed. Because body heat is easily lost it is important that the infant is examined in an atmosphere where cooling will not occur and coverings and clothing are removed for the minimum time. Only the area to be assessed is exposed. While hand washing precedes the assessment procedures, it is also important that the assessor's hands are warm. The infant should be touched and handled in a gentle manner, using smooth movements and supporting the head as the infant is moved. A soft, low voice is soothing. Procedures are best organised in a sequence so that the least disturbing or uncomfortable are carried out before those which are more so. A physical assessment should not be drawn out and all equipment should be readily at hand before the assessment begins.

MUSCULOSKELETAL SYSTEM

At birth the skeletal system is comprised more of cartilage than ossified bone, though shortly after birth ossification commences. The complement of muscle fibres is present at birth, having developed during gestation. Muscle growth after birth increases size rather than the number of fibres.[5]

Musculoskeletal assessment in the well newborn is based on the appearance of skeletal structures such as limbs, the contour and tone of muscles and the measurement of weight, height and head circumference. The assessment of muscle tone and head circumference is discussed in nervous system assessment. Weight for height measures give a correlated assessment of these growth measurements and are recommended. Even if the measurements are charted separately, reference to each will give a more accurate picture of the infant's growth and progress. To monitor growth during infancy, measurements of weight, length and head circumference should be taken at birth and 6 weeks. At 3 months, 6 months and 18 months, further measurements of weight and length are recommended.[6]

Posture

The newborn is typically in a position of flexion with the arms and legs flexed close to the body. The head and vertebral column are also flexed with the chin touching the upper chest and the spine held in a rounded shape. When the neonate is placed prone the spine appears straight and flat. At 3 months, with the development of head control, a further convex forward spinal curve develops in the cervical region. In keeping with the ability to sit and walk, a convex lumbar curve forms between 12 and 18 months.[2,5,7-9]

Joints and limbs

The limbs, shoulders and hips of the newborn and infant are symmetrical and joints firm but moveable. Feet are positioned in the midline or can easily be manipulated to the midline, even if they appear to turn inward.[2] Soles are usually flat. Hip joints are assessed for correct placement and that the femoral head is in the acetabulum. With the infant supine, legs are straightened and the level position of the knees and heels is noted. Legs are lifted to 90° and thigh creases and labia are inspected. The number of creases should be equal and the labia will appear in the midline. When the knees are bent and the feet placed flat, the knees should be level. Thigh creases, gluteal folds and the level position of knees and feet are further inspected with the infant in the prone position. With the infant supine, both legs are held at the knees and the thighs flexed to 90°. The thighs are fully abducted with very gentle backwards pressure. Any click, jerk or clunk is noted. This is the **Barlow test**. The **Ortolani test** may also be carried out. One leg at a time is held at the knee, flexed to 90°, the examiner's thumb over the lesser trochanter, the middle finger over the greater trochanter and the pelvis steadied by the other hand. The flexed thigh is abducted and adducted. During abduction the femur is gently rocked backwards and forwards on the pelvis and any movement noted. Again, any click, jerk or clunk as the head of the femur moves in or out of the acetabulum is noted.[5,10] Assessment of the hips using the Barlow and Ortolani tests should not be performed too vigorously in the 1st 2 days of life as the hip subluxes freely, and persistent dislocations can result. Tests should be carried out by those with experience[5] and training in order to distinguish between a harmless 'click', present in 5% to 10% of newborns, and the 'clunk' of the dislocated hip.[11] After 10 weeks the Ortolani sign disappears and the hips are then tested for limited abduction. Examination of the hips is carried out at birth, 6 weeks, 6 months and 12 months.[6,12]

Muscles and movement

The development of muscle groups and the quality of an infant's movements are important indicators of satisfactory musculoskeletal growth and development. The Meade Movement Checklist is used to screen young infants at four months for muscle development. The infant is observed in a range of positions for movement skills. The Meade Movement Checklist aims to determine muscle development before milestones are reached and detect problems before movement patterns are established.[13]

Weight

An assessment of the musculoskeletal system in the newborn will include weight and length measurements. These measurements reflect musculoskeletal growth and development and provide a baseline for the growth which will follow.

Birthweight is generally between 3 and 4 kg with the average for boys 3400 g and for girls 3200 g.[8] Newborns lose 5% to 10% of their birthweight in the 1st few days, but will have regained their birthweight by the 10th day. From birth to 6 months the average weekly gain is 150 to 210 g and from 6 to 18 months, 90 to 150 g.[5] Birthweight is usually doubled by 4 to 6 months and tripled at 12 months (Appendix A).[7]

Ideally, the infant is weighed without clothing. When this is not practicable, garments of similar weight should be worn for each weighing. If the infant's weight is to be carefully monitored, the measurement should be taken at the same time each day and with reference to the last feeding. It is also advisable to use the same weighing device. Before placing the infant on the scales, place a napkin or soft lining on the tray of the scales. Paper is sometimes used. The weight of the material is calculated and subtracted from the infant's weight or the scale is set on zero after the lining is placed on the tray. The scales may need to be balanced or calibrated. The infant is not touched at the moment of reading the weight, but by keeping a hand in position directly over the infant the nurse offers protection against an unexpected movement or fall. An infant is never left unattended on scales, even for a moment.

Length

Length from head to heel at birth is generally 48 to 53 cm. The average length for girls is 49.9 cm and for boys 50.5 cm. The crown to rump length (or sitting height) is sometimes used as a comparison with head circumference in the newborn. The 2 measurements are close to equal, with the crown to rump length ranging from 31 to 35 cm. From birth to 6 months body length increases at an average of 2.5 cm each month. The rate of growth in length slows to a monthly average of 1.25 cm between 6 and 18 months. At 12 months the length is about 50% greater than the length at birth (Appendix A).[5,8,10]

The length of the infant is measured with the infant supine, the head held straight with the crown touching a firm vertical surface. The legs are straightened and extended by gently pressing on the knees while the feet are held at a 90° angle. The distance from the top of the head to the heels is measured. It is recommended that the child be gently stretched using lengthwise traction applied by a second observer in order to obtain an accurate supine length measurement.[14] A measuring board with a sliding foot board is a useful device. If a tape is used, it should be made of non-stretch material.

Head

The head of the neonate and infant should be observed for shape and symmetry. Moulding of the head during birth may result in minor asymmetry, which has usually resolved by 4 months. The head is able to move freely in all directions, even though the neck is very short and creased with a number of skin folds.[2]

Head circumference at term averages 35 cm with a range of 32.5 to 36.5 cm.[15] There is an average increase of 2 cm per month in the 1st 3 months, 1 cm per month from 4 to 6 months and 0.5 cm per month from 6 to 12 months (Appendix A).[16] It is recommended that head circumference measures be taken at birth, 7 days and 6 weeks.[6]

The head is measured by placing a non-stretch tape around the area of greatest dimension commencing at the lower forehead just above the eyebrows and passing the tape over the pinnae and around the occiput. The head circumference measurement can be compared with the chest circumference for a relative estimation of growth. The chest circumference of the newborn is usually about 2–3 cm greater than the head circumference. By approximately 12 months the head and chest circumferences are equal.

The sutures of the neonate's head are felt as distinct ridges and may have overridden through moulding during birth. The suture lines will usually have flattened by 6 months. There are 6 fontanelles, but usually only the anterior and the posterior fontanelles are examined. They are flat or slightly concave, soft and can be seen to pulsate. The anterior fontanelle is diamond shaped and until 9 to 12 months measures from 1–5 cm in length and width. The posterior fontanelle closes at about 3 months and the anterior fontanelle is closed by 18 months.

Length, weight and head circumference measurements are recorded and graphed over time. Percentile charts which show expected growth within an established range are used for comparative reference and for the plotting of an individual infant's progress. (Appendix A)

NERVOUS SYSTEM

In the 1st weeks of the embryonic period the neural tube forms. This structure becomes the spinal canal and the ventricles of the brain. At 4 weeks parts of the neural tube close to form the brain and the spinal cord. By 5 weeks neuroblasts have differentiated to form the brain and the cranial nerves are present. Primitive nervous reflex activity is evident by 7 or 8 weeks. The ears develop mainly between 4 and 8 weeks while the structures of the eyes have developed by the 7th week. Nervous tissue, particularly the brain, is vulnerable to the effects of teratogenic agents in the critical period from the 10th to 30th days. The eye is susceptible to the effects of harmful agents between the 18th and 30th days. By 20 weeks myelination of the spinal cord has begun and at 28 weeks the nervous system is capable of regulating some functions.[2,17]

The nervous system continues to develop in infancy. Even though the full complement of nerve cells is present at birth, neurones continue to increase in size. Glial cells increase in size and number until about 4 years, while the dendrites increase in number and branchings and the axons in length. Myelination continues in infancy with the fibre tracts, in general, becoming myelinated in step with functional development. The brain increases rapidly in size from 325 g at birth to approximately 1000 g by 1 year.[1,7]

Reflexes

Reflex actions, which are not voluntarily controlled, are used to assess neurological status.

The **Moro reflex** is elicited by a sudden movement or change in equilibrium. To evoke the reflex the infant is firstly held and supported while lying on its back. The infant's head is allowed to extend by suddenly releasing support or the infant is lowered abruptly for about 15 cm. The infant responds with sudden abduction and extension of the arms with fanning of the fingers. The index finger and thumb form the shape of a C. The arms then adduct to the centre of body in an embrace-like movement with the hands clenched. Extension of the spine and legs occurs and may be followed by weak flexion of the legs. The infant may cry. There is a slow return to the flexed position. The Moro reflex is symmetrical, is usually strongest during the 1st 8 weeks and disappears by about 6 months.

The **startle reflex** is sometimes considered to be the same reflex as the Moro reflex. Following a loud noise or a sudden stimulus the arms abduct with flexion of the elbows. The hands remain clenched and the infant usually cries.

The **asymmetric tonic neck reflex** occurs when the infant's head is extended quickly to one side. The arm and leg on the same side will extend while the arm and leg on the other side will flex. This response is sometimes referred to as the 'fencing position' and prevents the infant from rolling over. It usually disappears by about 4 months.

The **grasp reflex** occurs both in hands and feet. When a finger or object is placed across the infant's palm at the base of the digits the palmar grasp reflex is elicited. The infant will grasp the object tightly and maintain the grip as he is pulled upwards. The strength of the grasp should be equal in both hands. The palmar grasp reflex decreases gradually and is weaker by about 3 months of age. The plantar grasp reflex occurs when pressure is applied to the soles of the feet at the base of the digits. The infant's toes will simultaneously flex. The plantar grasp reflex disappears by 12 months.

The **walking reflex** is elicited when the infant is held in an upright position with the soles of the feet placed on a firm surface. Rhythmic stepping-type movements will occur. The walking reflex is also known as the dance or step reflex and is lost after 2 months.

The **sucking reflex** is demonstrated when the infant responds with strong rhythmic sucking movements to the stimulus of a nipple or finger inserted into the mouth.

The **rooting reflex** is elicited with a light touch to one cheek near the mouth. The infant will turn towards the stimulus, the bottom lip lowers and sucking movements begin. The reflex usually disappears at about 4 months, but may persist for 12 months.

Gross motor skills

The movements of the newborn and infant will be symmetric, smooth and purposeful. The amount and range of limb movements will be equal on each side. While some jerkiness will be seen at times, especially in newborns, the body movements during infancy are smooth and become more so as the infant matures. Infants, even newborns, are able to make purposeful movements such as pulling away from an aversive stimulus or putting the fist in the mouth.[8]

The newborn can lift and turn the head from side to side when prone and can hold the head momentarily in line with the trunk when held horizontally in the prone position. There will be marked head lag, however, when the infant is pulled forward into a sitting position. Head lag diminishes until, at 3 months, it is minimal and the infant can hold the head with good control. At 2 months, the infant can raise his head to 45° when prone and by 3 months can raise the head by 90°. The infant can raise the head, chest and upper abdomen by 6 months and by 7 months can support the upper part of the body while bearing weight with one hand.

The infant is usually not able to roll from back to side until 4 months, but occasionally the younger infant may roll because of the rounded back. By 5 months the infant can roll from the abdomen to the back and by 6 months from the back to the abdomen.

As the back straightens the infant is able to sit, initially at 5 months with support, by 7 months alone and by 8 months alone and unaided.

Crawling can begin at 6 months with backward movements accomplished by pushing with both hands. Crawling, which may be backward at first, is often achieved by 9 months while forward crawling is usually established by 10 months. Standing follows the ability to bear weight on both legs which usually occurs at about 8 months. By 9 months the infant can pull himself into a standing position and remain standing while holding onto furniture. Walking with support or holding onto furniture is usually established by 11 months with independent walking established at 12 or 13 months. By 18 months walking up stairs while holding a hand and clumsy running is achieved.[5,8,10]

Fine motor skills

The hands of the newborn are tightly clenched with the thumb tucked under the folded fingers most of the time, though the hands will open and close at times, especially during feeding or when the back of the hand is stroked. By 3 months the hands are open most of the time and the infant will swipe at objects. The ability to hold an object placed in the hand and to reach for objects has been gained by about 4 months. Voluntary grasping of an object occurs at 5 months and by 6 months the infant can hold an object such as a bottle and grasp and handle small objects. By 7 months the infant is able to transfer an object from hand to hand and at 8 months has developed a crude pincer grasp using the 2nd and 3rd fingers in apposition with the base of the thumb. Finger-thumb apposition is refined by 12 months when the index finger and thumb are used in a fine pincer grasp. At 15 months the infant is able to place one block on another and hold a cup while at 18 months she can hold and drink from a cup, hold a spoon without rotation and remove her shoes and socks.[5]

Muscle tone

Muscle tone is assessed by the degree of resistance to passive movements. In the newborn the extremities should quickly return to their flexed position when the knees and elbows are extended. Muscle tone should be equal in both legs and both arms and can be assessed when extending the limbs from the flexed position. Muscle tone is also assessed by 'wrapping' the arm across the chest and around the neck. The elbow does not reach the midline of the chest and will not normally pass the nipple line on the side of the arm. This is known as the scarf sign and is recorded as negative with the above expected result.[2,5]

Alertness and responsiveness

The newborn sleeps about 16 hours per day though the amount of sleep ranges between 10 and 22 hours per day. As the infant grows the amount of sleep diminishes with the 4-month-old infant sleeping at night for up to 8 hours and having one or more periods of sleep during the day. When awake the infant is alert, is spontaneously active and responds to stimuli such as light and sound and later to familiar persons and objects.

The cry of the newborn is strong, lusty and medium pitched.[2] Crying in infancy is usually intense and accompanied by vigorous body movements. The face takes on a distressed grimace and becomes deeply flushed.[18]

The Glasgow Coma Scale is a standardised scale which assesses consciousness using 3 dimensions — eye opening, verbal response and motor response. The original scale, widely accepted, has been modified for infants. (Appendix B)

Eyes and vision

The eyes of the newborn are shut most of the time and may be difficult to inspect because of the strong reflex which resists separation of the eyelids. The eyes will open, allowing inspection, if the infant is held upright and gently tipped forward and backward or given a teat to suck.

The sclera is clear and usually has a bluish tinge. The pupils react to light and will be equal within a few weeks. The eyes are moist and shiny. Tears do not appear until 6 to 12 weeks. Absence of tears or inflammation of the lacrimal duct may indicate a blocked duct. The conjunctiva is pink and glistening. The permanent colour of the eyes is usually evident by 6 months and will be established by 12 months.

Disconjugate or wandering movements of the eyes may be noted in the 1st weeks, but disappear by about 4 weeks. The newborn will fix on objects within 20 cm and may follow a moving object briefly. It is recommended that soon after birth parents are questioned about any risk factors for visual disorders.[6] Between 6 to 8 weeks the infant consistently follows moving objects, will fix on a face and smile in response to a smile. At 6 weeks and 6 months parents are asked if they have any concerns, such as a lack of fixation or following. At 4 months the infant watches her own hands and by 6 months reaches for objects, sometimes quite small objects. By 9 months the infant watches people and moving objects with a held stare and reaches for minute objects. The infant at 14 months will point to objects and recognises people from a distance of 6 metres or more. Convergence is established by 18 months.

By the age of 4 months binocularity (the ability to fix on an object with both eyes simultaneously) is expected. Screening for non-binocular vision or squint (strabismus) is recommended at 6 months and 18 months.[6] The corneal light reflex test may be carried out to establish this alignment. With the infant looking straight ahead a light, at a distance of 30 cm, is pointed at the bridge of the nose. The light should be reflected at the same point in both pupils, that is, in the centre or just nasal to the centre if the eyes are looking straight ahead. Deviation from a symmetrical reflection may indicate strabismus. A cover test may be carried out to confirm strabismus. One eye is covered and the other eye is observed for movement towards fixation. Normally, there will be no deviation in either eye, but if there is a malalignment the weaker eye will move in an attempt to fix when the stronger eye is covered. An uncover test is used to observe for an intermittent strabismus such as may occur with fatigue. Each eye is covered in turn with the covered eye observed for movement just as the cover is removed. Ocular muscle function can also be tested by observing the infant's eye movements when the head is held in a forward-looking position. A bright, noisy object held at about 30 cm is moved to each side, up and down and across the field of vision. Movements of both eyes should be symmetrical. Infants with epicanthal folds of the upper lid which partly cover the inner canthus, or a broad nasal bridge may appear to have strabismus. The light reflex test and the cover test will establish whether alignment is correct or otherwise.[5]

Ears and hearing

The external ear or the pinna is placed and aligned at the side of the head with the top of the pinna lying in line with the outer angle of the eye along a horizontal plane to the occiput. The pinna is positioned at a vertical position which is not more than 10° from a vertical line set against the horizontal line from the eye to the occiput. The outer ears of the newborn are flattened against the head, but within a few weeks will sit slightly away from the head. Cerumen or ear wax is dark yellow and soft and is seen at the opening of the external canal.

The newborn has a startle reflex to a loud sound and will relax to mid-tone, rhythmic sounds. Within a few weeks the infant will stop crying at the sound of a voice and move in time with speech rhythms. By 6 months the infant will turn to a sound in an attempt to localise it. Babbling with a range of tones is evident by 7 months and by 10 months the infant responds to words and directions with appropriate behaviour.[5] It is recommended that screening for hearing be carried out at birth, six weeks, six months and 18 months.[6] A set of questions where parents record their observations of the infant's responses to sounds and early vocalisation is used to screen for hearing.[12]

Other sensory functions

The newborn demonstrates aversive behaviour to strong or unpleasant odours. Infants are also able to distinguish smells, especially the smell of the mother when she is lactating.

Sweet tastes are readily accepted by newborns and infants while unsweetened, strong tasting or salty substances are less acceptable. Sour and bitter tastes are rejected and will provoke facial grimacing and, sometimes, crying.

The newborn is sensitive to touch, even very light touch. Responses to painful and uncomfortable stimuli are usually brisk, aversive and followed by crying. Infants continue to be highly responsive to touch and will usually respond positively to stroking, patting and being held firmly.

Thermoregulation

While the newborn is capable of the production of body heat, heat conservation is not well established and is related to a number of factors. The relatively large surface area allows heat to be lost easily, even though the flexed position of the newborn decreases the exposed surface area. As well, the newborn has only a thin layer of subcutaneous fat and is not able to produce heat through shivering when there is a need for increased heat.[5] The ability to control body temperature becomes more efficient throughout infancy, though it remains necessary to keep the infant warm in cool conditions. Body temperature in the newborn ranges from 36.5 to 37°C[5] and during the 1st year ranges from 36 to 37.5°C.[19]

CIRCULATORY SYSTEM

Development before and after birth

In the 3rd week of gestation the heart develops as a single straight tube and begins to beat. During the 4th and 7th weeks the heart becomes partitioned into 4 chambers. The development of the heart, partitions and its associated vessels is complex and there are a number of critical events during development. The critical period for cardiac development is between 20 and 50 days of gestation. During fetal life the lungs are largely bypassed by shunts, which begin to close at birth.[1,7]

There are fundamental differences between fetal circulation and circulation after birth. In the fetus, blood is oxygenated in the placenta to a saturation of about 80%, passes along the umbilical vein to the inferior vena cava and thence to the heart. Most of this blood moves into the left atrium through the foramen ovale, a flapped opening between the right and left atria, and from there into the left ventricle, aorta and the arteries of the upper body. The lungs receive only a minimal flow of blood. A lesser amount of oxygenated blood flows into the right ventricle, mixes with blood which has less oxygen, and passes into the pulmonary artery, through the ductus arteriosus and into the aorta. This blood, saturated with oxygen at about 50%, is delivered to the lower body. Oxygen-reduced blood is transported to the placenta by the umbilical arteries which branch from the iliac arteries. In summary, fetal circulation involves oxygen-reduced blood passing through the placenta, being replenished with oxygen and nutrients and circulating through the heart and out to the body tissues.[17]

There are a number of dynamic circulatory changes immediately after birth. The expansion of the lungs and the increase in pulmonary arterial oxygen cause a reduction in pulmonary vascular resistance and an increase in the blood flow in the pulmonary system. The pressure in the right heart and the pulmonary arteries drops as the pulmonary blood vessels receive blood, while there is an increase in systemic vascular resistance and pressures in the left heart. As the blood flow responds to these pressure changes with blood flowing from areas of high pressure to areas of low pressure, the flow of blood through the fetal shunts is altered. The foramen ovale is functionally closed through the changes in pressure in the 2 atria soon after birth. Anatomical closure takes longer and is usually complete by 2 months. The ductus arteriosus, a structure which allows blood to pass between the pulmonary artery and the aorta, begins to close following the increase in oxygen pressure in the blood leaving the left heart. It remains patent for up to 3 days with complete closure taking up to several weeks. A ductal murmur may be heard in the period before closure. Other changes include an increase in the size of the inferior vena cava following the shift of blood from placental flow to systemic flow and an increase in the size of the aortic arch following the closure of the ductus arteriosus.[5,7,8,18]

Pulses

The pulse rate may rise to about 180 beats per minute at birth, then falls to a rate between 120 and 140 beats per minute, though any rate between 90 and 200 may be considered normal, depending on the infant's activity. Because the heart grows rapidly in infancy, doubling in size and weight in the 1st 12 months, there is an increase in the efficiency of contractions and therefore the rate slows as the infant grows.

The activity of the infant will vary the heart rate. When the infant is awake, feeding or crying the rate will increase and during periods of sleep the rate is decreased. During inspiration a small increase in rate and a small decrease during expiration is normal and is known as normal sinus arrhythmia. It is recommended that the pulse rate is counted before handling the infant in order to avoid the effects of stimulation and activity.

The apical pulse may be viewed, palpated and auscultated. In thinner infants the apical pulse may be seen as a visible pulsation.[7] Movements of the chest are best viewed by watching the anterior chest from an angle. The apical pulse may be palpated using the fingerpads across the anterior chest. The pulse will be felt at the apex or point of maximal impulse (PMI), which is found in the 3rd or 4th intercostal space just lateral to the left midclavicular line in the neonate. The apical pulse is felt in the 4th intercostal space along the left midclavicular (or nipple) line in infants. While the apical pulse may be observed or palpated, it is usually easier to locate and assess using a stethoscope placed over the PMI.

Other pulses will reflect cardiac function and vascular integrity. The radial, brachial, femoral, popliteal and dorsalis pedis pulses can be palpated for rate and volume. A light pressure is adequate. The blood vessels in the infant are soft and elastic and very firm pressure may obliterate the pulse. When assessing the radial pulse the point is found more easily if the infant's hand is held and slightly extended. The pulse is then palpated with the assessor's other hand.

Because pulse rates in newborns and infants are so susceptible to variation, the rate is counted over 1 minute. As it is often difficult to count for a full 60 seconds without interference, a sequence of counts over the minute, for example, 4 sequences of 15-second counts, can be more accurate and efficient.

Blood pressure

In the newborn the systolic blood pressure is low (70 to 78 mmHg), but rises as the left ventricle develops in size and contractile strength. By 12 months the systolic blood pressure is 90 to 96 mmHg. The blood pressure in infants will be increased by activity, anxiety and distress. Diurnal effects result in a slightly higher blood pressure during the day than in the evening and night. Up to 12 months of age, the blood pressure readings of infants are equal in the thigh and arm.[18] After 12 months the thigh pressure is between 10 and 30 mmHg higher.[8]

There are a number of methods for measuring the blood pressure. Ideally, measurement in the newborn is taken with oscillometry or a Doppler device. The oscillometer uses a pressure indicator to translate the pressures in the artery into a reading shown on a meter. The Doppler relays the sound of pressure changes in the artery and produces them audibly. The use of these devices is preferable for infants, but they may not always be available.

When the blood pressure is measured with the auscultation method, it is essential that an appropriate size cuff is used. A cuff that is too wide may produce low readings while a cuff that is too small may produce inaccurately high readings. The bladder in the cuff should be long enough to wrap around the arm without the bladder overlapping. A 2.5 to 4 cm cuff is used for newborns.[5] The cuff width should cover at least two-thirds of the upper arm or thigh on which the measurement is taken. A wider cuff is always preferable to a thin cuff.

The systolic reading is noted when the 1st clear sounds are heard. The diastolic is determined at the point of muffled sound, the 4th Korotkoff sound, even though the muffled sounds continue for some further beats and then disappear. The point of disappearance is the 5th Korotkoff sound. The 4th Korotkoff sound is used as the diastolic measure up to 12 years of age. It has been suggested that the blood pressure be recorded with both the 4th and 5th Korotkoff sounds, for example 100/60/54 mmHg.[9]

The systolic blood pressure may be obtained by palpation of the brachial or radial pulse using a technique similar to the auscultation method. The cuff is inflated approximately 20 mmHg above the obliteration of the pulse. The point at which the pulse is felt as the cuff is slowly deflated is recorded as the systolic blood pressure. Because a blood pressure reading using the radial palpation method will be approximately 10 mmHg lower than the arm pressure,[7] a palpation reading is considered to be an approximate mean pressure between the systolic and diastolic pressures.[20]

The flush method provides an estimated mean blood pressure reading and may be used when electronic methods are not available or auscultation is not successful. The cuff is applied to the arm or thigh just above the wrist or ankle. The extremity below the cuff is compressed, by squeezing with the operator's hand or by wrapping with an elastic bandage, in order to force blood from the extremity. The cuff is inflated to a point on the manometer above the expected systolic pressure[7] or about 100 mmHg.[20] The compression on the extremity is released and the cuff deflated slowly. The reading is taken when flushing is seen on the previously blanched extremity. Readings with the flush method tend to be lower than the actual blood pressure and do not have high accuracy or consistency.[21]

Pulse pressure, the difference between the systolic and diastolic pressures, is generally between 20 and 50 mmHg.[18]

Colour

The newborn may exhibit blue extremities and skin mottling, which are normal colour changes.[5] During the 1st month the cyanotic appearance of the feet, hands and lips, known as acrocyanosis, disappears as capillary function matures and responds to temperature changes.[8] In infancy, the nail beds, mouth, palms and soles are the preferred sites for colour assessment as these are the areas of least melanin production[5] and are pink in the healthy infant.

Capillary refill can be assessed by compressing a finger or toe at the tip until blanching occurs. When the compression is removed colour will return immediately.

Heart sounds

The 'lub' sound (S1), made by the closing of the atrioventricular valves and the 'dub' sound (S2), made by the closing of the semilunar valves, are the usual heart sounds. S1 has a longer and lower pitch than S2 and is usually heard as one sound even though the mitral valve closes slightly before the tricuspid valve. Occasionally an audible split may occur, the result of a slight asynchrony between the valves.[7] In infancy, S1 may be louder than S2[22] and is synchronous with the carotid pulse. Simultaneous palpation of the carotid pulse with auscultation will allow differentiation between S1 and S2, especially when the rate is rapid.[5] S2 is short and high pitched and may be split. Because the aortic valve closes before the pulmonic valve a distinguishable split, which widens with inspiration, may be heard.[5,8] The 1st sound is best heard with the bell of the stethoscope at the apex and the 2nd sound with the diaphragm at the base of the heart in the 2nd intercostal space.[22]

Murmurs are swishing sounds which are distinct from the normal heart sounds and are produced by the vibrations of turbulent blood flow in the heart chambers or in the major arteries.[5,8] Innocent murmurs are usually systolic, of short duration and found along the left sternal border at the 2nd or 3rd intercostal space. They are described as soft, low pitched, blowing, musical, groaning, vibratory or transient sounds. They may disappear or vary according to the infant's position, following exercise, crying or feeding, or may change during inspiration and expiration.[5,7,8,18,22] These murmurs do not increase over time or influence growth and development. Innocent murmurs are estimated to occur in 50% of children.[7,22]

GASTROINTESTINAL SYSTEM

Mouth and teeth

While the mouth of the newborn is short, the palate forms a high arch. The soft section of the palate is long in relation to the hard section. The tongue appears large in the short

Table 1.2 Eruption of the deciduous teeth

Deciduous teeth	Age of eruption (months)
Lower central incisors	6–10
Upper central incisors	8–12
Upper lateral incisors	9–13
Lower lateral incisors	10–16
First upper molars	13–19
First lower molars	14–18
Upper cuspids	16–22
Lower cuspids	17–23
Second lower molars	23–31
Second upper molars	25–33

mouth, but moves freely and upwards into the high roof. It has a smooth to rough texture. The gums are smooth with a raised line of tissue along the gum line. Small white, glistening raised specks, known as Epstein's or epithelial pearls,[21] may be seen along the gums[2] and the midline of the hard palate.[5] These will disappear by 1 or 2 months. Even though taste is immature, the neonate can discriminate between sweet and bitter. Taste is developed to an acute level of discrimination by 2 or 3 months. The lips are pink and the mouth a deeper pink. Round, thick areas, known as sucking blisters but which contain no fluid may be seen on the lips, particularly the mid-point of the upper lip.[21] Salivation is scant and is not established until about 3 months, when drooling begins. The extrusion reflex, a forward thrust of the tongue, is present until about 4 months. Forward and backward movements of the tongue are usually established by 6 months.

From 4 to 5 months the infant begins to show signs of teething. The gums over the erupting teeth are swollen, red and sensitive. The infant chews and bites and may be unsettled or irritable. Sleep patterns may be interrupted and the appetite may fluctuate.

Tooth eruption usually occurs in the following sequence so that at 1 year the infant can have 6 to 8 teeth and, by 18 months, 10 to 16 teeth. After the 1st tooth, the teeth erupt at intervals of approximately 1 to 2 months (**Table 1.2**).

Abdomen

The abdomen of the newborn is symmetric, cylindrical and protrudes slightly. It seems large in relation to the pelvis, appears distended after feeding and becomes more prominent as the infant grows. Bowel sounds are present and can be heard soon after birth. The cord begins to dry within 1 to 2 hours after birth, becoming dark and shrivelled by 2 or 3 days and sloughing off between 7 to 10 days.[2] A number of infants have an umbilical protrusion. This hernia closes spontaneously by 2 years in most instances.[7,18]

Ingestion and digestion

Because the muscle tone of the lower oesophageal sphincter is not fully functional until about 1 month, the young infant often regurgitates small amounts of milk after a feeding. Regurgitation of small amounts, known as possetting, may continue for several months in some infants. Intestinal peristalsis is rapid in the newborn and infant. The emptying time of the stomach is 2.5 to 3 hours in the newborn and 3 to 6 hours in infants and children. Stomach capacity rapidly increases from 10 to 20 mL in the newborn to 150 to 200 mL by 3 months.[5] The gastrocolic reflex is also rapid in newborns and infants. The frequency of stools in early infancy is related to the rapid progress of contents through the intestines.

Elimination

The buttocks are small in early infancy because the gluteal muscles only develop as a larger muscle mass when walking commences. The buttock creases should be symmetric.[9]

The anus in the newborn appears closed and its patency is confirmed by meconium, a dark greenish black, viscid substance, which is passed 24 to 48 hours after birth. Meconium continues for a couple of days and is replaced on the 3rd or 4th day with a stool which has a soft consistency and is light greenish brown in colour. The stools change colour as feeding becomes established. The breast fed infant produces stools which are yellow and scrambled looking with an acid odour while the stools of the artificially fed infant are pale yellow to light brown, more pasty and have a stronger odour. Infants who are artificially fed usually have fewer bowel actions per day. The stools of the breast fed infant are looser, smaller and more frequent, ranging from 3 to 6 per day. However, there is great variation in the colour, consistency and frequency of stools in infancy. Stools can be yellow, greenish or brown and be curd-like, pasty or softly formed. The frequency can range from 6 stools a day to stools every few days. As foods are introduced the stools will continue to change in colour, consistency and odour. By 12 months the number of stools has been reduced to 1 or 2 per day. The anus appears moist and hairless in infancy. The anal reflex can be elicited by stroking or gently pricking the anal area. The anus will contract quickly.[5,7,21,22]

Stool specimens can be obtained by catching faeces in a nappy lining. The nappy may be lined with plastic wrap or a plastic glove which is split part-way along the side edges and opened out.

RESPIRATORY SYSTEM

Respiration following birth

The collapsed alveoli of fetal life are expanded with the 1st breaths taken by the newborn. At birth, the alveoli are immature, duct-like structures,[18] the trachea is small with soft supporting cartilage and the accessory muscles are included in the respiratory effort.[8] The alveoli rapidly increase in number and size in the 1st 6 months. Newborns and infants have relatively large areas of anatomic dead space in the airways and high metabolic rates and, as a consequence, their respiratory rates are rapid.

Chest

In the newborn the chest is almost circular because of near equal front-to-back (anteroposterior) and side-to-side (lateral) diameters. Slight intercostal and sternal retractions are seen on inspiration.[5] The chest circumference, which ranges from 30.5 to 33 cm, is used as a comparison in the assessment of head circumference, which is usually 2 to 3 cm larger. Chest circumference is measured by placing a tape around the chest at the nipple line. It is recommended that 2 measurements be taken, during inspiration and during expiration and the mean of the measurements be recorded. It is not uncommon on the 3rd day for breast engorgement to develop. The enlargement is related to maternal hormones and usually subsides within a week or two.[21] With growth, the chest of the infant becomes more oval in shape with the lateral diameter becoming larger than anteroposterior. Chest circumference is generally equal to head circumference at 12 months.[5,8]

Breath sounds

Breath sounds will seem loud and harsh in the infant because of the thin chest wall.[7] In newborns and infants breath sounds are bronchovesicular with inspiration and expiration similar in pitch and duration.[21] Bronchovesicular breath sounds have a medium-to-high pitch, and a blowing muffled quality.[8] The breath sound of air entering the lungs will be bilaterally equal.[9]

Respirations

In newborns and infants respirations are diaphragmatic. The abdomen will be seen to rise with each inspiration and fall on expiration.[7] The rate and depth of the respirations are irregular.[9] Infants are obligatory nose breathers from birth until 3 or 4 months, though some infants continue to breathe only through the nose for as long as 8 or 9 months.[8]

After birth the respiratory rate ranges from 30 to 60 breaths per minute and decreases to a range of 30 to 40 breaths per minute as the infant grows.[8] The respiratory rate is very likely to be increased when the infant is awake and by activity, feeding, handling or discomfort. When assessing respirations it is better to count the rate before touching the infant in order to avoid the effect of these factors. The rate can be assessed by observing the rise and fall of the abdomen and counting the respiratory movements. Some nurses prefer to lightly place a hand across the abdomen and feel the movements of respiration. Because respiratory rates in infancy are irregular they are counted for a full minute for greater accuracy and are ideally taken when the infant is asleep.

GENITOURINARY SYSTEM

External genitalia

In the full-term female newborn the labia are usually oedematous with the labia majora large and prominent and covering the labia minora.[2] Vernix caseosa will be seen between the labia.[5] The labia should be symmetric and able to be separated. The labia minora become smaller in the 1st few weeks. The clitoris is usually enlarged after birth, related to the presence of female hormones. The urinary meatus is usually not visible, being located behind the clitoris, but the vaginal orifice can be seen and normally appears redder than the surrounding tissue.[18] There may be a mucoid, white or blood-stained vaginal discharge at or soon after birth. This discharge is also related to maternal hormones and generally disappears by the end of the 2nd week.[21]

The scrotum of the newborn is usually large and oedematous but should be symmetric and contain the testes. In some infants the testes descend in the 1st month or two after birth,[18] though in approximately 98% of male newborns the testes are present or can be easily manipulated into the scrotum.[21] A soft swelling around the testes which extends along the spermatic cord may be a congenital hydrocele. In most cases this will disappear spontaneously in the 1st year.[21]

The penis at birth is approximately 3 to 5 cm in length. The prepuce (foreskin) is adherent to the glans penis and cannot be retracted. Because the urinary meatus is generally not visible the urinary stream is observed for direction and force.[18]

Urinary function

The 1st voiding of urine normally occurs within 24 hours after birth. The bladder capacity of the newborn is only 15 mL and urine is involuntarily expelled when this amount collects in the urinary bladder. The amount of urine and the frequency of voidings increases during the 1st days after birth. By the end of the 1st week a urinary output of about 200 to 300 mL in 24 hours is expected. One study of breast-fed newborns recorded that the urinary output averaged 20 mL on the 1st day and rose to about 200 mL on the 10th day.[21] The infant voids up to 20 times a day. Because the immature kidneys of the infant are unable to concentrate urine it is colourless, odourless and has a specific gravity of about 1.008[8], with a range between 1.001 and 1.020.[5] The ability to concentrate urine increases over the 1st year as does the bladder capacity. The increase in bladder capacity is evidenced by fewer but wetter nappies by the end of the 1st year.[7] The average 24-hour urinary output at 6 months is 400 to 500 mL and ranges up to 700 mL by 2 years. Urinary output is assessed by the degree of saturation and number of wet nappies. A wet nappy with each feed is often used as a standard in the assessment of fluid status.

An adhesive urine collecting bag is applied to the infant when a specimen of urine is required. If a laboratory specimen is sought the genital area is washed and dried to ensure minimum contamination and to facilitate good adhesion of the bag. The infant is placed supine with the legs abducted. For girls, the lower adhesive part of the bag opening is placed onto the perineum before the rest of the adhesive section is applied. In boys, the bag opening is placed over the penis. Any wrinkles are smoothed out as the bag is applied in order to secure a leak-proof attachment. The nappy is applied loosely. The bag is removed gently and as soon as possible after the infant voids. If a laboratory test is required the urine is poured into a sterile container. Because the adhesive urine collector is irritant to the skin of the infant and can cause discomfort on removal, urine can be collected for non-laboratory testing in a plastic glove. The glove is split part-way along the side edges, opened out and placed as a liner in the nappy. Cotton balls are placed in several of the fingers of the glove. Urine collects in the fingers of the glove, is absorbed by the cotton balls and squeezed out for testing.

INTEGUMENTARY SYSTEM

In infancy, the skin is smooth and soft, warm to touch and should be intact. The skin of the newborn is thinner and more sensitive. Following birth, the skin is usually bright red, puffy and covered with vernix caseosa. Lanugo, soft downy hair, may be present on the forehead, cheeks, shoulders and back. There is some oedema of the face, especially around the eyes, and on the dorsal aspect of the hands and feet. By the 2nd or 3rd day the newborn's skin has become pink, dry and may peel. The skin flushes red when the infant cries. Occasionally, a skin flush occurs on one side of the body with a clear demarcation from the other side, which remains its normal colour. This is known as the harlequin change and is related to the lying position of the infant. The flush appears on the lower half of the body on which the infant lies.[5,21] Milia, tiny raised white spots, appear on and around the nose, cheeks and chin. In darker-skinned infants, areas of bluish black pigmentation, known as Mongolian spots, may be present across the sacral and gluteal areas and less commonly on the upper back and shoulders. Pink patches, superficial capillary haemangiomas, may be seen on the nape of the neck, eyelids and between the eyebrows above the nose. These are known as pressure marks, stork marks or salmon patches and occur in 15% to 30% of newborns.[17] Milia disappear in a few weeks, Mongolian blue spots fade during early childhood and often disappear spontaneously, and capillary haemangiomas fade within the 1st year. There is usually hair on the scalp in the newborn period, but it frequently falls out. It is gradually replaced during infancy with stronger and, sometimes, lighter toned hair.

Because the eccrine (small) sweat glands are functional the infant produces sweat, more noticeably in the palms, in response to temperature increase.

Body creases and folds are for the most part symmetrical. Flexion creases are evident on the palms and soles. There are normally 3 flexion creases on the palm.

Health Management

Anne Adams

Movement and activity

From birth the infant is active and highly responsive to movement. Kicking, stretching and reaching activities contribute to musculoskeletal and neuromuscular development. Physical activity is, however, closely related to social experience. From 3 months the infant kicks and squirms when freed from the napkin and at the same time will engage caregivers in social interaction by smiling and moving in response to their voice sounds and rhythms. Similarly, the vigorous activity often seen during bathing appears to delight the young infant. While it is often assumed that the caregiver initiates and controls such activities, it is the infant with his engaging responses who reinforces the caregiver to continue and repeat the activity.

Rhythmic movements are soothing to the infant and encourage sleep. Infants are particularly responsive to being held securely, patted and rocked. Rocking a crying infant at 60 rocks per minute at a travel of about 7.5 cm has been found to give maximum comfort.[23] Slings and pouches allow the young infant to rest against the warm body of the wearer and to hear heart beat and breathing sounds.[24]

Because infants are naturally active and mobile it is not usually necessary to encourage movement and activity. It is, however, necessary to provide an environment where activity which is safe, varied and develops gross motor skills can take place. Infants can move more easily on a firm surface such as the floor. Playpens are practical for the young infant, but with increasing mobility, such as crawling, opportunities to explore and move freely are desirable. Strollers, swings and walkers may restrict movement in the older infant. Walkers are not recommended in that they presume a level of motor development which may not have yet been reached.[25] Time out-of-doors can allow for further variety in activities, especially after the 1st year. Running, walking, climbing, pushing and scooting are a few examples.[5,8]

Stimulation

While the young infant has a great interest in everything around her, stimulation for optimal growth and development is needed. The infant is therefore dependent on caregivers

The infant in a pouch rests against the warm body of the wearer.

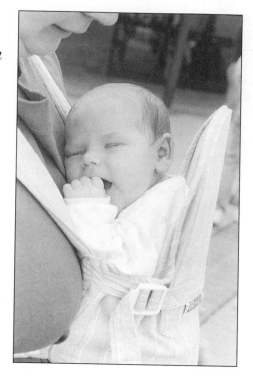

to provide a range of stimulating experiences which are appropriate to her age and experience. Stimulation can be visual, auditory, tactile or kinetic.[8] It may incorporate one or more of these components and is clearly linked with play. Combinations of two or more components can make an experience rich in stimulation.

Visually stimulating objects for the young infant include the use of shining, colourful and moving mobiles. The infant can be placed where he can see moving branches and leaves of trees, bright pictures, hangings and objects. It is the human face, however, which is particularly interesting to the young infant. The infant is highly attentive to a face which is close and accompanied by vocal stimuli. Changing the infant's position from cot or pram to bouncinette or infant seat can increase the range of visual experience. From 4 to 6 months the infant will look at his reflection in a mirror and can be placed where he can watch television. The older infant enjoys looking at pictures in books and magazines.

Auditory stimulation occurs with everyday sounds and voices. Toys which produce sounds, such as rattles, bells and squeaking objects catch and hold the attention of the young infant. Music, singing and rhythmic sounds are pleasurable. Music and rhythm may encourage sleep and relaxation in the young infant and, in the older infant, elicit movements and actions such as clapping and jigging in time with the rhythm. The human voice is the source of rich stimulation. Talking to the infant, making sounds, using and repeating his name, and later in infancy, repeating words provides auditory and social stimulation as well as the base for language.

Objects with a variety of textural qualities provide tactile stimulation. Some infants are particularly responsive to soft fabric objects such as cotton blankets, pillows, satin binding and soft, furry toys and may even develop strong attachments to them. So much so that removal of the object may cause intense distress. Most infants respond with pleasure and relaxation to experiences of touch and warmth where they are held, cuddled and fondled. On the other hand, some infants will cry when they are unwrapped or undressed. Massage, using warm oil, can provide a relaxing and soothing tactile experience. Infants can be massaged during bathing though the warm water of the bath alone provides a highly tactile experience. Water is also a satisfying play medium. Foods of varying textures can be given to older infants to handle and eat. Social play which includes holding, touching and tickling also provides tactile stimulation.

In the young infant, kinetic stimulation is achieved through movement such as rocking or riding in a capsule or pram. In the older infant any movement and activity provides kinetic stimulation. Play with toys which can be manipulated, stacked, pulled and pushed is particularly stimulating for the older infant.

Sleep

The newborn has a number of sleep periods in 24 hours, ranging from 30 minutes to 3 to 5 hours. Sleep usually follows feeding. At about 3 or 4 months the infant develops a nocturnal sleep pattern and begins to sleep for up to 8 hours during the night. Infants who are breast fed are more likely to wake during the night and sleep for shorter periods during the day.[5] At 4 or 5 months the infant has several sleep periods during the day of about 2 to 3 hours while the older infant may take only 1 or 2 naps during the day. It has been noted that individual patterns persist. For example, infants who sleep longer in the neonatal period continue to sleep more throughout infancy.[8] At 18 months the average night sleep period is 11 to 12 hours.

The infant will wake when hungry or uncomfortable. Sleep is promoted by feeding, warmth, secure wrapping, cuddling or rhythmic movement. Infants, for the most part, respond well to sleep time rituals, such as being tucked in for sleep, even while still awake.[5] It is recommended that infants should not be placed in the prone position for sleep but rather they should be placed on the side or back. The lower arm should be well forward to prevent the infant rolling onto the stomach. Infants sleeping in the prone position may have a higher risk for the sudden infant death syndrome (SIDS).[26] Parents have also been advised that infants should sleep next to or in the parents' bed for the 1st 12 months in order to meet the infant's needs for security and closeness[27] and to reduce the risk of sudden infant death syndrome.[28]

Nutrition

Human milk is the preferred food for infants. It is best suited to the biological needs of infants and the scientific evidence for its nutritional, immunological and antiallergic qualities is well established.[29]

Even so, for a number of economic, sociological and psychological reasons breast feeding in the western world has become a complex issue. While health education programs promote the benefits of breast feeding and more mothers begin to breast feed, the number of infants receiving artificial feedings remains high.[30] It would seem that preparation, encouragement and support are important factors in the success of breastfeeding and that nurses are able to help mothers through these activities.[31]

Commercially prepared human milk substitutes are recommended in preference to cow's milk feedings, even if diluted and modified, for infants who are not breast fed. It is further recommended that the human milk substitute be continued for 12 months and that cow's milk is not given until after the infant is 12 months of age.[10,32] The human milk substitutes, however, are derived from cow's milk which is modified to approximate the composition of human milk. These products are often described as humanised milks and include Nan, S26, Enfalac, Lactogen, Enfamil, and SMA. Follow-on formulae are marketed as milk feedings appropriate for infants from 6 months to 2 years. While these formulae have greater amounts of protein, electrolytes, minerals and vitamins and are preferable to cow's milk feedings, there seems small justification in changing from the humanised formula to a follow-on formula between 6 and 12 months.[32]

The fluid volume of feedings must meet the infant's fluid requirements and needs to be adjusted according to metabolic and growth needs. The newborn requires 80 mL/kg/day of fluid. This amount increases up to 150 mL/kg/day by the 8th day. Between 4 and 6 months, 150–180 mL/kg/day of fluid are needed by the infant while the amount decreases to about 120 mL/kg/day over the period between 6 months and 1 year. At 1 year approximately 100 mL/kg/day provides adequate fluid.[29,33]

The energy requirements for each day must be met by the infant's feedings. In the 1st 6 months the infant requires 460 kj per kg of body weight per day. By 6 months the energy requirement decreases to 420 kj/kg/day and further decreases to 378 kj/kg/day from 9 months to 12 months.[33]

There are a number of special-purpose milk preparations available for those infants who are in need of a formula which will meet nutritional requirements but avoid particular problems related to the intake of regular milk preparations. Soy-based preparations (Infasoy, Isomil, Prosobee) are used for infants who are intolerant of cow's milk. Infants who are sensitive to cow's milk protein, have lactose intolerance, are lactase deficient or have galactosaemia may be fed a soya bean based product which is as nutritionally adequate for infant needs as a milk-based preparation.

When an infant is lactose intolerant a lactose-free preparation is necessary. The soy-based preparations are suitable as are products where the lactose has been hydrolysed (Delact, Digestalact). Delact is suitable for infants up to 12 months and is a complete infant feeding. Digestalact is used after 12 months. Glucose Nutramigen and Pregestimil are lactose-free preparations with predigested casein and modified fat which allows for greater ease of digestion. They are often referred to as predigested milks.

Milk preparations which have modified fat and protein components (Alfare, Portagen, Tryglide) are used for infants with malabsorption syndromes such as those resulting from cystic fibrosis or biliary or liver disorders.

Special preparations for infants with metabolic disorders are available. Lofenalac is used for infants with phenylketonuria and Galactomin and Glucose Nutramigen for infants with galactosaemia. Lonalac is used for infants with congestive cardiac failure who require a reduced sodium preparation.

Infants who are pre-term or of low birth weight may require preparations which have increased energy, protein, calcium and electrolyte content. These formulae include Enfalac Premature, Enfamil Premature, Prenan, S26 (low birthweight) and Similac Special Care.[32–35]

While childbirth educators and midwives have important roles in the preparation, teaching and support of mothers who will breastfeed, nurses who care for infants in community and hospital settings have similar functions in helping mothers to establish and maintain lactation. Techniques for maintaining healthy and pain-free nipples, correct positioning for the mother and infant and the management of demand feeding are presented and discussed. The lactating mother needs adequate nutrition, fluids, rest and security. Successful breast feeding requires psychological acceptance and motivation, frequent sucking or expression of milk and a physical environment which allows breast feeding to be carried out frequently, in comfort and without haste. Nursing interventions which use collaboration and empowerment strategies are recommended.

When infants are artificially fed, accuracy and safety issues in relation to the feeding and its preparation must be considered. Hands are always washed before any of the procedures involved in preparation of an infant feed and before giving the feeding to an infant.

Bottles and teats must be sterile. This can be achieved through a system of central sterilisation within the hospital, by chemical sterilisation with hypochlorite solution or by boiling bottles, caps and jugs for 10 minutes and teats for 5 minutes.[24]

Preparation of infant feedings is relatively simple in a hospital where a centralised system of infant feed preparations is in operation and which uses prepacked products. Careful checking is undertaken to ensure that the correct feeding is given to each infant and that freshly prepared feedings have not been stored longer than 24 hours. Prepacked milk preparations are stored away from direct light. All feedings should be labelled with the name of the infant for whom they have been prepared.

Preparation of infant feedings using powdered and liquid products are undertaken according to the manufacturer's instructions which are included with the product.

Sterile teats are carefully applied to bottles with the aim of maintaining sterility. They are either applied directly to the bottle by stretching over the opening or by placing into a screw-on cap which in turn holds the teat onto the bottle. The choice of teat varies according to parental preference and the size and sucking ability of the infant. Teats designed to approximate the shape of the human nipple during sucking are popular. These orthodontic teats are soft with the hole placed slightly to the top of the teat at the tip. Silicone teats that are less degradable than rubber have been promoted for the stability of their material over repeated sterilisation. These teats are quite firm and do not permit milk to be shaken out in order to test the temperature of the feeding or for patency of the teat. The temperature of the feeding has to be assessed by feeling the bottle after shaking the contents well.

The manufacturers of prepacked milk preparations (usually prepared in 120 mL bottles) make the point that the feedings can be used at room temperature. Many nurses, however, prefer to warm the feeding, especially in cooler weather and when the feeding is for a small or hospitalised infant. The use of a microwave oven to heat feedings is potentially unsafe and not recommended.[24,36] The distribution of heat is uneven and the temperature of the bottle to touch may be less than the temperature of the milk.[37] The feeding can be warmed by standing the bottle in a container of hot water. The temperature of the feeding is tested by dropping a few drops onto the inner wrist. The amount of milk in the bottle is noted so the amount taken by the infant can be calculated. The time the feeding begins and the amount taken are recorded when it is necessary to monitor fluid intake and feeding behaviours.

Demand feeding is generally accepted as being preferable to regular schedule feeding because it acknowledges the immediate needs of the infant for both nutrition and comfort. Young infants respond to cues from the caregiver, particularly during feeding. Except in very hot weather, the infant seems more relaxed when wrapped firmly and held close when being fed. It is recommended that bottle fed babies be held in a semi-upright position, similar to the position of the breast fed infant during feeding. There is some evidence that bottle fed infants have more middle ear infections. From this, it has been concluded that the position of the breast fed infant during feeding prevents milk entering the Eustachian tube where inflammation and infection can develop in the presence of milk.[5] After feeding for 10 minutes or so most infants will signal when they are uncomfortable by refusing to suck or by squirming or grimacing. They can be sat forward in order to expel any swallowed air. Infants do not always have discomfort from wind, but gentle repositioning into an upright position will encourage burping. Patting and bumping on the back are not recommended and are likely to encourage regurgitation of milk. In normal circumstances the infant will decide when enough of the feeding has been taken. Breast fed infants will often continue to suck on the breast even when satiated. It is postulated that in this way comfort needs are met even when nutritional needs have been met. Infants fed from a bottle may use a dummy for sucking needs. Sleep most often follows feeding. The infant is best positioned on the right side with the lower arm placed forward and with some support behind the back to maintain the lateral position and on a slope of approximately 30 degrees with the head uppermost.

The introduction of solid foods before 4 to 6 months has not been shown to have any nutritional benefits. Some association with inappropriate early growth and increased frequencies of allergy and other adverse reactions have been reported with earlier introduction of solids. As well, the infant is not developmentally equipped to manage solid food in the mouth. The extrusion reflex fades at about 4 months and tongue movements, forwards and backwards, begin to develop. The gut has matured sufficiently by 4 to 6 months for the digestion and absorption of foods other than milk.[29] Solid food additions to the infant diet will supply the iron, trace elements, vitamins C and D and the extra energy needed after 4 months[29] and it is recommended they be prepared from the usual family foods.[38]

Rice cereal is often suggested as a 1st solid food because it contains iron, is highly digestible and gluten-free and therefore the least allergenic of the cereals. Cereal should be mixed with breast milk, formula milk or boiled water rather than cow's milk. Soft cooked fruits, mashed banana and strained vegetables are also suitable as 1st foods. It has been suggested that sweeter foods such as fruits be introduced several weeks after vegetables and meats because bland foods may not be readily accepted after exposure to sweeter tastes.[29] Because eggs may induce an allergic response, it is recommended they be introduced later — at about 9 to 12 months. Yolk is given first. Foods are introduced one at a time over a period of 3 to 7 days in order to establish whether each new food is tolerated.[10,29,39]

Opinion differs on the best way to introduce solids in relation to the milk feeding. It is often recommended that the solid food be given before the milk in order to encourage acceptance of the new food when the infant is hungry. Others suggest solid foods be given after the milk feeding to ensure adequate milk intake while yet others suggest solid food be given after part of the milk feeding and followed by the remainder of the milk or even between milk feedings.[10,23,39] It has also been recommended that solids are given after milk up to 6 months of age and that after 6 months solids can be given before the milk feeding.[36]

All authorities agree that salt and sugar should not be added to infant foods. Supplementary salt increases the renal solute load on the infant's immature kidneys, which have a limited ability to secrete excess sodium.[39] While inconclusive, studies have suggested an early sodium intake is related to essential hypertension in later life.[29,39] Sugars are related to tooth decay, may reduce the appetite and the acceptance of foods with greater nutritional value which in turn can predispose to later obesity. For these reasons, the addition of sugar, in any of its forms, is discouraged.[39]

Fruit juices, diluted with boiled water, are sometimes offered as a source of Vitamin C and extra fluid. Because breast-fed infants receive all their vitamin and dietary essentials, as do infants fed with breast milk substitutes, the offering of fruit juices is not a nutritional necessity. Commercially prepared juices or syrups with added Vitamin C may also contain high levels of sugar. Some infants are allergic to fruit juices. It has been recommended that juices are not introduced until about 8 months of age when the infant is able to take fluid from a cup,[39] or even later (at 12 months) in infants who are likely to have allergic responses.[8]

A variety of foods is introduced from about 6 months of age and includes broths, fish, chicken, cheese, cereals, vegetables and fruits. These foods are pureed or mashed and served very moist. Thicker and less smooth textures can be given as chewing develops. Finger foods are offered at about 8 months. At about 1 year the infant is eating a range of foods, most of which are prepared for the family. Some infants reduce their food intake about this time because of a slower growth rate and are more interested in small, frequent meals. At this age too, the infant will try to feed herself and is able to drink from a cup. Some infants will happily take milk from a cup rather than from a bottle, but others prefer to continue with bottle feeds. At 12 months the infant is having about 600 mL of milk each day. Some mothers continue with breast feeding beyond the 1st year. Foods not recommended include added salt and sugar, sweetened foods such as biscuits, cordials and sweet drinks and foods with high fat content. Prepared infant foods are convenient, but are not cost efficient and are limited in their range of taste, texture and appearance.[35]

Elimination

Because of the irritating effects of urine and faeces on skin and the general discomfort of a wet or soiled nappy, nappies need to be checked and changed frequently. The skin is cleansed and may be protected with lotions or creams. Skin cleansing can be carried out by washing with water and soap or by applying a lotion product which both cleans and protects the skin. The lotion is wiped over the nappy area, usually with cotton wool, at each nappy change and a residue of lotion is left on the skin though a wash with water and soap is recommended when faecal matter has made contact with the skin. Other skin protection products may be applied after washing and are designed to remain on the skin and form a protective barrier to the irritating effects of urine and faeces. Cleaning of the vulva is always done from the front to the back in order to keep faecal organisms away from the urethral opening. Talcum powder should be used with caution. The fine particles can be inhaled and the powder itself can cause irritation if it accumulates in skin creases. When moistened, powder will cake, causing friction and irritation. Some opinion holds that powder should not be used in infancy. Others maintain that if powder is shaken from the container away from the infant, applied sparingly and not allowed to collect in skin creases it is beneficial because of its drying, soothing and protective qualities.

Nappies commonly used in Australia are either disposable or made from washable cotton towelling. The washable nappy square is folded according to the size of the infant. Usually, the nappy is twice folded into a triangle shape and held with 1 pin for the young infant up to about 4 months. There are a variety of folds to suit the larger infant with the nappy held in place with 2 pins or a plastic clip.

Plastic pants and plastic-covered disposable nappies are efficient in protecting clothing and bedding from moisture. Frequent changing is particularly important when plastic products are used. Because the outside of the pants or nappy will not be wet to touch the need to change the nappy may not be obvious. The frequency of changing could be reduced. Prolonged contact with urine in a warm and contained environment predisposes the skin to irritation, discomfort and skin breakdown. Nappy products which draw urine away from the skin are useful. One-way nappy liners keep the skin dry. These liners allow urine to soak through into the nappy but do not retain moisture in the liner itself. Wool or thick-piled synthetic pants which absorb moisture reduce the amount of urine in contact with the infant's skin. Provided the atmospheric temperature is acceptable, the infant can be left without a nappy, which will expose the nappy area to the air and help keep skin dry and healthy.

Training the infant and young toddler to use a potty or toilet is a controversial issue. The psychobiological development of the young child offers a guide for when the ability to control elimination will be established. Many hold that only when this point of functional readiness has been reached should the child be introduced to toiletting. Other opinion holds that the child, through conditioning, can be successfully trained to respond to bodily sensations and consistent routines. This view claims that predictable elimination patterns can be established much earlier than if the child is allowed to develop toiletting behaviours in keeping with developmental abilities. The prevailing advice would seem to be based on either of these views, but it is essential to consider the individual response of the infant. Some infants and toddlers respond to a regular program where faecal elimination is expected and occurs at the same time each day. Others are unable to cooperate until their physiological development allows them to function predictably and with forewarning. Physiological readiness is related to the development of voluntary control of the anal sphincter. Such control usually does not occur until after 18 months and when walking is established.

Clothing and protection

Clothing for the young infant is primarily designed to maintain body heat and, when the infant is exposed to sunlight, to protect the skin.

The newborn is able to produce body heat but does not have an efficient ability to conserve it. While the choice of clothing will depend on atmospheric conditions, the newborn usually requires 2 layers of clothing and an outer wrap. Cotton singlets are favoured as a 1st layer though most infants object when the singlet is pulled over the head and face. Wide-necked garments are available and can reduce the infant's discomfort. The lower edge of the singlet may be folded back over the abdomen in order to prevent it becoming wet through contact with the nappy. Stretch suits, t-shirts and gowns are commonly used as a 2nd layer and a further warm garment may be added in cool weather. In cool and cold weather extra garments may be necessary. The newborn and young infants are particularly susceptible to heat loss from the head and extremities in low temperatures. Caps prevent heat loss from the head and bootees, socks and mittens provide extra warmth for the feet and hands. Front-fastening garments are convenient and easy to put on and remove. Garments made from cotton have advantages in that they are soft, absorb moisture and allow air to circulate. Wool garments have similar qualities but may cause skin irritation in some infants. Garments made from synthetics may be non-absorbent and trap heat in hot weather. Flame-resistant fabrics are highly recommended

The infant relaxes when gently massaged during the bath.

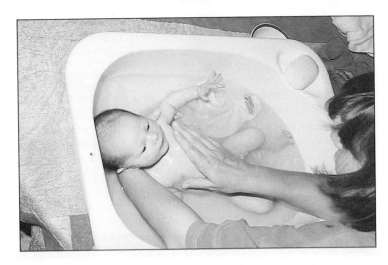

and are labelled in accordance with safe clothing standards. As the infant grows, larger sizes become necessary. Tight and restrictive garments should be replaced.

The infant who has achieved mobility should be clothed to allow for unimpeded movements and skin protection. When crawling, the infant needs his knees protected. When walking, he should be able to move without tripping or tangling.

The choice of clothing for the infant is related, not only to the physical needs of the infant, but to cultural, economic and safety factors.

Hygiene

The newborn is not necessarily bathed soon after birth. The 1st bath may be delayed for 24 hours or more. Vernix caseosa, which is absorbed within 24 hours, is thought to provide a protective layer through its insulating and lubricating qualities. A pH of about 4.95 on the skin of the newborn achieves a bacteriostatic effect.[5] For these reasons it is often recommended that plain, warm water is used for bathing or sponging in the 1st few days. It is often further recommended that the infant is not placed in water until the umbilical cord separates.[2]

The cord usually separates between 7 to 14 days and the stump takes a further few weeks to completely heal. Ideas about cord care vary. The regular application of methylated spirits has long been recommended for its drying qualities. More recent practice includes cleaning with cotton balls soaked in saline or merely keeping the site dry.

A tradition has built up in Anglo-Australian society that infants are bathed once a day and possibly more often. The young infant does not necessarily need to be bathed each day and in the early weeks sponging may be adequate. Many infants appear to relax when bathed, particularly if they are held confidently and massaged. Older infants may enjoy the bath, develop play activities and resist being taken out of the water. Bathing technique can vary but the sequence of cleaning the eyes and face and washing the hair before placing the infant into the bath is favoured by many nurses. The eyes are carefully wiped from the inner to the outer aspect. Cotton balls soaked in sterile water may be used in the 1st weeks, and a clean wet washer is suitable from then on. The face is gently wiped with a soap-free washer. The nose is cleaned if crusts are evident and the pinna of the ear is lightly wiped. When the infant is placed in the bath, skin folds and creases are carefully washed and the hands are gently opened out in the water. Thorough drying, especially of the skin folds and creases, is important. Milk or regurgitated milk and moisture can easily collect within the folds and creases. The infant should be kept warm throughout the bathing routine.

The hair is usually washed at the same time as the infant is bathed. Even with regular washing, seborrhoeic dermatitis (cradle cap) often appears. The thickened patches, composed of yellowish, oily scales, first appear across the top of the head and may extend over the whole scalp if not treated. The scales can be softened with shampoo, which is left on the scalp for a short while, or with oil which is left on overnight. When soft, the scales are lifted and removed with a soft brush or a fine-toothed comb. Thorough rinsing away of soap or shampoo seems to help prevent cradle cap. The reappearance of cradle cap is common in early infancy and removal of the scales will need to be repeated.

Finger nails and toe nails will be cleaned when hands and feet are immersed in the bath water, but nails will need to be trimmed from time to time.

Teeth cleaning begins as soon as the first teeth appear. It is recommended that the gums be gently rubbed with a finger at first, and then a small, soft toothbrush is used with water. A very small amount of fluoride toothpaste can be added later.[12]

Immunisation

Infants in the period from 2 months to 18 months should receive vaccinations for diptheria, tetanus and pertussis; poliomyelitis; *Haemophilus influenzae* type b; and mumps, measles and rubella.

The National Health and Medical Research Council immunisation schedule sets out the recommendations for immunisation of infants and children in Australia (Appendix C).[40]

At present hepatitis B vaccination is recommended only for those at particular risk, such as infants with carrier mothers and infants and young children in environments where there is a high hepatitis B carrier rate.[40]

Vaccination is available at local government clinics, through general medical practitioners and at outpatient clinics in paediatric and other hospitals. Parents must be given sufficient information about the effects of vaccines so that informed consent can be given. Vaccinations are recorded in the child's health record.

With the exception of Sabin vaccine, which is an oral vaccine, all vaccinations are achieved through an injection of vaccine. Vaccines contain antigens which are either live but altered organisms, killed organisms or the products of organisms (toxoids). Unfortunately, all vaccines may have untoward effects. Post-vaccinations reactions include local soreness, fever and general irritability and occur in approximately half the infants given triple antigen. Paracetamol is usually effective in reducing the infant's raised temperature and irritability.

The infant needs to be firmly held as the injection is given because she is very likely to move suddenly as the needle is inserted. Most parents are anxious about immunisation. They need clear and accurate information and support in their decision to have their infant immunised.

Safety

Keeping the infant safe becomes an important issue for all caregivers. The dependency and vulnerability of the young human means that infants are greatly at risk for physical harm.

The newborn needs adequate feeding, temperature maintenance, hygiene, sleep and loving physical contact in order to thrive. In meeting such needs there are safety considerations which must be acknowledged.

To keep the infant warm the provision of sufficient clothing and coverings is usually all that is required. If the atmospheric temperature is low, room heating will prevent body heat loss, especially when the infant is uncovered or unclothed. Even so, infants need to be covered quickly after bathing or examination. Hot water bottles to warm bedding or keep infants warm are no longer permitted in hospitals and are not advised in the home. Warming the clothing and covers before they placed on the infant assists in maintaining the infant's body temperature. Older infants may kick off covers and bedclothes. Bodysuits or sleeping bags are useful in keeping infants covered and warm. While it is important that newborns and infants are kept warm, it is also important that they do not become overheated. Too many clothes and coverings and the subsequent overheating of infants have been implicated in the sudden infant death syndrome.[41]

In hot weather infants need minimum clothing and extra fluids. In extreme heat conditions methods to reduce the atmospheric temperature around the infant are advised. Air conditioning, fans or draped wet sheeting will cool the immediate environment. Bathing and sponging with tepid water are effective in keeping the infant cool.

Clothing needs to be loose and the ties on jackets, bibs, caps, mittens and booties should be checked to ensure they do not constrict tissues and impair circulation. Bibs with ties are removed after the infant is fed. Mittens and booties should be examined on the inside for loose threads which could twist around a digit. Booties should be made without small holes through which toes could become entangled.

It is recommended that infants are placed on the right side after a feeding. A rolled rug placed behind the infant will maintain the position. At other times either side is recommended for sleeping. The prone position is to be avoided because of its relationship with the incidence of the sudden infant death syndrome.[41] The safety of the infant if left alone for any length of time has been questioned and recommendations that the infant be in physical contact with a caregiver for significant periods of time during the day have been made.[28]

Because infants can roll at about 4 months, they need to be safely contained in order to prevent falls. Cot sides are put up when the infant is in the cot, and restraining straps are necessary when the infant in placed in a pram, stroller, high chair or car seat. The car capsule is used until the infant is 6 months or 9 kilograms. The temperature of feedings and bath water is always carefully checked. Feedings are not warmed in microwave ovens and a sprinkling of milk should be comfortably warm to the inside of the wrist. Cold water should be run into the bath first so that the bathtub itself is not overly heated through direct contact with hot water. The temperature of the bath water, again, is tested at the wrist. The infant is never left unattended in water, even for a few moments. The often-advocated technique of soaping the infant before lifting into the bath is questioned. There is potential for body heat loss and the risk of losing hold of a slippery, moving infant with this technique.

Feeding equipment is kept sterile. Feeding utensils for the older infant should be unbreakable and without sharp edges or points. Teats and dummies should be inspected often and replaced when there are signs of deterioration.

The skin of the young infant is highly susceptible to the burning effects of sunlight. Protection, not only by keeping the infant in the shade, but also away from reflected light, is essential. It is recommended that sunscreen creams or lotions are not used on infants under 12 months.[24] Sunscreens with high sun protection factor of 15+ can be used on the young child. Those products with a titanium base are preferred.[42] There are some conditions, such as high temperatures, reflected light and hot wind, into which the young infant should not be taken if at all possible.

As the infant becomes more mobile and increasingly interacts with the environment the opportunity for harm and injury increase. In general, the infant and beginning toddler need constant and consistent supervision. Caregivers are required to be present, alert and aware of potential dangers and to provide a setting in which the infant can exist safely.

At the community level, safety issues have been the focus of educational programs, media campaigns and legislation. Relevant issues for the safety of the infant include car restraints, lead levels, swimming pool fencing, skin protection and immunisation.

ACKNOWLEDGEMENTS

Grateful acknowledgements are made to Gill Patterson, Linda Jones and Patricia Gornall, who supplied information for this section of the chapter.

Psychological Growth and Development

Sue Nagy

The term infancy is usually used to refer to the period from birth to approximately 18 months of age. Infants are born with little or no knowledge of the world. The impressions they receive in their 1st years have implications for their emotional and social adjustment for a long time, perhaps for their entire lives. By the end of the 1st year most infants have formed some feelings about the world, whether it is a place of relative safety, populated by generally benevolent people, or a place where they can not feel secure and confident that their needs will be met. By this time they will also have developed the ability to solve simple problems, such as searching for and finding a toy that has rolled out of sight.

Nurses can be very influential in the development of children for whom they care, as they are often involved in the major life events such as birth, death, severe illness and injury which have such formative influences on personality development. Nurses who have a sound understanding of the forces which influence normal development, are more able to help their patients during these potentially stressful times. They are also better equipped to identify developmentally delayed children, to implement suitable care and treatment and to refer them to other health professionals when appropriate.

A sound knowledge of normal development is critical to the ability to make accurate assessments of children in paediatric practice. Normal appearance and behaviour at one age may be abnormal at another. It is also important to keep in mind that the psychological development of human beings is an extremely complex process. A child's behaviour at any given time is the result of a complex set of interactions between her particular psychological make-up, her previous experiences, the influence of her family with all its individual characteristics, the influence of significant adults such as teachers, the culture in which she lives, and many other factors. As much psychological knowledge consists of descriptions of typical behaviour, textbooks are only able to provide guidelines for the

Table 1.3 Stages of development from infancy to adolescence

	Piaget	Freud	Erikson
Infancy	Sensorimotor	Oral	Trust vs mistrust
Toddlerhood	Sensorimotor	Anal	Autonomy vs shame and doubt
Preschool	Pre-operational	Phallic	Initiative vs guilt
School-age	Concrete operational	Latency	Industry vs inferiority
Adolescence	Formal operational	Genital	Identity vs role confusion

most common patterns of development. Most children are atypical in at least some as-pects. It is important, therefore, that caution is exercised when any assessments are made, and that conclusions are based on data of many types and from as many different sources as are available.

The process by which all this occurs forms the basis of this section, but first it is necessary to have a brief look at some of the concepts and theories that form the structure on which understanding of the process of human development can be based.

As we progress from completely dependent and helpless infants to fully functioning and autonomous adults, we develop in 4 main ways — physically, cognitively, emotionally and socially. Physically we develop our ability to move freely and competently, and to manipulate objects in our environment. As we develop cognitively we improve our ability to think in increasingly sophisticated ways, including our ability to reason logically and solve problems. Cognitive development also enables us to realise our full potential. As we develop emotionally we enhance our ability to maintain a sense of emotional well-being, to enjoy the pleasures that life offers and to find a degree of contentment with life. As we develop socially we learn to relate better to other people and to find satisfaction and enjoyment in our interpersonal relationships. People who relate well to others are more likely to attract the social support necessary to deal with the problems that inevitably arise during a lifetime.

THEORIES OF HUMAN DEVELOPMENT

A number of psychologists have observed people closely and have developed theories about the nature of psychological development. These theories provide an excellent start-ing point for the study of human development. The theorists whose ideas are considered in this book are Sigmund Freud, Erik Erikson and Jean Piaget (see **Table 1.3**).

Each of these theorists saw development as proceeding in a series of stages. Freud believed that sexual drives had an enormous influence on emotional development.[43] He described 5 psychosexual stages, each based on the body area which is the primary source of pleasure at a specific age. Erikson, while influenced by Freud's ideas, felt that development was also a function of one's social relationships.[44] He saw development as occurring in a series of 8 psychosocial stages. Erikson differed from the other 2 theorists in that he saw development as process that continues throughout life and into old age. Piaget focused on the development of cognition.[45] He described 4 stages in the develop-ment of thinking and reasoning abilities. These stages are summarised in **Table 1.3**. All of these theories offer different insights into the way we develop.

Freud's theory of psychosexual development

Sigmund Freud (1856–1939) lived in Europe. His theory is known as the psychoanalytic approach.[46] Although his ideas have been subjected to much criticism, he has been highly influential in the development of modern psychology.

Freud described different stages in the development of personality: oral, anal, phallic, latency and genital. He also believed there are 3 components of the personality — the id, the ego and the superego — which develop as the child matures. The id, which he also termed 'the pleasure principle', is that part of our personality which motivates us to seek pleasure and avoid pain. The id is well developed at birth and, in contrast to the more mature child, the id-dominated infant is motivated purely by the pleasure principle. He believed that infants primarily experience pleasure through oral stimulation — sucking, eating, drinking and generally placing all objects in their mouths. For this reason Freud described infancy as the oral stage of development.

During the 2nd year of life, the ego, or 'reality principle' gains strength. The ego is that part of our personality which helps us to be able to delay fulfilling our desire for pleasure because of the unpleasant consequences of unbridled id-motivated behaviour. Freud's observations lead him to believe that during the 2nd year, the source of the greatest sensual pleasure shifts from the oral to the anal area. He concluded that toddlers take pleasure in exercising voluntary control over the anal area by the expulsion or withholding of faeces.

The superego develops during early childhood. The superego also tends to discourage us from overindulgence in pleasure seeking, not because of the effects on ourselves, but because of the effects on others and on society in general. In other words, it plays the part of our conscience. At the time that the superego is developing, so is the focus of sensual pleasure again changing from the anal to the phallic areas. Freud observed that both male and female children begin to masturbate during this stage.

The id, ego and superego work together in a kind of psychic conflict, each aiming for expression. Freud emphasised the importance of these internal psychic conflicts for the development of personality. Ideally, the 'balance of power' between the personality components should be approximately equal, so that we are able to maintain a reasonable balance between serving our own needs and those of the society in which we live.

Erikson's theory of psychosocial development

Erik Erikson (1902–1994) was born in Germany and wrote his most important works around the middle of the 20th Century. He was influenced by Freud's ideas but departed from them with his emphasis on the importance of social relationships, as the basis of development, rather than psychosexual conflict. He believed that at each developmental stage the person must undertake a specific psychosocial task involving the relationship between the internal psychological self and the external social world. The crisis may be resolved positively or negatively. The more positive the outcome, the better equipped the person to negotiate the next stage.

Erikson believed that the young infant, born with no experience of the world and totally dependent on caregivers for survival, needs to develop a sense of trust that the world is basically a benevolent place where her needs will be met.[44] As the infant become a toddler and more physically able, she needs to test her abilities in order to develop a sense of autonomy and competence. By the age of three, when she has mastered most of the basic physical skills, she is ready to apply these skills to cope with new situations and so develop a sense of initiative. By the time the child is ready to attend school, ideally she has developed a sense of trust in the world, a strong sense of her own autonomy and is able to use her initiative to cope with new situations. She is, then, well placed to approach school with industry. An industrious child will learn the skills necessary to function effectively within her society. By adolescence, the child is ready to consider approaching adulthood and begin to prepare for the roles she will play as an adult, to develop the personality, values and beliefs that will constitute the kind of adult she will become. In other words she is ready to develop a sense of identity.

Piaget's theory of cognitive development

Jean Piaget (1896–1980) was a Swiss psychologist who was interested in the process of the development of thinking and reasoning and the effect of that development on the child's problem solving strategies.[47,48] His work is of great benefit in helping us understand the way in which children think. With the help of his wife, he closely observed the cognitive development of his 3 children, Jacqueline, Lucienne and Laurent, and it is largely on the basis of these observations that he built his theory. He described 4 stages which he believed characterised the progression of cognitive development from infancy to adulthood.

Piaget believed that intelligence is the ability to adapt to new experiences. He argued that people are continually trying to make sense of their experiences and achieving a state of mental equilibrium.[49] There are basically two ways that equilibrium can be achieved. First, one can interpret new experiences to fit with the way one already understands the world. Piaget called this process assimilation. For example, an infant may understand that most objects are food and so place all objects that come into his hand, into his mouth. However, it is also possible to change the way one thinks to accommodate new experiences. This process is known as accommodation. For example, the infant eventually recognises that some objects are more fun to play with than to eat (e.g., blocks) and others are better suited for eating (e.g., ice cream). So he has modified his thinking about the purpose of objects from his experience of them.

Piaget described 4 stages of cognitive development through which children, through the processes of assimilation and accommodation, understand their world (**Table 1.3**). Piaget believed that as children's mental structures develop, they continually reconstruct the way they understand the world until their understanding reaches the sophistication of adults. In this way they progress from the reflexive 'thinking' of infancy, to the logical and abstract thought of adulthood.

COGNITIVE DEVELOPMENT

Piaget's sensorimotor stage

The first of Piaget's stages of cognitive development is the sensorimotor stage which lasts from birth to approximately 2 years of age.[44] The very young infant does not 'think' in any conventional sense but rather reacts reflexively to the environment as perceived through her senses. However, as her mental structures mature and her experience of the world increases, the quality of her thinking will also change. She also comes to understand her own helplessness, and that her very survival is dependent on the care given by her parents. Infants learn to modify their thinking about the purposes of objects based upon their experiences of them.

Table 1.4 Substages of Piaget's sensorimotor stage of cognitive development

Substage	Age (months)	Major characteristics
1. Reflex activity	0–1	Reacts with a series of reflexive behaviours
2. Primary circular reactions	1–4	Repetition of behaviours that are pleasurable
3. Secondary circular reactions	4–10	Beginning of intentional behaviour
4. Coordination of secondary schemes	10–12	Development of concept of object permanence
5. Tertiary circular reactions	12–18	Actively experiments to find new ways of responding to environment
6. Mental combinations	18–24	Development of internal representations Beginning of thought

The sensorimotor stage has 6 substages which mark the infant's progression, from substage 1 when almost all her reactions to the world consist of a series of reflexes, to the beginning of true thinking in substage 6 (**Table 1.4**).

The infant's cognitive development is labelled 'sensorimotor' because infants largely gain knowledge of the world through their senses and respond with motor activity. There appears to be little or no true 'thinking' or 'reasoning' between the input from senses and the motor response. Neonates who respond almost entirely with reflexive activity (substage 1), will cry in response to discomfort, and will suck in response to a nipple being placed in their mouths. When their cheek is touched, they will reflexively turn towards the stimulus and try to suck. This has been termed the 'rooting reflex'. Such behaviour is 'intelligent' because, by reflexively sucking and placing objects in their mouths, infants ensure their own survival by feeding.

By the age of 1 month infants progress to substage 2 (primary circular reactions) and begin to show signs of more systematic responses to the world. Movements which seem to give pleasure, such as thumb sucking, become more repetitive and appear to be less random. At this age, however, infants do not appear to differentiate between their own bodies and the external world.

Between the ages of 4 and 10 months, infants demonstrate secondary circular reactions (substage 3). Signs of intentional behaviour become apparent, such as reaching out to hit a rattle strung over the cot. Now they are beginning to find solutions to simple problems and thus to exercise a degree of control over their world. Young infants do not understand that objects which are not directly visible nevertheless exist. When this understanding occurs, objects, events and people can be wanted, longed for and actively sought. Piaget called this the development of the understanding of object permanence. He believed that its development was a major cognitive task faced by infants. Some infants show the beginnings of object permanence by 4 months. Most have some understanding of it by 8 months although it is not normally fully developed until about 18 months.[50] The development of object permanence can be assessed by observing the child's behaviour. Before the age of 8 months, most infants will not search for an object which has obviously interested them but has been removed from sight.

Between 10 and 12 months, infants enter the 4th substage (coordination of secondary schemes). They now begin to experiment actively by coordinating behaviour to achieve desired results. Most infants will now search for a toy that is completely hidden. If the toy is subsequently hidden in a different place, the search tends to be directed to the original place, where the toy was last found.

The 5th substage (tertiary circular reactions) develops between the ages of 10 and 12 months. Infants now seem to understand that they can have more control over objects by using combinations of behaviours to bring about an event. They now seem to understand that it is necessary to search in a variety of places for a mislaid toy.

The development of object permanence is a critical point in the development of children's understanding of the world. Now that they understand that their mother still exists when she is out of sight, they can desire her presence and become anxious in her absence. This leads to the expressions of anxiety about separation from caregivers so frequently observed among older infants and toddlers.

A very conspicuous feature of the thinking and behaviour of children is egocentricity and it is most obvious in infants and toddlers. Because of their dependence on others they tend to be fully concerned with their own needs and to be unable to appreciate the needs of others. Egocentricity is reflected in their faulty reasoning. For example, when an infant's eyes are covered so that she cannot see the person with whom she is playing, she believes that she too is hidden. She seems to believe her view of the world (or lack of a view) is identical to that of others. Egocentricity is obvious in the young child who is talking on the phone and nods in answer to a question without also saying 'yes'.

LANGUAGE DEVELOPMENT

Language development is largely related to cognitive development. One of the tasks children normally accomplish during the sensorimotor period is the development of symbolic thought, which is the ability to understand that symbols, such as words, can be used to represent objects or people. Piaget called such symbols internal representations and believed that they are essential for remembering, for imagination and for language development. Symbolic thought may develop as early as 12 months and is usually fully developed by 18 months.[51]

Humans respond to language very early in life.[52] Infants as young as 3 days have been found to recognise their mother's voices.[53] Infants seem to be programmed to listen to their parents, especially their mothers, and to learn to speak their language.

Crying is the first attempt of young infants to communicate their various emotional states.[54] Communication between adults and infants begins with smiles, gestures and utterances that may or may not be linguistically correct, but it all helps to prepare the infant to develop her language skills. Adults seem, almost instinctively, to modify their speech and their voices when they speak to infants. For instance, they speak in shorter sentences, use much repetition, exaggerate the intonation and raise the pitch of their voices when speaking. Infants seem to prefer listening to higher pitched voices.[52,55]

By the age of nine months, infants of English-speaking mothers have been found to prefer the rhythm of their native language and will listen to it for longer than other languages.[56] More research is needed to establish whether this is true of all native languages.

A major step in language development occurs at about 4 weeks of age when infants begin uttering a series of vowel sounds, called 'cooing'. Perhaps fascinated by this new achievement, many infants seem to be entertaining themselves when they coo in their cribs.

Around the age of 5 months, most will be vocalising a mixture of vowel and consonant sounds known as 'babbling'. Infants may alternate listening to the speech of adults with some babbling of their own. Babbling frequently includes sounds, such as 'da-da' or 'ma-ma', which may be interpreted as words by adults. Around 7 months of age the babbling takes on a conversational quality. Some infants string together nonsense words with pauses, inflections and rhythms, so that they seem to be uttering sentences of unintelligible words. Babbling seems to be universal among children. Even deaf children begin babbling but do not continue to do so as long as hearing children because they cannot hear themselves.[57]

By 9 months most infants know their own names, imitate sounds of others (echolalia) and develop a basic repertoire of sounds ready for their 1st words. The ability to use internal representation usually occurs towards the end of the 1st year when many say their 1st word. Around 10 to 12 months, babbling starts to decrease and real words are substituted. At this time, infants are generally able to understand more than they can articulate. By 12 months, most infants have a vocabulary of about 3 to 5 words, although some will still not have spoken their 1st word.

Early in their 2nd year, 1 word sentences (holophrasing) start to appear such as 'Bottle!', (I want a bottle), 'Out!' (I want to go outside!), 'Doggie!' (Look! There's a dog!). At 18 months most toddlers have a vocabulary of 40 to 50 words.[58]

Parents often wonder if there are any potentially detrimental effects of 'baby talk' or 'motherese' as it is sometimes termed. Motherese consists of repetitive, grammatically simple sentences spoken in a higher than normal pitch. Research shows that infants prefer to listen to motherese,[55] so it probably is more effective in gaining their attention, and that it seems to actually facilitate language development.[59]

SOCIAL AND EMOTIONAL DEVELOPMENT

The psychoanalytic view of infancy

According to Freud and psychoanalysts, the id is that part of the personality which is present at birth. It is also known as the 'pleasure principle' as it urges us to gratify our desires. The id is not restricted by inhibitions or rules, it simply responds to the drive for desire gratification. Unsatisfied desires generate a degree of psychic tension. The id attempts to discharge this tension by motivating us to indulge in pleasurable activities.

Infants are almost completely motivated by the id and for them the main source of pleasure is the mouth. Freud therefore regarded infancy as the oral stage of development. Infants derive pleasure from sucking, feeding and sometimes from biting. In the very young infant, the urge to suck has a survival function but gradually oral activity becomes pleasurable for its own sake and becomes a source of comfort to the infant. The psychic tension generated by the need to seek oral pleasure will, if not discharged, result in an orally fixated personality. According to psychoanalytic theory, orally fixated individuals tend to become excessively passive, dependent, garrulous, bite their nails and over-eat.

Erikson's psychosocial view of infancy

Trust versus mistrust

In comparison with the young of almost any other species, one of the most conspicuous characteristics of human infants is their utter helplessness. For their very survival they must depend on others as they cannot find food, shelter or even maintain their body temperature without assistance. Crying is the means whereby the infant communicates her needs and ensures her survival.[60] When adults meet infants' needs for food, comfort, physical and mental stimulation and for relief from physical discomfort, they are reassured that the world is a safe and benevolent place. In this way, according to Erikson,[44] the infant negotiates the first psychosocial stage of trust versus mistrust.

The quality of care that infants receive has implications for their development at this stage and for subsequent stages. Infants who do not learn to trust will become emotionally insecure, and treat others with suspicion. They have learned to give priority to their own needs and are likely to grow up unable to give freely to others. As they fail to respond to others so others fail to respond to them. Their potential for developing satisfactory relationships is impaired.

The positive and negative outcomes of psychosocial crises occur on a continuum. No person becomes completely trustful or completely mistrustful, but well adjusted people are more trusting than mistrusting and establish a strong base from which to develop relationships with others throughout their lives. They tend to base their relationships with people on trust until the individual is proven to be untrustworthy, rather than suspicion until the person is shown to be trustworthy.

Nurses should be aware that infants cry to communicate their needs for comfort, food, liquids or pain relief to their caregivers. The old belief that infants will be spoiled if they are picked up when they cry is no longer accepted by most child psychologists. The crying of infants, who have been attended to promptly, has been found to decrease in intensity by age of 3 months.[60] Bell and Ainsworth found that by 12 months of age, infants whose mothers responded the most promptly to their cries, tended to cry less often and for shorter periods.[61] Those whose needs were attended to promptly in the 1st year of life, seemed to believe that help would come and had learned to be patient. The caregiver who responds promptly demonstrates a commitment to the infant and the infant will, in turn, develop an attachment to the caregiver.

Infants vary widely in the amount of time they sleep.[62] Infants who sleep less may also cry more often and for longer and caregivers may need help in managing infants' crying episodes.[63] Mothers who do not receive such help tend to be more anxious about their infants.[64] This may set up a pattern where parents becomes less responsive to infants' cries,[64] and infants become progressively less attached to their caregivers.

Bonding and attachment

Attachment between the child and caregiver is essential for infants' physical survival and for their long-term emotional, social, intellectual and physical health. Responsive caregivers are important for the development of trust during infancy and autonomy during the toddler years, thus laying the foundation for future development.

A child who is secure in its attachment has experienced the caregiver as a reliable source of comfort, as responsive to his/her needs and as available and sensitive.[65]

The terms 'bonding' and 'attachment', while often used interchangeably, are not synonymous. Bonding refers to the commitment that develops in the parents towards the child, whereas attachment refers to the reciprocal affection between parents and children. Bonding is a process that begins soon after birth. Infants usually show signs of attachment to their mothers at 6 months of age, and firm attachment by 8 months.

As most of the research has involved mothers, this section will focus mainly on bonding and attachment between mother and infant. This is not because it is seen as more important than the relationship between fathers and their infants, but because the development of this relationship is not as well understood.

There are many influences on the formation of attachment between mother and child. The child must learn to recognise the mother as the person who is most important for her survival and adults must feel a commitment to provide for the child. Infants are particularly well placed to learn to recognise their mothers. They like looking at human faces[66] and prefer to look at their mothers' faces rather than those of strangers.[67] While feeding, the mother's face is positioned at the infant's optimum focusing distance (about 20 cm). So feeding infants spend much time scanning the mother's face and by 3 months of age, many infants are able to recognise their mothers' faces.[67] Infants also seem to be attracted to the sound of human voices, particularly those with a higher pitch, and will synchronise their movements to its rhythm.[52] They quickly learn to recognise their mother's voice.[53] With the development of the concept of object permanence, children begin to understand that their mothers exist even when they are not in sight and it is at this time that the beginnings of object permanence can be seen.

The natural appeal that infants have for adults is an important feature of the bonding process. Large heads and eyes, soft rounded bodies, fat cheeks, prominent foreheads are characteristic of infants whether they are humans, ducklings or kittens and seem to trigger nurturant responses in adults.[68]

Klaus and Kennel argued that the initial contact between mothers and infants in the 1st few hours and days after birth are critical for the bonding of mother and child.[69] They found that mothers who had close skin-to-skin contact with their infants in the 1st 10–12 hours of life were more strongly attached than mothers whose initial contacts were delayed or abbreviated. Their conclusion was that the 1st few hours are a critical period for the development of the emotional bond between the mother and child. There has been much debate as to whether Klaus and Kennel were justified in drawing such conclusions and the extent to which the events of the 1st few weeks of life are critical to the mother–infant bond.[70] For instance, many adoptive parents bond to their children without any contact in the 1st few hours after birth as do many mothers who were separated from premature or sick neonates. In order to find some answers, researchers turned their attention to the effects of the separation of premature infants and their mothers.

There is evidence from United States, Britain and Australia that premature infants are more at risk of abuse than infants in general,[70] but this does not necessarily mean that separation in the early weeks of life is the cause. As premature infants are less physically attractive, it is possible that they are also less likely to elicit a nurturant response in their parents. The cries of premature infants are more high-pitched and irritating,[54,71] they are less likely to respond satisfactorily to their parents' efforts and they are generally more difficult to care for. This makes it harder for their parents to feel a success and abusive behaviour is more likely to occur. For example, mothers of infants who stiffen and are difficult to hold spend as much time in giving physical care but less time playing with them, than mothers of infants who mould themselves into the body of the person holding them.[72]

There are other factors which appear to influence bonding. Parental expectations of the relationship are an example. Adults who have been deprived of love, may have children in the expectation that they will fulfil this need. Such adults are often emotionally immature and have quite unrealistic expectations of their children's ability to be committed to their parents. The end result may be that the adult feels rejected, withdraws affection, and may neglect or even abuse the child.

Following unplanned pregnancies, parents may find it harder to develop an emotional bond. Matejcek, Dytrych and Schuller, compared children of mothers whose requests for abortion were refused with children whose mothers did not request an abortion.[73] They found that children of unplanned pregnancies tended to be hospitalised more frequently, to do less well in school, to have less stable family and peer relationships, and to be generally more irritable. It is, therefore, possible to conclude that bonding develops over many months and many events that occur during that time have an impact. Contact during the 1st few hours of life is probably important for the development of the mother–infant bond. However, it is unlikely that such contact is critical or that it is sufficient for bonding to occur.

On the basis of Klaus and Kennel's findings,[69] maternity hospitals changed their policies, allowing infants to be given to mothers as soon as they were born for cuddling and feeding, enabling fathers to be present, and for 'rooming in' of infants to occur. Nurses caring for young infants need to be aware that the early experiences outlined are at least influential, and may be critical for the future relationship between parents and children. It is therefore important to provide every opportunity for contact between the infant and mother and father, and to observe young families so that bonding difficulties may be detected early.

In an attempt to standardise nursing assessment of the mother's interactions with the infant during the immediate postnatal period, Salariya and Cater developed the First Scale.[74] However, there is presently no evidence that the Scale is able to predict later mother–child relationships.

The importance of secure attachment

The work of Mary Ainsworth[75] and others[76,77] has provided important insights into the relationship between mothers' behaviour towards their infants, the development of attachment and the child's emotional adjustment.

Ainsworth found the less mothers were sensitive to their infant's needs, especially in the 1st year, the less secure the child's attachment for the mother. She described 3 patterns of interaction between children and their mothers when separated in a 'strange situation', and subsequently reunited. The children were described as either securely attached, anxious-resistant or anxious-avoidant in their relationships with their mothers.

Securely attached children did not stay particularly close to their mothers, but would wander away a little to explore their environment. They tended to play comfortably with their toys and reacted positively to strangers who entered the room. When the mother left the room, they were obviously distressed and spent much less time playing with their toys. When their mothers returned, the children would go to them to be comforted and, when calmed, would resume playing. These children seemed to have secure and affectionate relationships with their mothers. They neither avoided their mothers nor resisted their mothers' attempts to provide comfort. In the long term, children who show secure attachment to their mothers in infancy tend to be generally happier, to be more socially and academically competent, more self-reliant and self-confident, than children who are less securely attached.[65] Their mothers were more sensitive to their infants' needs and less rejecting than mothers of insecure infants.[78]

Children who demonstrated an anxious–resistant form of attachment did not seem to be as interested in their environment as the securely attached children. They were more uncomfortable with strangers, even in the presence of their mothers. They were also quite upset when their mothers left the room and appeared to be more ambivalent when they returned. They would approach their mothers, and alternately seek comfort, resist it when it was offered and they expressed greater anger towards their mothers. For example, a child may run to her mother, reach out to be picked up, and then struggle to get down, stiffening and crying angrily. Anxious–resistant children tended not to resume playing, but remained near their mothers, glancing at them frequently, but still resisting contact. In short, they appeared as if they did not trust their mothers. Research into mothers of anxious–resistant children[75,77] has shown that during the 1st year of the children's lives, the mothers seemed to lack understanding of their infants' needs and did not respond consistently to them. Maternal attention seemed to depend more on the mother's mood than on the children's needs. Early in their infants' lives, these mothers have also been found to be more rejecting of their infants than mothers of secure infants.[78]

The 3rd pattern of attachment observed by Ainsworth was that of anxious–avoidant attachment. Anxious—avoidant children tended to avoid or ignore their mothers and were relatively unaffected by the presence of strangers. They were not willing to explore. They did not appear to be particularly distressed when their mothers left and were as easily comforted by a stranger. A study of the secretion of salivary stress hormones of infants in strange situations showed that the infants were actually quite distressed, even though they appeared to be emotionally unaffected.[79] However, the children tended not to run to their mothers when they returned or did so tentatively.

Generally, anxious–avoidant children seemed to have little ability to form close relationships. Investigations of the parenting patterns of these mothers suggest that they are both relatively insensitive and unresponsive to their infants' needs.[78] They seem to dislike physical contact and pick up the infants only when it is necessary.[77]

Separation anxiety

The fear that is most frequently observed in older infants is that they will be separated from the person on whom they have come to rely virtually for their survival. This fear is known as 'separation anxiety'. When separation is enforced, most children become very distressed. Their responses tend to occur in a series of stages described by Robertson[80] and Bowlby.[81] These stages are discussed in detail in Chapter 9.

Body image development

Body image is the perception of the appearance, function and structure of one's body. It involves notions of the body's completeness, its boundaries and a sense of being in control of body functions.[82] These perceptions contribute to the person's self-esteem. Self-esteem is the value that one places in one's self as a whole and includes the value one places on one's body.

Infants' concept of their body image is largely undeveloped. They learn about their bodies through being handled, through their own movements and through such somatic experiences as hunger, thirst, comfort, discomfort and pain. For instance, young infants do not understand the limits of their body boundaries, they gaze at their hands in the same way as they do at a mobile above the crib. The sense of being separate from their surroundings is learned during the 1st year of life, probably through moving, through being handled and through observing the departure and return of others. Through such experiences, infants begin to conceptualise themselves as having a separate existence. By the age of 13 months, most infants have developed sufficient understanding of their own and their mothers' bodies to use their mothers as 'tools' to achieve their goals. An infant, for example, may guide her mother's hand to reach a ball or to wind up a toy car.[56]

Nurses can contribute to the development of a healthy body image by responding to the infant's need for tactile stimulation. For example, when feeding milk or solids, it is better if infants can be fed on the nurse's lap rather than lying in their cots or propped in a chair. Of course, there are times when this is either not practicable or desirable.

By the end of the 1st year, most children appear to have a sense of their separateness, but as their understanding is not yet complete, misconceptions frequently occur. It is not until 18 months of age that a toddler seems to recognise herself as the image seen in the mirror.[83] Children who are upset at having their fingernails or hair cut, or who seem frightened at seeing their faeces flushed down the toilet, are probably having trouble in distinguishing between dispensable and indispensable body parts. Nurses who understand such misconceptions can more readily predict and respond to associated fears.

The development of self-esteem

Children learn self-esteem when significant others relate to them as important people, attend to their needs, play with them and generally indicate that they are worthy of the attentions of another. Their body image, self-concept and ultimately their relationships with others are influenced by the extent to which their needs are met.

When the demands of daily living exceed resources parents may have difficulty in providing their children with sufficient attention for the development of a strong sense of self-esteem. Such parents should be referred to a social worker or another appropriate professional. They may be able to be helped to manage better the stresses of family life.

Hospitalised infants may not receive sufficient attention, especially in a busy ward when their parents are not able to stay with them. Nurses who have a sound understanding of the importance of adequate attention will be more motivated to include playing with the infant as an essential component of nursing care.

The development of a concept of death

To fully comprehend the meaning of the word 'death', children must be able to understand its universality, permanence and inevitability. Although infants cannot understand what death means, they can be very much affected by a death in the family. If parents are grieving, infants can detect their sadness and be affected by it. If the child's mother dies, particularly if it was unexpected, there will be some disruption to mothering until the family can reorganise itself.

To experience grief, infants must have developed the concept of object permanence and be capable of experiencing separation anxiety. They may therefore be capable of grieving long before they can fully understand the concept of death or are able to verbalise their distress. Infants or toddlers may look for their mother. They may search for her particularly in places where she might normally be seen, or was last seen. If old enough to talk a toddler may ask for her mother. Small children may be regarded as too young to be affected and their need for support and comfort may not be recognised by adults who are also highly distressed, and the child may be left with some unresolved grief.[84]

Responses that have been observed in bereaved infants and toddlers include exaggerated separation responses such as clinging, screaming, refusing to let other attachment figures out of their sight; disturbances of sleep and eating; and regressive behaviour such as curling into the fetal position, increased thumb-sucking or even loss of speech.[84]

Coping

As infants have not yet developed the sophisticated coping of adults, their strategies tend to be more primitive and most respond well to physical comforting and soothing. Comfort can be especially effective when provided by the parents or other people to whom the child is attached. Unless the child is acutely distressed, a dummy is often a useful means of providing comfort. Some infants will not accept a dummy and prefer to suck their thumbs.

Psychosocial assessment

Assessment is more successful if it is done with the cooperation of the child. This can be achieved by being sensitive to the child's needs, establishing rapport with both the child and her parents, gaining her trust and confidence before attempting any examination, and assessing as far as possible while the mother holds the child. Assessment of infants works best when it becomes part of a game. Allowing infants time to become more familiar with staff by talking and playing with them is usually worth the time and effort.

There are several critical issues that must be kept in mind when making an assessment of any child's developmental status.

1. It is essential to recognise the value of the mothers' reports. Significant information can be gained by seriously listening to what she has to say, and by asking relevant questions.
2. It is important to recognise that no individual tool or method of assessment alone can be relied upon to give an accurate picture of the child's developmental status. A general picture must be assembled gradually from a variety of sources of information.
3. The wide variation in normal development must be recognised.
4. If any doubt exists about a child's progress, she should be referred to a child development centre, or to a paediatrician via her local doctor.

A FINAL NOTE

Children are on the whole emotionally resilient and one can make mistakes when caring for them without doing much damage. In fact, it is likely that the child will learn that circumstances do not always go smoothly and develop a degree of coping ability. It is the child whose needs are consistently not met, who does not develop a sense of security about the world or a sense of her own self-worth that is likely to be emotionally damaged. Nevertheless, there is some evidence that the damage done by poor parenting early in life can be reduced by positive experiences in later life.[51]

REFERENCES

1. Moore KL. *The developing human: clinically oriented embryology*. 3rd ed. Philadelphia: W.B. Saunders, 1982.
2. Ladewing PA, London ML, Olds SB. *Essentials of maternal-newborn nursing*. 2nd ed. Menlo Park: Addison-Wesley, 1990.
3. Marlow DR, Redding BA. *Textbook of pediatric nursing*. 6th ed. Philadelphia: WB Saunders, 1988.
4. Apgar V. The newborn (Apgar) scoring system, reflections and advice. *Pediatr Clin North Am* 1966; 13: 645.

5. Wong DL. *Whaley and Wong's nursing care of infants and children.* 5th ed. St Louis: Mosby, 1995.

6. National Health and Medical Research Council. *Screening and health care of children.* Canberra: AGPS, 1993.

7. Engel J. *Pocket guide to pediatric assessment.* St Louis: Mosby, 1989.

8. Mott SR, James SR, Sperhac AM. *Nursing care of children and families.* 2nd ed. Redwood City: Addison-Wesley, 1990.

9. Wong DL, Whaley LF. *Clinical manual of pediatric nursing.* 3rd ed. St Louis: Mosby, 1990.

10. Department of Health, New South Wales, Western Metropolitan Health Region. *Developmental paediatric manual.* Sydney: The Department of Health, 1987.

11. Carmichael A, Parry T, Vimpani G. Health of the under 5s. *In:* Vimpani G, Parry T, eds. *Community child health: an Australian perspective.* Melbourne: Churchill Livingstone, 1989.

12. Department of Health, New South Wales. *Personal health record.* 2nd ed. Sydney: State Health Publications, 1990.

13. Australian Physiotherapy Association. Physiotherapist develops screening to detect movement problems in four-month-old babies. *Physiotherapy Today* 1986; 1: 1–2.

14. Silink M. Normal growth. *In:* Buchanan N. ed. *Child and adolescent health for practitioners.* Sydney: Williams and Wilkins, 1987.

15. Tan D. Normal development. *In:* Clements A. ed. *Infant and family health in Australia: a textbook for community health workers.* 2nd ed. Melbourne: Churchill Livingstone, 1992.

16. Department of Community Services and Health. *NCHS Growth Percentiles.* Canberra: AGPS, 1986.

17. Beischer NA, Mackay EV. *Obstetrics and the newborn.* 2nd ed. Sydney: WB Saunders, 1984.

18. Scipien GM, Chard MA, Howe J, Barnard MU. *Pediatric nursing care.* St Louis: Mosby, 1990.

19. Johnson A. Examination of infants and young children. *In:* Clements A. ed. *Infant and family health in Australia: a textbook for community health workers.* 2nd ed. Melbourne: Churchill Livingstone, 1992.

20. King EM, Wieck L, Dyer M. (Adapted for the United Kingdom by Weller BF.) *Paediatric nursing practice and techniques.* London: Harper and Row, 1979.

21. Vulliamy DG. *The newborn child.* Edinburgh: Churchill Livingstone, 1982.

22. Gill D, O'Brien N. *Paediatric clinical examination.* Edinburgh: Churchill Livingstone, 1988.

23. Leach P. *Baby and child: from birth to age five.* 2nd ed. Harmondsworth: Penguin, 1989.

24. Karitane Mothercraft Society. *The baby book: a practical guide to caring for your young child.* Sydney: Doubleday, 1990.

25. Cohen D, Kilham H, Oates K. *The complete book of child safety.* Sydney: Simon and Schuster, 1989.

26. National Health and Medical Research Council. *Risk factors associated with sudden infant death syndrome.* Canberra: AGPS, 1991.

27. Jackson D. *3 in a bed: why you should sleep with your baby.* London: Bloomsbury, 1989.

28. Barker W. Cot deaths: no longer a mystery? *Empowerment* 1989; 1: 1–5.

29. Bohane TD. Current thoughts on infant feeding. *In:* Buchanan N. ed. *Child and adolescent health for practitioners.* Sydney: Williams and Wilkins, 1987.

30. Hitchcock NE, Coy JF. Infant-feeding practices in Western Australia and Tasmania: a joint survey 1984–1985. *Med J Aust* 1988; 148: 114–117.

31. Solberg SM. Indicators of successful breast feeding. *In:* Houston MJ, ed. *Maternal and infant health care: recent advances in nursing 9.* Edinburgh: Churchill Livingstone, 1984.

32. Thompson S. Infant feeding. *In:* Procopis PG, Kewley GD. *Current paediatric practice.* Sydney: Harcourt Brace Jovanovich, 1991.

33. Richardson C. Artificial feeding. *In:* Clements A, ed. *Infant and family health in Australia: a textbook for community health workers.* 2nd ed. Melbourne: Churchill Livingstone, 1992.

34. Harris M. *Textbook of child care and health.* Sydney: Science Press, 1988.

35. Allen J, Coyne T, Dumbrell S, Fairbairn A, Marr C, Mason T, Vermeesch M. *A new look at infant feeding.* Sydney: Science Press, 1981.

36. Thompson S. *A healthy start for kids: how to convince your children to eat well*. Sydney: Simon and Schuster, 1991.

37. Sando WC, Gallaher KJ, Rogers BM. Risk factor for microwave scald injuries in infants. *J Pediatr* 1984; 105: 864–867.

38. National Health and Medical Research Council. *Nutrition policy statements*. Canberra: AGPS, 1990.

39. Delatycki J. Developing food patterns in infancy and early childhood. *In:* Clements A, ed. *Infant and family health in Australia: a textbook for community health workers*. 2nd ed. Melbourne: Churchill Livingstone, 1992.

40. National Health and Medical Research Council. *The Australian immunisation handbook*. 5th ed. Canberra: AGPS, 1994.

41. Fleming PJ, Gilbert R, Azaz Y, Berry PJ, Rudd PT, Stewart A, Hall E. Interaction between bedding and sleep position in the sudden death infant death syndrome: a population based control study. *BMJ* 1990; 301: 85–89.

42. Cancer Council of NSW. *Sun protection for babies*. Sydney: Cancer Council of NSW, 1993.

43. Freud S. *An outline of pychoanalysis*. London: Hogarth Press, 1964.

44. Erikson EH. *Childhood and society*. New York: Norton, 1963.

45. Piaget J. *The construction of reality in the child*. New York: Basic Books, 1954.

46. Hall CS. *A primer of Freudian psychology*. New York: New American Library, 1979.

47. Piaget J, Inhelder B. *The psychology of the child*. London: Routledge Kegan & Paul, 1969.

48. Flavell JH. *The developmental psychology of Jean Piaget*. New York: Van Nostrand, 1963.)

49. Bemporad JR. Theories of development. *In:* Bemporad JR, ed. *Child development in normality and psychopathology*. New York: Brunner/Mazel, 1980.

50. Diamond N. Cognitive theory. *In:* Wolman BB, ed. *Handbook of developmental psychology*. New Jersey: Prentice-Hall, 1982.

51. Phillips S. *Do babies think? How do babies think?* Foundation for Child and Youth *Studies*. Selected paper No. 23. 1982.

52. Rosenthal M. Vocal dialogues in the neonatal period. *Dev Psychol* 1982; 18: 17–21.

53. DeCasper AJ, Fifer WP. Of human bonding: newborns prefer their mothers' voices. *Science* 1980; 208: 1174–1176.

54. Zeskind PS. Adult responses to the cries of high and low risk neonates. *Infant Behav Dev* 1980; 3: 167–177.

55. Fernald A. Four month old infants prefer to listen to motherese. *Infant Behav Dev* 1985; 8: 181–195.

56. Jusczyk PW, Cutler A, Redanz NJ. Infants' preference for the predominant stress patterns of English words. *Child Dev* 1994; 64: 675–687.

57. Clifton C. Language acquisition. *In*: Spencer T, Kass N, eds. *Perspectives in child psychology*. New York: McGraw-Hill, 1970.

58. Bee H. *The developing child*. 5th ed. New York: Harper & Rowe, 1989.

59. Mussen PH, Conger JJ, Kagan J, Huston AC. *Child development and personality*. 7th ed. New York: Harper and Rowe, 1990.

60. Hope M. *Understanding crying in infancy*. Paper no. 43. Kensington: Foundation for Child and Youth Studies, 1986.

61. Bell SM, Ainsworth MDS. Infant crying and maternal responsiveness. *Child Dev* 1972; 43: 1170–1190.

62. Wooding AR, Boyd J, Geddis DC. Sleep patterns of New Zealand infants during the first 12 months of life. *J Paediatr Child Health* 1990; 26: 85–88.

63. Michelsson K, Rinne A, Paajanen S. Crying, feeding and sleeping patterns in 1 to 12-month old infants. *Child Care Health Dev* 1990; 16: 99–111.

64. Downey J, Bidder RT. Perinatal information on children crying. *Child Care Health Dev* 1990; 16: 112–113.

65. Sroufe LA. The coherence of individual development: Early care and subsequent developmental issues. *Am Psychologist* 1979; 34: 834–841.

66. Fantz RL. The origin of form perception. *Scientific American* 1961; 204: 66–72.
67. Barrera ME, Maurer D. Recognition of mother's photographed face by the three-month-old infant. *Child Dev* 1981; 52: 714–716.
68. Eibl-Eibesfeldt I. *Ethology: the biology of behaviour*. New York: Holt, Rinehart & Winston, 1975.
69. Klaus MH, Kennel JH. *Maternal-infant bonding*. St Louis: Mosby, 1976.
70. James D. *Bonding: mothering magic or pseudo science*. Selected paper no. 40. Kensington, NSW: Foundation for Child and Youth Studies, 1985.
71. Zeskind PS, Lester BM. Acoustic features and auditory perceptions of the cries of newborns with prenatal and perinatal complications. *Child Dev* 1978; 49: 580–589.
72. Shaffer D. *Social and personality development*. California: Brooks/Cole, 1985.
73. Matejcek Z, Dytrych Z, Schuller V. The Prague study of children born from unwanted pregnancies. *Int J Mental Health* 1979; 7: 63–74.
74. Salariya EM, Cater JI. Mother-child relationship. *J Advanced Nursing* 1984; 9: 589–595.
75. Ainsworth M. Infant-mother attachment. *Am Psychologist* 1979; 34: 932–937.
76. Belsky J, Rovine M, Taylor D. The Pennsylvania infant and family development Project III: the origins of individual differences in infant-mother attachment: maternal and infant contributions. *Child Dev* 1984; 55: 718–728.
77. Egeland B, Farber EA. Infant-mother attachment: factors related to its development and changes over time. *Child Dev* 1984; 55: 753–771.
78. Isabella RA. Origins of attachment: maternal interactive behavior across the first year. *Child Dev* 1993; 64: 605–621.
79. Spangler G, Grossman KE. Biobehavioral organization in securely and insecurely attached infants. *Child Dev* 1993; 64. 1439–1450.
80. Robertson J. *Young children in hospital*. 2nd ed. London: Tavistock Publications, 1970.
81. Bowlby J. *Attachment and loss, Volume II. Separation: anxiety and anger*. Middlesex, UK: Penguin Books, 1975.
82. Blaesing S, Brockhaus J. The development of body image in the child. *Nursing Clin North Am* 1972; 7: 597–607.
83. Lewis M, Brooks J. Self, other and fear: infants' reactions to people. *In:* Lewis H, Rosenblum L, eds. *The origins of fear: the origins of behaviour*. Vol. 2. New York: Wiley, 1974.
84. Raphael B. *The anatomy of bereavement*. London: Hutchinson, 1984.

Chapter 2

Growth and Development: 18 Months to 5 Years

Physical Growth and Development

Anne Adams

ASSESSMENT OF TODDLERS AND PRESCHOOLERS

For the purpose of this chapter, toddlers are defined as those children aged between 18 months and 3 years and preschoolers refers to children between 3 and 5 years of age.

The physical assessment of young children in these age groups requires a sensitive approach and a knowledge of the developmental abilities and responses of toddlers and preschoolers. Young children may be apprehensive about being approached, touched and examined by an unfamiliar adult. Time should be allowed for the child to become accepting of the nurse. Friendly and relaxed conversation with parents, addressing the child calmly and with genuine interest, using distraction techniques such as play and maintaining honesty are methods of gaining the confidence of a young child. The presence of a parent or parents is preferred with the child, in most instances, sitting on the lap of a parent. While an examination is best carried out in a logical sequence, such as from head to toe, some areas of assessment are left until the end of the examination. Testing for reflexes, examining the ears or inspecting the genital area are examples where the young child may become uneasy or uncooperative.

MUSCULOSKELETAL SYSTEM

The ossification process advances in these early years with the demands of activity and, in particular, weight bearing and walking, which stimulate the increase in bone size and density.[1] Muscle growth continues, but at a slower rate than during infancy and muscle tone increases.[2] Bones and muscles, however, are still immature despite the obvious increases in strength and physical ability.[3]

Assessment of musculoskeletal growth and function is based on the measurement of increases in musculoskeletal tissue and the ability of the child to move and use his body. Body weight and height are the main parameters by which musculoskeletal growth is assessed. Weight for height measures are recommended as more accurate estimations of growth than measures of weight and height interpreted singly. It is the ratio of the two dimensions and their pattern of growth over time which give the most accurate assessment of growth.

Posture

The convex forward curve of the lumbar spine and the somewhat undeveloped abdominal muscles give the toddler a rounded, pot-bellied appearance.[3] The lumbar spine curve becomes even more exaggerated as the child starts to walk, but gradually during the toddler and preschool years an upright and straighter posture is attained. The preschooler, between 4 and 5 years, has achieved an erect posture and become more slender in shape.[3]

Joints and limbs

Joints are easily moveable, both passively and actively, through a full range of movements. Toddlers have a broad-based gait, but as the legs strengthen and straighten the feet come closer together and the gait becomes more refined.[4]

The legs are often curved or bowed in the 2nd year because of the relatively large weight of the trunk,[3] but by the time the child has been walking for 12 months the legs have become much straighter.[5] By 2 years the distance between the knees when the child stands with the medial malleoli touching each other should be less than 5 cm.[4] Knock-knees, where the knees touch and there is a distance greater than 7.5 cm between the malleoli, is common after 2 years of age.[3] Despite these stages in leg growth, most children have straight legs by about 5 years.[5]

Weight

The average gain in weight during toddlerhood is about 2.25 kg per year with an average weight at 2 years of 12.3 kg. Birthweight is quadrupled by 30 months.[3] Between 3 and 5 years the average weight gain is about 2 kg per year. The average weight at 3 years is 14.5 kg, at 4 years 16.5 kg and at 5 years 18.2 kg (Appendix A).[3]

Weight measurements in early childhood are ideally taken with the child undressed. However, young children and even toddlers may protest at the removal of their clothing, so minimal underwear may be retained. It is suggested that 0.1 kg be subtracted when this is done.[6] During hospitalisation the young child will need to be weighed and may have attachments such as monitoring electrodes, drainage devices, limb boards or splints. The presence of attachments is usually noted alongside the recorded weight or the weight of the attachment may be determined and subtracted from the weight reading. If possible, the bladder should be emptied before the child is weighed.

Length and height

The increase in weight and height in the toddler and preschooler continues in a step-like fashion rather than a regular curve and slows as the child gets older. The anticipated growth rate per year for height between 12 months and 2 years is about 11.5 cm. Between 3 and 5 years the rate has fallen to about 7 cm per year. There is greater growth in the legs than in the trunk. The average height at 2 years is 86 cm (Appendix A) and is approximately half the final adult height. The crown to rump length at 2 years is 60% of the total length.[7] By about 4 years the length at birth has doubled.[2,4] Familial effects should be considered when assessing height against percentile chart figures. Tall parents are more likely to have long and tall children while short parents are more likely to have children with a shorter stature than the 50th percentile.

It has been recommended that recumbent length be taken until 3 years.[8] Height is measured with the child standing without shoes, with the head in the midline and the eyes looking directly ahead. The head should be positioned so that a line from the external meatus of the ear to the outer angle of the eye is parallel to the floor. Because height measurements taken at the end of the day will be less than those taken early in the day some gentle stretching of the head is advised.[9] The back, heels and buttocks should touch a flat surface such as a wall with a measuring scale. Legs, knees and shoulders should be as upright as possible and the feet should remain flat on the floor. A firm, flat surface is placed across the crown of the head at a right angle to the wall. The point of the right angle on the scale is the height. Occasionally the sitting height is measured. The child sits against a wall and the distance between the crown and the flat sitting surface is measured. Sitting height at 2 years accounts for 60% of the total height.[3]

Head

While the head continues to grow, the rate of increase in the head circumference slows during early childhood. There is an increase in circumference of about 2.5 cm in the 2nd year. Head circumference is equal to the chest circumference between 1 and 2 years.[3] The head may be measured until 2 years,[7] although it is the pattern of growth in the first year and, in particular, the first months, which is most important. By 5 years the rate of increase has slowed to about 1.25 cm per year.[3]

The head is measured by placing a non-stretch tape around the most prominent part of the occiput with the tape placed just above the eyebrows and the pinnae. The measurement is taken to the nearest 0.1 cm.[8]

NERVOUS SYSTEM

Nerve tissue continues to grow rapidly in early childhood. The brain, by 2 years, is 90% of adult size[2] and, by 5 or 6 years, has tripled in weight.[3] As the brain grows and develops, the reflex activity of infancy is increasingly replaced by controlled activity, the result of a maturing nervous system.[3] Cerebral dominance is established in preschoolers at about 4.5 years, with hand preference becoming evident.[2]

The assessment of the nervous system in early childhood involves a wide range of growth and development observations taken over time. Because all human function is dependent on neurological activity, a full neurological assessment will include physical and behavioural assessments. The main activities of a physical assessment are described in this section as they would be undertaken in a nursing assessment of the nervous system in the young child. While the assessment of a number of functions related to the cranial nerves is included, details of full cranial nerve assessment can be found in the next chapter.

Reflexes

Both superficial and deep tendon reflexes are present in these early years. While the assessment of the reflexes is described, they are not usually tested in toddlerhood or early childhood unless there are indications of dysfunction. Young children may become alarmed at the testing procedures.

Superficial reflexes are present at a number of sites in the young child. These are the abdominal, cremasteric, anal and plantar reflexes. The **abdominal reflex** is elicited when the skin is scratched or stroked towards the umbilicus. The umbilicus will deviate towards the stimulus or quadrant of stimulation. When the inner aspect of the thigh is stroked the **cremasteric reflex** of the male child is demonstrated. The testes, on the side of the stimulus, will rise within the scrotum or even into the inguinal canal. The **anal reflex** is seen when the anus quickly contracts in response to stroking or gently scratching around the anal area. The toes or the whole foot will point downwards when the **plantar reflex** is present. The reflex is stimulated by pressing the thumb against the lateral sole of the foot, moving along the sole towards the little toe and then across the foot to the big toe.[2,3,7]

Deep tendon reflexes are the stretch reflexes of muscle which are elicited at points on the limbs. These reflexes can be stimulated by tapping the tendon when it is slightly stretched with a reflex hammer or the side of the hand. The reflexes are usually graded according to the response.

Grade 4 = ++++ hyperactive or clonus
Grade 3 = +++ brisker than normal
Grade 2 = ++ normal
Grade 1 = + diminished
Grade 0 = 0 absent, no response

The **biceps reflex** is demonstrated by partial flexion of the forearm at the elbow when the tendon in the antecubital space is tapped. The child's arm is held at the elbow with the examiner's thumb over the antecubital space. The examiner's thumbnail is struck with the reflex hammer and presses down in the tendon. The triceps tendon is struck above the elbow when the child's arm is supported at the upper arm or the palm of the hand by the examiner or is resting over the child's chest when the child is in the supine position. The forearm will partially extend. The **brachioradialis reflex** is tested by placing the child's forearm on the abdomen or lap with the elbow flexed and the palm down. The radius is struck about 2.5 cm above the styloid process of the wrist. The arm will flex at the elbow and the palm will turn upward. To test for the **patellar reflex** the child needs to be sitting with the legs flexed at the knee and hanging freely. When the patellar tendon is tapped just below the kneecap the lower leg will partially extend. The same position is used for the **Achilles reflex.** The foot is lightly supported in the hand of the examiner while the Achilles tendon is tapped. The foot will point downwards in plantar extension.

Two further reflexes, which are normally absent, may be tested for. When the child is supine and the head and neck are quickly flexed forward the knees and hips will flex involuntarily in the presence of meningeal irritation. This is the Brudzinski sign. The Kernig sign is also elicited in the presence of meningeal irritation. The hip and knee are flexed while the child is supine and if there is pain and resistance to knee extension the Kernig sign is said to be positive.[2,3]

Gross motor skills

The increase in gross motor ability is closely related to neuromuscular development. In the toddler years and early childhood such development is demonstrated by increased agility and locomotion.

The toddler, by 2 years, is walking independently, can run with good coordination and walk up and down stairs with two feet to a step. Falls are less frequent in the 2nd year. By 2.5 years the toddler can jump with both feet and throw and kick a ball. The 3-year-old child can walk on tiptoe, stand on one foot, climb stairs with alternate feet and pedal a tricycle.[3,5,10,11] At 4 years, the child can catch a ball, skip and hop on one foot. Skipping on alternate feet, climbing, walking upstairs without holding the hand rail and walking backwards are usually achieved by the 5 year old.

Fine motor skills

The ability to grasp is the main fine motor skill of the early years, reflecting the development of fine muscle coordination. At 2 years, the toddler can turn the pages of a book, hold and use a spoon, manage a cup with one hand, stack 4 to 6 blocks and grasping a crayon or pen, draw circular scribbles. By 3 years the child is able to stack 8 or 9 blocks, copy a circle, can undress with help with fastenings, use a fork and spoon and string large beads. The 4 year old can cut with scissors, copy figures and printing, draw pictures of 3 or more details, and dress herself. Five year olds can use a knife, copy a triangle and a square and other shapes, print their own name and other letters and draw recognisable objects.[11,12]

Muscle tone

The muscles in early childhood, developing through growth and activity, are firm and symmetric and should demonstrate equal strength in matched muscle groups. Tone is estimated by feeling the muscle when it is both relaxed and tightened. Muscle strength can be assessed by observing the child's movements and resistance to an opposing force. The child can also be asked to push and press against an object or person and to grasp and squeeze the assessor's hand.

Alertness and responsiveness

The fully alert and responsive child is interested in her surroundings, is active and moves easily with brisk movements and responds to a wide range of environmental stimuli.

Sleep patterns vary for individual children. Toddlers sleep between 10 and 14 hours each night with most 2 year olds needing a late morning sleep of 1 to 2 hours. In the preschool years, sleep needs decrease, though most young children sleep between 10 and 12 hours at night. Many 3 year olds still need a daytime nap for about an hour or so but daytime sleep can be given up anytime between 18 months and 5 years. Sometimes on awakening from daytime sleep, children may be irritable and seem disoriented. It is not uncommon for toddlers and young children to wake during the night.[2,3,5,7]

Consciousness is assessed according to levels of alertness and responsiveness. Levels of altered consciousness include sleep, confusion or coma. These terms can be used as early criteria for the assessment of consciousness. The Glasgow Coma Scale is a more precise tool used to assess levels of consciousness where an alteration to consciousness is suspected or has occurred. Some modifications to the scale have been made for paediatric use (Appendix B).[2,3]

Eyes and vision

The eyes are clear and look moist. The distance between eyes is approximately 4.5 to 5.5 cm between the pupils and 2.5 cm between each inner canthus. There is symmetry for the shape of the eyelids, iris and pupil. The pupils will constrict with light and relax when the light source is removed.[13] The conjunctiva lining the eyelids is smooth, pink and shiny.

Between 2.5 and 3.5 years it is recommended that the eyes are examined for fixation and following and parents are questioned about any concerns they may have. It is further recommended that visual acuity (the ability to see close and distance objects clearly) be screened at 4 to 5 years with formal visual acuity tests.[14] The Sheridan-Gardiner test requires the child to point to a matching letter on a card when shown the letter by the examiner. The test is carried out at 6 metres with the examiner's letters held at the level of the child's eyes. The E test (or variant) uses a similar technique. The child holds a plastic 'E' and moves it to match the position of the examiner's 'E', which is held pointing up, down or sideways.[13] The eyes are tested together and separately in both these tests. Suggestions for covering one eye include using a card, the hand of a helper or parent or a folded tissue held over the child's eye.[13] Visual acuity is recorded as a fraction. The numerator (top figure) is the distance in metres from the child to the image, the denominator (figure below the line) is the size given to the smallest letter able to be identified which is, in fact, the distance in metres at which the majority of the population of normally sighted persons can recognise that letter. Seeing at 6/6 is normal sight and is usually reached in the toddler years.[2,3] In both tests, 3/6 or 6/9 is an acceptable pass.[13]

The light reflex test and the cover test (Chapter 1) may be carried out in early childhood in order to establish binocularity.[15]

Peripheral vision, or the visual field, may be tested in early childhood but is dependent on the child's ability to understand and cooperate. The child is required to stare at a fixed point or object directly ahead. An object is brought from out of the field of vision towards the fixed point and the child tells when it is seen. This is done for each eye and for each quadrant. The angle between the straight line of vision and the point where the object is seen is estimated. Children can see about 50° upwards, 70° downwards, 60° nasally and 90° temporally.[3]

Colour vision can be assessed in early childhood once colours can be identified. The child is asked to name the colours of objects. If there is doubt about the child's ability to discriminate colours, further testing with colour plates may be undertaken. A symbol or number printed in dots is placed on a field of dots of a different colour. Children with full colour vision will recognise the symbol or number.

Ears and hearing

The external ear is placed with the top of the pinna meeting or crossing a line from the outer eye to the occiput. Cerumen may be present at the meatus of the external canal. When the middle ear is examined it will be necessary for the young child to be held in such as way that a sudden movement when the otoscope is inserted into the ear is not possible. The parent may firmly hold the child's head across the forehead as it rests against the parent while the child sits on the parent's lap. The child's arms are constrained by the parent's other arm. In the child under 3 years the pinna is gently pulled downward and backward in order to straighten the upward curving canal and allow visualisation of the middle ear structures. In children 3 years and older the canal slopes downwards and forwards and the pinna is pulled upwards and backwards.[3] A full description of the otoscopic examination is given in Chapter 3.

It is recommended that screening for hearing be carried out before school entry. Testing with sweep audiometry is used. The child, wearing headphones, responds verbally or by action to each sound heard.[14]

Audiometric testing can be used for children after 4 years if there are concerns about hearing.[16] Assessment where the nurse seeks parental accounts of hearing and speech are undertaken throughout early childhood.

Other sensory functions

The young child can discriminate between the touch of different objects when his eyes are closed. Superficial sensation can be established by touching the skin at points of the body with a wisp of cotton wool and asking the child to say where the sensation is felt or point to the touched area.[2] The young child can also discriminate for temperature and the differences between hard or soft, blunt or sharp, thick or thin, rough or smooth objects. The sense of smell is well established in early childhood. The young child can identify familiar odours such as peanut butter when his eyes are closed.[7] Taste is also a well established sense in early childhood. The toddler and young child will accept pleasant tastes and reject strong or unusual tastes.

Balance and coordination

Balance and coordination are cerebellar functions and continue to develop during toddlerhood and early childhood. Testing of the young child is not easily accomplished, but the preschooler can usually stand balanced on one foot for 5 seconds and, by 5 years, walk heel to toe along a straight line.[10,17]

Coordination can be assessed by observing the child carrying out fine motor skills relevant to her age (see section above) and other activities such as dressing and undressing. The preschooler can usually bring his finger to within 5 to 7.5 cm of his nose when his eyes are shut.[3]

Body temperature

Body temperature falls slightly throughout early childhood as a result of the child's overall growth and the consequent reduction in the metabolic rate. The average body temperature at 3 years is 37.2°C and by 5 years is 37°C.[3]

A mercury or electronic thermometer is used to measure body temperature. The axillary route is used in early childhood but may necessitate retaining the mercury thermometer for several minutes in order to achieve an accurate reading. The electronic thermometer will usually reach the maximum reading within a minute. Temperature recording strips which are placed on the child's forehead are useful devices for parents, though accuracy has not been established for this method.[3] The child is not left during the measurement of his body temperature. Young children often register irritation when the thermometer is placed under the arm. Friendly interaction and distraction can help the child tolerate the thermometer for the required time. The thermometer is cleansed with an alcohol wipe after each use. More recently, the tympanic membrane sensor has become available. The probe of the sensor is carefully inserted into the ear canal and a temperature reading is displayed within 1 second. Temperature readings are recorded and may be graphed when there is a need to monitor changes and trends in body temperature over time.

CIRCULATORY SYSTEM

The cardiovascular system continues to mature during early childhood and with increases in muscle mass and blood volume the heart becomes more efficient at contracting and maintaining an adequate blood flow. As the stroke volume increases the heart rate decreases. Even so, the growth of the heart is slower than overall growth in this period.[2]

Pulses

Auscultation of the apical pulse at the fourth left intercostal space a little medial of the midclavicular line is frequently used to assess the heart rate in the toddler and young child, though as the child grows, assessment of a pulse by palpation becomes easier and may be more practical. The radial pulse is the most commonly palpated pulse. The carotid, femoral, brachial, popliteal and dorsalis pedis pulses may also be palpated in the assessment of rate, rhythm, volume and quality of the pulse.

While the pulse rate decreases as the child grows, the rate in the young child is strongly influenced by activity, emotion and other environmental factors. In the presence of such factors the rate is likely to increase. The average pulse rate in early childhood when the child is resting and awake is about 105 beats per minute, but can range from 80 to 130 beats per minute. Because the blood vessels of the young child are soft and easily compressed, light and steady pressure is required when palpating the pulse. The rate is counted over a full minute and other qualities, such as volume and rhythm, are assessed at the same time.

Blood pressure

The blood pressure increases in early childhood in keeping with an increased cardiac output and stroke volume. Girls at 2 years have an average systolic blood pressure of 90 mmHg with an average diastolic blood pressure of 56 mmHg. By 4 years the average systolic pressure is 92 mmHg with the diastolic pressure remaining at 56 mmHg. The average systolic blood pressure is higher by 1 mmHg for boys, though the diastolic readings are the same as for girls. A quick general guide for expected blood pressure measurements between 1 and 5 years is to add the age of the child to 90 for an estimate of the systolic pressure. The diastolic blood pressure remains constant at 56 mmHg.[18]

Blood pressure is measured with a sphygmomanometer or an electronic device such as an oscillometer or Doppler which transmit arterial pressures to a readable scale, display or sound. With each method a cuff is required which is wrapped around a limb, preferably the left upper arm. The width of the cuff should be no less than half or more than two-thirds of the chosen part of the limb.[3] Some authorities recommend cuff width cover 75% of the upper part of the limb.[3] A cuff which is too wide or too narrow will distort the reading so that a falsely low measurement will result with a cuff which is too wide and a falsely high measurement will result with a cuff which is too small. As a guide, cuff sizes 6 or 7 cm are used for toddlers and preschoolers up to 4 years and cuff sizes 8 to 10 cm from 5 to 10 years.[2] The bladder within the cuff should be long enough to encircle the limb. The diastolic blood pressure is recorded at the fourth Korotkoff sound where the sounds become muffled. The fifth Korotkoff sound is noted at the point where the sound can no longer be heard. The fourth Korotkoff sound is used for the diastolic reading in young children.[7]

Some authorities recommend that blood pressure be recorded each year in early childhood from 3 years,[3] or at every health assessment throughout childhood.[2,19]

The pulse pressure in childhood ranges between 20 and 50 mmHg. The pulse pressure is widened with an increase in stroke volume and/or decreased peripheral resistance. A narrowed pulse pressure is related to increased peripheral resistance or a decrease in stroke volume or blood volume.[7]

Colour

While skin colour in the young child is dependent on inheritance, an assessment of skin colour provides information about circulation and oxygen levels in the blood. In children with light skin, colour is normally white, creamy yellow or beige with pink tones. Children with dark skins have lighter palms of the hands and soles of the feet. The oral mucosa is dark pink in all children. Because pallor and cyanosis, indicators of circulatory change, are not easily distinguished in children with dark skin, colour is more readily assessed by inspecting the mouth, palms, soles, nails and sclera.

The time it takes for normal skin colour to return to an area where pressure has produced blanching is known as the capillary refill or filling time. Capillary refill should take 1 to 2 seconds.[2] In children with dark skin, blanching may be produced on the lips, gums and nails. This test is a useful and quick method for estimating peripheral circulation.

Heart sounds

The heart sounds, S1 and S2, are best heard at the apex and base of the heart respectively. A further heart sound, S3, may be heard in some children. The sound is caused by vibrations produced during ventricular filling and is heard, like S1, at the apical point, the 5th intercostal space on the midclavicular line. The base of the heart where S2 is heard is auscultated at the 2nd intercostal space, close to the sternum on either side. Another sound, S4, which occurs just before S1 is sometimes heard in a normal healthy heart, but should be further investigated if detected. This sound is the result of vibrations between the chambers after atrial contraction and could be the result of ventricular overload.[2,3] (For further details about heart sounds, see Chapter 1.)

Heart sounds are assessed for rate, rhythm and quality. Sinus arrhythmia may be present in some young children and is related to the respiratory cycle. The rate increases during inspiration and slows during expiration. Sinus arrhythmia is confirmed if the rate remains constant when the child holds his breath.[3] This arrhythmia is not considered abnormal.

GASTROINTESTINAL SYSTEM

The processes of digestion reach maturation in early childhood. Salivary glands are adult size and initiate the digestive processes. The young child is able to swallow saliva and has muscular control of mouth movements. In the stomach, hydrochloric acid secretion increases during early childhood further facilitating digestion.[2] The stomach, round in shape during infancy, grows into a more elongated shape during early childhood.[3] Because the young child is able to digest most foods and efficiently reabsorb water in the large intestine, the frequency of bowel movements is decreased and the consistency of the stool is increased.[2]

Mouth and teeth

The lips are symmetrical and deeper pink than the surrounding skin in light-skinned children and similar to the surrounding skin in dark-skinned children. The skin of the lips is intact though dryness and flaking may be present if the child has been in the sunlight or wind or when hydration is less than optimal.

The mucous membranes lining the mouth are dark pink, smooth and moist. The breath is non-odorous. Saliva production is well established in toddlerhood, but without the drooling of infancy. The hard and soft palates are intact and the uvula hangs in the midline. The palatine tonsils are large in early childhood, are visible and the same colour as the surrounding mucous membranes. The tongue is pink to red with the rough texture of the papillae on the upper surface. The gums are slightly more yellow-pink than the surrounding pink of the membrane. A brown line along the gum line may be seen in dark-skinned children.

The 20 deciduous teeth are usually present by 33 months (see Chapter 1 for eruption schedule). A guide for estimating the expected number of teeth in the child under 2 years is to take the age of the child in months and subtract 6 for the number of teeth expected for age.[3] The teeth are white, usually even and without caries.

Many young children find it difficult to cooperate with an assessment of the mouth. A mouth spatula should be reserved for the final part of the inspection and placed across the tongue at 45° rather than along its length, which will elicit the gag reflex.[7]

Abdomen

The abdomen in early childhood is symmetric, cylindrical and until about 4 or 5 years is prominent when the child is standing. The skin is smooth and in light-skinned children the blue pattern of superficial veins can be seen.[3] The umbilicus is inverted and dry. Occasionally umbilical protrusion is seen. Umbilical herniation usually resolves by 2 years, but in a number of children can take up to 3 years. The abdomen moves with respiration throughout early childhood. Bowel sounds are heard through a stethoscope and occur about every 10–30 seconds.[2]

Ingestion and digestion

The stomach capacity increases to 500–600 mL in early childhood, which means a three-meal-a-day pattern of eating can be accommodated. Extra food between meals, however, may be needed. The high rate of metabolism in the young child requires that the blood sugar level be maintained. The child may become hungry if protein has not been eaten or there is a long period between food intake. By 2.5 years the ability to chew with a rotary movement has been achieved and the child is able to masticate fibrous foods and muscle meats quite well.[2]

Elimination

During the 2nd year, voluntary control of the anal sphincter is gained, but many children are not ready for full control of bowel function until the 3rd year. Bowel training usually precedes bladder control because of the stronger sensations, regularity and predictability related to bowel elimination.[3] The stools are soft and mid-brown. Patterns of elimination vary from 1 to 2 stools a day to every 2 or 3 days.[20] The lower limits for frequency are 6 bowel movements a week for toddlers and 4 a week for children over 3 years.[3]

RESPIRATORY SYSTEM

Along with the general growth in early childhood, the structures of the respiratory system increase in size. Thoracic volume is increased and the respiratory rate decreases.[12]

Chest

The shape of the chest in early childhood changes from the round shape seen in infancy to an oval shape where the lateral diameter is greater than the anteroposterior diameter. As well, the chest circumference becomes greater than the head circumference by about 5 to 7 cm.[2,3]

The bony structures of the chest are the markers for the assessment of the chest and its contents. The nipples are usually placed at the 4th intercostal space. The apical heartbeat is heard in the 5th intercostal space at the midclavicular line. The costal angle, the angle between the lower costal margin and the sternum, is about 45°.

The sides of the chest and the movements of the chest during respiration are symmetric. The abdominal breathing pattern of infancy is retained in the toddler and young child.

Breath sounds

Breath sounds in young children are usually loud and easily heard with a stethoscope and are described as vesicular, bronchovesicular and bronchial. Vesicular sounds are heard over most of the lung area as soft swishing sounds. They are louder, longer and higher on inspiration than on expiration. Bronchovesicular sounds are heard over the upper intrascapular area and manubrium as muffled blowing sounds and are almost equal in intensity, duration and pitch during inspiration and expiration. These are the main breath sounds in childhood. Bronchial sounds are harsh sounds heard only over the trachea near the suprasternal notch. The sounds on expiration are louder, longer and higher than those of inspiration.[2,3,7] The toddler or young child can be asked to blow on an object such as a tissue to achieve the deep breathing necessary for satisfactory auscultation of the chest. Because breath sounds are the sounds of air moving in and out of the airways, any absence or alteration to normal sound or additional noises indicate altered function and require further investigation.

Respirations

The respiratory rate slows as the child grows and tends to be more regular, though the rate will increase noticeably under the influence of emotion, exercise or fever. The rate is between 20 and 30 breaths per minute from 2 to 4 years[2] with an average rate of 22 breaths per minute for the 5 year old. Breathing is normally quiet, involuntary and without effort.[18] Abdominal breathing persists throughout early childhood though there will be some movement of the chest during inspiration and expiration.[12]

An assessment of respirations will include observations of the rate, rhythm and quality. The rate should be counted over a full minute. There is usually a ratio of 1 breath to 4 heartbeats in early childhood.[3] Respiratory movements and vibrations may be felt by placing both hands on the chest or on the back with the thumbs in the midline along the costal margins. The respiratory effort can be assessed by the amount of movement as the child breathes. Respiratory rates and movements are often best assessed when the child is not aware that observations of respiratory function are being taken.

GENITOURINARY SYSTEM

External genitalia

The genitalia in the female toddler and preschooler are usually only examined externally and by inspection. Inspection may be undertaken during hygiene procedures such as nappy changing or bathing. Encouraging the child to sit with the soles of her feet together in order to allow visualisation of the structures which lie behind the labia majora has been recommended.[3] The labia majora in early childhood have a full appearance and are the colour and texture of the surrounding skin. The labia minora are small and thin and well covered by the labia majora. The labia are symmetric with the inner surfaces deep pink and moist. The clitoris is small and covered with a small hood of tissue. The urethral meatus and vaginal opening are visible, though if it is necessary to establish the position of the urethral meatus it may be more easily identified by wiping downwards from below the clitoris towards the vaginal opening. The meatus can be seen as a V-shaped slit.[3] The vaginal opening is darker than the surrounding tissue.[2,3,7]

The external genitalia of the male toddler and preschooler are inspected and gently palpated. The penis is usually small. The foreskin should not be forced back and will become retractable in the period from 1 to 3 years. The urethral meatus is normally at the centre of the tip of the penis. The skin of the scrotum is slightly darker than the surrounding skin and is wrinkled. The testes can be felt in the scrotum though the cremasteric reflex may cause the testes to move up into the inguinal canal. Light digital pressure on the inguinal canal will prevent such movement during palpation of the scrotum. It is also suggested that having the child sit with his legs crossed or in a warm bath will facilitate the presence of testes in the scrotum.[7] The testes are equal in size and freely moveable.[2,3,7]

Urinary function

The ability to remain dry and control urinary elimination develops during toddlerhood and by 3 years most young children are dry during the day. By 5 years, 90% are dry during the night.[21] The 2 year old is able to hold urine for up to 2 hours or more. This ability is related to greater sphincter control and an increased capacity of the bladder. The capacity of the urinary bladder triples by 2.5 years, when approximately 85 mL can be held.[2] Urinary output in 24 hours is between 600 and 800 mL in children between 2 and 5 years.[7] By 5 years the young child is voiding between 4 and 6 times during waking hours.[22] The urinary stream is straight, quite forceful and finer in boys.

Urine is collected for testing according to the child's ability to assist in catching a specimen. For toddlers who are still wearing nappies, urine is collected in the same manner as for infants (Chapter 1). Preschoolers can usually indicate when they are ready to void and allow the urine to be caught in a container, though they generally prefer the parent to manage the procedure. If urine is to be sent to the laboratory for testing the procedure aims to collect a specimen which is as uncontaminated as can possibly be managed. Such a specimen is often referred to as a 'clean catch'. The area around the urethral meatus is washed with warm water and soap, rinsed well and dried thoroughly as close to the time of collecting the urine as possible.

The pH of urine is usually acidic, from 5.0 to 6.0, but can become more alkaline when dairy foods are part of the diet.[7] Early morning urine, which is usually concentrated, has a specific gravity between 1.024 and 1.030,[7] though the lower level may drop to 1.002[2] at other times. Urine analysis carried out with a dipstick should reveal an absence of protein, glucose, ketones, blood or bilinogen. Urobilinogen is normally present at 1%.

INTEGUMENTARY SYSTEM

During these early years the skin becomes tougher and more mature, though it is thinner than in later childhood. The sweat glands produce sweat but only in small amounts. The

The joints of the young child are easily moveable.

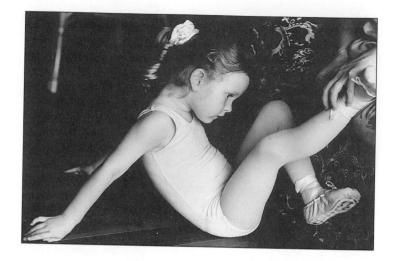

skin of the young child easily becomes dry because of a low level of sebaceous gland secretion. Fine hair appears on the forearms and lower legs. The skin of the toddler and preschooler is firm but elastic, smooth, clear, warm and dry to touch. Good turgor and elasticity is evident when gently pinched skin quickly returns to its normal shape. Mucous membranes are deep pink and moist.[2,3]

The condition of the skin is an indicator of nutritional and fluid status and can give cues about the levels of care and hygiene the child receives. Temporary colour changes of the skin reflect activity, environmental and body temperature and circulation. The child may become flushed when very active, febrile or during hot conditions. In very cold conditions the child may be pale with blue fingers, toes and lips. The young child who is ill or nauseous may also exhibit noticeable pallor.

Health Management

Anne Adams

Movement and activity

Toddlers and preschoolers are highly active and are capable of an increasing range of physical movements which become more sophisticated as the growth and development of the musculoskeletal and neurological systems continues. Vigorous activity is undertaken spontaneously and includes running, climbing, jumping and hopping. Young children greatly enjoy physical exercise such as skipping, hopping, sliding, pedalling, swinging or scooting and participate in these activites with enthusiasm. Physical activity in early childhood contributes to bone and muscle growth, the development of neurological functions such as balance and coordination and the healthy function of body systems.[2]

Movement and activity are frequently undertaken as part of the toddler's play. Toys which can be moved about by pushing, pulling or wheeling encourage activity as do toys which can be rocked, ridden or rolled. As the preschooler develops socially and is able to interact with other children in associative and cooperative play, equipment which allows for physical activity can be provided. Exercise with outdoor and adventure playground facilities, wheeled toys for riding or scooting and the activities of outdoor trips are some ways whereby physical activities can be experienced.

Young children need periods of rest or quieter activity between energetic and boisterous activities[20] and before bedtime. Quiet activites often need the participation of a caregiver because the toddler and the young child are not always able to remain quietly involved without company. Reading stories or looking at picture books is particularly enjoyed by most young children and can be carried out while the child is held or cuddled, adding an affective dimension to the activity. Other quiet activities include role playing ('pretend games'), playing with toys which require organising or building, watching television or video film, manipulating electronic and computer games, listening and joining in with music and experimenting with art.

Stimulation

As the toddler and preschooler become more proficient in exploring and managing the environment the need to actively provide stimulation becomes less. The visual, auditory, tactile and kinetic senses of the young child constantly receive stimuli through everyday activities. Even so, stimulatory experiences for the young child can be devised and serve to optimise development and enrich experience. Social activity with peers can be gained through playgroups, day-care centres and kindergartens. Interactions with caregivers and other adults offer social, language and behavioural experiences. Play provides stimulation but some games and activities have particularly stimulatory features. These include games and activities with verbal interactions and 'helping' with adult tasks by toddlers. For preschoolers, games and activities such as matching, comparing, counting and recognition of objects encourage identification and discrimination abilities.[7]

Sleep

While sleep is a necessity in the toddler and preschool years, it is common for the young child to resist sleep and for conflict to develop with parents and caregivers over sleep routines. An established routine and the expectation that sleep will be taken seems to be the most successful approach to the young child's sleep needs. Toddlers, who usually need a daytime nap, are responsive to rituals where a predictable set of events occurs at a similar time each day. For example, sleeping in the same place with particular objects such as a rug, pillow and soft toys, establishes the pattern for a daytime sleep.

It is often recommended that, before bedtime and in order to prepare for sleep, the young child has quiet activities rather than any which will arouse and excite him. If the child is attached to a toy or object it will be needed for him to feel relaxed and comforted enough for sleep. Many young children are able to settle to sleep if a soft light is visible and they have confidence in a parent's presence. Other comfort measures such as warmth in cold weather, coolness in hot conditions and attention to fluid and elimination requirements should be considered when preparing the young child for sleep.

Young children may wake during the night and need to be made comfortable by a change of nappy, a drink, covering, touching and soothing. The issue of whether it is better for the child to remain in his own bed is often debated. Many parents have found that when the child is placed in bed with them he is able to return to sleep quickly, while others, who maintain that their child must stay in his own bed, have established ways to soothe their child back to sleep while in his own bed. Regardless of the method by which the awake child is helped to return to sleep, contact and comfort are usually required.

Nutrition

Adequate nutrition for the young child plays an essential part in healthy growth and development but in order to fully appreciate the management of nutrition in toddlers and preschoolers behavioural and developmental aspects of early childhood must be considered.

The toddler, in learning to gain control, both of himself and his environment, will often behave in negative and resistive ways. As well, after 18 months, when the toddler's nutritional needs begin to decrease in line with metabolic and growth demands, the desire for and interest in food begins to fluctuate. Toddlers may become highly selective about which foods they will eat and, at the same time, have marked variation in appetite from one day to the next. The management of the fussy and disinterested toddler's nutrition requires a calm and imaginative approach together with a good knowledge of the nutritional requirements of the young child.

Toddlers and preschoolers are able to eat most of the foods eaten by the rest of the family. An optimum diet is described according to the types and proportions of foods as set out in the Healthy Diet Pyramid.[23] Within this model of nutrition it is recommended that vegetables, cereals, bread and fruit are eaten in the largest quantities, meat, chicken, fish, eggs, milk and milk products in moderate quantities and fats and sugar are to be eaten in small amounts. Salt should not be added and salted foods avoided.

Young children generally accept foods in small portions and at frequent intervals. Between meal snacks are therefore a good strategy for maintaining an adequate food intake and nutritional requirements. Servings at meals should be in proportion to the child's age and requirements. A guide for the serving size of foods recommends a tablespoon of solid food for each year of age or a quarter to one-third of the adult serving. It is further suggested that the tablespoon guide be used with easily measured foods such as vegetables and that the fraction guide be used for foods such as bread and milk.[3]

It is generally recommended that toddlers have about 600 mL of milk per day and preschooler a little less, about 400–500 mL. Some toddlers, particularly those who are attached to their bottles, may have a higher milk intake and as a consequence, their intake of other foods is reduced. These toddlers could be at risk for deficiencies in iron and other nutrients and for dental decay. Encouraging the use of a cup and reducing the amount of milk is desirable. Fruit juice is usually favoured by young children but also needs to be limited. About 200 mL per day is adequate. A higher intake can cause intestinal irritation and reduce the amount of water the child will accept. Fruit juices should not have added sugar.

Elimination

Toilet training is achieved when the young child is physically and psychologically ready. This means she is able to recognise the sensations related to the need to eliminate, to signal this need and is prepared to use the toilet or potty. Excretory control is ideally achieved in a harmonious atmosphere and with acknowledgement of the child's ability to participate.

The discomfort of a wet or soiled nappy and the observation of toilet use by others are often related to the toddler's wish to wear pants and use the toilet. Pants can be worn during the day even though the toddler may not always be able to keep dry. Many parents continue to use nappies at night until the child has demonstrated overnight urine control. Once a young child has dispensed with nappies they should not, for the most part, be reintroduced, even during periods of illness or hospitalisation.

While the toddler may be ready and cooperative with the use of the toilet, help with removing and replacing clothing, getting into position, using toilet paper, cleaning and hand washing will be required. The preschooler will become more adept with these tasks, but will need to be taught cleaning procedures, how to flush the toilet and hand washing routines. Girls will need to be taught to wipe toilet paper from front to back. Girls should also be taught to blot with toilet paper after urinating so the genital area and underclothing remain dry. The surrounding skin will be less likely to become irritated or excoriated. Boys are usually able to keep dry if they are taught to shake off the last remaining drops of urine when voiding is complete.

The young child will, of course, experience times when full control of bladder and bowel is not maintained. Such 'accidents' can be distressing for the young child and should be managed with minimum fuss, reassurance and, if appropriate, a sense of humour.

The frequency and appearance of the stools of the young child should be noted. The frequency of urination should also be noted as well as any uncomfortable sensations during urination. Stinging during urination may be caused by tissue irritation in the immediate area, but further opinion should be sought for any discomfort.

Clothing and protection

While the function of clothing is to protect skin, provide warmth and contribute to hygiene there are functional and aesthetic factors to be considered in the choice and management of clothing for the young child.

Ideally, clothing for toddlers should be easy to put on and take off, sturdy and easy to care for. Toddlers are attracted to bright colours and often have favourite garments. Synthetic fabrics are not recommended because they restrict the circulation of air and are a risk with fire. Cotton and cotton blends are preferred in warm and hot weather. Wool is safe and warm in colder weather, but is not as fuss-free to launder and dry as winter-weight cotton.

Clothing for the preschooler should be easy for the child to put on and take off, especially pants and underpants. Preschoolers are more aware of their clothing and that worn by their peers and may want their clothing to be the same or similar.

The young child's clothing should not be constricting and should allow for free movements. At the same time, roomy clothing should not cause the child to trip or get easily caught on furniture or outdoor objects. As the child grows, elastic casings, edges and fastenings on garments may become tight and should be replaced or the garment no longer worn. Spills, play and toilet accidents mean that the young child needs a supply of clean clothes and may require several changes in a day. Clean clothes, however, should not be the priority when play and healthy activity is undertaken. Summer clothing should allow the child to keep cool and in winter, sufficient warm clothing will be needed. Extra outdoor clothing is needed in cold windy conditions. The head of the young child is still capable of considerable heat loss. For this reason, and for comfort, a warm cap which covers the head and ears should be worn. In summer, protective clothing such as shirts and hats with brims and neck shades, is necessary when the child is in strong sunlight.

Clothing and, in particular, the nightwear of young children should be chosen with reference to the hazards of fire and the risk for burns. It is recommended that long, loose, frilled nightwear and readily flammable material in children's clothing be avoided and that clothing which is labelled flame-resistant and close fitting is chosen.[24] Shoes should allow enough room around the toes and be replaced as the feet grow. Laces should be tied firmly so the child will not trip. Socks should also allow enough space for movement of the toes and be replaced when they become tight.

Hygiene

It is common practice in most parts of Australia for young children to be bathed each day, and in extreme heat conditions, more often. For toddlers and preschoolers bathtime is generally enjoyable, a time of play and social interaction with parents and siblings. Showering the young child is not so easily managed and most caregivers find bathing a more convenient procedure. Cold water should be run into the bath initially to prevent overheating the floor of the bath and the final temperature of the bath water must be carefully checked. It has been recommended that bubble bath solution is not used routinely because of its potential to irritate the external genitalia, which can predispose to urinary tract infection.[2,7,12] A suction mat in the bottom of the bath will prevent slippery falls. Young children must not be left unattended in the bath for even the shortest period.

Hair needs to be washed at least weekly, though some parents prefer to do it more frequently. Shampoo which does not sting the eyes should be used. Young children, on the whole, do not like the sensation of having water poured over the head and down the face. Protecting the face with a washer, tipping the head backwards and lying face-up in the bath are some ways this problem can be avoided.

Teeth hygiene begins in infancy but it is in toddlerhood that the young child begins to participate in cleaning her own teeth. A small toothbrush and pleasant tasting toothpaste are used. Parents will clean the teeth at first, but the toddler can practise the actions and gradually become proficient. It is also recommended that parents floss the teeth with dental floss at least once a day.[3] At first, the toddler is not able to rinse the mouth and spit out. Teeth should be cleaned after each meal and the young child should go to bed each night with a clean mouth. Rinsing and swishing the mouth with tap water is suggested for those times when regular teeth cleaning is not possible. From 2.5 years the first visit to the dentist for a dental check is recommended.[25] This visit is also to introduce the toddler to the idea of visiting the dentist and should be a friendly and happy experience. Dental checks are continued each year until school age.

Though fingernails may become dirty during play activities, nails will usually be kept clean with daily bathing and a number of hand washes during the day. Nails need to be trimmed at regular intervals. Toenails should be cut straight across while an emery board may be preferred for fingernails.

Immunisation

The recommended immunisation schedule is maintained in the period from 18 months to 5 years (Appendix C). At 18 months a further injection of triple antigen, which immunises for diphtheria, tetanus and pertussis, is given. The *Haemophilus influenzae* type b (Hib) Schedule 1 vaccination is also given at 18 months. At 5 years or before commencing school the child is given a triple antigen injection and a further oral dose of Sabin vaccine. While the immunisation schedule should be maintained, the child should not receive a vaccine if he has an acute illness with a fever. The vaccination is delayed until the child is well.

Safety

Toddlers and preschoolers are the most vulnerable group for accidents during childhood.[24,26] Falls, emersion, motor vehicle accidents, burns, and ingestion of poisonous substances are common occurrences in early childhood and are related to the child's mobility and inability to anticipate danger.

Adult supervision and awareness, together with product standards, child safety legislation and community education are the measures by which early childhood trauma can be prevented and reduced.

The presence of an informed and alert adult is the best prevention for accidents, but because there are a number of factors at play in any situation of risk, a safe environment can also reduce the potential for accidental injury to the young child. Supervision should prevent the young child from falls, in that climbing and exploring is restricted to safe and appropriate settings, but play equipment and the surface beneath it should be designed to minimise the effect of a fall. Because swimming pools are a recognised hazard to the toddler, safety fencing is a requirement for home pools. There remains, however, the risk to the young child of drowning, if other sources of emersion, such as garden ponds and wading pools, are overlooked, and if swimming pool users neglect to secure the gate in a safety fence. Legislation in Australia requires that children be secured in automobiles. Toddlers and preschoolers up to 4 years should be accommodated in a child safety seat. From 4 years the child can sit in a booster cushion held in place by a seat belt[26] or a harness. Young children should not be left in cars, even for the shortest time.

The kitchen and bathroom are potentially dangerous to young children because of food preparation and the use of hot water. Cooking implements, hot substances and fluids should be inaccessible to young children. Matches and other flame-producing equipment should be stored away from children's reach, as should flammable fluids. Such fluids, and others such as cleaning solutions, should be labelled and stored in childproof containers. Tablets and medications are particularly attractive to young children and should be kept in locked and out of reach storage in childproof containers. Many medications are dispensed in blister packs in order to make it more difficult for young children to remove them. Such packs still need to be stored safely away from children. Some foods are unsafe for young children and should not be accessible to them. These include peanuts, other nuts and hard sweets which could be inhaled, and alcohol.

Other safety measures which should be taken in order to have a safe environment for the young child include guarding sources of heat such as fires or heaters, placing blank non-removable plugs and circuit breakers in power sockets and using short or curly cords for electrical appliances. Locks or catches can be placed on cupboard doors, room barricades can keep the child away from areas of risk, transfers or 'dots' should be placed on glass doors at children's eye level and safety gates positioned around the home.

Skin protection in sunlight remains important for the toddler and preschooler. Protective clothing and shady head coverings are necessary when outdoors, especially in summer. Sunscreen creams should be applied to skin areas not covered by clothing.

First aid training is another way in which parents and caregivers can contribute to the safety of young children. It still remains, however, that close and vigilant supervision by an adult is the best means by which toddlers and preschoolers can be kept safe.

The nurse's role in contributing to the safety of the young child is expressed in two ways. Firstly, through giving information to parents about safety issues and secondly, when undertaking care of the young child, to offer care which is safe and informed.

Psychological Growth and Development

Sue Nagy

During early childhood, children make the transition from the end of infancy, when they are just beginning to explore their environment, to becoming toddlers and 'school kids' and learning the skills that are important for life in their culture. A significant amount of development takes place during this time.

COGNITIVE DEVELOPMENT DURING EARLY CHILDHOOD

Piaget's preoperational stage

Young children think in a qualitatively different way to adults. Understanding the thought processes of young children is critical to communicating with them effectively. Indeed, it is fundamental to understanding almost everything about them . . . their play, the way they deal with stressful situations, their understanding of the way their bodies work and how they become sick, how they conceptualise death and how they understand the difference between right and wrong. To communicate effectively with a child, an adult needs to understand the way the child interprets what is happening to him. This involves not only understanding how children make sense of the world, but also any limitations on their thinking ability.

Early childhood involves the second of Piaget's stages of cognitive development, the preoperational stage.[27,28] Preoperational thinking is characterised by certain features which account for many of the misconceptions that young children have about events in the world.

Preoperational children have difficulty in understanding that objects can change their appearances but not change their nature, such as believing that a boy who wears a dress is a girl. They also have difficulty understanding the concept of time. A child of my acquaintance celebrated his 4th birthday at preschool and then had a party at home the following weekend. When a party guest inquired about his age, he replied that he was 5. He had calculated that he turned 4 on his birthday at school and 5 on his next 'birthday' on the weekend! Most young children have some idea of the concepts of 'past' and 'future', but they are not well developed. Preschool children may refer to events that happened at any time in the past as happening 'yesterday'. A nurse who tells such a child that he will have his plaster removed 'tomorrow' may be communicating only that it will happen some time in the future.

A striking characteristic of preoperational thinking is centration.[29] This refers to the tendency of the child to 'centre' his attention on one, usually the most obvious, aspect of a situation, and to ignore all the other aspects. He may believe that 20 cents is more valuable than $2, because it is bigger or that a tall person is older than a short person. A young child may believe that there is less orange juice in a wide, short glass than a tall thin glass, even when both glasses contain the same volume of orange juice. He may focus on only the height of the orange juice, and not consider any change in width. Accordingly, a child whose fluids are restricted may be more satisfied if he is given fluids in a tall thin glass. He may similarly believe that he has more beans to eat if they are served on a small plate than if the same amount of beans is placed on a large plate. A child who has a small appetite may respond better to food served on a large plate. Centration makes it difficult for the child to understand that while an injection may hurt, it will also help make him better. He is likely to focus only on the 'hurting' aspect and be unmoved by a nurse's explanations of its necessity.

The reasoning patterns of adults commonly take 3 main forms: inductive reasoning (i.e., deriving general rules from specific cases); deductive reasoning (i.e., applying general rules to specific cases); and hypothetico-deductive reasoning (formulating hypotheses and testing them systematically). In contrast, young children reason transductively, that is they tend to reason from specific cases to specific cases.[29] In the process they may come to believe that events which occur together are related, and may even have caused each other. A child may reason, for example, 'I wished that my brother would get sick and he did. I made him sick!' or 'I played under the apple tree and I got sick. The apple tree made me sick!' or 'The nurse was angry with me and gave me an injection. She gave me the injection because she was angry.'

Young children's difficulty with deductive reasoning provides some insight into why they have problems playing games according to rules. Rules are based on the application of the general concept of the rights of individuals to specific instances (deductive reasoning). While young children may be able to restrain themselves from some prohibited behaviours, they often have difficulty in grasping the principles behind rules and in the application of the principle to a new circumstance. A child may not, for example, understand that everybody is entitled to take a turn throwing the dice in a board game and therefore try to take a turn every time they can grab the dice.

The egocentricity of their thinking prevents them from coping with rules which are for the benefit of all. Egocentricity leads them to believe that the world exists for their benefit. They may believe that the sun rises so they can play and that it sets so they can sleep. It also limits their ability to understand the point of view of other people. Because they are so focused on their own needs, hospitalised children may not respond to exhortations to stop screaming because they are upsetting other children in the ward. They often have problems understanding that the thoughts of others are different to theirs. Many children seem to believe that adults automatically know what they are thinking and feeling, so there is no need to explain. For instance, a child may not feel it is necessary to explain that he wants to wait until his mother arrives before his wound is dressed or his sutures removed. He may believe that the nurse knows this and if she does not wait until his mother arrives, it is because she doesn't care. Young children believe that adults have enormous power and can make anything happen if they want to. If the adults do not intervene, it is because they do not want to, not because they can't. A hospitalised child, whose mother is unable to be present, may plead with a nurse 'Please, get my mummy' and not have any doubts about the nurse's ability to do so.

Evidence of the young child's egocentric view of the world can be seen in many daily interactions — referring to a woman's husband as her 'daddy' or nodding during a phone conversation instead of answering 'yes'. Egocentric thinking can be demonstrated in the following way. Ask a 3- or 4-year-old child with a same sexed sibling, 'Do you have a brother (or sister)?' When the child answers 'Yes,' ask him 'Does your brother have a brother?' Most children of this age will have difficulty in seeing the relationship from a sibling's point of view and will answer 'No.'

It is through sharing of thoughts with others that children begin to understand that their thoughts are uniquely theirs, and that others have different points of view. While this normally does not happen until the child is 6 or 7,[30] there is limited evidence that it could begin as early as 4 years. Shatz and Gelman, found that as 4 year olds spoke in more complex sentences when talking to adults than when they spoke to toddlers, they concluded that these children understood the need to adjust their speech to the capacity of the listener to understand them.[31]

Animism is a tendency to endow inanimate objects with the characteristics of animals and people. A very small child may believe that most objects have life and can therefore feel. Gradually he will come to modify this view to believe that only objects that move are alive, such as toy cars and a jack-in-the-box. Later he will come to believe that only objects that move of their own accord are alive, such as the wind and the moon. Finally, the child achieves the full realisation that only people, animals and plants are alive.

An understanding of the limits of children's cognitive ability is fundamental to their nursing care.[32] Because children often misunderstand situations, it is important to check their perceptions of what is happening and correct any misconceptions. When children must undergo painful procedures, comforting young children may be more effective than trying to provide reasons for the procedure. As most children believe that adults are very powerful, they will feel more secure if they believe that the adult truly has their welfare at heart. Simply worded explanations may help the child understand what is happening and explanations work better if they are phrased in terms of familiar, daily events. 'We will take the plaster off your arm in the morning after you have your breakfast'.

MORAL DEVELOPMENT

A major developmental task faced by children is learning the difference between right and wrong. Many psychological theories have tried to explain the process of moral development.

According to **psychoanalytic theory** children initially learn moral behaviour because of a fear of punishment. This is an ego response based on the 'reality principle'. However, as the superego becomes stronger, children begin to internalise their parents' sanctions and prohibitions and so develop a sense of guilt and shame when they misbehave. Guilt and shame are sufficiently painful to be strong motivators of virtuous behaviour.[33]

Social learning theorists believe that children initially learn to behave morally because they are rewarded for good behaviour and punished for bad. Eventually children come to reward themselves with feelings of virtuousness so that they behave morally even when an authority figure is not present. Social learning theorists have also argued that children imitate adults whom they see rewarded. As virtuous behaviour is more likely to be rewarded, children have another means of learning to behave morally.

Lawrence Kohlberg developed a theory of moral development that has been arguably the most influential.[34] He based his ideas on those of Piaget and focused on the rationale behind moral judgements, rather than the actual decision. His research involved the use of a series of hypothetical moral dilemmas, the most well known of which surrounds 2 people, Heinz, a man whose wife is dying of cancer, and a chemist who has developed a drug that could cure her. The chemist is demanding an exorbitant price for the drug

Table 2.1 Kohlberg's levels of moral reasoning

Level 1	Preconventional morality: Moral judgments are based on the consequences for the person making the judgment
	Stage 1 Moral behaviour is that which avoids punishment
	Stage 2 Moral behaviour is that which is rewarded

Level 2	Conventional morality: Moral judgments are based on social conventions
	Stage 3 Moral behaviour is that which is approved of by others
	Stage 4 Moral behaviour is that which is sanctioned by legitimate authorities

Level 3	Moral judgments are based on ethical principles
	Stage 5 Moral behaviour is that which provides the greatest good for the greatest number
	Stage 6 Moral behaviour is that which is governed by universal ethical principles The person conforms to avoid personal censure

which Heinz cannot afford. Research participants are asked to indicate whether or not Heinz should steal the drug and to give reasons for their answer. From the answers, Kohlberg identified 3 levels of moral reasoning. Within each level are 2 stages (**see Table 2.1**).

He found that children initially judge the morality of behaviour by its consequences and called this the 'preconventional' stage of moral development. The greater the damage caused by a person, the naughtier they are. Such beliefs can be illustrated by the answers of young children to the following story.

Jack was helping with the washing up and accidentally broke 5 cups. Joshua was stealing some sweets from a kitchen cupboard and accidentally broke one cup. Who was the naughtiest of the two children?

Preconventional children regard the child who broke 5 cups as naughtier than the child who broke 1 cup. It is not until later that the intentions of the person are taken into account.

Around the age of 4, children begin to behave, not only to avoid punishment but also for the rewards that are dispensed to the 'good' child. The preschool child will, therefore, generally behave morally to avoid punishment and to gain rewards.

LANGUAGE DEVELOPMENT

Children's ability to use language develops along with their ability to think. Toddlers typically speak in short sentences consisting of 1 to 3 words, and frequently become frustrated as they struggle to communicate ideas. By the age of 2 most toddlers have learned the meaning of the verbal symbol 'Bedtime!' and are able to respond with another symbol, the word 'No!'. However, to reach such a point in language development, they must first be exposed to much verbal interaction with caregivers. During the preschool years, children learn to construct increasingly more complex sentences. They learn to include articles, and auxiliary verbs, to change the tenses and use singular and plural number appropriately. The average 6-year-old child can construct grammatically correct sentences almost as well as an adult.

By the age of 2, the average child has a vocabulary of about 300 words. By 3 years of age, most children have a vocabulary of between 900 and 1000 words, 50% to 75% of which is understood by the child's family; also they can construct 3 to 4 word sentences. By 4 years of age their vocabulary consists of about 1500 words and sentences comprise 5 to 6 words. Most 5 year olds have a vocabulary of about 2500 words, almost all of which is understood by people outside the family and by the age of 6 they have a vocabulary of about 14 000 words.[35]

Preschool children tend to understand the meaning of sentences by the sequence of the ideas within them. Sentences constructed in the passive voice may be misunderstood.[36,37] A child may, for example, interpret the sentence 'Fiona was hit by Joanne' to mean that Fiona did the hitting. Similarly, the statement 'You can have breakfast after your operation' may be interpreted to mean that the child can have breakfast before the operation as it preceded the word 'operation' in the sentence.

Adults play a vital role in helping children develop their language skills. Children learn by imitating the speech of adults around them.[36] Most adults seem to instinctively adapt their speech to the level of the child's understanding. When children use incorrect grammar, rather than overtly correcting them, adults seem to instinctively repeat the sentence correctly. By naming objects in the environment, repeating sentences correctly when the child makes mistakes, expanding sentences beyond telegraphic language, and by reading stories aloud, adults can provide models for children to imitate.[36]

It is important to note that children of parents whose native language is other than English may be slightly delayed in their language development. Minor delays are not serious as most children catch up eventually[35] and a minor delay is more than compensated for by their bilingual skills.

SOCIAL AND EMOTIONAL DEVELOPMENT

During early childhood, the progression is made from the dependence and separation anxiety of toddlerhood, to being able to attend school all day without their mothers; from having little idea of how to conform to the expectations of society, to being generally able to behave in socially acceptable ways; and from having little idea of the differences between the sexes, to having a strong sense of gender identity. The ideas of Freud and Erikson provide a framework for understanding how these changes come about.

The psychoanalytic view of early childhood

During the 2nd and 3rd years of life, the child's id or pleasure seeking impulses come to be modified by the development of the ego. The ego is also known as the 'reality principle' because of its direct connection with the realities of the external world. The ego, aware of the consequences of unrestrained self-indulgence, attempts to restrain the id. Id impulses may be prevented from being expressed or delayed until a more appropriate time. Through id/ego conflict the child begins to respond to the control exerted on him by the external world, but only in so far as his behaviour has consequences for himself.

During the 4th and 5th years, the child's superego, or conscience, begins to develop. It is now that they begin to realise that behaviour can be 'right' or 'wrong'. Preschool children frequently express shock at the 'bad' behaviour of other children. In this way, they learn to apply the moral values of their culture and make judgements about the 'goodness' or 'badness' of behaviour. They are now beginning to internalise the values of their family and of the wider society. Internal psychic conflicts now begin to involve consideration of the consequences of behaviour for others.

The anal stage

The anal stage of development occurs during the toddler years. As children develop some control over their bodily functions, the focus of their sensual pleasure changes from oral activities such as sucking and eating to anal activity and elimination. They must now learn to manage the conflict between their desire to expel faeces (pleasure principle), and the demands of society that they only do so in certain places (reality principle). Toilet training may become a focus for the expression of children's need for autonomy and a means of exercising a degree of control over their relationship with their parents. They may withhold faeces if they wish to exercise autonomy or may please their parents by using the toilet. During toddlerhood, relationships between parents and children have the potential to develop into a power struggle.

Freud believed that the way that parents manage toilet training has implications for personality development. Parents who are highly controlling inadvertently encourage a behaviour pattern where the child withholds her faeces. This behaviour may extend into other areas of their lives resulting in adults who hoard their possessions just as they once withheld their faeces. They may become possessive, mean and obstinate and defiantly messy.[38] On the other hand, toddlers who are allowed to control the situation while parents lavish excessive praise on them for proper bowel habits, may, as adults, seek to buy love by giving presents as they once earned their parents approval with their faeces. They may also become obsessively clean and neat.[39]

The phallic stage

Most children, by the time they have reached the age of 3, are beginning to be aware of the differences between boys and girls. Initially they tend to identify the gender of people by such outward appearances as dress or hair style. Later they are aware of the anatomical differences. By the age of 6 or 7, when they reach the end of the phallic stage, most will have developed a strong sense of sex role identity.

Freud believed that small girls unconsciously envy boys their penises and feel that they have lost part of their anatomy. On the other hand, boys have an unconscious belief that girls have had their penises cut off and consequently feel anxious the same may happen to them. Small boys' anxiety about their penises forms the basis for Freud's explanation of the process by which boys come to make the transition from using their mother as a role model to identifying with their fathers and so develop a sense of gender identity. Freud called this process the Oedipus complex. He argued that small boys unconsciously see their fathers as rivals for their mother's affection, but they also see their fathers as having a great deal of power. When a boy becomes anxious about losing his penis, he believes that his father has the power to castrate him. He attempts to appease his father by trying to be like him in behaviour, attitudes, dress etc. In this way he comes to use his father rather than his mother as a role model.

During the Oedipal stage, small boys may react with great anxiety to genital surgery such as hypospadias and epispadias repair. By understanding the source of this anxiety and by providing reassurance, nurses can help the child to cope with it. Parents may also need reassurance that their son's reaction is normal and healthy.

Preschoolers' curiosity about genitals and sexual matters needs to be addressed by adults. It is important to answer their questions truthfully and not to include more information than the child can deal with. A good rule of thumb is to answer the question that the child asked without giving excessive detail that the child has not requested.[39,40]

Erikson's psychosocial view of early childhood

Autonomy versus shame and doubt

Freud's anal stage corresponds with Erikson's 'autonomy versus shame and doubt' stage of development. Erikson argued that, equipped with the security that comes from acquiring a sense of trust, toddlers begin to establish the foundations of autonomous behaviour.[41] To accomplish this, they need ample opportunity to explore the world and to try out what they can do for themselves. By exploring their environment and testing their motor abilities they develop an appreciation of their own competence. With competence comes a sense of self-control, a realistic appreciation of their abilities, a sense of pride in their accomplishments and the foundation of a sense of self-esteem. The child's struggle for autonomy may result in frustration and temper tantrums, a common phenomen among 2 year olds. 'No' is the word most often used by toddlers as they insist on carrying out tasks for themselves, irrespective of whether they can manage or not. Many parents are forced to watch wilful toddlers making futile attempts to tie their shoelaces, or sweep the floor, refusing all offers of help. Parents may become concerned about their uncooperative child who is exerting her will and feel that they should 'control' her before she becomes completely 'out of hand'. In other words, parents may see this stage as a power struggle and they must win. The work of Diana Baumrind has shown that highly restrictive and controlling parents tended to produce children who lack autonomy,[42] perhaps because of reduced opportunities for learning self-direction. Paradoxically, permissive parents who were unwilling to set limits also had children who were highly dependent. Baumrind found that parents who had high expectations of their children's behaviour, but also encouraged their efforts, produced the most autonomous and self-reliant children.[42]

As toddlers do not have the wisdom or discrimination to know what behaviours are acceptable or unacceptable, parents need to provide guidance. A badly behaved child may perceive that she is arousing overt or veiled hostility from adults, but not know what to do. If limits are not set children may feel that no one cares. If children continually find themselves left to cope with tasks that are beyond their capacity they may doubt their ability and feel ashamed that they encounter so many difficulties. Toddlers need to be helped to discriminate safe from unsafe situations. By doing this parents helps to convince their children that they are worth the attention of the parent, increasing their sense of self-esteem. Adults who ridicule children or are excessively critical of their efforts foster a sense of shame and doubt.

Nurses can help parents to deal with the behaviour of toddlers by explaining that this is a normal part of development and that it is best handled by allowing children to try out their abilities, while the parents maintain close supervision and set reasonable limits on their children's behaviour. For example, diversional tactics may defuse a temper tantrum which has not fully developed. Calmly removing the child to a quiet, but not frightening place for a very short time (2 or 3 minutes) is often a more effective way of dealing with a very furious small child.

*Sibling relation-
ships are often
ambivalent.*

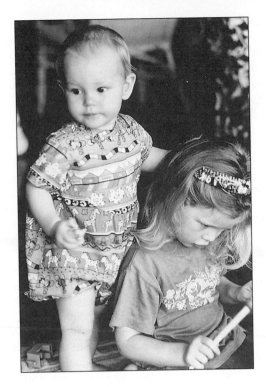

Initiative versus guilt

By the age of 4, most children have a good sense of their physical abilities. Naturally curious about the world and wanting to pursue new interests and activities, they are now ready to apply these abilities to new situations and so develop a sense of initiative. Inevitably, their attempts to initiate new activities bring them into conflict with their parents. If their behaviour is strongly disapproved of and criticised, they may develop a sense of guilt and be inhibited from showing much initiative. On the other hand, if they are allowed opportunities to experiment and are secure in the knowledge that their parents will protect them by providing guidance and setting reasonable limits on their behaviour, they will develop a sense of initiative without excessive guilt.

It is important for young children that the adults provide opportunities for them to plan and carry out their own activities. The child's efforts should be encouraged and excessive ridicule or criticism should be avoided. Fear of doing the wrong thing may result in the child being inhibited and severely restricting his own activities. In this way, initiative will be impeded and guilt will be fostered.

Sibling relationships

The relationships that a child has with his siblings contributes to the quality of his life. Sibling relationships vary from very close relationships where the children play together and share a great many experiences to relationships where the siblings have relatively little contact with each other. Children are more likely to have close affectionate relationships with siblings who are the same sex and who are close in age.[43] Sibling relationships are often ambivalent. Siblings may show great affection towards each other but at other times fight with each other and compete for the attention of their parents.[43] Research has shown that the degree of conflict between siblings is related to the rivalry that exists between them and that fighting is more likely to occur when their mother is present.[43] Parents who are concerned by the amount of fighting among their children may try to share their attentions as equally as possible, but this may be especially difficult if one sibling has a chronic illness or a disability.

Play

Maria Montessori, a great educationalist, summarised the importance of play when she said that 'play is the work of childhood'. Play is not a frivolous pastime but is one of the main ways that children learn and develop. Through play, children develop and practise their motor skills, and improve their physical coordination. They learn the art of negotiation with peers and so improve their social skills.[44] Play helps develop their cognitive abilities by improving their understanding of the world and the behaviour of different materials. It also fosters emotional development. By re-enacting real life, children express emotions, act out situations that are worrying them and develop ways of dealing with them. Play, therefore, may also be a form of stress management for children.

Play can be classified according to the type of activity.[3] When adults play with babies, they tend to use social affective play. They smile at them, tickle them, and talk to them. From this kind of play, infants learn to respond to adults and to attract their attention by calling, smiling and even initiating games. Sense–pleasure play consists of playing with different materials such as sand, water, clay, mud and food. It involves feeling, observing and learning how these materials behave. It includes trying new body movements such as swinging, bouncing and rocking. Any or all of the senses may be involved. Skill play involves the exercise of new-found motor abilities by repeating the action over and over. It can cause the child some frustration when he tries new and underdeveloped skills. Examples of skill play are piling blocks, walking, pulling things apart, putting things together, throwing, jumping, climbing, riding a bike, or riding a skateboard. Dramatic play is seen in toddlers, but is more evident in early childhood and in young school-age children. It consists of acting out fantasies. Children take on the roles and identities of family members, school teachers, shopkeepers, nurses, doctors, policemen, robbers, cowboys, astronauts, Indians and so on. The dramatic play of the preschooler may reflect her new awareness of gender differences. For example, when playing mothers and fathers, father must be played by a boy and mother must be played by a girl. Toys representing the tools of other roles are useful at this age. Ritualistic play consists of games such as 'Ring-a-Ring-a-Rosie', 'The Farmer in the Dell', 'Oranges and Lemons', which are popular among school children. The repetitive nature and consequent predictability of ritualistic play seems to provide a means of managing the stresses encountered during childhood.

As children develop, their play becomes more social. Infants' play does not involve other children, but the play of school-age children is often quite socially involved. It is through play that children learn to interact with their peers. Through play children's social skills improve and the amount of conflict between them decreases.[45]

Play, therefore, can also be categorised according to the quality of the social interaction involved in it.[46] Onlooker play involves merely observing the play of other children without actually participating in it. Solitary play consists of engrossed but independent play with toys. Minimal attention is given to other children. It is essentially egocentric in nature as the child is only interested in his own activity. Although children of any age can play alone, solitary play is more characteristic of older infants. Parallel play involves 2 or more children who, side by side, engage in similar activities, seem to be aware of the other children but, apart from occasional interactions, play largely by themselves. It is typical of toddlers and occasionally is seen in preschool children. In associative play, children play together, borrowing and exchanging toys but do not share goals. Group goals require the acceptance of rules that regulate cooperation. As preschool children do not fully comprehend the principles behind rules, they do not cooperate well in achieving common goals.

THE DEVELOPMENT OF THE UNDERSTANDING OF DEATH

Two early studies[47,48] showed that the development of the child's understanding of death changes according both to the child's level of cognitive development, and to their experiences. Children who have had close experience with death or life-threatening illnesses may have a more advanced concept of death.

While young children do not fully understand the concept, they tend to have many 'death words' in their vocabularies. By the age 2.5 years, the vocabulary of many children includes the words 'die' and by the age of 3 includes 'live'. Between the ages of 3 and 5, children begin to use the terms 'death' and 'dead'.

There are 3 characteristics of death that children must understand before they can understand its full meaning. Death is: permanent or irreversible; inevitable or universal; and it is an absolute state, one cannot be partially dead.

Young children have difficulty in understanding that death is irreversible and may believe that the dead person has only departed temporarily. They may, therefore, have trouble accepting that a deceased grandparent will not return. This idea is perpetuated by cartoons such as 'The Road Runner', where a character may be totally destroyed in one scene and reconstituted in the next. Many young children regard death as something that happens only to old people and believe that children do not die.[49] They may also have trouble conceptualising death as an absolute state and believe that people may be 'a little dead'.

Generally, children's concepts of death develop on a continuum from infancy, when they have no understanding of death to around the ages of 8 or 9, when there is full comprehension. Some studies have shown that full understanding can occur as early as 4[50] or 5.[51] The age at which a child develops a full understanding may depend on several factors, such as their previous experience of death, their experience of discussions about death and their level of cognitive development.

Research has shown that children can conceptualise death in many different ways. Many children under 5 seem to conceptualise death as similar, yet somehow different to living. For some children it may be a form of sleep, but different to normal sleep. For others, death is equated with lack of movement. This is the natural converse of the children's animistic beliefs. Live things move, dead things are still. Others seem to believe that the dead grow, walk about, get hungry and eat. They breathe and they feel, but only when no one is looking.[52] For others, being dead seems to mean not being fully alive. For example, a child declared that a dead person may feel 'a tiny little bit, but when he is quite dead he won't feel anything'.[53]

Many young children seem to believe that dead people can wake up, especially if a powerful adult such as a doctor or a parent wishes it. Some see death as caused by the person's own behaviour and may even believe it to be a punishment. For example, a child may believe that a person died because he ate something dirty or because he was naughty. A 5-year-old boy believed that his mother was dead because the day that she died he had told her he hated her.[54]

While young children may not fully comprehend death, they are frightened by it.[55] The death of a close family member may precipitate symptoms of anxiety such as enuresis, stammering,[56] regressive behaviour, diffuse distress and disturbances of sleep and eating.[57]

Children can be helped to understand and cope with their fear of death if it is freely discussed and they are encouraged to talk about it and ask questions.[57] Questions should be answered honestly and clearly. Euphemisms such as 'Granny has gone away on a big ship' or 'Grandpa is having a long sleep' only serve to confuse the child and block effective discussion.

THE DEVELOPMENT OF BODY IMAGE

In early childhood, children become more aware of their bodies. They begin to notice the physical differences between boys and girls and between children and adults. Sexual curiosity can be quite strong and can lead to a preoccupation with sexual and elimination matters. Through exploration of their own bodies, most preschool children discover the pleasures of masturbation.[58] Excessively shocked and angry reactions from adults may inculcate in the child a sense of shame and guilt about sexual matters. This may have profound effects on the development of the child's personality. By dealing matter-of-factly with children's curiosity and masturbation practices, and gently encouraging appropriate behaviour, adults can help them make a more satisfactory transition from infancy to an emotionally stable childhood.

As children develop their sex role identity, they learn to behave as society expects of their gender role.[59] A sense of moderation, however, is desirable. Boys should be discouraged from excessively macho and perhaps violent behaviour and girls should be discouraged from behaving as passive and dependent individuals. Nonetheless, encouraging unisex behaviours may have negative effects if it is taken too far. Children ultimately have to function in a society that has differing expectations of boys and girls, and to do so they need to have a healthy sex role identification. If they are unduly discouraged from behaving in a manner that is consistent with their gender identity, they may develop shame about their gender and have difficulty in adjusting to the development of secondary sex characteristics during adolescence.

Toddlers may have difficulty in understanding the relationship between their bodies and other objects. For instance, they may cry when the plug in the bath is removed and appear terrified of being washed down the plughole with the bath water.

By the end of the 2nd year, most toddlers have learned relatively good control over their gross muscles and are ready to test their physical competence. As they succeed or fail in various motor tasks, their body image is continually being modified and evaluated. Parents have an influence on body image development by helping their children to develop a realistic image of their body's abilities and appearance. A sense of shame and doubt in their abilities and a loss of self-esteem is likely to result from continual attempts at tasks which they will inevitably fail, or when they fail to take on tasks at which they could have succeeded. Ignoring or ridiculing their efforts may contribute to the development of unrealistic ideas of their abilities. By encouraging and praising their children's efforts, parents can gently help them to realise their limitations and their strengths.

At this age, children are prone to many misconceptions about their bodies, which can lead to irrational fears. For instance, preschool children may believe that if they are injured, their insides will spill out, just as teddy's stuffing spills out. Preschool children's misconceptions of their body's structure and function, together with their limited grasp of the meanings of words, has implications for the ways that adults communicate with them. Young children often have difficulty in understanding words that have multiple meanings.[60] They may be frightened when nurses explain 'I am going to take your temperature', because taking their 'temperature away' might be painful. They may believe that a limb that is covered in plaster has disappeared, or that is terribly mutilated beneath the plaster. A 4-year-old girl may believe that her broken leg has snapped in half in the same way as her doll's leg broke. The use of the word 'dye' to explain the process of an intravenous pyelogram may be confused with 'die'; organs may be mistaken for musical instruments; a medical 'test' may invoke images of 'passing' or 'failing'.

Children can be helped to deal with their fears when adults are willing to spend time questioning and talking to them, allowing them to express their concerns, and correcting their misconceptions. To do this effectively, however, adults need to be able to understand the way the child construes the world.

BELIEFS ABOUT HEALTH, ILLNESS AND PAIN

Beliefs about the causes of health and illness

Children's understanding of the nature of health, illness and pain appear to follow developmental sequences that are consistent with Piaget's stages of cognitive development.[61,62]

Preoperational children are beginning to understand that health is a desirable state and generates a feeling of well-being. Health is therefore associated with feeling good and being able to carry out desired activities. Being sick is being unable or not wanting to play or not feeling good.[63,64]

Preschool children have limited views on healthy lifestyle behaviours. Studies have found that preschool children place much emphasis on eating well but also include such activities as having enough sleep and exercise, not having too many sweets, brushing their teeth and visiting the doctor.[64,65] Some children regard nurses as important for keeping children healthy and believe that they do so by hugging them, by 'holding' them and by generally 'taking care' of them.[65]

Many ill and hospitalised children believe that illness is a direct result of their own behaviour, especially eating. Some children seem to believe that illness is a punishment for bad behaviour.[66] This is especially true of sick children.[66]

Bibace and Walsh asked 180 well children to tell them what makes people get colds.[61] They found that they could categorise the responses in a developmental sequence that was consistent with Piaget's stages. The explanations of preoperational children could be grouped into 2 categories, phenomenism and contagion.

Phenomenism is the most developmentally immature explanation of the causes of illness. In the child's view, illness is caused by concrete phenomena (such as the sun, the moon, or trees) that are present at the time that the person becomes ill, but remote, in terms of time and space, from the illness. While children connect the cause and the illness, they are unable to explain the process. For example, a child may claim that a person caught a cold from the trees, but cannot explain how a tree could give someone a cold. Similarly, children of this age may know that a treatment is effective, but cannot say how it works. Harbord et al found that preoperational children with cystic fibrosis were only able to say that pancreatic enzymes and antibiotics 'work because you swallow them' and a bronchodilator works because 'it fixes the chest'.[67]

As children become more mature, they may believe that illness can be caused by objects that are near but not actually touching the person.[68] This is the contagion stage. A rudimentary explanation of how objects can cause illness is now beginning to emerge. At this stage, it is the nearness of the object or its magic that makes the person sick.

Just as young children have misconceptions about death and body functions, so are they prone to develop misconceptions about health, illness and its causes. Many children believe that when they get sick it is because they did not practice healthy behaviours and may, therefore, feel guilty about being ill.[69] Neuhaser et al found that healthy preschool children were able to understand tangible changes in their health status, such as a cut, but had greater difficulty in grasping the more abstract concept of 'illness' where there were no visible cues to suggest that anything was amiss.[70] Steward and Steward wrote about a 4-year-old victim of a motor vehicle accident who believed that the cut on his arm was his most serious injury. It was the only one he could see.[71] Young children may see blood as a non-renewable body resource and believe that repeated venipunctures for blood tests could cause them to run out of blood.[71]

When correcting children's misconceptions or explaining about health and illness and medical procedures, it is important to use appropriate language that can be understood by the child. To understand illness, children have to imagine what is going on inside them. Young children need very concrete cues to enable them to understand. When explaining illness to a child it is useful to use concrete and familiar analogies. For example, to explain the need for blood transfusions to a young child with leukaemia, a nurse might show the child pictures of bad white cells which are trying to rid the body of its good red cells. If the cells have faces and arms and legs, the nurse is able to make use of the child's animistic thinking to promote further understanding. With a little ingenuity and thought, models can be constructed out of readily available materials. A broken tongue depressor wrapped in a handkerchief can be used to simulate a broken leg. Layers of tissues can represent skin layers to explain skin grafts. Balloons filled with air can simulate lungs, and when filled with water can simulate the bladder. Puppets, dolls and drawings can all be used to make explanations more concrete and therefore more comprehensible to the young child. They can also be used to enable the child to demonstrate what she thinks is going to happen so that misconceptions can be identified.

Beliefs about pain

A large study by Gaffney and Dunne found that preoperational children have a very simple concept of pain and lack the verbal fluency to communicate adequately their painful experiences.[72] Pain is simply 'something that hurts' and occurs mainly in the tummy, arms, legs or head. Gaffney and Dunne's study provided some insights on the meaning of pain for children. Pain was perceived as an unpleasant experience which is associated with illness. Boys were more likely than girls to believe that pain can be a direct outcome of the child's behaviour and boys were also more likely to regard pain as a punishment for past misdeeds. The children's responses showed that they saw themselves as having little control of pain and that they did not appreciate its warning nature.

A later study by Harbeck and Peterson showed that young children had difficulty describing their pain.[73] They tended to answer in terms of the way they would react to an injury rather than describe the type or intensity of the pain. However, when asked 'Why does pain hurt?', older preoperational children answered by describing the pain (e.g., because it stings). Younger preoperational children were unable to understand the question sufficiently to formulate an answer.

FEARS IN EARLY CHILDHOOD

As each child is unique, so are their fears. There are, however, some fears from which almost all children suffer. Around 2 years of age, fears of separation from parents begin to decline and fears of ghosts, bogey men, animals or darkness begin to appear.[74] The child's tendency to animism can promote fears of inanimate objects as they become endowed with the characteristics of animals. These fears may last for several years before they subside.[75]

The predominant fear of preschool children is of physical injury, which may range from fears of relatively minor invasive procedures such as injections[76] to fears of major disruptions to the integrity of their bodies. At this age children become more aware of their bodies. It is the age of Freudian castration anxiety and penis envy. It is not surprising then that fears of injury and mutilation are foremost in the child's mind. Their reactions to relatively minor procedures, such as injections, may be utterly out of proportion to the extent of trauma.

Such anxieties are common at this age, and decline as the child grows older.[77] Whenever possible, elective surgery should be delayed until the child is older. This is especially true for genital surgery in boys as they are at the Oedipal stage of development.

Children who must undergo invasive procedures, need the constant support and reassurance of their parents and of nursing and medical staff. The fears of preschool children may seem to be totally illogical and perhaps may not be taken seriously by adults. For example, adults may be amused by the small child who is terrified that he will be sucked down the drain hole when the bath water is emptied. Simple strategies may be very effective in helping children cope. Bandaids, for example, seem to help children cope with minor injuries such as cuts, abrasions and scratches. They seem to serve to reduce anxiety by covering the injury from sight and by 'sealing a leak' and preventing the loss of internal body parts and fluids.

COPING STRATEGIES IN EARLY CHILDHOOD

Toddlerhood is the age for the development of autonomy, which in itself can provide a degree of stress reduction. For example, although exhausted, a distressed hospitalised toddler may refuse to lie down, and stand at the end of the cot falling asleep. Attempts by nurses to lie her down may be resisted. She may literally be falling asleep on her feet. Allowing toddlers to explore the environment under the eye of a sympathetic adult seems to help them deal with their anxiety, especially when the environment is unfamiliar.

Preschoolers' responses to stress include whining, crying, clinging, sleep problems, aggression towards other children, and blaming themselves. Their egocentric view of the world makes it more likely that they will see the source of the stress as arising from their own behaviour.

Young children use a variety of coping strategies such as denial and regression.[78] Young children seem to be better at denial than older children.[79] It is important to evaluate the value of the child's denial in helping him cope and allow the child to use it until he is able to confront the source of the fear. The child who regresses may behave in ways typical of a younger age group, such as thumb-sucking or bed-wetting or having tantrums.[80]

Children can be helped best if they are allowed to deal with their fears in their own time and with the support of significant adults. They may be helped to face the object of their fears in a safe environment with a supportive adult. Forcing children to confront their fears may be counterproductive. It is especially important for adults to avoid humiliating children for being afraid or make fun of them.

Boys are more likely than girls to be encouraged to be brave, while girls are allowed to cry and express their fears. Condry and Condry found that adults tended to label an emotional response as anger when it came from a boy and fear when it came from a girl.[59] Nurses can help boys to express their fears by telling them that children are allowed to yell if they are frightened and to cry if they are sad.

Play can help children to express and confront their fears. Fears can be acted out in dramatic play. Children, for example, may play games which involve a bogey-man or werewolf or some other frightening creature. Nurses can help children act out their fears of hospital by providing them with empty syringes (no needles) or stethoscopes and allowing them to listen to teddy's chest or give him an injection. With imagination, many games can be created where the child's fears can be managed more effectively.

ASSESSMENT OF DEVELOPMENT

Assessment of the young child should be calm and unhurried. It is important to spend time getting the child's confidence. Children will often become uncooperative if an adult, especially a stranger, is attempting to force or hurry them into compliant behaviour. Children are more likely to attend if the adult talks to them on their level — physically, by kneeling or sitting and cognitively, by using language which is consistent with his ability to understand. Warn him when you are going to interrupt his play. Explain what you are going to do. Praise him when he cooperates.

In making an assessment of the child's psychological development, it is important to base assessment on as many different sources as possible. Observation of the child's behaviour, setting the Piagetian type tasks, and assessment tools such as the Denver Developmental Screening Test can all help build up a picture of the child's developmental status. When assessing a child's cognitive development, it should be recognised that as the child learns new behaviours, many of the old are still being used and this does not mean that the child is delayed.

REFERENCES

1. Tan D. Normal development. *In:* Clements A, ed. *Infant and family health in Australia: a textbook for community health workers.* 2nd ed. Melbourne: Churchill Livingstone, 1992.
2. Mott SR, James SR, Sperhac AM. *Nursing care of children and families.* 2nd ed. Redwood City: Addison-Wesley, 1990.
3. Wong DL. *Whaley and Wong's nursing care of infants and children.* 5th ed. St Louis: Mosby, 1995.
4. Wong DL, Whaley LF. *Clinical manual of pediatric nursing.* 3rd ed. St Louis: Mosby, 1990.
5. Harris M. *Textbook of child care and health.* Sydney: Science Press, 1988.

6. Silink M. Normal growth. *In:* Buchanan N, ed. *Child and adolescent health for practitioners.* Sydney: Williams and Wilkins, 1987.

7. Scipien GM, Chard MA, Howe J, Barnard MU. *Pediatric nursing care.* St Louis: Mosby, 1990.

8. Department of Endocrinology, The Adelaide Children's Hospital. *Length, weight, head circumference, post natal 0–3 years.* Adelaide: The Hospital, 1989.

9. Aynsley-Green A. An approach to the child with abnormal stature. *In:* Buchanan N, ed. *Child and adolescent health for practitioners.* Sydney: Williams and Wilkins, 1987.

10. Johnson A. Examination of infants and young children. *In:* Clements A, ed. *Infant and family health in Australia: a textbook for community health workers.* 2nd ed. Melbourne: Churchill Livingstone, 1992.

11. Brunner LS, Suddarth DS. *The Lippincott manual of paediatric nursing.* 3rd ed. Adapted by BF Weller. London: Harper and Row, 1991.

12. Marlow DR, Redding BA. *Textbook of pediatric nursing.* 6th ed. Philadephia: Saunders, 1988.

13. Maclean H, Edwards G. Vision and hearing. *In:* Clements A, ed. *Infant and family health in Australia: a textbook for community health workers.* 2nd ed. Melbourne: Churchill Livingstone, 1992.

14. National Health and Medical Research Council. *Screening and health care of children.* Canberra: AGPS, 1993.

15. Hutchins P. Developmental assessment. *In:* Buchanan N, ed. *Child and adolescent health for practitioners.* Sydney: Williams and Wilkins, 1987.

16. Carmichael A, Parry T, Vimpani G. Health of the under 5s. *In:* Vimpani G, Parry T, eds. *Community child health: an Australian perspective.* Melbourne: Churchill Livingstone, 1989.

17. Frankenburg WK. *Denver Development Screening Test — Revised.* Denver: University of Colorado Medical Centre, 1978.

18. Wong DL. *Pediatric quick reference.* St Louis: Mosby, 1995.

19. Robinson MJ, ed. *Practical paediatrics.* Melbourne: Churchill Livingstone, 1986.

20. Leach P. *Baby and child: from birth to age five.* 2nd ed. Harmondsworth: Penguin, 1989.

21. Roy LP. Enuresis. *In:* Procopis PG, Kewley GD, eds. *Current paediatric practice.* Sydney: Harcourt Brace Jovanovich, 1991.

22. Chinn PL, Leitch CJ. *Child health maintenance: a guide to clinical assessment.* 2nd ed. St Louis: Mosby, 1979.

23. Thompson S. *A healthy start for kids: how to convince your children to eat well.* Sydney: Simon and Schuster, 1991.

24. Cohen D, Kilham H, Oates K. *The complete book of child safety.* Sydney: Simon and Schuster, 1989.

25. Department of Health New South Wales. *Personal health record.* 2nd ed. Sydney: State Health Publications, 1990.

26. Pearn JH. Accidents and their prevention in childhood and adolescence. *In:* Buchanan N, ed. *Child and adolescent health for practitioners.* Sydney: Williams and Wilkins, 1987.

27. Piaget J. *The construction of reality in the child.* New York: Basic Books, 1954.

28. Piaget J, Inhelder B. *The psychology of the child.* London: Routledge Kegan & Paul, 1969.

29. Flavell JH. *The developmental psychology of Jean Piaget.* New York: Van Nostrand, 1963.

30. Philips S. *Self concept and self esteem. Infancy to adolescence.* Selected paper no 27. Kensington, NSW: Foundation for Child and Youth Studies, 1983.

31. Shatz M, Gelman R. The development of communication skills: modifications of the speech of young children as a function of the listener. *Monographs of the Society for Research in Child Development, 38* (Serial No. 152) 1973.

32. Hauck MR. Cognitive abilities of preschool children: implications for nurses working with young children. *J Pediatr Nursing* 1991; 6: 230–235.

33. Hall CS. *A primer of Freudian psychology.* New York: New American Library, 1979.

34. Kohlberg L. The development of moral character and moral ideology. *In:* Hoffman ML, Hoffman LW, eds. *Review of child development research.* Vol. 1. New York: Russell Sage, 1964.

35. Bee H. *The developing child.* 5th ed. New York: Harper & Rowe, 1989.
36. Kaplan PS. *The human odyssey: life span development.* St Paul: West Publishing, 1988.
37. de Villiers JG, de Villiers PA. *Language acquisition.* Massachusetts: Harvard University Press, 1978.
38. Hjelle LA, Ziegler DJ. *Personality theories: basic assumptions, research, and applications.* New York: McGraw-Hill, 1976.
39. Bemporad JR. Theories of development. *In:* Bemporad JR, ed. *Child development in normality and psychopathology.* New York: Brunner/Mazel, 1980: 3–42.
40. Bretherton D. *Emotional development in children.* Kew: IECD, 1976.
41. Erikson EH. *Childhood and society.* New York: Norton, 1963.
42. Baumrind D. Current patterns of parental authority. *Developmental Psychology Monographs 4, (1) Part 2.* 1971.
43. Furman W, Buhrmester D. Children's perceptions of the qualities of sibling relationships. *Child Dev* 1985; 56: 448–461.
44. Odom SL, McConnell SR, McEvoy MA, eds. *Social competence of young children with disabilities.* Baltimore: Paul H Brookes, 1992.
45. Stewart A, Perlmutter M, Friedman S. *Lifelong human development.* New York: Wiley, 1988.
46. Parten M. Social participation among preschool children. *J Abnormal Soc Psychol* 1932; 27: 243–269.
47. Nagy M. The child's theory concerning death. *J Genetics Psychol* 1948; 73: 3–27.
48. Anthony S. *The discovery of death in childhood.* New York: Basic Books, 1972.
49. Lonetto R. *Children's conceptions of death.* New York: Springer, 1980.
50. Bluebond-Langer M. *The private worlds of dying children.* New Jersey: Princeton University Press, 1978.
51. Landsdown R, Benjamin G. The development of the concept of death in children aged 5–9 years. *Child Care Health Dev* 1985; 11: 13–20.
52. Codden P. The meaning of death for parents and the child. *Maternal-Child Nursing J* 1977; 6: 9–16.
53. Krause DM. Children's concepts of death. *In:* Martinson IM, ed. *Home care for the dying child: professional and family perspective.* New York: Appleton-Century-Crofts, 1976.
54. Johnson-Soderberg S. The development of a child's concept of death. *Oncology Nursing Forum* 1981; 8: 23–26.
55. Raphael B. *Anatomy of bereavement.* London: Hutchinson, 1984.
56. Stapleton T. Mourning in childhood. *Aust Paediatr J* 1965; 1: 39–41.
57. Waechter E. Children's awareness of fatal illness. *Am J Nursing* 1971; 6: 1168–1172.
58. Blaesing S, Brockhaus J. The development of body image in the child. *Nursing Clin North Am* 1972; 7: 597–607.
59. Condry J, Condry S. Sex differences: a study of the eye of the beholder. *Child Dev* 1976; 47: 812–819.
60. Dorn LD. Children's concepts of illness: clinical applications. *Pediatr Nursing* 1984; 10: 325–327.
61. Bibace R, Walsh ME. Children's conceptions of illness. *In:* Bibace R, Walsh ME, eds. *Children's conceptions of health, illness and bodily functions.* San Francisco: Jossey-Bass, 1981.
62. Walsh M, Bibace R. Children's conceptions of AIDS: a developmental analysis. *J Pediatr Psychol* 1991; 16: 273–285.
63. Natapoff JN. Children's views of health: a developmental study. *Am J Public Health* 1978; 10: 995–1000.
64. Robinson CA. Preschool children's conceptualisations of health and illness. *Children's Health Care* 1987; 16: 89–96.
65. Flaherty M. Preschool children's conceptions of health and health behaviours. Monograph 16, *Maternal-Child Nursing J* 1986; V15.
66. Gratz RR, Piliavin JA. What makes kids sick: Children's beliefs about the causative factors of illness. *Children's Health Care* 1984; 12: 156–162.

67. Harbord MG, Cross DG, Botica F, Martin AJ. Children's understanding of cystic fibrosis. *Aust Paediatr J* 1987; 23: 241–244.
68. Osborne ML, Kistner JA, Helgemo B. Developmental progression in children's knowledge of AIDS: implications for education and attitude change. *J Pediatr Psychol* 1993; 18: 177–192.
69. Brewster AB. Chronically ill hospitalised children's concepts of their illness. *Pediatrics* 1982; 69: 355–362.
70. Neuhauser C, Amsterdam B, Hines P, Steward M. Children's concepts of healing: Cognitive development and locus of control factors. *Am J Orthopsychiatry* 1978; 48: 335–341.
71. Steward MS, Steward DS. Children's conceptions of medical procedures. *In:* Bibace R, Walsh ME, eds. *Children's conceptions of health, illness and bodily functions.* San Francisco: Jossey-Bass, 1981.
72. Gaffney A, Dunne EA. Developmental aspects of children's definitions of pain. *Pain* 1986; 26: 105–117.
73. Harbeck C, Peterson L. Elephants dancing in my head: a developmental approach to children's concepts of specific pains. *Child Dev* 1992; 63: 138–149.
74. Bauer D. An exploratory study of developmental changes in children's fears. *J Child Psychol Psychiatry* 1976; 17: 69–74.
75. Murphy DM. Fears in preschool-age children. *Child Care Q* 1985; 14: 171–189.
76. Fassler D. The fear of needles in children. *Am J Orthopsychiatry* 1985; 53: 371–377.
77. Dolgin MJ, Phipps S, Harow E, Zeltzer LK. Parental management of fear in chronically ill and healthy children. *J Pediatr Psychol* 1990; 15: 733–744.
78. Armstrong-Dailey A, Goltzer SZ, eds. *Hospice care for children.* New York: Oxford University Press, 1993.
79. Mischel W. *Introduction to personality.* New York: Holt, Rinehart and Winston, 1976.
80. Smitherman C. *Nursing actions for health promotion.* Philadelphia: FA Davis, 1981.

Chapter 3

Growth and Development: 5 to 12 Years

Physical Growth and Development

Anne Adams

ASSESSMENT OF SCHOOL-AGE CHILDREN

The physical assessment of the school-age child requires a sensitive and imaginative approach based on knowledge of anticipated growth and the developmental stages of children in this period. Some children will be apprehensive about a physical examination while others will be curious and sociable. School-age children are highly distractable and may enjoy taking an active part in the procedures of a physical assessment. Most children will be modest, prefer to retain their clothing and require privacy. A positive and friendly approach which incorporates interest in the child's world and honesty about the steps of the assessment will help gain confidence and cooperation. Praise, encouragement and rewards usually have positive effects and help to make the assessment a pleasant and interactive experience. Children usually prefer a parent or parents to be present, though in later childhood there may be a preference for one or both parents to wait outside while the assessment takes place. When parents are present it is important to communicate directly with the child rather than through the parents. Clear explanations and answers about findings are appreciated by children and parents.

There is no prescribed sequence for a physical assessment though many nurses find the logical sequence of the head to toe approach works well. Assessment of the genitals, an area which may be causing a health problem or any procedure which may be uncomfortable may be left until the end of the examination.

MUSCULOSKELETAL SYSTEM

The ossification of bones continues during middle childhood, but full mineralisation is not yet established. The bones and muscles of the school-age child, while increasing in size and strength, are still not able to completely withstand force and stretch. Proportions within the musculoskeletal system change in this period with head circumference and waist measurement decreasing in relation to height and the face becoming larger in proportion to the remainder of the head. Cranial growth is minimal, but the increased length and width of the mandible and the development of the chin results in the face of the 6 year old growing to about 80% of the final adult size.[1] The increase in height is a reflection of bone lengthening, particularly in the legs, which occurs alongside an increase in muscle tissue. The increase in weight in middle childhood is primarily the result of musculoskeletal growth. Fat is replaced by muscle and bone tissue replaces cartilage.[1] These increases produce an overall increase in strength and coordination.[2]

Posture

The school-age child is more slender and poised than the younger child. As the pelvis tips backward and the abdominal muscles strengthen posture improves,[1] giving a taller, straighter appearance. As well, standing posture is steadier and movements are smoother. Together with a lower centre of gravity these changes not only produce an improved posture but allow the child to increase her range of movements and physical abilities.[2]

Joints and limbs

Joints move freely and such ease of movement is noticeable as the child walks and runs in a balanced, agile and supple way. Children in this period will often appear to have large elbow and knee joints, but these have to be assessed in the light of rapidly growing long bones and the relative slenderness of the limbs of school-age children.

Growth in the legs is most pronounced in this period of childhood. The limbs are longer and stronger. Legs and arms should be symmetric and equal in length, shape and strength.

Weight

Weight continues to increase in middle childhood but at a slower pace, with an average gain of about 2.3 kg per year.[1] The average weight at 6 years is 21 kg and at 12 years, 40 kg. Boys tend to be a little heavier than girls in the early part of this period but the difference is small.[2] At 5 years weight is about twice that of the weight at 1 year and at 7 years the weight is about 7 times the birthweight.[1] Weight gain in late childhood may be a sign of approaching puberty. Girls have a growth spurt about 18 months to 2 years before boys with sharper increases in weight and height commencing at about 9.5 years. The growth spurt continues into the adolescent period.[2] (Appendix A.)

While it is recommended that the child should be nude for the recording of weight, children in this period usually prefer to keep some clothing on. If underwear such as a singlet and pants or a surgical gown is worn, 0.1 kg is subtracted before the weight is recorded.[3] Because it is recommended that the bladder should be empty the child is requested to void before the weight is taken. When the child is weighed during a period of hospitalisation any attachments, such as a drainage device or an arm board or splint, which cannot be removed, are taken into consideration. The weight of the attachment can be estimated and subtracted from the child's weight or the presence of the attachment is simply noted on the weight chart for consideration when the chart is read.

Height

While the rate of increase in height per year continues to decrease there is an overall growth in height throughout middle childhood. Growth, however, occurs in bursts with the child remaining at a near-constant height for a time followed by a quick and noticeable increase. The average height increase per year is about 5 cm.[1] At 6 years the average height is 116 cm and at 12 years the average height is 150 cm.[2] Boys are a little taller until late in middle childhood when the growth in girls exceeds that of boys.[2] The growth spurt associated with the onset of puberty in girls will bring about an increase in height from 5 to 20 cm.[2] (Appendix A.)

Height is measured with the child standing, without footwear, against an upright surface such as a wall. The heels and back should touch the wall and the child should look directly ahead. It is recommended that in order to maintain the head in the correct position the lower borders of the eye sockets should be on a horizontal line with the external auditory meati. The child is asked to stretch but not to let her heels leave the floor. To help the child stretch, gentle upward pressure can be applied under the mastoid processes. These stretching measures aim to minimise the variation in height from early to late in the day.[3] The height is recorded at the point on a scale where a right-angled flat surface meets the top of the child's head. By 10 years the proportion of sitting height to total height has reduced to 52%.[2,4] The sitting height may sometimes need to be assessed. This measurement is taken with the child sitting on a firm surface. The distance from the top of the head to the point where the buttocks touch the surface is measured.[4]

Head

While the head continues to grow during middle childhood, the rate of growth is much slower. When head circumference is compared with chest circumference the change in proportional growth is evident. During this period head circumference becomes less than the chest circumference with the difference ranging from 5 to 7 cm.[1,5]

A non-stretch tape is passed around the head from over the eyebrows, above the pinnae and around the occiput at the most prominent point. The head circumference is not usually measured in a physical assessment or health screening in middle childhood.

NERVOUS SYSTEM

After the rapid increase in brain volume in infancy and the steady growth in early childhood brain growth continues, but at a slower rate, during middle childhood. As a result of the maturing nervous system, children in this period are able to carry out more complex and refined activities with greater control and perception.[1] As myelination proceeds and the conduction of nerve impulses becomes more efficient the child, by the end of middle childhood, is dextrous and skillful.[1] It is estimated that by 7 years, the nervous system has achieved nine-tenths of its growth[4] and that by 10 years the nervous system is essentially mature.[6]

As in early childhood, the assessment of the nervous system in middle childhood involves a range of growth and development observations taken over time. Assessment will take into consideration the child's age and the expected level of nervous system development. The main activities of a physical assessment were described in Chapter 2, and are relevant to the assessment of children in middle childhood. This chapter includes the assessment of the cranial nerves which is applicable to nervous system assessment in both early and middle childhood.

Reflexes

The assessment of superficial and deep tendon reflexes is outlined in Chapter 2. Reflexes are tested for presence, power and symmetry. The presence of the deep tendon reflexes indicates that the reflex arc is intact and there is normal involvement of sensory nerve endings in the tendon, nerve fibres, spinal cord, motor neuron and muscle.[6] If the child is anxious and unable to relax her muscles, the reflex may be inhibited.[2,6] It has been suggested that the child's attention be diverted by asking her to grasp her hands together at the front and to try to pull them apart while the testing takes place.[2]

Gross motor skills

As neuromuscular development continues the child demonstrates increased and more complex gross motor capabilities.

At the beginning of middle childhood the child is usually in motion and has achieved greater control over physical activities. Balance, coordination and dexterity are improved so that motor skills become more refined. These gains, together with the growth in musculoskeletal strength, mean the child is able to ride a bicycle, climb, skate, use a bat, throw objects with momentum and take part in ball games.

In the latter part of middle childhood, physical skills have become even more refined, not only through on-going development, but also through repeated and earnest practice which, in late childhood, is often a characteristic behaviour. As well, strength and endurance increase. Between 10 and 12 years, activities such as gymnastics, target and team sports, athletics, ballet and dance are often taken up. In these activities gross motor skills are at a high level of precision and refinement. Many children in this period compete with themselves and each other. They may work at refining a particular skill, develop individual variations and train for competitive events.[1]

Fine motor skills

Further evidence of the maturing central nervous system is seen in the child's ability to carry out more complex fine motor skills with better control and finer dexterity.

At 5 years, the child can tie knots, manage buttons and fasteners, use scissors and tools with some precision and use a hair comb and toothbrush. The child is also able to write numbers, letters and some words and make drawings which contain details such as eyes, ears and main parts of the human body. By 6 years the child is using writing equipment, tools and cutlery. While there is still some awkwardness the child is eager to manipulate materials and generally carries out activities quickly with good coordination between the eyes and hands. The 7 year old can compose and write letters using words and numbers. Pencils and writing equipment are held in a firm grasp, giving greater control and refinement to writing and drawing. Seven year olds can draw a triangle and 8 year olds can draw a diamond.[1]

In later childhood the coordination between eye and hand has further developed and fine motor activities become more smooth, rapid and accurate. The child may write rather than print with the writing becoming smaller. The ability to master complex board and video games, model construction, sewing, drawings, fine crafts and musical instruments develops.[1]

Muscle tone

As the muscle mass increases through growth and the replacement of fat with muscle, the muscles become stronger and firmer. The increase in muscle tone can be easily felt when the muscles are tensed. The strength of muscles is assessed by observing the child pulling away and pushing onto an object or person. Corresponding muscles are symmetric and matched for size, tone and strength.

The development of fine motor skills allows a child to make drawings.

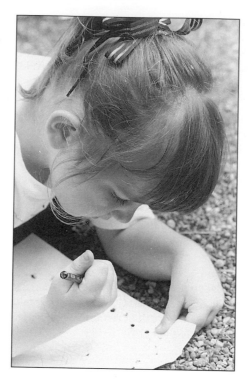

Alertness and responsiveness

The school-age child is normally alert, aware and highly responsive to external and internal stimuli. There are high levels of curiosity and activity. In addition, there is an increasing ability to concentrate for longer periods with greater retention of information and recall of experience.

Less sleep is required in middle childhood and the amount of sleep continues to vary for individual children. In the early part of this period about 12 hours' sleep each night is needed, by 8 years 10 or 11 hours may be sufficient and at 12 years the child may be having 8 hours or so, an amount similar to that required by adults.[1] It is not uncommon for children in middle childhood to resist sleep and bedtime. Some children may also need time to wake in the morning. They may be drowsy, unable to concentrate, slow and disorganised until fully awake.[1]

Consciousness is assessed by, firstly, observing the child's levels of alertness, responsiveness and activity. School-age children can answer questions about time and place to establish their levels of orientation. Assessment for levels of altered consciousness begins by determining if the child is asleep, confused or comatose. The Glasgow Coma Scale is used to assess and monitor the child's level of consciousness over time when there is reason to suspect an alteration has taken place (Appendix B).

Eyes and vision

Vision develops during middle childhood and becomes less hyperopic (far-sighted). The fovea, the part of the retina where vision is sharpest, matures by about 6 to 7 years.

Before 6 years the child needs large print reading material because of far-sightedness which makes it difficult to focus on near objects. Normal vision is further enhanced by the development of the ocular muscles and the child's ability to control eye movements. School-age children use their improved visual ability to advantage. Because they are able to focus more efficiently, they visually observe and explore and are able to find and identify objects within complicated contexts.[1]

The eyes are clear and shining. The lashes lie outward, the lids are clean and can be blinked and closed easily. When the upper lid is open its lower margin lies at some point between the pupil and upper iris. Epicanthal folds, vertical skin folds of skin which cover the inner canthus, are more prominent in Asian children and children with Down's syndrome. The palpebral conjunctiva, which lines the upper and lower lids, is pink, smooth and moist. The bulbar conjunctiva, which covers the eye except for the cornea, is moist and transparent with the sclera readily seen beneath it. The sclera is usually white and clear. Pupils are round, equal and will constrict in bright light or when a light is directed into the eye.[1]

The assessment of visual acuity, where the ability of the child to see objects clearly whether close or far is tested, is described in Chapter 2. School-age children are tested with the Snellen Alphabet Chart and are asked to read lines of letters which are increasingly smaller.[1] The child looks at a chart which is 6 m away, placed at eye level, and reads each line starting from the top line. The eyes are tested together and separately. If the child can read line 7, she has 6/6 vision, which is the standard for normal vision. The Snellen Chart is also used to test for myopia (nearsight) and hyperopia (farsight). Testing for binocularity (see Chapter 1), visual field and colour vision (see Chapter 2) are also carried out with school-age children. Screening for visual acuity is recommended between 10 and 13 years.[7]

Ears and hearing

The external ear is skin tone in colour though often pinker along its edges. The external auditory canal is clean and dry though fresh, slightly moist cerumen may be visible.

The middle ear can be inspected with an otoscope using the relevant size speculum. Insertion of the speculum will be more easily accomplished if the speculum is warm. Children in this period are usually cooperative. The head is tilted away from the examiner towards the child's further shoulder. The ear canal is about 2.5 cm in length and curves downward in middle childhood. The pinna is pulled up and back in order to examine the canal. The canal is deep pink throughout and smooth, except where fine hairs appear in the outer part of the canal. The tympanic membrane is pearly gray or pink and translucent. The light reflex can be seen as a triangular cone-shaped reflection at the 5 to 7 o'clock position on the membrane. Landmarks, the umbo and the short and long processes, are visible as they are attached to the other side of the tympanic membrane.[1,2,4]

While there is no reason to screen school-age children for hearing, audiometric testing may be undertaken in children with hearing or behaviour problems.[8]

Other sensory functions

Touch is readily assessable in school-age children who can differentiate between pain, temperature and pressure and verbalise about these sensations. Superficial pain can be evaluated by asking the child to close her eyes and identify when a sharp point or a blunt object is pressed onto various parts of the body in random sequence. Temperature can be identified by handling containers of cold and warm fluids. Pressure can be applied to the limb muscles and the child is asked to evaluate the amount of squeezing. Matching parts of the body are tested for comparison of response and symmetric sensation.[1] The sense of smell is acute in middle childhood with children able to differentiate between pleasant and unpleasant odours. Taste perception continues to be sensitive. Children have strong responses to taste and may vigorously reject new or strong tasting substances.[1]

Balance and coordination

Balance is more finely developed in middle childhood with the child able to carry out a range of activites which demonstrate this development. Balance is assessed by asking the child to stand independently with the feet together when the eyes are open and when the eyes are closed. A slight sway is normal when the eyes are closed. This is the Romberg test and if the child wobbles, leans to one side or falls the sign is positive and is an abnormal finding.[6] In this period the child can also stand on one foot for at least 15 seconds and hop on one leg in one place and remain balanced.[1]

The coordination of the school-age child can be assessed by observing the child's ability to manipulate objects and other fine motor skills. The finger-to-nose test is commonly used to assess coordination. In this test the child is asked to touch the tip of the nose with the index finger of each hand in turn, with the eyes open and then closed. Other tests for coordination include the ability to touch the thumb with each finger of the same hand in rapid succession and the heel-to-shin test. In the heel-to-shin test the child is asked to move the heel down the anterior tibia of the opposite leg while standing, with the eyes open and with the eyes shut.

Children over 6 years are usually able to complete these tests. When the eyes are closed it is mainly the sense of position being assessed and when they are open, mainly coordination is being assessed.[2,6]

Cranial nerves

The 12 cranial nerves have motor, sensory and mixed nerve functions and are more easily assessed in middle childhood than in earlier periods of childhood. The nerves, their function and methods of assessment are listed in **Table 3.1**.

Body temperature

In keeping with the reduction in the metabolic rate throughout childhood, the mean body temperature drops by approximately 0.3°C between 5 and 12 years. At 5 years the temperature is 37°C and at 11 years, 36.7°C.[2] Temperature readings are taken with a mercury or electronic thermometer. As a safety measure the axillary route rather than the oral route is used in childhood even though the child is able to understand the principles of body temperature and its measurement. The nurse remains with the child while the thermometer is in position. The tympanic membrane sensor is a more acceptable to children as a method of measuring body temperature. Temperature readings are recorded and, if a series of readings is taken, plotted on a graph in order to display the pattern of body temperature over time.

Table 3.1 Assessment of the cranial nerves

Cranial nerve	Function	Assessment
I Olfactory	controls the sense of smell	with eyes closed child to identify common odours such as coffee, peanut butter
II Optic	visual acuity, colour and peripheral vision	check for light perception, visual acuity and fields, colour vision and normal optic disc
III Oculomotor	controls eyelid movements, eye movements	check lid position have child move eyes and follow object in all directions with the head still
	pupil reactivity	check for reaction to light
IV Trochlear	controls eye movements down and out	ask child to look down
V Trigeminal	controls muscles of mastication	ask child to bite hard on object and open jaw, check for strength and symmetry
	sensation to face, scalp, nose and mouth, sensation to cornea	ask child to identify touch to face test corneal and blink reflex by light touch with wisp of cotton wool
VI Abducens	moves the eye laterally	ask child to look towards the right and then the left
VII Facial	controls facial movements	ask child to make a face and observe for symmetry and muscle strength
	transmits taste sensations from front two thirds of tongue	ask child to identify sweet and salty tastes
VIII Acoustic	governs hearing and balance	assess hearing, assess balance
IX Glossopharyngeal	functions in tongue and pharynx in swallowing, transmits taste sensation from posterior 3rd of tongue	ask the child to swallow, test for gag reflex, test sour or bitter taste on back of tongue
X Vagus	controls muscles of pharynx	check for gag reflex and swallowing
	controls muscles of larynx responsible for smooth muscle movement in heart, lung and some gastrointestinal organs	observe for hoarseness of voice

Table 3.1 (*continued*)

Cranial nerve	Function	Assessment
XI Accessory	controls movement of head and shoulder through sternocleid-omastoid and trapezius muscle contraction	ask child to shrug shoulders against downward pressure and turn head from side to side against opposition
XII Hypoglossal	controls muscles of tongue	ask child to put tongue out as far as possible, move it in all directions and push object away with tongue

CIRCULATORY SYSTEM

By middle childhood the heart lies in a more vertical position because of the development of the left ventricle and the more downward position of the diaphragm.[6] Because the rate of growth of the heart is much slower in this period, the size of the heart relative to the body is smaller in middle childhood than any other period.[2] Even so, at 5 years the heart is 4 times the size at birth and by 7 years the left ventricle is as thick as the adult ventricle.[1] At 9 years the heart is 6 times its weight at birth.[1]

Pulses

The apical pulse is auscultated at the 5th left intercostal space at the midclavicular line in middle childhood. Palpation of pulses becomes easier in the school-age child because of the increased dimensions of the blood vessels, a greater blood volume and a slower cardiac rate. The radial pulse continues to be the most commonly used pulse point for palpation. Children in middle childhood are usually curious and cooperative when pulses are auscultated and palpated. They may want to listen to their apical pulse and learn to locate and feel their pulses. Palpation can be carried out on the carotid, femoral, brachial, popliteal, and dorsalis pedis pulses.

The pulse rate continues to decrease as the child grows. The average resting pulse at 6 years is about 95 beats per minute with a range from 75 to 115 beats per minute. By 10 years the average resting pulse has fallen to about 90 beats per minute with the range between 70 to 110 beats per minute. Exercise, activity and emotion will cause the pulse rate to increase while the rate usually drops during sleep. Steady but gentle pressure is applied to the pulse point while the rate, rhythm and volume are assessed. The rate is counted over 1 minute, though the estimation may have to be made over segments of time and calculated for the full minute.

Blood pressure

While the blood pressure continues to rise during middle childhood there will be variability among children in this period according to age, weight and height.[8] The small difference for mean blood pressure values between girls and boys in early childhood virtually disappears in middle childhood. The average systolic blood pressure for 6 year olds is 96 mmHg and the average diastolic blood pressure is 57 mmHg. By 10 years the average systolic blood pressure is 102 mmHg and the average diastolic blood pressure is 62 mmHg.

As a quick general guide, blood pressure in children from 6 years can be estimated by doubling the child's age and adding the result to 83 for the systolic reading and adding the child's age to 52 for the diastolic reading.[5]

The selection of cuff size remains an important issue in the accurate measurement of blood pressure. As a general rule the cuff width should cover about two-thirds of the upper arm. There are benefits in estimating the appropriate cuff size with a calculation based on the upper arm circumference. The circumference is measured at the midpoint of the upper arm and the cuff width should measure between 40% and 50% of the arm circumference. Cuffs selected according to this calculation will measure blood pressure more accurately because arm size and the pressure needed to compress the artery have been taken into consideration.[2] The same size cuff should be used each time the blood pressure is measured. Between 5 and 10 years the cuff size is usually between 8 and 10 cm.[1] The 4th Korotkoff sound is taken as the diastolic pressure during middle childhood though it is recommended that the 5th Korotkoff sound is recorded as well.[2] See Chapter 2 for methods of blood pressure measurement in children.

The pulse pressure, the difference between the systolic and diastolic blood pressure, is usually between 20 mmHg and 50 mmHg throughout childhood.[6]

Colour

Skin colour is assessed because of the information it provides about circulation and blood oxygen levels. To a lesser extent skin colour can indicate the child's nutritional status and the movement of fluid within the body spaces. Light-skinned children have warm tones with a soft pink flush to the face. Children with darker skins have pinkish palms and soles. The oral mucosa is deep pink.

Heart sounds

The heart sounds are auscultated in order to assess the quality, rate, intensity and rhythm and to pick up any deviation from normal. The sounds should be clear and well-defined, not muffled or distant. The rate of the heart is related to the child's age and is expected to be relatively consistent even though activity and emotion will produce temporary increases. When the stethoscope is placed at the apex, that is, the 5th left intercostal space in the midclavicular line, S1 is louder than S2. S2 will be more intense at the base of the heart and is heard at the 2nd intercostal space on either side of the sternum. The rhythm should be regular with the 'lub dub' sound and the interval between heard in an even pattern. Any heart sounds which do not meet these normal standards require further investigation. It is generally recommended that heart sounds are auscultated with the child in 2 positions, sitting and lying.[2,6]

About half the children in middle childhood have innocent heart murmurs with the incidence highest between 6 and 9 years.[1] The murmurs are heard most commonly in the 2nd, 3rd or 4th intercostal space at the left sternal border. They may cease to be heard when the child changes position and do not signify cardiac problems.[4] (See Chapters 1 and 2 for further details about heart sounds).

GASTROINTESTINAL SYSTEM

During middle childhood the stomach attains a capacity of about half to two-thirds of the adult capacity. After about 7 years the position of the stomach is more upright and the

Table 3.2 Eruption of the permanent teeth

Permanent teeth	Age at eruption (years)
First upper and lower molars	6–7
Lower central incisors	6–7
Upper central incisors	7–8
Lower lateral incisors	7–8
Upper lateral incisors	8–9
Lower cuspids	9–10
First upper bicuspids	10–11
First lower bicuspids	10–12
Second upper bicuspids	10–12
Upper cuspids	11–12
Second lower molars	11–13
Second upper molars	12–13

shape is straighter than the elongated shape assumed during early childhood.[2] From about 10 years the stomach assumes the adult shape and by late childhood mature gastrointestinal function has been achieved. The length of the small intestine at birth has doubled by late childhood and the ascending colon is adult size.[1]

Mouth and teeth

The mucous membranes of the mouth are moist and smooth and like the lips, deep pink. The arch is dome shaped and the number of teeth present will be related to the progression of tooth loss and replacement.

In middle childhood the deciduous teeth are replaced by permanent teeth. The process begins at about 6 years when the central incisors are lost and is largely completed by about 12 years. Because the permanent teeth are bigger than the deciduous teeth they appear very large, but as the facial bones grow the teeth assume a more proportional appearance. Malocclusion is not uncommon.[1] The first of the permanent teeth to erupt are the 6-year molars, which appear behind the deciduous molars. The rest of the permanent teeth generally erupt in the same sequence as the deciduous teeth.[2]

Abdomen

The abdomen is symmetric and smooth. The contour is dependent on the fat layer and muscle development and is inspected while the child is standing and lying. When standing, the abdomen in thin children will be concave while in fatter children it may remain prominent. When supine the abdomen is flat. The umbilicus is inverted in most instances.[1] Bowel sounds are heard when the diaphragm of the stethoscope is placed firmly over the abdominal wall. Rubbing a fingernail across the abdominal surface may stimulate peristalsis and permit bowel sounds to be heard. The abdomen continues to move with respirations up to about 7 years.[6]

Ingestion and digestion

By 10 years the stomach capacity has increased to between 750 to 900 mL. This increased capacity means the school-age child is able to ingest more food and reduce the frequency of eating. Chewing ability in school-age children is more efficient because of the increase in bone and muscle strength. Children in this period are usually very active and may eat quickly with minimal chewing. An increased range of different foods is tolerated, but the lining of the tract is still sensitive to irritating substances.[1] By late childhood digestion and absorption have reached adult levels of function and the tolerance for different foods has been further extended.[1]

Elimination

Children have gained, on the whole, good control of faecal elimination by the time they start school. Stools throughout childhood are soft, brown and formed and should be passed without straining. The number and frequency of stools vary, but 1 or 2 stools each day is common.[1] It has been suggested that the lower limit for frequency of stools is 4 per week.[2] Occasionally, the school-age child may become constipated. Constipation may result from lack of fibre, fluid or exercise. Children in this period will resist the sensation which requires them to visit the toilet because they are too busy or absorbed in other activities. Some children, especially those who have just started school, may avoid using the school toilets. Constipation may result from holding-on behaviour, particularly if the behaviour becomes established.

RESPIRATORY SYSTEM

The thoracic cavity enlarges with the overall growth of the school-age child and the lungs continue to descend in the cavity. The increase in the number of alveoli is probably complete by about 8 years and from then the alveoli increase in size. These increases produce a more mature and efficient lung function. Because the tidal volume and the vital capacity are increased, school-age children are able to carry out and sustain more physically demanding activities. The respiratory rate decreases in keeping with these functional changes. Breathing becomes more thoracic than abdominal as the costal muscles become more involved.[1]

Chest

The chest continues to change shape during middle childhood, becoming wider from side to side. The anteroposterior diameter, while enlarging with growth, is noticeably less than the transverse diameter and gives the chest an increasingly oval shape.[2] The chest and its bony markers are symmetric. Symmetry is also evident in the respiratory movements of the chest.

The first signs of breast development may appear at about 10 years in girls. Breast buds appear and are the most visible signs of approaching puberty. A small elevation develops around the papilla and the areola enlarges.[2] One breast may develop before another and some breast bud development occurs in boys.[1]

Breath sounds

Breath sounds are heard through a stethescope as air flows through the pharynx and large airways and are most easily heard over the trachea. The sounds are changed as they are transmitted through the smaller airways and lung tissue.[6] There are 3 main breath sounds. These are classified as vesicular, bronchovesicular and bronchial, and are heard at different points over the thoracic cavity. (See Chapter 2, for a description of the breath sounds in childhood.)

Voice sounds can also be heard through the stethoscope as the chest is auscultated. The resonance of the voice is heard as a muffled sound though words or syllables cannot be distinguished.[6] Resonance sounds are low pitched, loud in intensity and have a long duration.[1]

Respirations

With growth the lungs become more efficient in their ventilatory function and the respiratory rate decreases. The average quiet breathing rate during middle childhood is about 20 to 24 breaths per minute.[1] By late childhood the rate has decreased further to between 17 to 22 breaths per minute.[1] Even so, children will breathe more quickly under the influence of emotion, activity or an elevated temperature. The ratio of breaths to heartbeats is usually 1:4.[2]

Respirations are assessed for their rate, rhythm, depth and quality, and, as with the smaller child, are best taken when the child is not aware that they are being assessed. Between 6 and 7 years respiratory movements will be seen more clearly in the chest while younger children will still exhibit abdominal breathing. The rate is counted over a full minute. Breathing is quiet and without effort and usually regular.

GENITOURINARY SYSTEM

External genitalia

As for the younger girl, the genitalia of the school-age girl are usually only examined externally and by inspection. The location of the structures can be checked with the child lying supine with the knees bent and the upper legs laterally extended.

The mons pubis and labia majora have a full, rounded appearance during middle childhood. In later childhood the labia majora become thicker and the labia minora fill out.[4] Soft downy hair along the labia majora is an early sign of approaching puberty.[2] Each pair of labia are symmetric. The inner surfaces are deep pink and moist. The urethral meatus and the vaginal orifice are usually visible in the area between the 2 labia minora. If the position of the urethral meatus is not easily established it can be more readily identified by wiping downwards from the clitoris. The meatus will appear as a V-shaped slit.[2] The hymen, a thin membrane, covers part of the vaginal opening, giving the orifice a small appearance.[4]

The external male genitalia are inspected and may be palpated if further assessment is required. The penis remains relatively small during middle childhood. The foreskin can be easily pushed back and the glans penis and surrounding tissue inspected. The skin of the scrotum is wrinkled and, because the left spermatic cord is longer than the right, the left side of the scrotum hangs slightly lower than the right.[2] Testes can be felt in the scrotum on both sides and are about 1.5 to 2 cm in size throughout childhood.

Urinary function

The structures of the urinary system increase in size and weight during middle childhood. By late childhood the length of the kidneys is double that at birth[1] and the capacity of the bladder is increased. Girls have slightly larger bladders than boys.[1] The volume of urine produced per day is between 700 and 1000 mL,[6] although the amount is influenced by fluid intake, activity and environmental conditions. School-age children are, for the most part, continent during the night. Most children who have been incontinent at night are dry by 6 years.[1]

Urine specimens are usually collected from school-age children without difficulty. Most children will cooperate by voiding into a container but may not be able to void immediately on request. Many prefer a parent to catch the specimen or be present during the collection. If an uncontaminated specimen is required for testing in the laboratory the urethral meatus is cleaned before the child voids. (See Chapter 2, for cleansing procedure). The child is asked to begin voiding. After the first few seconds the container is positioned under the urinary stream until the required amount is collected. The container and lid are handled in such as way as to prevent contamination. The specimen is despatched quickly for testing.

The specific gravity and components of urine are similar to adult values.[1] The specific gravity with a normal fluid intake is between 1.016 and 1.022. Urine is usually acidic with an average pH of 6, within a pH range of 4.8 and 7.8.[2] Urine analysis, using a dipstick, will reveal the presence of abnormal constituents and abnormal levels of expected constituents. Normal urine will contain no protein, glucose, ketones, blood or bilirubin and 1% of urobilinogen on a dipstick test.

INTEGUMENTARY SYSTEM

The appearance of the skin does not change significantly during middle childhood, although it continues to become tougher. The skin is smooth, soft and elastic.[4] Light-skinned children may show evidence of sun exposure with tanning and freckling. In late childhood the activity of the sebaceous glands is more active. Involuntary blushing may occur because the vasomotor response is not yet stabilised.[1]

Health Management

Anne Adams

Movement and activity

During middle childhood the child has greater control over body movements and gains a wider repertoire of physical skills. School-age children are usually enthusiastic about games and activities which involve coordination and the continued refinement of skills. A greater range of individual activity and exercise is undertaken such as running, hopping, skipping, climbing, acrobatics and swimming. Activities with equipment such as bicycle riding, skating and bat and ball games are appealing because they give the child the experience of consciously aiming for and achieving competence.

School-age children are very active and invariably on the move. Many find it difficult to remain still or in one place for any length of time. The requirements for sitting and attending in the first years of school may be quite demanding. As well, children in this period are not always able to achieve a balance between intense exercise and quieter activities.[1] Caregivers need to help children arrange their activities in order to gain this balance.

Much of the physical activity in the school-age years is carried out in the company of peers, where the drive to practise and become adept is reinforced by social interaction. Team games are popular in middle childhood and provide children with experience in group membership where cooperation with each other and the striving for a common goal are expected. As well, sport and exercise facilitate large muscle growth and the development of balance and coordination.

Stimulation and learning

While the world of the school-age child is rich in stimulatory experiences, there are particular activities which have the capacity to stimulate the senses, promote learning and encourage development.

The visual, auditory, tactile and kinetic senses receive stimuli through the everyday activities of the child at home, school and in other social contexts. School-age children have reading and writing skills and are usually fascinated by television, video and computer programs. Painting, drawing and artwork are generally enjoyed and may give insight into the child's perceptions of his world. Colouring-in pre-drawn forms is not encouraged by educationalists because this may stifle the child's expressive and creative activity. While music and singing are usually included in school curricula, their place in the child's experience can be enhanced by organising opportunities to listen to music and to participate in musical activities. Tactile and kinetic stimulation is afforded through play, games and interaction with others. Many children in this period still enjoy the feel of soft toys, while pets are good sources of stimulation and pleasure. Pets also provide the child with learning experiences related to personal responsibility and caring.[2]

Sleep

As the rate of growth slows during middle childhood the child's energy requirements and amount of sleep are reduced. Twelve hours of sleep each night is generally held to be the required amount in the middle childhood years,[1] although the amount of sleep required by school-age children and their bedtime schedules vary according to age, the time of arising, activity and individual differences. Some children wake early and are ready to go to bed early in the evening, while others tend to sleep later and not want to go to bed till later. Children in the early school years frequently become very tired after a full school day and need an early bedtime. By late childhood the amount of sleep is close to that of adult requirements and bedtime has been pushed back to the middle of the evening.

In the early school-age years children may need quiet and comforting strategies to help them go to sleep. Older children may read, play or listen to the radio or music before sleeping at night. Most children will settle to sleep more easily if there is a light source and they are not left in complete darkness. Sleep is sometimes disturbed during the night because of a full bladder or a frightening dream.

Children in middle childhood may resist bedtime. They may not feel particularly tired or they may wish to continue with interesting activities when they are expected to go to bed. Conflict between parents and children may result with resistance and disagreements becoming a feature of each evening. Consistency in expectations and some pleasant and interactive experiences before bedtime can reduce the levels of argument and help the child achieve adequate restful sleep. Some parents have found that accompanying the child to the bedroom and spending some time together as the child settles, rather than sending the child to bed, is a useful and preferable strategy.

Nutrition

Nutrition in middle childhood, while continuing to play a central part in the growth and development of the child, has to be considered in the social context of the child's world and the influences encountered therein. The school-age child has moved beyond the bounds of home and spends a large proportion of time at school, in social interactions with children and teachers. Children in this period experience contact with the wider community through involvement with sport groups and other organisations. In addition, they are the direct recipients of advertising and media communication which is designed to target them as an market audience.[9] It has been observed that children, early in this period, have developed ideas about body image and the desirability of being slim.[10] Each of these influences can be instrumental in the child's food preferences, eating pattern and nutritional status.

While children in middle childhood are more likely to try different tastes and accept a wider range of foods than they may have in early childhood, they are usually selective in the foods they will eat. Among the commonly accepted foods are the fast foods which, unfortunately, are likely to be high in fat, salt or sugar. Children in this period usually receive pocket money and have opportunities to purchase food items at school or local shops. Potato crisps, chips and other savoury snack foods, soft drinks and confections are favoured. Parents, teachers and health care staff face a particular challenge in teaching and convincing children about the benefits of the Healthy Diet Pyramid as a model for nutrition. The rule-bound thinking of the school-age child means, however, that the child is receptive to morally justified recommendations and that health teaching in middle childhood can be effective and influence behaviour. Healthy eating does not mean occasional treats are forbidden. It has been suggested that there is room each day for 1 or 2 indulgences without negating the effects of a healthy eating plan.[10]

Milk and milk products are important during middle childhood because they are the main source of calcium. There is a range of dairy foods which, with milk, can supply the 6 serves of milk or milk products recommended for school-age children each day. Cheese, yoghurt and ice cream are examples. One serve is 100 mL of milk.[10] Milk need not be high in fat as there are a number of fat-modified milks available which can be given to children in this age group. Fruit juice, while a good source of fluid and vitamin C, does not need to be the only other fluid offered to children. About 200 mL of fruit juice per day has been recommended.[10] Children can be offered water and become accustomed to drinking it as the most readily available and acceptable drink.

In accordance with the recommendations of the Healthy Diet Pyramid model, the child's diet will include fruit, vegetables, cereals and bread in the largest quantities. The recommended amounts for school-age children are 4 serves of fruit and vegetables and 4 serves of cereal and bread. Examples of a serve are 1 medium-sized piece of fruit, a potato or half a cup of vegetables, 1 slice of bread or half a cup of cooked rice or pasta.[10] Protein, such as meat, chicken and fish, is recommended in moderate amounts, that is, 3 servings per day. Fats and sugar are eaten in small amounts. Extra salt, added to cooking or sprinkled on food, should not be included in a child's diet.

Children often have preferences and aversions for particular foods which at times can be very strong. These likes and dislikes can also change. There is little point in allowing conflict to develop over food when an eating plan which provides the necessary nutrients can be devised with some thought and imagination. The organisation of food which takes into account the child's daily program and its social pressures is a further consideration.

School-age children are often too busy and absorbed to eat. It is common for children at school to miss eating lunch because of the playground activity. Swapping foods at school is also common, with children developing firm ideas about what foods are most desirable. A number of children are inclined to skip breakfast. Their appetite is at a low point in the early morning and they are busily getting ready for school. Parents can set expectations that some foods are eaten for breakfast and can negotiate a plan for eating at school. Some children, for example, are more willing to eat at the mid-morning break than at lunch time. Schools often organise the classes of younger children so that play does not begin until lunch is eaten.

Elimination

While school-age children are continent during the day they may still have occasional elimination 'accidents'. Night bed wetting is the most common. It seems that some children on occasions are unable to inhibit bladder emptying while they are asleep. In other circumstances school-age children may wet or soil if they are unwell, stressed or delay toiletting beyond their level of control. Children may be immensely distressed by these events and require a calm and positive approach. As the child progresses through the school years the likelihood of incontinent episodes becomes less.

During middle childhood the pattern of elimination varies for individual children and can be related to external factors such as environmental temperature, the child's activity, diet, fluid intake and emotional state. Generally, however, school-age children will void up to 6 times a day and have 1 or 2 bowel motions on each or alternate days. Urine should be passed with a strong stream and without discomfort. The stools are formed but soft, brown and easily passed. Children have to manage their toiletting and are taught how to clean themselves and to wash their hands. Both girls and boys can make sure the area surrounding the urinary meatus is dried after urination. Girls are taught to wipe toilet paper from front to back in order to reduce the risk of urinary tract infection through contamination by faecal organisms. Cotton underpants are preferred because of their absorbent qualities. Bathing with bubble bath solution may contribute to the incidence of urinary tract infection in girls. Bubble bath solution should be used sparingly and infrequently.

Clothing and protection

Clothing in middle childhood has both functional and social aspects. The functions of clothing for the school-age child are to provide warmth or allow the child to keep cool, protect the skin and tissues from sunlight, moisture and friction, and permit safe and unimpeded movement. The social considerations for the school-age child's clothing are related to gender, the pervading culture and the setting in which the child is required to function.

Clothes should be so designed that the child can manage dressing, undressing and toiletting, particularly in the early school-age years. It is important that garments accommodate the energetic activity of school-age children by allowing free movements. Clothing should be comfortable, not tight or constrictive. Replacement of clothing with larger garments is needed following a period of growth. Cotton and cotton blend fabrics are favoured because of their versatility in being warm in cool temperatures and cool in warm weather as well as their easy care and good wearing qualities. Wool and wool blends are good for supplying warmth though not as easy to launder and maintain.

Garments made from these fabrics are preferred over synthetics because they allow circulation of air, are absorbent and are less flammable. As for the younger child, nightwear that is close fitting and made with flame-resistance fabric is recommended for children in this period.

Shoes need to be checked regularly for size so that feet are not cramped and subject to distortions of growth through pressure from tight shoes. Socks and the feet of tights also need to be checked for size even though the fabric will have some degree of stretch. Footwear needs frequent replacement because of the rate of growth.

Because school-age children become absorbed in their immediate activities they may need to be reminded to add clothing in cold weather to maintain warmth and in hot weather to wear enough clothing to protect them from sunlight.

Clothing begins to take on social properties during childhood. School uniform may be worn and uniformity may be required for sport and group activities. The cultural and social characteristics of the family will influence clothing choices. Children's clothing is also influenced by fashion and popular trends. The school-age child becomes increasingly aware of appearance and will often place demands on parents to supply clothing which they believe to be situation appropriate and up-to-date. Some children show marked preference for gender specific clothing in middle childhood while others are unconcerned and opt for garments which are intended for either girls or boys.

Hygiene

A daily bath is usually necessary for school-age children. The range of activities, both indoors and out-of-doors, undertaken in this period usually means the child has had contact with other children, animals, food, play equipment, games areas and craft materials. In most instances by the end of the day, particularly in hot weather, the child will need a bath or shower. Younger children continue to have a bath and need help and supervision until about 9 years, after which they may bath themselves or manage with a shower. School-age children may try to avoid their daily bath or shower because time is taken from other activities. Supervision is needed to make sure all body surfaces are thoroughly washed. Soap is effective for cleansing purposes but should be rinsed from the skin. It is not recommended that soap is used on the child's face. Soap has a drying effect on sensitive facial skin and it may inadvertently enter the eyes and cause intense discomfort.

Bathroom safety remains an issue even though children in this age group have become more aware of safety matters. Younger children should not use the hot water taps. Adult supervision is required to establish that cold water is run into the bath tub before hot water and that the bath water is the correct temperature. Thermostatically controlled taps are recommended in homes with young children. To prevent slipping, children need some help to step out of the bath and a mat can be placed on the floor. Children are not left unattended in the bathroom though towards the end of childhood they may prefer to bath or shower in privacy. In this circumstance caregivers need to monitor the time in the bathroom and listen for the sounds of safe progress.

The hair is washed at least weekly. Some children do not like having their hair washed. They particularly object to having their hair rinsed by pouring water over the head and face and having shampoo or soap sting their eyes. A washer can be placed over the face and eyes and the child can lie back in the bath as the hair is rinsed. Many children, even younger children, find the shower is easier for hair washing, particularly if a moveable shower head is available. Shampoo which does not sting the eyes and is marketed for children's use is recommended. Hair conditioner, while not necessary for hair care in childhood, reduces knots and tangles in longer hair and can make hair grooming less troublesome.

School-age children are able to clean their teeth though they do not have the fine motor skills to brush teeth effectively until about 7 years[2] or even later.[11] A soft-bristled toothbrush and fluoride toothpaste is used. Children are taught to brush all tooth surfaces with up-and-down and rotary movements and to include the gumline when brushing. It has been noted that while a number of methods of brushing teeth have been advocated it is the thoroughness of the cleaning which is the important factor.[2] Brushing teeth is ideally carried out after each meal and before bedtime. It is not always possible for children to brush their teeth after eating during the day, but they can be taught to rinse out their mouths with water after eating. Children can also be taught how to floss between the teeth, though they are not usually able to manipulate the flossing techniques until about 9 years,[1] Brushing and flossing should be carried out each evening. Younger children will need parental help. Regular checks by the dentist are maintained every 6 months.

Fingernails and toenails will, in most instances, be adequately cleaned during the daily bath or shower. If there is an accumulation of dirt or debris under the nails, brushing with a nail brush and soap will be necessary. Nails are kept trimmed.

Immunisation

There is one further vaccine given in middle childhood in accordance with the National Health and Medical Research Council immunisation schedule (Appendix C).[12] Children aged between 10 and 16 years are offered measles, mumps and rubella vaccine, which is given as an intramuscular or deep subcutaneous injection. It is important that the uptake of rubella vaccination is high. Vaccination protects those who are vaccinated and, as well, affords protection against infection for seronegative women. If the child has a febrile illness, vaccination is delayed.[12]

Safety

Throughout middle childhood the potential for harm is high and is related to the child's inexperience, susceptibility to distraction and growing independence. The mortality and morbidity rates for school-age children reveal the major causes of death and injury. Mortality rates for school-age children from 5 years show that transport-related deaths rank first among the major causes of death. Further analysis shows that transport accidents for children in the 5 to 9 years group are mostly pedestrian deaths while in the 10 to 14 year age group it is passenger deaths which are the most common. Transport accidents, as measured by hospital separations, are surpassed by falls as the major cause of injury for children in the same period.[13,14] The school-age child is also vulnerable to drowning, suffocation and trauma through being struck, cut or pierced. Boys are more likely to suffer injury than girls in middle childhood. The context in which injury occurs changes with the child's age. As the age of the child increases so does the likelihood of injury away from the home.[14]

It has been proposed that injury prevention is achieved through education, better design and legislation.[13] Education, directed to the community, is designed to inform, increase awareness and influence the behaviour of members of the community who have contact with and the care of children.

School-age children can also be the recipients of education which aims to increase their knowledge about dangerous circumstances and reduce risky behaviour. Teaching about road safety begins in early childhood but, because in these middle years children move around the community by themselves, instructions need to be clarified and reinforced. Road safety rules should be taught, routes to school and other destinations planned with as few crossings as possible and the legal requirements for helmet wear by bicycle riders be observed. Protective clothing for children who use skateboards or skates can reduce the effects of falls and children must be taught about safe areas for these and other outdoor activities[15] Parents and other adults must insist on the use of seat belts in vehicles.

While school-age children need to be taught about their own behaviour in preventing injury, the primary responsibility for the safety of children in this period remains with adults. School-age children must be supervised when in or near water. By middle childhood many children have learned to swim but some will need to learn in this period. Teaching at home and school about fire and flammable liquids, safe handling of gas and electrical heaters and appliances, hot water and domestic equipment such as knives is important. Children need to be reminded about careful behaviours on stairs and with doors, especially glass doors, when running and climbing in areas where they may harm themselves, riding bicycles and using wheeled equipment at speed and with the use of balls and other projectiles. In keeping with their developing abilities, school-age children want to experiment, use equipment or undertake activities, many of which have the potential to cause injury. In such instances adult supervision is essential. Equipment and substances, such as firearms, medicines, alcohol, poisons and tools which have the capacity to harm children must be securely stored and children taught that they must not access them. Children will often challenge safety measures. Caregivers need to be consistent and resolute about injury prevention and the requirements they place on children. For example, some parents refuse to start the car unless seat belts are fastened.

Psychological Growth and Development

Sue Nagy

In Australia, most children begin school at the age of 5 years. By this time, they have well developed gross motor skills, and they are beginning to develop their fine motor skills. Their social skills are improving by interaction with peers, their thinking is becoming less egocentric and they are beginning to reason with simple logic. By the time puberty starts and they enter high school, their motor and cognitive capacity will be similar to that of adults.

COGNITIVE DEVELOPMENT

During middle childhood, cognitive development makes a gradual transition to the concrete operational stage.[16,17] During the development of concrete operations, children learn to communicate with others on quite a sophisticated level and to solve a range of simple, and sometimes not so simple, problems. In contrast with the pre-operational child who relies more on transductive reasoning (see Chapter One), concrete operational children begin to use inductive reasoning to understand the world. Inductive reasoning involves the development of general principles from the observation of specific instances. Observing the study patterns of friends, for example, may lead a 10 year old to conclude that consistent study is more likely to result in high grades than last minute cramming.

The reasoning ability of concrete operational children is strongly linked to their own experiences. They are not very good at imagining events or situations that they have never experienced. Concrete operational reasoning, therefore has elements of logic, providing it is applied to concrete situations that the child has experienced and not to the understanding of abstract concepts. By the age of 8, most children have well established concrete operational thinking.

In the previous chapter, the discussion of cognitive development in early childhood focused mostly on the child's incapacity to understand certain concepts. By contrast, in middle childhood cognitive development progresses to such an extent that it is more a story of children's capacities. Thinking becomes less magical and more logical. They can now decentre and thus consider many elements of a situation at once. They can mentally reverse operations so that when situations or objects change, they visualise them as they were. Not only can they conserve, they can also explain why materials remain quantitatively the same when their shape is changed. They can understand why 200 mL of orange juice in a short, fat glass is the same as 200 mL in a tall thin glass. They are now able to understand that an object can be classified into more than one category. For example, if a 4 year old and a 9 year old child are each given a bag of 20 lollies, 5 of which are bull's eyes and 15 of which are jelly beans, and are asked if there are more jelly beans or more sweets, the 4-year-old pre-operational child, is more likely to focus on the most salient characteristic and reply that there are more jelly beans. The 9-year-old concrete operational child will most likely answer that there are more lollies. She may also count them before she answers.

A major feature of cognitive development during middle childhood is a marked reduction in egocentric thinking and an increasing ability to understand that their own views are not necessarily those of others.[18] This is the beginning of the development of empathy. Children may, however, have trouble in understanding situations that are outside their own experiences. They may feel sympathy, for instance, for someone who is distressed, if they have been distressed in similar circumstances, but may have difficulty empathising with a person who is in a predicament with which they are totally unfamiliar.

The thinking of school-age children develops to such an extent that they can understand and apply elementary principles of logic to make simple deductions and judgments about situations. School-age children, for example, can reason that it is necessary to eat a balanced diet to be healthy. Eliza eats a lot of junk food, therefore Eliza is not healthy.

They may, however, have trouble distinguishing hypotheses from reality and therefore, on the basis of anecdotal evidence, make unwarranted assumptions about the general nature of the world. Such distinctions require the ability to reason hypothetico-deductively, which is not mastered until at least adolescence and sometimes even later.[19]

During middle childhood, understanding of relational concepts improves. School-age children can now understand that while that person is 'my mummy', she is also 'Grandma's daughter'. A preschool child may have difficulty understanding that a person can be at the same time taller than one person and shorter than another. Most concrete operational children can solve the following problem provided they have graphic representation of each person; 'If Jane is taller than Melissa and Penny is shorter than Jane, who is the tallest?'

Another major feature of concrete operation thinking is appreciation of the concept of rules and their application to specific instances.[19] Because of this new skill, they are able to learn valuable new skills, such as elementary mathematics. As they understand rules, they can also adhere to them. Indeed, young school children are very likely to take an inflexible and rigid view of rules and be quite shocked when another child breaks one. They may not, however, practise what they preach and may take a more lenient view of their own behaviour. By the age of 11 or 12, the child has a complete grasp of the nature of rules and can fully participate in cooperative play that relies on rules to regulate behaviour. Children can play as a group to achieve a common goal, such as in the games of hopscotch and Monopoly. Such understanding forms the basis for the development of moral reasoning ability.

MORAL DEVELOPMENT

According to Kohlberg, school children progress to a higher level of moral reasoning than pre-schoolers who are mostly motivated by the prospect of gaining a reward or avoiding punishment.[20] During school age, most children progress to Kohlberg's Level Two, the stage of conventional morality. At this level, they start to consider the intentions of the person when making moral judgments, rather than making them purely on the basis of outcomes of behaviour. They are also influenced by the reactions of others around them and behave morally more to gain social approval than to achieve material rewards or avoid punishment. Good behaviour is judged as that which incurs the approval of others in the immediate environment, such as parents and teachers. Gradually children learn to conform also to the regulations of legitimate but relatively anonymous authorities such as the police. In this way children come to regulate their behaviour because they recognise the need for social order.

Social learning theorists believe that children initially behave in the way expected by their parents to earn rewards and to avoid punishment. During middle childhood, children learn to behave morally as they identify with powerful and nurturant parents, model themselves on their parents and adopt their attitudes about right and wrong.[21,22] The child eventually internalises these attitudes, which become so deeply entrenched that they continue to exist regardless of any external reinforcements.[21]

LANGUAGE DEVELOPMENT

During the primary school years, most children become very proficient in the use of language and understand subtleties that had escaped them during their pre-school years. They appreciate jokes based on puns, and they use scientific and technical language even though they may not fully understand the meaning. Vocabulary increases and sentence construction becomes more complex. School-age children can detect grammatical differences that affect the meaning of sentences. They can, for example, understand which noun is the subject in passive sentence forms so that when told that 'Lucy was hugged by Jane' they know that it was Jane, not Lucy, who did the hugging.

Language development is influenced by children's exposure to others' use of language. Bernstein studied the use of language in economically advantaged and disadvantaged families.[23] He found variations in the language pattern used by mothers of different socioeconomic classes when interacting with their children. Economically disadvantaged mothers tended to use a 'restricted language code' which consisted of short, simply constructed and easily understood sentences that refer to present events. Additional meaning was often conveyed by intonation and gestures. Middle-class mothers were more likely to address their children with an 'elaborated language code' which consisted of explanations framed in more complex sentences with a richer vocabulary. Exposure to richer and more complex language helps explain why they tend to do better academically than children from more disadvantaged homes.[24]

SOCIAL AND EMOTIONAL DEVELOPMENT

Freud's latency stage

Freud regarded the period from about 6 years to puberty as a time of sexual latency, when the sexual concerns that preoccupy pre-schoolers and adolescents are put aside so that the child's energy can be directed towards learning the skills necessary for adulthood. Support for Freud's ideas is evidenced by school-age and early adolescent children's preferences for interactions with same-sex peers.[25] However, as school-age children masturbate and show curiosity in sexual matters, they are probably not as sexually latent as Freud believed.[26] Perhaps they have merely learned to be more circumspect in their sexual interest and inquiry.

Erikson's industry versus inferiority stage

Erikson agreed with Freud that school-age children need time to learn and indeed, regarded learning as critical for the development during middle childhood.[27] The important psychosocial task of middle childhood is the development of a sense of industry rather than a sense of inferiority. As school-age children succeed in meeting the expectations of themselves and others, they become increasingly industrious and competent. Continual failure and excessive criticism lead to feelings of inferiority that threaten to stay with them and jeopardise their future emotional and social development. Erikson believed that school children are ready to learn the pleasure that comes from effort, perseverance and achievement. They are beginning to use other children as a yardstick in order to develop a more accurate picture of their own competencies.[28] These comparisons form the basis for the development of a sense of self-esteem during childhood, and of identity during adolescence.

Adults can help the child become industrious, competent and develop a high self-esteem in a number of ways. They can help children not only to set realistic goals at which they have a reasonable chance of succeeding, but to encounter challenging opportunities. Unreasonably high aspirations may lead to feelings of failure and incompetence. Expectations that are too low, do not allow children to feel the satisfaction that comes from mastering a challenge. Adults can provide guidance, instruction and encouragement to help children to achieve their goals. Encouragement is more effective when it focuses on praise of successes rather than excessive criticism of failures. Excessive criticism accentuates children's disappointment in their own progress and can increase their feelings of inadequacy. All children sometimes fail at tasks, but by encouraging and praising the child's effort the child can be encouraged to keep trying. Children who are thus supported are more likely to develop a strong sense of self-esteem.

The development of self-esteem

Children now begin to develop, not only a sense of who they are, but also a sense of what they might be. They can now see a discrepancy between their real self and ideal self. The

smaller this discrepancy, the greater the self-esteem.[29] Children begin to develop competencies in many areas. As they succeed in their aspirations, they become better equipped
to cope with times of failure. As they accept both their strengths and their weaknesses,
they develop a realistic self-concept.

Significant adults, such as parents, teachers and nurses, have an important role to
play in the development of the child's self-esteem.[30] Those who show their confidence in
the child's ability by having reasonably high expectations, who show that the child is
sufficiently worthwhile to merit attention and support and who praise the child's achievements, make an important contribution to the development of self-esteem.[28,30,31]

Socialisation within the family

Parents may need help in providing for the psychological needs of their children, especially when their own needs have not been met. For example, parents who are in conflict
with each other may not be able to foster their children's development as well as parents
who are supportive of each other.[32-34] For this reason, it is important for paediatric nurses
to include an evaluation of the family in their assessment of the child. It is all very well
to identify a child who is in need of support and encouragement from her parents, but
this is to little avail if the parents are unable to supply it. Parents may also need support
and encouragement so that they can effectively meet the needs of their children.

Most children have times when they feel neglected within the family and resort to
attention-seeking behaviours. When a pattern of neglect is established, the children may
try to seek attention by whining, rebellious behaviour and develop into passive, solitary
individuals.[35] Parents who reassure their children that they are loved and wanted can
reduce unpleasant, attention-seeking behaviours.

The aims of discipline are twofold. First, to inhibit annoying and socially unacceptable behaviour, and second, to develop a conscience in the child so that socially desirable
behaviour will occur whether or not parents are present to enforce it. Some forms of
discipline are better at achieving the first aim and others the second. Some forms of
discipline seem to foster self-esteem and self-reliance in children and others do not.
Many studies have been made of the different discipline patterns that are used by parents
and of their effect on children. Freiburg describes 3 types of discipline; power-assertive,
love-withdrawal and inductive.[36]

Power-assertive discipline involves the use of physical punishment or threat to enforce
obedience. It tends to be effective in achieving short-term control over the child's behaviour, but ineffective in producing children who have a high self-esteem, are self-reliant
and who have a strong social conscience.

Parents who make their love contingent on the child's behaviour are using love-
withdrawal discipline. Regular use of love-withdrawal discipline tends to produce resentful
children who are anxious about losing love and affection. They tend to behave morally
to earn the affection of others rather than from motives of social responsibility.

Parents who use inductive discipline explain to their children why behaviours are
expected and point out the consequences of the child's behaviour for other people.
It is the most effective form of discipline.[37] Children whose parents rely on inductive
discipline tend to be more able to empathise with others and to have a strong social
conscience.

Diana Baumrind also studied the different types of discipline commonly used by
parents and their effects on the children within the family.[38] She found that child-rearing
practices could be classified as either authoritarian, authoritative or permissive.

Authoritarian parents tend to make many rules and rigidly insist that the children conform to them. They are reluctant to enter into discussion of their rules, and believe that the children should accept them unquestioningly. They seem to operate from a belief that it is necessary to coerce children into good behaviour and often use punitive methods. Children may be obedient but are often unhappy, have average social and cognitive competencies, they tend to be distrustful, uncomfortable in social situations and lack independence.

Permissive parents make few demands on their children, and do not seem to have high expectations of them. Very little discipline is exercised, and the children are often left to make decisions for themselves. Parents who exercise this type of child rearing pattern seem to be conveying to their children that they are not worthy of the attention and guidance of a more experienced adult. Consequently their children tend to have a low self-esteem. It also places a responsibility on children to make decisions that require a wisdom beyond their years. Perhaps this is why children of permissive parents were found to be unhappier than children of parents using either of the other types of discipline. They were also the least self-reliant and self-controlled.

Authoritative parents set limits on their children's behaviour, but keep them to a minimum. Those that are set, however, are enforced. Children have the right to present another viewpoint which is listened to but parents reserve the right to be the final arbiters. Parents recognise that they have more competence than the child but are also not infallible, so that they take the child's viewpoint into account. Discipline therefore is more democratic. Children of authoritative parents are more likely to be happy with themselves, generous with others, and to be more socially competent. They were also found to be high achievers and demonstrated a high degree of independence and self-reliance.

Maccoby and Martin analysed the effects of parenting styles according to (a) the warmth of parents' responsiveness to their children and (b) to parental expectations of their children.[39] Parents who had few expectations and were least responsive had the poorest outcome in terms of the children's behaviour. Their children tended to be aggressive, impulsive and to have poor self-control. Those who had high expectations of their children but were also responsive and warm were most likely to have children who had a high self-esteem and good self-control, and were self-reliant and responsible.

In summary, it seems that the most effective parenting styles are those where parents have high expectations of their children, and also help them to meet those expectations. The most damage arises from parent's failure to convince the children that they are worthy of parental love, respect and attention. Such children seem to have difficulty in convincing themselves and others of their own worth. Children who are harshly disciplined seem to learn obedience providing the disciplinarian is present, but fail to learn personal responsibility for their behaviour. They learn to be aggressive, probably because their parents model aggressive behaviour and because resentment is a natural reaction to the harsh treatment they have received. Effective parents are warm, responsive and respectful to their children and they demonstrate their respect by explaining the reasons behind parental requests and decisions. They also demonstrate that their love is enduring and is not contingent on the children's compliance with their parents' wishes.

Relationships with siblings

Siblings can be a major source of support for each other and help provide an environment for learning many of the skills associated with normal development.[40,41] Relationships

*The relationship
between siblings
may be warm and
supportive.*

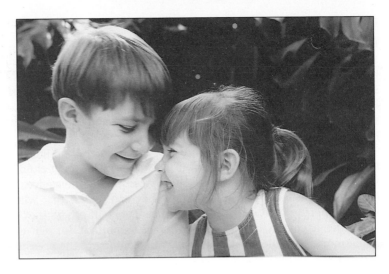

between them may be warm and supportive or competitive and quarrelsome, but most involve a mixture of positive and negative aspects. Sibling relationships are therefore complex, but as they seem to be highly influential in the development of children within the family, it is important that the positive aspects be developed as far as possible.

The quality of sibling relationships is established early in life and tends to persist.[42] Relationships depend on a number of factors, including the age of the children, and the position of the children in the family, the gender of the siblings, and parental influences.

The birth of a new baby can be a difficult time for a child who previously has had his parents to himself and now finds that his mother's attention is often diverted to the new baby.[42] Relationships between siblings can be especially strained if there is less than 2 years difference between their ages.[43] Toddlers are in a stage of development where they are still very dependent on their parents but, at the same time, are trying to exert their autonomy. When the children and parents are interacting, parents seem to naturally focus their attention on the younger child.[44] A new brother or sister makes demands on their parents' attention at a time when the toddler also needs much attention and understanding. Mothers find it especially difficult to meet the needs of both a toddler and a new baby.[45]

First-born children are more likely to resent the attention given to younger siblings and younger siblings are more likely to resent the extra freedom and autonomy of the older child. There are, however, many positive effects of the relationship of closely spaced siblings[44] They are more likely to have strong feelings of closeness and warmth towards each other, and especially when they are of the same gender, to have less conflict.[43]

Parents can help their children adjust to the birth of a new sibling by adequately preparing them for changes that will be associated with the arrival of the baby. Parents need to be warned that some changes in the behaviour of the older child are likely, particularly sleep disturbances and regressive and attention-seeking behaviour. When the baby arrives, involving older children in the care of the baby and setting aside time to be spent with the older child, and without the baby, can reduce feelings of neglect. It is easy for parents to reinforce negative behaviour unwittingly if they wait until the child demands attention before giving it.

Relationships with peers

During middle childhood, dependence on parents decreases and children become more open to the influence of peers and rely on them more for support.[46-48] Friendships become more enduring than they were in early childhood.[49] This enables children to take a further step towards the autonomy and emancipation from the family that is necessary for full adulthood.[30] With peers, children learn to relate to others on a more reciprocal basis,[50] rather than one in which they are protected and expected to obey. Peer interaction, therefore, teaches self-reliance.

In middle childhood, peers are more likely to mix in single-sexed groups.[51] Perhaps this has a functional value in that it allows the developing child better opportunity to develop appropriate sex-role behaviour. By comparing themselves with their peers, children can develop a realistic sense of self. They can realise that while in some respects they may not perform as well as some of their peers, in others they may do as well or better.

Being accepted by the peer group is important for self-esteem and psychological adjustment.[52] Middle childhood sees the beginning of the pressure to conform to the peer group expectations that are so characteristic of early adolescent relationships. Indeed, warnings about the negative social effects of poor health practices may be more effective in gaining children's cooperation than warnings about negative effects on their health.[53]

Children who are chronically ill, disabled, disfigured or members of minority racial groups may be at a disadvantage. Prejudices may have already been learned from parents. Being unable to participate in certain activities, being different from others, bringing different foods to school, may all invite ridiculing and teasing from other children.

Play during middle childhood

During middle childhood, play becomes more structured and cooperative. Cooperative play is a highly organised activity involving rules by which children cooperate to reach group goals. In some instances, leaders who direct the activities of others are chosen or emerge. As children begin to learn to relate better to peers, and as they develop the cognitive maturity to understand the need for rules, they are able to play more cooperatively. Marbles, jacks, board games and team games are examples of cooperative play based on the understanding and observance of rules. Cooperative play helps children learn social skills, elementary negotiation and conflict resolution skills and appropriate sex-role behaviour. (See Chapter Two for a more detailed discussion of the development of the social content of play.)

Play is also therapeutic. It provides a means of expressing pent-up energies and frustration. It gives children ways of dealing with fears and promoting feelings of control. Ritualistic games such as avoiding cracks in the footpath and its associated rhyme 'Don't step on a crack or you'll break your mother's back' may help children develop a sense of control over the fear of losing their mother. Games such as cops and robbers or cowboys and Indians may help them to master their fears of death. The use of play to help children deal with the anxieties associated with illness and hospitalisation is discussed in Chapter Nine.

THE DEVELOPMENT OF THE CONCEPT OF DEATH

To understand the meaning of death fully, it is necessary to understand that it is universal, irreversible and absolute. Research has shown that children progress through a number of stages before reaching full understanding of the concept.[54-57] During the early school years, children may have many fantasies about death which may cause them to develop fears of being in situations that are associated with the fantasies. Some children conceptualise death as a distinct personality such as a bogey-man or a skeleton. They may believe that dying means being carried off by 'the deathman' and this may lead to fears of being carried off in the middle of the night. Explanations that 'God loved Grandma so much that He took her to live with him' may result in anxiety and sleep disturbance. Fears of being alone in the dark may also be heightened for other children who believe that death usually occurs at night, in the dark when no-one can see. If death is equated with sleep, others may go through a stage of being afraid to go to sleep. Some school-age children seem to see death as punishment for bad behaviour, believing, for example, that 'Granny died because I was angry with her'.

Older children may accept the finality and universality of death for all but themselves. 'Old people die, but not children' or 'I might die one day, but not until I am very old.' This belief may persist well into adolescence.

Children seem to vary on the age at which they reach complete understanding. Lansdown and Benjamin[58] found that 60% of 5 year olds and almost all 9 year olds fully understood the concept of death, while Childers and Wimmer[59] found 10 year olds who did not and Bluebond-Langer[56] found 4 year olds who did. The differences may be related to the child's previous experiences of the deaths of family members or pets.

When trying to help a school-age child understand death it is wise to find out the parent's beliefs about death and an after-life. While pointing out that people have different beliefs about death and what happens after it,[60] it is important not to undermine children's relationships with their parents. Children should be allowed to grieve and to express their grief in any way that they are able, depending on their personality and developmental level. It is important that children's grief is not denied and that it is allowed full expression, irrespective of their age. Their grief is just as real as that of adults.

THE DEVELOPMENT OF BODY IMAGE

During school-age the sex role development which started in early childhood becomes more firmly established. Physical competence involves more than the gross motor skills of running, jumping, or riding a bike, as fine motor abilities are now becoming increasingly important to their sense of competence. Concepts of body boundaries are now fully developed. Children are able to evaluate themselves and their bodies in relationship to those of others, particularly the same sex. It is in this way they develop a realistic sense of their own body image.

The vulnerability of school-age children to feelings of inferiority is obvious. They need help to see themselves as individuals with their own unique set of competencies, strengths, weaknesses and limitations.

Although most concrete operational children are beginning to have some idea of their body's interior,[61] they still have problems understanding what they cannot see, hear or feel. So they often have trouble in conceptualising the changes that occur under bandages, dressings and plaster casts or inside their bodies. Children's drawings of themselves can provide insights into their body image development. Drawings of the insides of their bodies typically show body parts that can be discerned from the outside (such as bones), or substances they have seen going in or coming out of the body (such as food and faeces).[62] Children's attitudes about their bodies are often reflected in their drawings and can be a useful assessment tool. Schizophrenic children, for example, tend to draw themselves with shadowy, almost ghostly outlines that appear to reflect their perceptions of themselves as lacking reality.[63] Children with a satisfactory body image tend to draw detailed pictures of themselves of a realistic size and with definite boundaries.[64] Satisfactory sex role identification is often reflected in drawings which clearly indicate the child's sex.[63]

BELIEFS ABOUT HEALTH, ILLNESS AND PAIN

Beliefs about the causes of health and illness

School-age children tend to place a great deal of emphasis on the value of a healthy diet, but know very little else about healthy behaviour.[65,66] While they entertain a lingering belief that illness is a form of punishment for wrong doing,[65,67] they are beginning to understand that illness does not 'just happen' and that the environment plays a role in the development of illness.

School-age children are likely to have difficulty distinguishing the risk factors for different types of illness. For example, Sigelman et al found that 9 year olds believed that needle-sharing, blood exchange and sex were as likely to cause colds as they were to cause AIDS.[68]

Bibace and Walsh found that during the concrete operational period,[69] children began to be aware that the body has an interior as well as an exterior environment and that this awareness is reflected in their understanding of the causes of illness. Younger concrete operational children tended to see illness as a result of contamination by external factors that act upon the body in some way to cause illness.[66,67,69] The most commonly mentioned external causes of disease are germs[66,67,71] misbehaviour[66,67] animals, food and being in a particular place.[66] The following quotation from a concrete operational child illustrates the contamination explanation.

'What is a cold?'
'It's like in the winter time.'
'How do people get colds?'
'You're outside with a hat and you start sneezing. Your head would get cold, the cold would touch it and it would go all over your body.'[69]

Older concrete operational children understand that illness is caused by external factors that must somehow enter the body to cause harm. Bibace and Walsh termed this type of explanation as internalisation.

'What is a cold?'
'You sneeze a lot, you talk funny and your nose is clogged up.'
'How do people get colds?'
'In winter they breathe in too much air into their nose, and it blocks up the nose.'
'How does this cause colds?'
'The bacteria gets in by breathing. Then the lungs get too soft [child exhales], and it goes to the nose.'
'How does it get better?'
'Hot fresh air, it gets in the nose and pushes the cold air back.'[69]

Bibace and Walsh based their conclusions on the responses of well children.[69] This raises the issue of the influence of illness experience on children's conceptions of illness causation. Williams studied hospitalised children and found that although they were better informed about illness, they did not have any better understanding of the disease process than well children.[61] She also found that while well children were more likely to believe that illness is caused by natural phenomena (sun, wind, cold etc.), hospitalised children were more likely to include germs and contagion. Eiser and Patterson found that diabetic children could accurately describe the causes of their own disease, but were not any better informed about other diseases.[72]

Beliefs about pain

Just as the children's conception of health, illness and death becomes more sophisticated as they mature, so does their understanding of painful experiences. Just as children begin to understand that germs enter the body to cause disease, so do they begin to see pain as an internal phenomenon.[73] Pain is seen as 'a feeling' that can occur anywhere in the body. They can now comprehend that different types of pain can cause different sensations and use quite graphic analogies to describe them, such as, 'It's like someone twisted a burning knife inside you'.

However, while concrete operational children can describe their pain,[74] including its intensity, location and duration, they have difficulty distinguishing different types of pain, such as stinging and aching.[75]

While egocentric preschoolers may believe that doctors and nurses automatically know when a child is in pain, school-age children feel that it is necessary to communicate pain by crying.[76] Gaffney and Dunne, however, found that boys were more likely than girls to feel it was necessary to conceal that they were in pain.[73]

STRESS AND COPING

The fears which tend to haunt school-age children reflect the developmental demands of the age group. Fears of loss of function and self-control are common.[77] Common childhood dreams about losing control such as trying to escape a car and one's legs won't move or having bowel or bladder 'accidents' at school, reflect these fears.

The child's repertoire of coping strategies increases during middle childhood. Regression, denial, escape and avoidance are used by school-age children. Positive self-talk is a common and effective strategy.[78] Brown et al found that a common but not very effective response of school-age children was to 'catastrophise' by 'focusing on or magnifying the negative aspects of the event'.[78] Typical catastrophising thoughts were 'I'm going to bleed all over the place,' 'What if the doctor is a meany'.

School-age children need support from significant adults and the support of friends is becoming increasingly important.[36] As the child grows older, his social network grows smaller and he tends to develop fewer but closer friendships.[79] Recognising children's need for their friends' support can be important in helping them deal with stress.

Relaxation training has been found to be effective in helping school-age children cope with stress.[80] Stories which use relaxing images and guide the child in muscle relaxation can be effectively used by nurses.

Paediatric nurses can facilitate coping in school-age children by recognising their need to regain or maintain control, by supporting effective coping strategies and teaching the child new ways to deal with stress. Opportunities should be provided for the child to improve her personal competence and her efforts should be encouraged and praised. Incidents involving loss of bowel and bladder control should be handled sensitively.

REFERENCES

1. Mott SR, James SR, Sperhac AM. *Nursing care of children and families.* 2nd ed. Redwood City: Addison-Wesley, 1990.
2. Wong DL. *Whaley and Wong's nursing care of infants and children.* 5th ed. St Louis: Mosby, 1995.
3. Royal Alexandra Hospital for Children, Sydney. *Length, weight, head circumference, males and females 2–18.* Designed by the Department of Endocrinology, The Adelaide Children's Hospital, 1991.
4. Scipien GM, Chard MA, Howe J, Barnard MU. *Pediatric nursing care.* St Louis: Mosby, 1990.
5. Wong DL. *Quick pediatric reference.* St Louis: Mosby, 1995.
6. Marlow DR, Redding BA. *Textbook of pediatric nursing.* 6th ed. Philadelphia: Saunders, 1988.
7. National Health and Medical Research Council. *Review of Child Health Surveillance and Screening.* Canberra: AGPS, 1993.
8. Brunner LS, Suddarth DS. *The Lippincott manual of paediatric nursing.* 3rd ed. Adapted for the UK by BF Weller. London: Harper Collins, 1991.
9. Vimpani G. Contemporary influences upon child health. *In:* Vimpani G, Parry T, eds. *Community child health: an Australian perspective.* Melbourne: Churchill Livingstone, 1989.
10. Thompson S. *A health start for kids: how to convince your children to eat well.* Sydney: Simon and Schuster, 1991.
11. Craig G. Dental health. *In:* Clements A, ed. *Infant and family health in Australia.* 2nd ed. Melbourne: Churchill Livingstone, 1995.
12. National Health and Medical Research Council. *The Australian immunisation handbook.* 5th ed. Canberra: AGPS, 1994.
13. Pearn J, Vimpani G. Promoting healthy and safe physical environments. *In:* Vimpani G, Parry T, eds. *Community child health: an Australian perspective.* Melbourne: Churchill Livingstone, 1989.
14. New South Wales Health Department. *Childsafe NSW Report No. 1: childhood injury in NSW, 1980s.* Sydney: The Health Promotion Unit, NSW Health Department, 1991.
15. Cohen D, Kilham H, Oates K. *The complete book of child safety.* Sydney: Simon and Schuster, 1989.
16. Piaget J. *The construction of reality in the child.* New York: Basic Books, 1954.
17. Piaget J, Inhelder B. *The psychology of the child.* London: Routledge Kegan & Paul, 1969.
18. Lucco AA. Assessment of the school-age child. *Families in Society* 1991; 72: 394–408.
19. Flavell JH. *The developmental psychology of Jean Piaget.* New York: Van Nostrand, 1963.
20. Kohlberg L. The development of moral character and moral ideology. *In:* Hoffman ML, Hoffman LW, eds. *Review of child development research.* Vol. 1. New York: Russell Sage, 1964.
21. Bandura A. *Social learning theory.* New Jersey: Prentice-Hall, 1977.
22. Sears RR, Rau L, Alpert R. *Identification and child rearing.* California: Stanford University Press, 1965.
23. Bernstein B. A sociolinguistic approach to socialization: with some reference to educability. *In:* Williams F, ed. *Language and poverty: perspectives on a theme.* Chicago: Markham, 1970.
24. Templin MC. *Certain language skills in children.* Institute of Child Welfare Monograph, Serial No. 26. Minneapolis: University of Minnesota Press, 1957.
25. Dunphy D. The social structure of urban adolescent peer groups. *In:* Collins J, ed. *Studies of the Australian adolescent.* Melbourne: Cassell, 1975.
26. Goldman RJ, Goldman DG. The prevalence and nature of child sexual abuse in Australia. *Aust J Sex, Marriage Family* 1988; 9: 94–106.

27. Erikson EH. *Childhood and Society.* New York: Norton, 1963.
28. Philips S. *Self concept and self esteem. Infancy to adolescence.* Selected paper No 27, Kensington, NSW: Foundation for Child and Youth Studies, 1983.
29. Rogers C. *On becoming a person.* Boston: Houghton-Mifflin, 1961.
30. Howes C, Hamilton CE, Matheson CC. Children's relationships with peers: differential associations with aspects of the teacher–child relationship. *Child Dev* 1994; 65: 253–263.
31. Coopersmith S. *The antecedents of self-esteem.* San Francisco: Freeman, 1967.
32. Vuchinich S, Vuchinich R, Wood B. The interparental relationship and family problem solving with preadolescent males. *Child Dev* 1993; 64: 1389–1400.
33. Grych JH, Fincham FD. Marital conflict and children's adjustment: a cognitive–contextual framework. *Psychol Bull* 1990; 108: 267–290.
34. Buchanan CM, Macoby EE, Dornbusch SM. Caught between parents: adolescents' experience in divorced homes. *Child Dev* 1991; 62: 1008–1029.
35. Dreikurs R, Solz V. *Children: the challenge.* New York: Hawthorn, 1964.
36. Freiberg KL. *Human development: a life span approach.* Boston: Jones and Bartlett, 1987.
37. Bearison DJ, Cassel TZ. Cognitive concentration and social codes. Communication effectiveness in young children from differing family contexts. *Dev Psychol* 1975; 11: 29–36.
38. Baumrind D. Current practices of parental authority. (Monograph 1) *Dev Psychol* 1971; 4: 1–103.
39. Maccoby EE, Martin JA. Socialisation in the context of the family : parent-child interaction. *In:* Mussen PH ed. *Handbook of child psychology: socialization, personality and social development.* Vol. 4, 4th ed. New York: Wiley, 1983.
40. Lamb ME. Sibling relationships across the lifespan. *In:* Lamb ME, Sutton-Smith B, eds. *Sibling relationships.* New Jersey: Erlbaum, 1982.
41. Cicirelli VG. Family structure and interactions: sibling effects on socialisation. *In:* McMillan M, Sergio M, eds. *Child psychiatry: treatment and research.* New York: Brunner/Mazel, 1977.
42. Dunn J, Kendrick C. Siblings and their mothers: developing relationships within the family. *In:* Lamb ME, Sutton-Smith B, eds. *Sibling relationships.* New Jersey: Erlbaum, 1982.
43. Minnett AM, Vandell DL, Santrock JW. The effects of sibling status on sibling interaction: influence of birth order, age, spacing, sex of child, and sex of sibling. *Child Dev* 1983; 54: 1064–1072.
44. Bryant BK. Sibling relationships in middle childhood. *In:* Lamb ME, Sutton-Smith B, eds. *Sibling relationships.* New Jersey: Erlbaum, 1982.
45. Lynch A. Maternal stress following the birth of a second child. *In:* Klaus MH, Robertson MO, eds. *Birth, interaction and attachment: Pediatric Round Table; 6.* New Jersey: Johnson and Johnson, 1982.
46. Nelson-Le Gall SA, Gumerman RA. Children's perceptions of helpers and helper motivation. *J Applied Dev Psychol* 1984; 5: 1–12.
47. Furman W, Bierman KL. Children's conceptions of friendships: a multimethod study of developmental changes. *Dev Psychol* 1984; 20: 925–932.
48. Berndt TJ, Perry TB. Children's perceptions of friendships as supportive relationships. *Dev Psychol* 1986; 22: 640–648.
49. Berndt TJ, Hoyle SG. Stability and change in childhood and adolescent friendships. *Dev Psychol* 1985; 21: 1007–1015.
50. Bigelow BJ. Children's friendship expectations A cognitive developmental study. *Child Dev* 1977; 48: 246–253.
51. Hartup WW. Peer relations. *In:* Hetherington EM, ed. *Handbook of child psychology: socialization, personality and social development* Vol. 4, 4th ed. New York: Wiley, 1983.
52. Coie JD, Kupersmidt J. A behavioural analysis of emerging social status in boys' groups. *Child Dev* 1983; 54: 1400–1416.
53. Knapp LG. Effects of type of value appealed to and valence of appeal on children's dental health behavior. *J Pediatr Psychol* 1991; 16: 675–686.
54. Nagy M. The child's theory concerning death. *J Genetics Psychol* 1948; 73: 3–27.

55. Anthony S. *The discovery of death in childhood.* New York: Basic Books, 1972.
56. Bluebond-Langner M. *The private worlds of dying children.* New Jersey: Princeton University Press, 1978.
57. Lonetto R. *Children's conceptions of death.* New York: Springer, 1980.
58. Landsdown R, Benjamin G. The development of the concept of death in children aged 5–9 years. *Child Care, Health Dev* 1985; 11: 13–20.
59. Childers P, Wimmer M. The concept of death in early childhood. *Child Dev* 1971; 42: 1299–1301.
60. Grollman EA. *Explaining death to children.* Boston: Beacon Press, 1967.
61. Williams PD. Children's concepts of illness and internal body parts. *Maternal-Child Nursing J* 1979; 8: 115–123.
62. Pantell RH, Lewis CC. Communicating with children in hospital. *In:* Thornton S, Frankenburg W, eds. Child health care communication. New York: Johnson and Johnson, 1983.
63. Blaesing S, Brockhaus J. The development of body image in the child. *Nursing Clin North Am* 1972; 7: 597–607.
64. Spinetta JJ, McLaren HH, Fox RW, Sparta SN. The kinetic family drawing in childhood cancer. *In:* Spinetta J, Deasy-Spinetta P, eds. *Living with childhood cancer.* St Louis: Mosby, 1981.
65. Eiser C, Patterson D, Eiser JR. Children's knowledge of health and illness: implications for health education. *Child Care Health Dev* 1983; 9: 233–240.
66. Gratz RR, Piliavin JA. What makes kids sick: children's beliefs about the causative factors of illness. *Children's Health Care* 1984; 12: 156–162.
67. Wood SP. School age children's perceptions of the causes of illness. *Pediatric Nursing* 1983; 9: 101–104.
68. Sigelman C, Maddock A, Epstein J, Carpenter W. Age differences in understandings of disease casuality: AIDS, colds and cancer. *Child Dev* 1993; 64: 272–284.
69. Bibace R, Walsh ME. Children's conceptions of illness. *In:* Bibace R, Walsh ME, eds. *Children's conceptions of health, illness and bodily functions.* San Francisco: Jossey-Bass, 1981.
70. Osborne ML, Kistner JA, Helgemo B. Developmental progression in children's knowledge of AIDS: implications for education and attitude change. *J Pediatr Psychol* 1993; 18: 177–192.
71. Perrin E, Gerrity P. There's a demon in your belly: children's understanding of illness. *Pediatrics* 1981; 67: 841–849.
72. Eiser C, Patterson D. 'Slugs and snails and puppy dogs tails' — children's ideas about the insides of their bodies. *Child Care Health Dev* 1983; 9: 233–240.
73. Gaffney A, Dunne EA. Developmental aspects of children's definitions of pain. *Pain* 1986; 26: 105–117.
74. Ely EA. The experience of pain for school-age children: Blood, band-aids and feelings. *Children's Health Care* 1992; 21: 168–176.
75. Harbeck C, Peterson L. Elephants dancing in my head: a developmental approach to children's concepts of specific pains. *Child Dev* 1992; 63: 138–149.
76. Pantell RH, Lewis CC. Communicating with children in hospital. *In:* Thornton S, Frankenburg W, eds. *Child health care communication.* New York: Johnson and Johnson, 1983.
77. Adams M. A hospital play program: helping children with serious illness. *Am J Orthopsychiatry* 1976; 46: 416–424.
78. Brown JM, O'Keefe J, Sanders S, Baker B. Developmental changes in children's cognition to stressful and painful situations. *J Pediatr Psychol* 1986; 11: 343–357.
79. Berger K. *The developing person through the life span.* New York: Worth, 1988.
80. LaMontagne LL. Facilitating children's coping. *AORN Journal* 1985; 42: 718–723.

Chapter 4

Growth and Development: 12 Years to Early Adulthood

Physical Growth and Development

Anne Adams

ASSESSMENT OF ADOLESCENTS

The physical assessment of the adolescent requires a particularly sensitive approach. The growth and development of adolescence means there are significant physical, social, psychological and emotional changes to be negotiated by the adolescent. The teenager may have some confused feelings about these changes and can be uncomfortable and uncertain about the experience of a physical assessment.

Adolescents value clear explanations and honest answers to their questions. They may, however, have difficulty in articulating their concerns and the questions they wish to ask unless a rapport has been established with the nurse. An empathic approach is essential for creating a comfortable relationship and helping the nurse understand any issues of concern to the teenager.

Privacy and confidentiality are of central importance to the adolescent. Teenagers are usually very modest and should retain their clothing or wear a gown. They should remain covered except for the area of the body which is being assessed and should not be exposed for any longer than is necessary. Adolescents may prefer parents not to be present. Special consideration must be given to those adolescents and their families whose culture places a high value on female modesty and requires that females will examine the female adolescent.

MUSCULOSKELETAL SYSTEM

Adolescence is marked by a striking increase in growth. This growth spurt takes place over a 2 to 3 year period and may begin in late childhood.[1] Skeletal growth in adolescence is influenced by the hormones which are activated at puberty. Girls and boys have different patterns of skeletal growth. Bone growth in girls is controlled by epiphyseal closure of the long bones under the influence of oestrogen. Boys are taller with longer limbs because of the longer period of growth of long bones before epiphyseal closure takes place. Boys have wider shoulders while the pelvic girdle is wider in girls. Accentuated muscle growth follows the skeletal growth spurt and is more pronounced in boys. The growth and development of both skeletal and muscle tissue is influenced by androgenic hormones in boys and results in denser bone and muscle.[1,2]

Posture

Posture undergoes a series of characteristic changes during adolescence. In early adolescence teenagers have a gangly appearance because the limbs and neck lengthen before the trunk but with the lengthening of the trunk in middle adolescence the teenager assumes adult proportions.[3] Teenagers may adopt a forward slump and a round-shouldered appearance where the distance between the shoulder blades will be wider than normal. A slight kyphosis may develop.[4] This posture is related to the pattern of the growth spurt where the rapid growth in height and the gain in weight precedes an increase in muscle strength.[5] Poor posture may also be related to an intense awareness and sensitivity experienced by some teenagers about their growing and changing body. In an effort not to be noticed the teenager may slouch and hold his head down.

Posture is assessed by observing the adolescent from the side. Good posture is present when the head is held in such way that a vertical line from the ear would pass through the shoulder, hip and ankle. The shoulders are level.[4]

Scoliosis, a lateral S-shaped deviation of the vertebral column, can occur in adolescence, mainly in girls. The curve is more often convex to the right.[5] To test for scoliosis the adolescent is asked to remove clothing from above the waist so the whole of the back can be seen. Girls may prefer to retain their brassiere. The back is studied from behind, firstly, while the adolescent remains standing. There should be symmetry of the hips and shoulders and the spine should be straight.[4] The adolescent is then asked to bend well forward with both arms freely hanging. The contour of the back is studied for any elevation of the ribs on one side.[5]

Joints and limbs

There is free and easy movement of joints which allows the adolescent to participate in a range of physical activities and to develop refined and skillful movements such as those required for gymnastics, dancing and sport. The limbs lengthen to their ultimate adult size and are straight with each pair equal and symmetric. Arms and legs become stronger and have greater power and endurance for physical activity.

Late in puberty the angle of the neck of the femur becomes more acute in girls. This change is known as 'sculpting' and causes a widening of the pelvic outlet and changes the gait of older adolescent girls.[6]

Weight

The growth spurt of adolescence produces a dramatic increase in weight which is greater in boys than girls. The average weight gain in girls is between 7 and 25 kg and in boys is between 7 and 30 kg.[1] The average weight for girls at 12 years is 41.5 kg, at 15 years 53.5 kg and at 18 years 56.8 kg. The average weight for boys at 12 years is 39.5 kg, at 15 years 56.5 kg and at 18 years 69 kg (Appendix A). While weight gain is directly related to growth there are characteristic differences in the pattern of tissue growth in girls and boys. In boys the increase in the amount and density of muscle is greater. For both girls and boys there is a steady increase in adipose tissue, but in girls the deposition of fat is more pronounced, especially over the hips, thighs, buttocks and the breasts.[1]

Adolescents are ideally weighed with minimal clothing, such as underwear or a hospital gown. It is, however, acceptable in most instances to weigh the adolescent without removing clothes provided the clothing is light. The difference light clothing would make to the weight reading is small and the embarrassment many teenagers feel at undressing in front of others is avoided. Adolescents can be weighed in garments of similar weight if the weight is to be monitored over time. Shoes and heavy outer garments are, of course, removed.

Height

The increase in height associated with the growth spurt is more dramatic than the increase in weight. Growth in the length of the trunk is fastest and accounts for 60% of the increase in height during adolescence.[2] The average increase in height for girls is between 5 and 20 cm and for boys, between 10 and 30 cm.[1] The average height for girls at 12 years is 151.5 cm, at 15 years 161.6 cm and at 18 years 163.5 cm. Boys on average at 12 years are 149.3 cm, at 15 years 168.5 cm and at 18 years are 176.8 cm (Appendix A). Girls cease growing in height at about 16 or 17 years while boys continue to gain height until 18 or 20 years.[1] The difference in the pattern and extent of the increase in height between girls and boys is marked. Girls begin and complete the growth spurt about two years before boys, while boys have a substantially greater increase in both height and weight.

The height of the teenager is determined by measuring the vertical distance between the top of the head and the soles of the feet when the teenager stands upright against a wall or measuring device. The teenager is asked to stand tall, look directly ahead with bare feet firmly on the floor, and the back and heels touching the upright surface. The height is taken where a flat surface placed across the top of the head touches the wall or measuring scale.

Head

While the head is not usually measured in adolescence there are distinctive changes to the dimensions of the face and head. The face becomes longer with a higher and wider forehead, a longer and more prominent nose and a larger jaw. As the teenager assumes adult proportions the head becomes relatively smaller to the body than in childhood when the head is large in proportion to the body size.[1] The changes in facial proportions are more marked in boys.[2]

NERVOUS SYSTEM

By adolescence, the nervous system is mature and the teenager is able to demonstrate behaviour and performance which is essentially adult.

The assessment of the nervous system has been described in Chapter 2, where the main activities of physical assessment are given and in Chapter 3, where assessment of the cranial nerves is included.

Reflexes

In adolescence, the assessment of reflexes is facilitated by the ability of the teenager to understand the purpose of the assessment and to cooperate with the various test procedures. Adolescents are more able to accept the use of the reflex hammer to elicit the tendon reflexes. Even so, some adolescents may be anxious about reflex testing and will require clear explanation about the purpose of the tests and the sensations they are likely to experience. The superficial reflexes, i.e., the abdominal, cremasteric, anal and plantar reflexes, are not tested unless there is a requirement for this level of assessment. The testing of the biceps, triceps, brachioradialis, patellar and Achilles reflexes, the five tendon reflexes which are usually tested, is described in Chapter 2. Positive results for deep tendon reflexes indicate that the reflex arc is intact and that the sensory nerve endings in tendons, nerve fibres, motor neurones, muscles and the spinal cord are present.[4]

Gross motor skills

With improvements in coordination and muscle control the adolescent's gross motor skills reach adult level. Many adolescents work hard at refining their gross motor skills and spend long hours in practice and training. Team games and individual activities such as sport, martial arts, dancing and running are popular. There are gender differences in physical abilities related to the greater growth and strength of muscles in males. Boys are more able to perform activities such as lifting and running with greater physical ability. Even so, both girls and boys are able to improve physical performance with regular exercise and activity.

Fine motor skills

Maturation of the nervous system enables the adolescent to carry out fine motor tasks with accuracy and dexterity. The control, coordination and precision of movements are well developed, especially in late adolescence, allowing the adolescent to undertake craftwork and artistic activities such as musicianship, model building, textiles craft and artwork with success.[2] Handwriting reaches an adult level of refinement.[2] Teenagers are often interested in technology and the working parts of equipment and become adept in carrying out fine adjustments and repairs or even creating new devices.

Alertness and responsiveness

Normally, adolescents are alert, aware of themselves and their surroundings and respond in a way which is relevant to the immediate context. Adolescents, however, may have periods of daydreaming where their attention is diverted from the immediate environment. Daydreaming is considered a useful activity provided it does not lead to over-absorption in fantasy or withdrawal from the activities of everyday life.[2]

While less sleep is needed in adolescence than in late childhood, the adolescent still needs about eight hours' sleep. During periods of intense physical, cognitive and emotional output, longer periods of sleep may be needed.

The conscious state of the adolescent is assessed, in the first instance, by observing levels of alertness, responsiveness and activity. The teenager can be asked about time and place in order to establish her orientation. Altered levels of consciousness are manifest by drowsiness, unclear speech, confusion or incoordination. Substance use, likely in adolescence, needs to be considered when alterations to consciousness are found. When there is reason to suspect an alteration to consciousness, further assessment is made using the Glasgow Coma Scale (Appendix B).

New activities which require the aquisition of skills may be taken up.

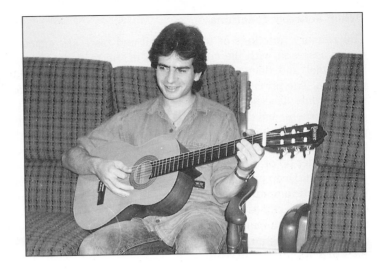

Eyes and vision

The eyeball lengthens during periods of growth and by adolescence has gained adult dimensions. The visual abilities to fix and focus are well established by adolescence and the process of fusion whereby fixation and focusing are combined to produce mature visual function is completed.[2]

The eyes will look bright, moist and clear. The structures of the external eyes are symmetric and the pupils will react to bright light by constricting briskly. The eyelids and lashes are clean and move freely. Teenagers who keep late hours and are tired may show signs of sleep deprivation such as reddened eyes and drooping eyelids.

It may be necessary to assess visual acuity, because of the incidence of refractive errors in adolescence. It is estimated that the incidence of binocular myopia increases from 1% at 6 years to 20% at 16 years.[7] Testing for visual acuity is described in **Chapter 3**. Normal visual acuity of 6/6 is anticipated in adolescence. It is recommended that secondary students be given information about colour vision.[8]

Ears and hearing

The external ear increases in size in keeping with the rapid growth of the teenager. Cerumen is produced and may be visible at the meatus of the auditory canal. Many teenagers choose to have the lobes of the ears pierced. Healthy pierced sites will be dry and clean. Examination of the middle ear can be carried out with an otoscope with the appropriately sized speculum. The pinna is pulled back and upwards in order to straighten the canal and permit visualisation of the structures. The procedure is described in **Chapter 3**.

While hearing is well established in childhood, the process by which hearing matures continues into adolescence.[5] The improved hearing of the teenager is also related to the ability to concentrate attention and to discriminate between different sounds.[2] On the other hand, there is a risk of hearing loss among adolescents because of their exposure to loud sounds and music, especially with the use of earphones. It is likely that, as hearing loss occurs, the volume of sound will be increased causing further damage to hearing.[3] Testing with pure tone audiometry may be indicated in those teenagers with suspected hearing loss.

Other sensory functions

The sensory functions of touch, smell and taste are intact in adolescence and can be easily assessed with the collaboration of the teenager. Touch can be assessed through superficial and deep sensations. Superficial sensations include pain, temperature and pressure. The procedures for assessment are described in **Chapter 3**. Deep sensation is usually only assessed when there are clinical signs of dysfunction, such as decreased consciousness, and can include assessment for vibration perception, position sense, deeper pain and discrimination. Vibratory perception is assessed with a tuning fork placed over prominences such as the knees or elbows. Position sense is assessed by moving the distal toe or finger up or down and asking the adolescent, with closed eyes, to state the position of the digit. Deep pain can be assessed by applying strong pressure to limb muscles while discrimination testing includes the identification of objects placed in the hand, numbers drawn on the skin and the quality and location of touch.[1,2,4] Smell and taste can be assessed by introducing substances to be smelt and tasted or through the teenager's report.

Balance and coordination

Adolescents demonstrate good balance and coordination, though coordination is not fully refined until the mid-teens.[4] Balance and coordination are assessed through a series of activities which include heel-to-toe walking and standing unsupported, feet together and with the eyes open and closed. Coordination testing activities include finger-to-nose, fingers-to-thumb, heel-to-shin movements carried out at increasing speed (**see Chapter 3**) and rapid alternate turning of the hands from supine to prone.[2]

Cranial nerves

The cranial nerves have motor, sensory and mixed nerve functions which are described, together with assessment procedures, in **Chapter 3**.

Body temperature

Body temperature continues to decline in adolescence, though at about 12 years normothermic measurements in girls are relatively stable. In boys, body temperature continues to fall for several more years.[1] In practice, a temperature reading in the range between 36°C and 37.1°C is considered normal. Readings are usually taken with a mercury or electronic thermometer. The axillary route is favoured, though the oral route can usually be safely used if it is preferred. A tympanic membrane sensor if available is preferred because it is less intrusive and gives a better result.

CIRCULATORY SYSTEM

Though the heart and lungs grow more slowly than other body systems in adolescence,[4] the size and functional ability of the heart continues to increase during early and mid adolescence until adult dimensions are reached. It has been estimated that the heart nearly doubles in weight during puberty.[9] Systolic blood pressure and blood volume are also increased. Boys have a higher blood volume than girls, a difference thought to be related to the increased muscle development in boys.[1] The larger, stronger heart contracts at a slower rate. There is an increase in the number of red blood cells and the level of haemoglobin though the increase is greater in boys because of the influence of testosterone. In girls, lower red blood cell and haemoglobin levels are influenced by the onset of menstruation.[2]

Pulses

Throughout adolescence the pulse rate slows, tending to be slightly slower in boys.[2] The average resting pulse in early adolescence is about 85 beats per minute and later in adolescence falls to about 80 beats per minute. The range is between 60 and 110 beats per minute. Very fit adolescents will have pulse rates lower than the average.

The pulse is usually taken at the radial point in adolescence and is regular, soft and moderately strong on palpation. Assessment of other pulses may be carried out by palpating the carotid, femoral, brachial, popliteal and dorsalis pedis pulses. Steady and moderately firm pressure is maintained over the pulse point and the rate, rhythm and volume are assessed over one minute. Teenagers can usually remain still while their pulse is palpated, permitting an uninterrupted count. The apical pulse may be auscultated at the 5th left intercostal space at the midclavicular line, though the modesty of the teenager may make this route the least preferred. Teenagers will be eager to know if their pulse is normal and the result of the rate count. They may be aware of rate norms for their age. The rate may be falsely elevated in teenagers who are anxious. Sometimes this response occurs simply because the teenager is disconcerted at having the pulse taken. Friendly conversation will relax and distract the teenager and help establish the rate at its true level.

Blood pressure

Blood pressure increases during adolescence and by late adolescence has reached adult levels. Boys have a slightly higher systolic pressure than girls though there is no significant gender difference for the diastolic pressure.[2] The average systolic blood pressure for boys and girls at 12 years is 107 mmHg and the average diastolic blood pressure is between 64 and 66 mmHg. At 15 years the average systolic blood pressure in boys has increased to 114 mmHg and the average diastolic blood pressure is 65 mmHg while in girls the average systolic blood pressure is 111 mmHg and the average diastolic blood pressure is 67 mmHg. Average readings for systolic blood pressure at 18 years are 121 mmHg in boys and 112 mmHg in girls and for diastolic blood pressure are 70 mmHg in boys and 66 mmHg in girls.[1]

The measurement of blood pressure in adolescence is, for the most part, carried out using the auscultation method and the same-sized equipment as for adults. The cuff should cover about two-thirds of the upper arm and the same-sized cuff should be used for subsequent measurements. From 12 years of age the diastolic blood pressure is recorded at the 5th Korotkoff sound, the point where sound is no longer heard.[1] Adolescents, particularly those who are unfamiliar with the blood pressure measurement procedure, may be apprehensive about the measurement of their blood pressure and as a result the measurement may be artificially elevated. Clear explanations and friendly talk can help the teenager relax and allow an accurate measurement to be taken.

Colour

The colour of the skin and mucosa is assessed in order to make an early estimation of oxygen uptake and circulatory function. Skin colour in adolescence is related to hereditary factors, the condition of the skin and nutritional status as well as haemodynamic function. Generally, however, adolescents with dark skins will have pink palms of the hands and soles of the feet and the oral mucosa will be deep pink. Adolescents with lighter skins will have soft pink tones on the face. Blushing across the face and the neck is likely to occur and is related to an unstable vasomotor response and the increased self-consciousness of adolescents.

Heart sounds

Heart sounds are auscultated to assess for quality, rate, intensity and rhythm and to identify any variation from normal sounds. Details of the procedure are given in **Chapter 3**.

Heart sounds are distinct and easy to locate and hear. Murmurs may be heard as the heart and chest is auscultated. The most common innocent murmurs in adolescence are a vibratory murmur which is heard at the left sternal border and an ejection murmur heard in the left second intercostal space.[10] Pregnant teenagers may also exhibit an exaggerated ejection murmur, which is related to the increase in blood volume during pregnancy.[11]

GASTROINTESTINAL SYSTEM

The gastrointestinal system functions well in adolescence though the growth spurt brings with it certain effects. The intestine undergoes a period of accelerated growth during the adolescent growth spurt. The capacity of the stomach reaches approximately 1500 mL at 16 years and is approximately 2000 mL by the end of adolescence.[1] In addition, there is an increase in free hydrochloric acid, more so in boys. These increases, in stomach and intestinal size and digestive function, are related to the rise in food consumption by teenagers in this period.

Mouth and teeth

The healthy mouth of the teenager is moist and the tongue pink and uncoated. The mucosa and lips are deep pink. Teenagers who spend periods of time outdoors may have dry skin on the lips.

With the appearance of the 2nd permanent molars between 11 and 13 years, the adolescent has a full complement of teeth except, for the 3rd permanent molars. These final molars or wisdom teeth do not erupt until sometime between 18 and 25 years or even later. In keeping with the sex-related pattern of growth in adolescence, the permanent teeth appear earlier in girls than in boys.[1] Dental caries are more likely to develop between 14 and 17 years. The changes associated with maturation are thought to be related to this increase.[2]

Abdomen

The abdomen is symmetric in form and usually concave when the teenager is supine. The calibre of the abdominal muscle layer ranges from soft to hard and is related to physical fitness and the type and amount of exercise undertaken by the teenager. Pubic hair may be present across the pubis, upper thigh and lower abdomen, depending on the stage of pubertal development. Bowel sounds are present. By late adolescence the abdomen has taken on an adult shape, especially noticeable in girls.[1]

Ingestion and digestion

The substantial increase in stomach capacity permits the teenager to consume more food at a time of rapid growth and energy demand. Ingestion is efficient with chewing facilitated by the large permanent molars. Digestion is aided by increased amounts of gastric secretion and both digestion and absorption are fully mature.

Elimination

By adolescence, faecal elimination has, for the most part, taken on a regular daily pattern for the number of stools and the time when elimination takes place. Some adolescents may experience constipation, which is usually related to diet and exercise. High-fat snacks and fast foods may lessen the intake of a more balanced diet. As part of the teenager's move to independence the foods promoted as healthy or those offered by the family may be given a secondary place in the diet. Girls may reduce their food intake and their active involvement in sport in a response to social pressures related to body image and sex role.

RESPIRATORY SYSTEM

The respiratory structures undergo growth as part of the overall growth in adolesence. The larger structures such as the bronchial tree and lungs enlarge with the expansion of the trunk and there is also an increase in the size of the smaller structures such as the alveoli. There are associated increases in lung capacity and ventilation efficiency. As a result of improved ventilatory function the respiratory rate decreases to between 15 to 20 breaths per minute.[2] Tidal volumes and the vital capacity increase with the vital capacity for boys averaging about 6% more than for girls.[2] Boys have a greater respiratory capacity than girls because of their larger lungs, which develop as a result of larger chest and shoulder dimensions.[1]

Chest

There are two marked developments in the chest during adolescence which need to be considered when assessing the chest. The growth spurt results in a chest with adult dimensions such as a long trunk and a broader, deeper chest. These changes in chest size occur in a characteristic sequence. Increases in the breadth of the chest take place a few months after the lengthening of the extremities. There is an increase in the width of the shoulders after another few months and then the trunk lengthens and the chest increases in the depth.[1]

Breast development in girls is the second important development to be considered in assessment of the chest during adolescence. Following the appearance of breast buds in late childhood, further enlargement of the breasts and the areolae takes place. This enlargement occurs in a distinctive pattern of development which has been described in 5 stages. The 1st stage is the prepubertal change where elevation of the papilla (nipple) occurs. The breast buds appear at the 2nd stage. The area around the papilla becomes elevated and the areolar diameter increases. In the 3rd stage the breast and areola enlarge, but the papilla does not yet protrude. By the 4th stage the papilla and the areola project and the breast has further enlarged. The adult configuration, where the papilla protrudes and the areola flattens to follow the general breast contour, is the 5th and final stage. The breasts in this stage have enlarged to their mature size.[1] There is great variation in the size of the breasts in a given population of adolescent girls. In individuals breasts will be of similar shape and appearance though it is not uncommon for one breast to be slightly larger than the other.

The 1st and 2nd stages of breast development occur in about 40 per cent of boys.[2] This is a transient gynaecomastia and usually lasts less than a year.[1] Late in adolescence many boys will have hair growth on the chest. There is variation in the amount, colour and texture of body hair according to hereditary influences.[1]

Breath sounds

Breath sounds are clear without rales (rattling sounds), rhonchi (snoring-like sounds) or wheezes and are auscultated with the diaphragm of the stethoscope. The sound of air moving in and out of the airways has distinctive qualities which differ according to the area of auscultation. Breath sounds, their qualities and sites of auscultation are described in **Chapter 2**. The teenager will usually assist in the assessment of breath sounds by inspiring deeply and vocalising when requested.

Respirations

The respiratory rate slows throughout adolescence as the thoracic cavity and structures expand until adult values are reached. Average respiratory rates over 1 minute, combined for both sexes, are 18 breaths at 14 years, 17 breaths at 16 years and 16 to 18 breaths at 18 years.[1]

Assessment of respirations for rate, rhythm, depth and quality is carried out by observing the chest movements. The rate may increase in the sensitive and aware teenager who realises that the chest is being observed. Assessment is most accurate when the teenager's attention is diverted. Many nurses observe the chest movements while continuing to palpate the pulse, creating the impression that assessment of the pulse is continuing. The rate is counted for a minute. Respirations are normally regular, quiet and without effort.

URINARY SYSTEM

As the structures of the urinary system reach adult dimensions the capacity of the urinary bladder to hold urine is further increased. The daily urinary output during adolescence is between 700 and 1400 mL and from thereon the output for males is between 800 and 1800 mL and for females between 600 and 1600 mL.[1]

Adolescents will usually participate in a helpful way with the collection of urine for analysis. Provided privacy is assured the teenager will void into a container. If the specimen is for laboratory testing and required to be uncontaminated, the teenager will need to be instructed about the steps in midstream urine collection. The urethral meatus and surrounding area is washed with soap and water, rinsed well and dried carefully. After the first few seconds of the urinary flow a sterile container is moved into the urinary stream in order to collect the desired amount of urine. On some occasions the teenager may prefer the nurse or parent to assist her in collecting a midstream urine specimen. Uncontaminated urine specimens are often required because there is an increased incidence of urinary tract infection in adolescence, particularly in girls and those who are are sexually active.[1]

The characteristics of urine are similar to those of the adult and are described in **Chapter 2**. If blood is detected in the urine of the adolescent girl the nurse needs to establish whether menstruation could be the source.

REPRODUCTIVE SYSTEM

Pubertal changes

Puberty refers to the attainment of sexual maturity. The period in which puberty occurs is characterised by dramatic physical growth and distinctive development. The reproductive system undergoes a series of changes which lead to sexual and reproductive maturation. These changes occur in a sequence over several years and have been plotted according to identifiable stages in breast, genital and pubic hair development. There are marked differences between girls and boys and between individuals in the timing of the onset of puberty and the length of the pubertal process. In girls, puberty begins about 18 months to 2 years earlier than in boys. The duration of puberty ranges from 2.5 to 4 years.[12]

The onset of puberty in girls occurs between 8 and 14 years and usually takes 3 years to complete.[1] The first change of puberty is an increase in the size of the ovaries, while the first visible sign of puberty is breast enlargement. There is accelerated growth of the uterus and vagina about the same time and the first appearance of pubic hair occurs soon afterwards.[12] Menarche occurs approximately 2.5 years after the onset of puberty.[1] The average age for menarche is estimated at 12.7 years.[7]

The first sign of puberty in boys is testicular growth, which begins between 9.5 and 16 years. There is enlargement of the scrotum with changes to the scrotal skin.[1] The scrotum in adolescence is wider at the distal portion than the proximal portion.[4] The skin assumes a darker colour, becomes coarser and more wrinkled. These changes in the testes and scrotum are followed by lengthening of the penis. Ejaculation usually occurs within a year of the first signs of penile growth.[12] Further growth of the penis with development of the glans follows.[13] In the final stage of growth, there is further darkening of the skin of the scrotum and the penis increases in length and width to reach adult dimensions.[1,2]

Pubic hair growth is also described in stages. The 1st stage is the prepubertal stage where no pubic hair is seen. In girls, pubic hair usually first appears about 6 months after the breast bud stage, though in about one-third of girls, pubic hair precedes breast buds.[14] This pubic hair is fine, long and straight and appears mainly on the sides of the labia. In the 3rd stage the hair is darker, thicker and curled and is spread sparsely over the pubis in the inverted triangle pattern of the female. The hair continues to grow and covers the pubic area more densely in the 4th stage. By the 5th stage, pubic hair is dense, curled and has spread to the inner thighs and perianal area.[1,2] Pubic hair growth and distribution in boys first appears as fine, straight, downy hair at the base of the penis. The pubic hair becomes darker, thicker and curled in the 3rd stage and begins to extend beyond the base of the penis over the whole pubis. By the 4th stage hair fully covers the pubic area and at the 5th stage has extended to the thighs and upwards along the linea alba in the characteristic diamond-shaped distribution of pubic hair in males.[1]

Axillary hair and in boys, facial hair, does not appear until about 2 years after the 1st signs of pubic hair.[12]

External genitalia

Assessment of the genitalia is usually only carried out when there is some concern about development or healthy function. An initial assessment will include external inspection and examination. Clear explanations about the purpose and steps in the assessment are essential.

The normal external genital structures are described in **Chapter 3**. Girls and boys during adolescence will exhibit some degree of pubic hair growth. Assessment in girls will need to take into account the onset of menstruation and the menstrual history.

The female genitalia is inspected for labial symmetry, moist inner surfaces of the labia, the position of the urethral meatus and the size and shape of the vaginal opening. The male genitalia will be assessed for evidence of scrotal and penile growth, the presence of testes in the scrotum, the easy retraction of the foreskin with dry, clear skin at the base of the glans and the position of the urethral meatus.

INTEGUMENTARY SYSTEM

The skin of the adolescent is subjected to a number of changes during puberty. Under the influence of oestrogen the skin in girls becomes soft and smooth, but with a thicker texture, while androgens cause the skin to become slightly darker and thicker in both girls and boys.[1] This effect of androgens is more pronounced in boys. In addition, there are increases in sweat and sebaceous gland activity.[2]

There are 2 types of sweat glands and both become fully functional during puberty. The eccrine sweat glands are located throughout the skin and produce sweat in response to heat and emotion. The apocrine glands are larger than the eccrine glands and are found in areas of hair growth such as the axilla and genital area. These glands produce a thick secretion in response to emotion.[1]

The sebaceous glands, especially those at the genital area, the face, shoulders and upper back, are highly active during adolescence.[1] Teenagers may develop acne because of the increased secretion of sebum and plugging of the sebaceous follicles. It has been estimated that about 90% of adolescents have acne of different degrees of severity.[3]

Health Management

Anne Adams

Movement and activity

Many adolescents are active and spend time participating in sports and group activities. These activities may be modified over time so that an enthusiastic involvement in sport and exercise in early and middle adolescence may give way to a spectator role by late adolescence. In general, however, the early teenager is eager to participate in sports and will practise determinedly to reach the required standard of fitness or skill. In middle adolescence there is often a strong competitive drive for team sports or individual excellence. This, in turn, may be replaced towards the end of the adolescent period by a more limited involvement in team activities. These activities are often gender differentiated with boys being more likely to take part in energetic outdoor activities than girls. Teenagers often enjoy dancing and participate with great energy. Dancing, while having social and emotional functions, is a good source of physical exercise.

The benefits of exercise should be promoted to adolescents. Girls, in particular, need encouragement and recognition for their participation in sport and physical activity. Growth and development are enhanced through exercise. For example, muscles will increase in size and weight with exercise once puberty has begun.[12] Regular exercise in adolescence is held to enhance learning and can also establish a life-long pattern of healthy physical activity.[2]

Stimulation and learning

The adolescent is exposed to a varied, challenging and exciting world which provides numerous stimuli for intellectual and emotional growth. Rather than having to be provided with stimulatory experiences, adolescents are more likely to need guidelines, limits and support as they explore their environment and learn to manage their daily lives.

Most adolescents are responsive and curious and, as they move towards independence, keen to make choices about their learning and activities. When teenagers are given opportunities to make their own decisions they are provided with practice for the future role of adult. School, interest groups and peers are important agencies of learning and social experience.

Learning in adolescence is facilitated by the involvement of others and the personal experience of achievement. The interest and encouragement of the family and an experience of schooling which emphasises self-development as well as performance can increase learning outcomes, confidence and self esteem.

The adolescent may continue with interests and activities which began in childhood, such as crafts, sport, music, pets and community group membership. As well, new activities which demand mastery and skill acquisition may begin. Because they are becoming more independent, teenagers want to try new and different experiences, but may still need help in maintaining a balance between family life, school, friendships and community interests.

Sleep

At times teenagers may appear tired and lethargic. They may be unwilling to involve themselves in family activities or with chores and occupy themselves in passive activities such as watching television or videos and listening to music. On other occasions, the teenager may become so absorbed in physical, social or study activities that the amount of rest and sleep is seriously reduced. A balanced mix of sufficient sleep and exercise is necessary for healthy physical and emotional development. While the overall amount of sleep may be decreased in adolescence, the teenager usually needs approximately 8 hours' sleep each night. Teenagers may need to be encouraged to plan their activities so they have sufficient sleep and exercise in proportion to their study and sedentary activities. Some families manage the sleep needs of the teenager by setting requirements for sleep and rest during the week and agreeing to a more flexible arrangement at weekends and holidays.

Nutrition

The quality of the diet is an important issue in adolescence, a time of rapid growth and development with high energy demands. It is, however, not possible to consider nutritional needs without reference to the social context of the adolescent. As the adolescent becomes more self-directed and interacts with the environment beyond the family home, he is subjected to a number of influences which can shape his dietary behaviour. The impact of marketing, designed to convince the teenager that he should consume particular food products, cannot be underestimated. Group influences and fads can be strong and may override healthy patterns of eating. In addition, the teenager usually has available money and can exercise choice about how it will be spent.

While many adolescents are interested in health and fitness and recognise the association between good nutrition and a healthy body, some particular stresses of adolescence can interfere with the intake of a healthy diet. The risk-taking behaviour of adolescents, which is a manifestation of the need to explore and challenge in order to become independent, can result in a disregard for healthy nutrition. Another important issue for the adolescent is the development of a body image which is in keeping with cultural values. An unsatisfactory body image can induce the teenager to adopt eating behaviours which are designed to improve physical attractiveness, but which may result in an inadequate level of nutrition and may even threaten overall health and well-being.

By adolescence, the gastrointestinal function is mature and functions efficiently and most teenagers enjoy a varied diet and will accept a range of foods. Health teaching for the adolescent about nutrition is based on nutritional recommendations as set out in the Healthy Diet Pyramid (**Chapter 2**). The Dietary Guidelines for Australians, which were drawn up with the aim of reducing morbidity and mortality in the population and to improve the health of Australians, can serve as guidelines for teenagers as well as for adults. The guidelines recommend that a nutritious diet be chosen from a variety of foods, weight be controlled, too much fat and sugar are to be avoided, more wholegrain breads, cereals, vegetables and fruits are to be eaten, alcohol intake is to be limited and that less salt is used.[15] Teaching adolescents about nutrition needs to be an interactive undertaking, where teenagers' opinions, ideas and questions are received in an accepting way and their ability for self-care reinforced.

The intake of food is regulated by the energy demand and will be greatly increased during the growth spurt. The appetite increases, especially in boys. It has been estimated that nutritional requirements are doubled in the 18 to 24 months of the growth spurt.[3] Energy requirements are also governed by the activity level of the teenager. Active teenagers will need a greater intake of protein and energy producing foods while those who are inactive may be prone to obesity. Calcium, iron and zinc are essential for optimum growth and are the minerals most likely to be inadequate in the adolescent's diet. The need for calcium, which contributes to skeletal growth, is increased by 50% in adolescence.[3] Australian recommendations for the daily intake of calcium for girls and boys between 12 and 15 years are 1000 mg for girls and 1200 mg for boys. Between 16 and 18 years, 800 mg is recommended for girls and 1000 mg for boys.[15] Milk and milk products should feature in the adolescent diet because of the high calcium content in these foods. Two cups of milk and 30 g of cheese contain 800 mg of calcium. Reduced-fat dairy products are good sources of calcium and contain as much calcium as full cream products.[15] Red meat, green vegetables, cereals, dried beans and fruits, eggs and seafood are good sources of iron and zinc.[1]

As well as learning about nutrition, the adolescent will benefit from developing skills in selecting and preparing food. Many teenagers find cooking an interesting activity while the attainment of food preparation skills is another step towards the self-sufficiency of adulthood.

Elimination

Having achieved maturity of gastrointestinal and urinary functions, elimination is not usually an issue in adolescence. Most teenagers have a natural and individual routine with a bowel motion or two every day or every other day. Constipation may result from a diet low in fibre or from inadequate exercise. Some teenagers experience bowel changes with diarrhoea-like motions or constipation at times of stress and emotion. When the tension is reduced the bowel function returns to its usual pattern.

Urinary elimination assumes an adult pattern where voiding is required up to 4 to 6 times in 24 hours. The urinary stream is strong and urine is passed without discomfort. Girls are reminded about the importance is wiping with toilet paper from front to back in order to prevent contamination and subsequent infection of the urinary tract.

Health teaching in relation to elimination includes teaching about the place of a high-fibre diet in the production of normal, soft and frequent stools. Teenagers should be encouraged not to delay their visits to the toilet. Holding-on behaviours may predispose to constipation and urinary tract infection. The importance of an adequate fluid intake should be emphasised. Fluids need to be increased in hot weather and when the teenager is physically active.

Contraception

Approaches by adolescents to contraception can range from denial, where the likelihood of pregnancy resulting from sexual intercourse is denied, to an informed decision about the need to prevent an unwanted pregnancy. There may be differences between girls and boys in the acceptance of responsibility for the outcomes of sexual activity. The use of contraception by adolescents is influenced by the amount and quality of knowledge about sexual behaviour and contraception, accessibility to information and services, financial resources, religious and family beliefs and, for girls in particular, a concern that the use of contraception is premeditated and commits them to sexual activity when they may have uncertainties about their wish to participate.

While not all adolescents are sexually active, it is clear that a high proportion of adolescents engage in sexual behaviour which includes sexual intercourse[1,16] and that more younger adolescents are engaging in sexual intercourse.[7] Adolescents have been found to be unreliable users of contraception and may have been sexually active for some time before seeking advice about contraception.[1,16]

Oral contraception is the preferred method for adolescents.[16] It is a safe and effective method and is the choice of most teenagers, though oral contraceptives are not advised until ovulation and the menstrual cycle are established.[1] It is recommended that there be good follow-up and monitoring once oral contraceptives are prescribed. There is a high dropout rate in the first 2 months.[16] Oral contraception places the responsibility for prevention of pregnancy on the girl. The requirement for consultations and health screening and the cost of oral contraceptives are seen as deterrents by some adolescents to the use of this method.

The use of condoms has been promoted in recent years as protection against sexually transmitted diseases as well as for contraceptive purposes. Condoms are readily available, easy to use but unless used correctly, do not have a good record for effectiveness. Condoms can be carried by girls and boys, but the boy has to take responsibility for using this method of contraception and using it correctly.

The provision of information about sexuality and contraception is essential in adolescence. While teenagers are generally exposed to information about sexuality and reproduction, they may not be fully informed. Teaching should include the topics of menstruation and the menstrual cycle, sexual activity and conception and types of contraception. Many teenagers choose community services where information, health care and contraceptives are available. Nurses who are engaged in this area of practice are aware of how highly the teenager values confidentiality, privacy and the opportunity to relate to an empathic informant.

Clothing and protection

Clothing in adolescence has more social and personal significance than in childhood, when clothing is primarily functional. Teenagers readily adopt codes of dressing which are linked to the determination of group, sex and personal identities. The adolescent will usually exhibit a strong preference for particular styles of clothing. Conflict between adolescents and their parents and other authority figures can develop over the choice of clothing.

The need for skin protection remains important in adolescence and teenagers need to be reminded of skin cancer prevention. Skin which is exposed to sunlight should be protected with clothing. While a number of teenagers may disregard advice about skin covering, many are adopting protective habits such as adding a T-shirt when swimming and wearing a hat in sunlight.

The choice of footwear is also subject to popular preferences. On the whole, recent trends in shoe design for the young are for comfortable and non-constricting shoes which are not detrimental to foot development. Foot size increases rapidly during the growth spurt and necessitates frequent purchases of larger-sized footwear. Protective clothing for outdoor activities, sports and work may be required. Adolescents who are frequently unable to appreciate the risks or long-term effects of environmental hazards need to be informed about possible risks and the protection certain clothing can afford. Examples of activites where teenagers may need to wear protective clothing include water sports, team games and work environments where chemicals are in use.

Hygiene

The adolescent, in taking responsibility for self-care, will manage his own hygiene. Daily showering is common practice in Australia and many teenagers will shower or bath more than once a day in hot conditions or if they have been very active. The increase in sebaceous and sweat gland activity makes showering and bathing a necessity. Because of the increased production of body oil, teenagers find they need to wash their hair more frequently. Deodorants are favoured and serve to resassure teenagers about body odour. Adolescents are highly aware of their physical presentation and are motivated to be accepted by peers and others and be as attractive as possible. Adolescent girls may become very interested in cosmetics, hair styles and body care. Boys begin to shave and may also take an increased interest in their physical appearance and grooming.

The appearance of acne causes considerable concern in the adolescent. The affected areas should be kept clean with regular washing. Cleansing with soap and water or a mild cleanser once or twice a day is recommended.[1,13] Oily creams are discouraged and girls are advised to use only those cosmetics which have a light base or are especially formulated for adolescent use. Some teenagers find that certain foods such as chocolate will provoke an outbreak of spots. If acne is troublesome, medical treatment may be necessary.

With the onset of menstruation, the adolescent girl has to manage her menstrual flow and maintain hygiene. There are 2 main types of absorbent products which are used during menstruation. Tampons are inserted into the vagina and sanitary pads are worn externally. A wide range of products for internal or external use is available and adolescents will choose according to personal preference and the advice of family, peers or health care providers. Information about the safe handling of tampons should be provided. Girls are taught to wash hands before handling a tampon, to minimise handling of the tampon and how to insert a tampon. Tampons should be changed frequently and some authorities recommend that pads are worn overnight[2] to minimise the risk for toxic shock syndrome. Extra cleansing of the vulva is necessary during menstruation and can be achieved with additional bathing, showering or washing of the area. It can also be suggested to the teenage girl that she be prepared for unexpected bleeding, especially in the first months after menstruation begins, when a regular cycle may not yet be established.

While dental care and teeth cleaning routines are usually established by adolescence, teenagers may need encouragement to maintain regular dental checks. A number of adolescents will require orthdontic treatment which may be physically uncomfortable and a source of embarrassment. Teeth should be cleaned after meals and before bed. Flossing should be included in the care of the teeth.

The adolescent is usually able to maintain her own hygiene, though in early adolescence, encouragement and reinforcement may be needed from time to time. Health teaching can refer to the desirable results of body care and health routines. Adolescents are keenly interested in looking and feeling attractive. Self-esteem and body image are strengthened when the adolescent feels positive about her appearance.

Immunisation

There are 2 further routine vaccinations during adolescence. The measles, mumps and rubella (MMR) vaccine is given between 10 and 16 years, preferably in the last primary school year or the first year at high school. This vaccination is given in a single dose by intramuscular or deep subcutaneous injection and is offered in clinics at schools or community centres. Vaccination is postponed if the adolescent has a febrile illness and is given on recovery. MMR vaccine must not be given to a girl who is pregnant or thinks she might be pregnant. Girls are advised that they should not become pregnant for 2 months after vaccination.[17] The aim of rubella vaccination is to increase immunity levels for rubella in the whole community.

At 15 years or before leaving school, reinforcing doses of the adult diphtheria and tetanus vaccine (ADT) and Sabin vaccine for poliomyelitis are given. The adolescent is advised to have a booster dose of tetanus vaccine or ADT in 10 years in order to maintain immunity (Appendix C).[17]

Safety

Safety is an important issue during adolesence. There is a substantial potential for harm in active and independent teenagers who have only a short experience in managing themselves in the community. In addition, adolescents tend to believe that they are immune to the consequences of their behaviour, even high-risk activity.

While adolescence is generally a healthy period with early adolescents having the lowest mortality and hospital admission rates of any group[7] there is a trend for the incidence of motor vehicle accidents to increase throughout adolescence. Males between 15 and 19 years have the highest incidence of motor vehicle and other accidents with male: female mortality rates 3:1.[18] The motor vehicle accident rate is related to the teenager being able to drive a car or ride a motorcycle. Teenagers, especially boys, are prone to risk-taking behaviours. As drivers and riders they are particularly vulnerable to injury through errors of judgement and hazardous behaviours. Alcohol use can be a factor in dangerous driving.

Sports injuries are not uncommon in adolescence and can involve the head, spine and limbs. Teenagers need to be instructed about the use of safe equipment and practices and they should be restrained from recommencing sport too soon after an injury.[5]

The use of alcohol and drugs in adolescence can seriously threaten the well-being of the teenager. It has been proposed that there are three patterns of drug use in adolescence. Experimentation with chemical substances such as over-the-counter drugs, sedatives, narcotics, stimulants and alcohol, is not uncommon in the adolescent years. Many teenagers experiment as part of their exploration of the adult world, using chemicals once or intermittently. Others use chemical substances more often, even regularly. A smaller group becomes addicted and is compulsive in the use of drugs.[5] This group is at risk for breaking the law and having to endure the consequences. Information about the use and misuse of chemical substances is essential in health education programs.

Smoking has become a health issue among Australian adolescents. A large proportion have smoked by 17 years and there is a trend for younger adolescents to smoke. Girls are more likely to start smoking.[18]

Adolescent girls are at risk for sexual assault, particularly from middle to late adolescence. A high proportion of assaults are perpetrated by a person known to the victim. Other attacks are carried out by a stranger and seem to be related to the vulnerablility of the adolescent girl. Incest, particularly between fathers or father-figures and girls, has been recognised as a significant form of sexual abuse in adolescence.[1] Adolescent boys are also at risk for sexual assault, although the incidence is not as great.

Protective strategies for adolescents include the provision of information, interactive learning experiences and the maintenance of a secure and supportive family environment.

Health education programs can supply information which aims to convince teenagers about the benefits of safe and healthy behaviours. Information about chemical substances, smoking, the effects of sunlight, breast and testicular examination, road and driving safety, sports injuries, safe sexual practices and the risks of sexual assault is relevant and necessary in order to give adolescents a sound base from which to make decisions. Interactive learning in adolescence is an effective form of education. Group experiences allow teenagers not only to gain information, but to process and analyse it within a safe context. Because so many of the threats to safety in adolescence are related to the social and emotional development of adolescents, an understanding and supporting family is probably the most important factor in helping to keep teenagers safe and able to progress through adolescence without undue physical or emotional trauma. Parents of adolescents are often uncertain and anxious about the management of their teenager, particularly when there is a continuing need for parental care while at the same time the teenager has a strong need to become independent. Parent programs can give parents the knowledge, skills and confidence which can assist them in their task and, in turn, facilitate the adolescent's safe progression though adolescence.

Psychological Growth and Development

Sue Nagy

Adolescence marks the transition from childhood to maturity. It can be roughly divided into 3 stages: early adolescence from puberty to about 14 years of age; mid-adolescence from approximately 15 to 17 years of age, and late adolescence from 18 years of age to the beginning of adulthood. Puberty is usually regarded as the beginning of adolescence, but there is no agreement about the end of adolescence and the beginning of adulthood. Airline companies, for example, define adulthood as commencing at 12 years of age, for public transport operators it is 14 years, for employment purposes it is 15 years, to be legally able to give consent for sexual intercourse it is 16 years, to leave home without parental permission, or give permission for an invasive medical procedures it is 16 years, but to give permission for one's child to have a medical procedure it is 14 years. Legally, adulthood begins at 18 years. Some argue that the end of adolescence occurs at the end of the teenage years, while others believe it ends when a person has accomplished most of the tasks of adolescence.[19]

Havighurst described certain physical, cognitive and psychological tasks that he believed must be learned in order 'to achieve healthy and satisfactory growth in our society'.[19] His ideas are particularly useful as a guide to the expectations that society has of adolescents. He grouped the tasks of adolescence into 3 categories: the development of mature social relationships, the development of personal independence and the development of a philosophy of life.

The development of mature social relationships

1. Achieving new and more mature relations with age-mates of both sexes.
2. Achieving a masculine or feminine social role.
3. Preparing for intimate personal relationships and for family life.

The development of personal independence

4. Accepting one's physique and using the body effectively.
5. Achieving emotional independence of parents and other adults.
6. Achieving assurance of economic independence.
7. Selecting and preparing for an adult occupation.
8. Developing the intellectual skills and concepts necessary for civic competence.

The development of a philosophy of life

9. Desiring and achieving socially responsible behaviour.
10. Acquiring a set of values and an ethical system as a guide to behaviour.

COGNITIVE DEVELOPMENT

During early adolescence a qualitative change in thinking ability occurs and marks the beginning of the stage of formal operations.[20] Formal, or abstract, thought involves the ability to manipulate ideas and abstract concepts, to understand not only the 'actual', but also the 'possible' or the 'hypothetical'. It can be described as the ability to 'think about thinking'. Abstract thought develops over the adolescent period, with 12 year olds capable of limited abstract thinking, and 20 year olds able to apply far more formal operational strategies to a range of problems.[21,22]

While the capacity for inductive reasoning (generating general rules from the examination of many individual experiences) develops during the concrete operational period, the formal operational adolescent is developing the ability to reason deductively. This entails the application of general rules to specific instances. The ability to reason deductively is an important cognitive achievement because it enables adolescents to make predictions about the outcome of events that they have not directly experienced. They can imagine new experiences and situations, anticipate problems, and find solutions in advance. They can, for example, understand the danger of speeding on a motor bike, even though they have never had an accident or even known anyone who has had an accident. An adolescent may, nevertheless, continue to speed on his motor bike, not because he cannot understand, but because he believes that 'it won't happen to me'.

During adolescence, children become more aware of the thoughts, feelings and attitudes of those around them. They are now developing a capacity for empathy. They can understand the predicament of another person even though it may be outside their own experience. So while they may only have lived during a period of world peace, they are able to imagine some of the anguish of citizens caught up in a world war.

An interesting example of the development of formal thought comes from the work of Rosenberg, who asked children ranging from 8 to 16 years 'What would a person who knows you best know about you that other people would not know?'.[23] While younger children referred to concrete, external characteristics and observable behaviours (such as hair colour or sporting skill), older children were more likely to focus on more abstract personality characteristics or innermost thoughts and feelings.

Adolescents are capable of scientific reasoning or, as Piaget called it, 'hypothetico-deductive reasoning'. They can formulate hypotheses and test them systematically. They have the cognitive capacity to solve problems in an orderly and systematic way rather than the 'hit and miss' pattern of concrete operational children. Piaget and his colleague, Barbel Inhelder, tested hypothetico-deductive reasoning ability by presenting children with 5 jars of colourless liquid, 2 of which would combine to change the colour of the liquid to yellow.[24] The children were asked to identify the 2 jars. Concrete operational children tried to solve the problem by randomly mixing the contents of the jars. Initially, many adolescents also tried to solve the problem haphazardly, but eventually, most were able systematically to try each combination and thereby solve the problem. The game of '20 questions' can also be used to demonstrate hypothetico-deductive reasoning. Children are shown pictures of fruit, vegetables, machines, people and so on, and are asked to work out which of the pictures the experimenter is thinking about. Only questions may be asked of the experimenter to which only the answers 'yes' or 'no' may be given. Concrete operational children are most likely to try to solve the problem by guessing, by asking, for example, 'Is it the dog?', 'Is it the train?' Formal operational children are more likely to try to narrow down the categories by asking, 'Is it an animal?', 'Is it a machine?', 'Is it used for transport?'

In order to construct personal ideologies and develop an 'ethical system',[19] adolescents tend to spend time thinking about questions regarding the nature of the world and grappling with political, social and religious issues. Their questioning of previously unquestioned values sometimes brings them into conflict with parents and other authority figures. Because they are able to differentiate the actual from the possible, they can, for example, find discrepancies between the actual parent and the possible parent.[25] Similarly, they may find discrepancies between the ideologies and behaviour of their parents and accuse them of hypocrisy.

While adolescents are capable of formal thought, their reasoning is often immature and they often make ill-considered judgements. There is still an egocentric quality in adolescent thinking, although it is different to the egocentric thinking of the pre-school child. While they are now able to see matters from a number of different perspectives, their egocentrism is such that they tend to believe that others are as interested in issues that they find absorbing. They tend to be more focused on their own thoughts than those of others. This tendency is reflected in the old story of the 15 year old who accused his father of being hopelessly out of date and of 'not knowing anything'. Five years later he was heard to say that he was astonished at how much his father had learned in 5 years! Egocentrism may be adaptive for adolescents, in the sense that it can help reduce the uncertainty that would otherwise accompany intense questioning of established practices. In the long term, it may facilitate the adolescent's search for an adult identity.

One may ask, if adolescents are capable of such sophisticated reasoning and problem solving, why do they make so many foolish decisions? There are a number of reasons why advanced cognitive ability is not a sufficient condition for wisdom. First, adolescents are sometimes more cognitively advanced than they are emotionally mature. Second, a great deal of life experience is needed for astute decision making. Third, an even greater degree of self-discipline is required for the implementation of many decisions over long-term issues. Emotional maturity, life experience and self-discipline improve as the person grows older.

MORAL DEVELOPMENT

Kohlberg believed that formal operational thinking is necessary for his 3rd level of moral development which he termed 'post-conventional morality'.[26] Post-conventional reasoning involves the recognition that people in authority do not necessarily make laws based on sound ethical principles. At stage 5, moral judgements are made on the basis of the 'greatest good for the greatest number'. By stage 6, the most advanced stage of all, people begin to establish for themselves a set of moral principles by which they evaluate their own behaviour and that of others. Kohlberg, however, believed that few adults reach the 3rd level of moral development or make moral judgments beyond level 2, stage 4 (the law and order orientation).

Research into Kohlberg's stages has produced inconsistent results.[27,28] Some of the inconsistency may arise from the methodology used to measure reasoning. Researchers who used examples of dilemmas actually experienced by the participants, found higher levels of moral reasoning than Kohlberg found when he used hypothetical dilemmas.[29]

Gilligan has criticised Kohlberg for basing most of his studies on male participants and applying the results to females.[27] She studied the reasoning behind women's moral judgements and argued that the processes that males and females experience to achieve gender identity affect their outlook on moral issues. To achieve a sense of gender identity, men must separate themselves from their mothers, while women develop a sense of individuality within the context of their attachment to their mothers. The sex role identity of males, therefore, is threatened by intimacy and that of females by separation. While men are more likely to focus on issues of justice and fairness, women are more likely to incorporate issues surrounding the maintenance of relationships in their moral judgements. As Kohlberg developed his theory primarily from research on males,[30] reasoning from a male perspective produces higher scores than that based on a female perspective. Subsequent research, however, has not produced consistent evidence in support of Gilligan's contention. Women seem to score as highly as men on Kohlberg's levels of moral development.[28,31]

SOCIAL AND EMOTIONAL DEVELOPMENT

The psychoanalytic view of adolescence

The genital stage

According to Freud, sexual urges lie dormant during late childhood while the skills are learned that are necessary to function as adult members of their societies. As children mature physically, sex drive or libido becomes more intense and Freud's 'genital stage' begins.

As many children relate more comfortably with others of the same sex, they may initially experience a type of 'homosexual' stage where they become infatuated with a person of the same sex. The person may be a peer, a teacher, or a friend. Eventually, however, most adolescents begin to their focus their energies on the opposite sex. According to Freud, the major aim of the genital stage is to form mature sexual relationships.

Erikson's psychosocial view

Identity versus role confusion

Erikson believed satisfactory development during adolescence requires more than mature heterosexual relationships. He thought that Freud had under-emphasised the importance of social influences on adolescent development. He believed that adolescence is a time when the people begin to develop a sense of who they are and of their own individuality. This sense of personal uniqueness is what he meant by the development of identity versus role confusion. He also believed that this was accomplished largely in response to the cultural and social influences. Identity involves an integration of one's physical appearance, competencies, values and ideals into a total self-concept. Self-understanding requires an ability to see oneself from the point of view of others. Adolescents, therefore, are cognitively well placed to enhance the self-understanding necessary for identity development.

The negative outcome of this stage is role confusion. Role-confused people have difficulty in discovering a sense of identity. They have not developed a strong sense of personal values and ideals that might guide them in their dealings with others. They have difficulty in feeling a sense of personal pride and therefore are likely to suffer from low self-esteem. They become particularly impressionable and open to negative influences from others. Delinquent behaviour may be the consequence.

Erikson believed that adolescents who have successfully negotiated all previous crises would be in a better position to resolve the identity crisis.[32] Those who have a basic sense of security have confidence in their ability to make their own decisions and to initiate their own activities, and have learned the satisfaction of personal achievement, are in an ideal position to increase their understanding of themselves. Those who had not resolved such previous developmental crises would need to put additional effort into dealing with them during their adolescent years. Perhaps this explains why some adolescents seem to regress and have a more turbulent adolescence than others.

The development of identity requires adolescents to have the freedom to experiment with many different social and personal roles, and to explore a variety of attitudes and behaviours in the safety of their families and peer groups. They use their family and friends as audiences on whom they try out different roles. In this way, they make the transition from childhood to the sense of ego identity that is necessary for full, independent adulthood.

According to Erikson,[32] the person who is unable to resolve his identity crisis becomes unable to make a commitment to himself, to an occupational choice or to relate intimately to another. Support for this argument comes from the increased frequency of breakdown in young marriages.[33] Erikson argued that intimate relationships require the partners to submerge their individuality and to construct a joint identity. This is more difficult when the partners have difficulty in understanding their own motives or formulating their own goals.

Erikson, however, applied this more stringently to males then to females. He argued that while resolution of the identity crisis is important for males, he also believed that an adolescent girl should keep part of her identity, especially occupational identity, 'open' until married so that she is able to base some of her identity on that of her husband.[34,35] For this reason he has often been accused of sexism. His assertion has not been supported by the literature. The findings of Kahn et al., for example, show that the marriages of women who have not developed a strong sense of identity are more prone to break down.[36]

Identity status

James Marcia described 4 possible outcomes of the adolescent identity crisis.[37] He argued that as adolescents achieve identity by actively experimenting with different ideologies and identities, identity crisis resolution occurs when the adolescents make a commitment to a value system that forms the foundation of their character.

Identity achievement is the most psychologically healthy outcome. Those who achieve a strong sense of identity have a positive and stable self-concept. They have invested time and energy in thinking and sorting out issues that are important to them and have come to an understanding of where they stand on these issues. So they have made a commitment to certain beliefs and values that will provide direction for their future activities. They also have sufficient flexibility to be able to modify their existing belief systems as they evaluate new ideas.

The adolescent who is in the process of developing a sense of identity is in a state of moratorium. The adolescent in moratorium is postponing the adoption of any firm identity. He is actively experimenting, but has still not made a commitment.

Identity diffusion is the least psychologically healthy outcome. Identity-diffused people have not thought through important issues and so lack a commitment to any value system. They have given up considering these issues, and therefore lack self direction. Such people are highly susceptible to the influence of others and tend to adopt temporarily whatever identity is required at the time.

Identity foreclosure is characteristic of people who have made a commitment to an identity, but rather than basing this commitment on their own thoughts and values, they have based in on those of others. They tend to have little conflict with parents and other authorities. They often appear to have made an easy transition to adulthood and to be satisfied with it.

An additional identity status known as negative identity has been used to describe the behaviour of the adolescent who feels under pressure to adopt the beliefs, values and behaviour of significant adults and resists by behaving in the opposite way.[38] A child of conservative parents, for example, may adopt a punk appearance, mores and behaviour.

A firm sense of identity is not always established during adolescence. Indeed, Meilman found that little more than half the 24 year olds studied could be classified as having achieved a sense of identity.[39] What factors help the development of a healthy identity? It seems that parents and peer groups are both important elements.

The influence of parents starts to decline during middle childhood and that of peers increases. Adolescent is a period when most people form closer friendships. The ability to empathise is an important condition for the development of close friendships. During adolescence, both parents and peers are influential, but in different areas. For the development of basic values or advice on major life decisions such as career choice, adolescents turn to their parents. For advice on social behaviour they rely more on the advice of peers.[40,41]

The role of parents in adolescent development

Adolescents' relationships with their families reflect their transitionary status. While they need to emancipate themselves from their families and take responsibility for themselves, they also have a need for support and guidance from their families, especially during early adolescence.[42,43]

Parents can help their children negotiate the tasks of adolescence by allowing them the freedom to experiment with ideas, roles and behaviours. When parents try to project their own unfulfilled ambitions onto their children or place undue pressure on them to conform to the wills of others, it is harder for adolescents to discover ways of behaving and thinking that make sense to them as individuals.

While adolescents have developed the cognitive ability to problem solve, they do not have the life experience to always make wise choices and their immaturity may lead them into inappropriate or even dangerous decisions. They tend to make decisions that result in short-term but not long-term gains, for example, leaving school prematurely for a seemingly high-paying job. They need, therefore, to have their parents listen to them, set reasonable limits on their behaviour and provide them with advice and guidance.[44] Parents who monitor their adolescents' behaviour, but are also accepting of them, are likely to have children who are both competent and self-disciplined.[45] Limits should gradually be lifted as the adolescent becomes more skilled at mature decision making. Parents and adolescents may disagree about the age at which, and the issues about which, parents would allow their children greater autonomy.[46] Parents who make arbitrary rules in a heavy-handed manner, are likely to invoke rebellion in their children whereas parents who are over-permissive and do not set limits or provide support and guidance are likely to be regarded by their children as uninterested or even rejecting. Parents, for example, who are uninvolved with their children are more likely to have adolescents who use drugs.[47,48]

The authoritative parenting pattern seems to provide ideal circumstances for the development of a strong identity[49] and high psychosocial adjustment.[43] Authoritative parents who use reasoning and persuasion and are willing to take the child's viewpoint into consideration, are more likely to foster independence and self-reliance and a mature identity.[43,49,50] Such families are more likely to foster family discussion and to listen to adolescents' points of view on issues of interest. Adolescents may not always accept parental limit setting with good grace, but nevertheless, it is an indication of their parents' esteem and respect for them and has the effect of increasing their self-esteem.[51,52]

The fine line between granting sufficient freedom and setting appropriate limits is not always easy for parents to achieve. They may allow their children as much latitude as possible, but then feel rejected when their children consider and adopt contrary

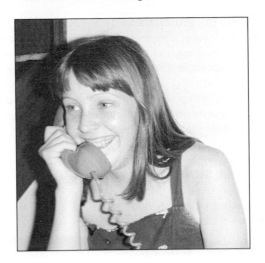

Discussions between close friends are important for the development of self-understanding.

viewpoints and behaviours, and become critical of their parents' views and behaviours. It may be of some comfort to parents to know that Erikson argued that as questioning is important for identity development, parents ought to be more concerned if their adolescent is not critical of them.[53]

The role of peers in adolescent adjustment

Much of the adolescent experimentation with different identities and ideologies takes place within the peer group. Here, with the support of others who are in similar circumstances, they explore different ideas and behaviours.[44] Discussions between close friends are an important forum for the development of the self-understanding of both.[51] Relationships with peers tend to be more on a shared basis, whereas parents are more directive. Interactions with peers foster social competence, particularly as peers tend to be less forgiving than families. On the other hand, children from unduly restrictive or rejecting families, may find acceptance among their peers that they have rarely found at home.[42,54]

The peer group provides opportunities for adolescents to manage the world which they are entering, rather than the world in which their parents grew up. Adolescents, for example, who are trying to cope with the drug culture, or with fears of not finding a job, or with more open attitudes towards sexual experimentation, may find greater understanding among their contemporaries who are battling the same problems than with their parents who faced different problems. The relative strength of parental and peer group influence seems to vary. As adolescents tend to associate with peers who hold similar values to their parents, parents appear to retain at least an indirect influence over their children's peer group affiliations.[55] Hundleby and Mercer, however, found that peers were a much greater influence than parents on adolescent decisions to use alcohol, marijuana and tobacco.[47]

The adolescent peer group can provide an environment for the improvement of coping strategies. Adolescents who are able to benefit from the sympathetic support of peers and the accumulated wisdom of their parents are probably in the best position to resolve these conflicts.

Dunphy's classic Australian study showed how the structure of peer groups develops throughout adolescence.[56] Early adolescents tend to mix in isolated unisexual groups.

During middle adolescence, the group gradually becomes more heterosexual and, with the support of closely knit 'cliques', members learn to get along with opposite-sex peers. During late adolescence, when required role behaviours have been mastered, members tended to mix in loosely associated groups of couples. This is the final stage before the selection of a marriage partner.

During early adolescence, group membership is largely based on conformity to group standards. Throughout, emphasis on conformity gradually decreases as late adolescence approaches, and the person develops the greater individuality of young adulthood.[54]

THE DEVELOPMENT OF A SENSE OF BODY IMAGE

Accepting one's physique and using the body effectively is an important task of adolescence and there is a strong relationship between adolescents' satisfaction with their body image and their self-esteem.[40] The relationship is stronger in females than in males.[57,58] Girls' self-esteem depends more on their physical attractiveness, while boys' self-esteem is more dependent on physical competence.[59] Body build is important to boys as it contributes to their masculinity.[60] Body image concerns of adolescent boys are likely to focus on the size and development of genitalia, and the embarrassment of spontaneous erections.[61]

Most teenagers are dissatisfied with some aspect of their bodies.[40] Body satisfaction in girls tends to decline during teenage years. Most adolescent girls are concerned about being overweight,[62,63] even when their weight is normal or they are underweight.[64] Girls who feel fat are more likely to feel shy, lonely, hopeless,[64] depressed and have a lower self-esteem[65] than girls who are satisfied with their weight.[64] Hip measurements seem to cause girls more concern than other parts of their bodies.[66] Girls who perceive themselves as overweight tend to centre their body dissatisfaction on their waist and hips, whereas girls who see themselves as underweight tend to centre their dissatisfaction on their bust measurements.[66] The ideal seems to be a large bust and small hips.

The rate at which adolescents mature not only affects the way they see themselves, but also the way others relate to them. Adolescents tend to be treated according to the way they look, rather than their age. The rate at which they mature therefore influences their social relationships. Early maturing males fit more closely the ideal of the tall and physically well developed 'macho' male. They also perform better in athletics than their peers. They tend to be more satisfied with their bodies and to have a higher self-esteem.[67] There is evidence that early maturing boys are more likely to be perceived in a positive light by others. They are more likely to have greater leadership abilities,[68] to be more popular and more confident[69] Late maturing boys are likely to look and to be treated as younger than they really are. Their small stature is more likely to elicit scorn from other boys and to provide problems attracting the interest of girls. Thus they are likely to have greater self-esteem problems.[69,70]

The effect of maturation rate on girls is less clear cut. While some studies have found no difference in popularity of early and late maturing girls,[71] others have found that early maturing girls are less well adjusted and less popular with their peers[72] and still others have found this to be true of late maturing girls.[73] Early maturing girls look older than their peers, and are likely to want to date earlier. As girls develop, on average, 2 years earlier than boys, early maturing girls are more likely to date much older boys. Parental concern that their daughter is neglecting her school work, and wanting to date older boys at an earlier age than the majority of her classmates, may result in increased family conflict.

THE DEVELOPMENT OF A CONCEPT OF DEATH

Adolescents have a full concept of the universality and finality of death,[74-76] but seem to believe that death is something that happens to others and will not happen to them, at least until they are much older. This seems to represent a belief in one's own immortality. Elkind, described this belief as a 'personal fable', that many adolescents behave as if they believe they have a kind of 'guardian angel' whose role it is to protect them from harm.[77] Protected by such beliefs, they act out behaviours such as substance abuse and reckless driving. It is exemplified in 'Superman' stories where Lois Lane and Jimmy Olsen often seem to rush recklessly into ill-conceived schemes because they know that at the end of the episode Superman will rescue them.

ADOLESCENT BELIEFS ABOUT HEALTH, ILLNESS AND PAIN

Beliefs about the causes of health and illness

Adolescents develop the potential to understand fully the cause of illness. Bibace and Walsh found that young adolescents are able to conceptualise illness as physiological disruption, but in later adolescence they also acknowledge the role of psychological processes in the development of illness.[78]

They are now able fully to comprehend the implications of illness. However, Wilkinson found that adolescents are more likely to worry about the immediate, rather than the long-term, effects of illness.[79] This has important implications for the health education of adolescents. Educators would do better to relate the effects of unhealthy behaviour, where possible, to the way it affects present feelings of well-being. Harbord et al., for example, found that adolescents felt that the worst part of having cystic fibrosis was the restriction it placed on their freedom, and the way it made them feel different from others at school.[80] They found little evidence of adolescents' concern for the future.

Beliefs about pain

The adolescent is able to comprehend the warning nature of pain and therefore, to be concerned with the implications of persistent pain.[81,82] The young child's passive acceptance of pain has given way to a more active view in which the adolescent recognises that pain must be managed or endured. However, adolescents may still be frightened by the prospect of even relatively minor painful experiences. Favaloro and Touzel, for example, found that some adolescents may refuse pain medication because they do not want an injection.[83] Awareness of the impact of socialisation on males and females is also important when assessing the pain of adolescents as males may be less likely to admit pain than females for fear of appearing weak.[83] Adolescents need to be encouraged to report their pain and to accept appropriate pain relief.

COPING IN ADOLESCENCE

People who develop a wide repertoire of coping strategies tend to be better equipped to manage stressful events in their lives than those who rely on a more limited range.

Adolescents' newly developed cognitive abilities allow them to use strategies that were previously unavailable to them. Denial and intellectualisation, for example, are often used by adolescents as defences against anxiety. Discussions of anxiety-laden issues by brighter and better-educated adolescents may appear, at times, to be particularly intellectual and impersonal.[35] It is possible that intellectualisation not only allows them the protection of detachment, it probably also serves the additional purpose of providing adolescents with 'important practice in thinking abstractly and formulating and testing hypotheses'.[84] While denial can be a useful method of coping with stress, it can also lead to dangerous behaviour such as failing to practice safe sex or use contraceptives.[85]

Frydenberg and Lewis studied the differences in coping strategies used by adolescent males and females.[86] Girls tended to use social support whereas boys, were more likely to 'keep others from knowing how bad things were'. Girls were more likely to daydream and 'hope for a miracle' and boys 'make light of the situation' and to 'stand my ground since nothing can be done'.

Adolescence has been described as an emotionally turbulent time, when the person makes a difficult transition from childhood to adulthood. There is no doubt that this is true for some people. However, it also seems that many adolescents experience this time as one of emotional stability and satisfaction.[87]

REFERENCES

1. Wong DL. *Whaley and Wong's nursing care of infants and children*. 5th ed. St Louis: Mosby, 1995.
2. Mott SR, James SR, Sperhac AM. *Nursing care of children and families*. 2nd ed. Redwood City: Addison-Wesley, 1990.
3. Scipien GM, Chard MA, Howe J, Barnard MU. *Pediatric nursing care*. St Louis: Mosby, 1990.
4. Marlow DR, Redding BA. *Textbook of pediatric nursing*. 6th ed. Philadelphia: Saunders, 1988.
5. Edelman CL, Mandle CL. *Health promotion throughout the lifespan*. St Louis: Mosby, 1990.
6. Wolfish MG. Normal adolescent development. *In:* Buchanan N, ed. *Child and adolescent health for practitioners*. Sydney: Williams and Wilkins, 1987.
7. Robertson SI. Health of young people. *In:* Vimpani G, Parry T, eds. *Community child health: an Australian perspective*. Melbourne: Churchill Livingstone, 1989.
8. National Health and Medical Research Council. *Review of Child Health Surveillance and Screening*. Canberra: AGPS, 1993.
9. Coleman JC, Hendry L. *The nature of adolescence*. 2nd ed. London: Routledge, 1990.
10. Bennett D. Medical assessment of the adolescent. *In:* Procopis PG, Kewley GD, eds. *Current paediatric practice*. Sydney: Harcourt Brace Jovanovich, 1991.
11. Beischer NA, Mackay EV. *Obstetrics and the newborn*. 2nd ed. Sydney: Saunders, 1984.
12. Sinclair D. *Human growth after birth*. 5th ed. Oxford: Oxford University Press, 1989 .
13. Brook CGD. *All about adolescence*. Chichester: John Wiley and Sons, 1985.
14. Tanner JM. *Foetus into man: physical growth from conception to maturity*. 2nd ed. Ware: Castlemead Publications, 1989.
15. National Health and Medical Research Council. *Nutrition policy statements*. Canberra: AGPS, 1990.
16. Parcel GS, Finkelstein JW. Adolescent sexuality. *In:* Buchanan N, ed. *Child and adolescent health for practitioners*. Sydney: Williams and Wilkins, 1987.
17. National Health and Medical Research Council. *The Australian immunisation procedures handbook*. 5th ed. Canberra: AGPS, 1994.
18. Stanley FJ, Williams HE. Morbidity and mortality patterns. *In:* Vimpani G, Parry T, eds. *Community child health: an Australian perspective*. Melbourne: Churchill Livingstone, 1989.

19. Havighurst RJ. *Human development and education.* New York: Longmans, Green and Co., 1953.
20. Martorano SC. A developmental analysis of performance on Piaget's formal operations tasks. *Dev Psychol* 1977; 13: 666–672.
21. Neimark ED. Adolescent thought: transition to formal operations. *In:* Wolman BB, ed. *Handbook of developmental psychology.* Englewood Cliffs, NJ: Prentice-Hall, 1982.
22. Marini Z, Case R. The development of abstract thinking about the physical and social world. *Child Dev* 1994; 65: 147–159.
23. Rosenberg M. *Conceiving the self.* New York: Basic Books, 1979.
24. Piaget J, Inhelder B. *The psychology of the child.* London: Routledge Kegan & Paul, 1969.
25. Elkind D. Cognitive development in adolescence. *In:* Adams JF, ed. *Understanding adolescence.* Boston: Allyn & Bacon, 1968.
26. Kohlberg L. The development of moral character and moral ideology. *In:* Hoffman ML, Hoffman LW, eds. *Review of child development research.* Vol. 1. New York: Russell Sage, 1964.
27. Gilligan C. *In a different voice.* Cambridge, Mass: Harvard University Press, 1982.
28. Rest JR. *Moral development: advances in research and theory.* New York: Praeger, 1986.
29. Berger KS. *The developing person through the life span.* New York: Worth Publishers, 1988.
30. Colby A, Kohlberg L, Gibbs J, Lieberman M. *A longitudinal study of moral development.* Monographs of the Society for Research in Child Development, 48 (1) Serial No. 200, 1983.
31. Walker LJ. Sex differences in the development of moral reasoning: a critical review. *Child Dev* 1984; 57: 677–691.
32. Erikson EH. The problem of ego identity. *In:* Gold M, Douvan E, eds. *Adolescent development. Readings in research and theory.* Boston: Allyn & Bacon, 1969.
33. Mussen PH, Conger JJ, Kagan J, Huston AE. *Child development and personality.* 7th ed. New York: Harper & Rowe, 1990.
34. Freiberg KL. *Human Development. A life span approach.* 4th ed. Boston: Jones & Bartlett, 1992.
35. Philips S. *Self concept and self esteem: infancy to adolescence.* Selected paper no 27. Kensington, NSW: Foundation for Child and Youth Studies, 1983.
36. Kahn S, Zimmerman G, Csikszentmihalyi M, Getzels JW. Relations between identity in young adulthood and intimacy at midlife. *J Personality Soc Psychol* 1985; 49: 1316–1322.
37. Marcia J. Identity in adolescence. *In:* Adelson J, ed. *Handbook of adolescent psychology.* New York: Wiley, 1980.
38. Erikson EH. *Identity and the life cycle: selected papers.* Psychological Issues, Monograph 1.1. 1959.
39. Meilman PW. Cross-sectional changes in identity during adolescence. *Dev Psychol* 1979; 15: 230–231.
40. Kaplan PS. *The human odyssey.* St Paul: West Publishing, 1988.
41. Wilks J. The relative importance of parents and friends in adolescent decision making. *J Youth Adolescence* 1986; 15: 323–334.
42. Hoelter J, Harper L. Structural and interpersonal influences of adolescent self-conception. *J Marriage Family* 1987; 249: 129–139.
43. Steinberg L, Lamborn SD, Darling N, Mounts NS, Dornsbusch SM. Over-time changes in adjustment and competence among adolescents from authoritative, authoritarian, indulgent and neglectful families. *Child Dev* 1994; 65: 754–770.
44. Youniss J, Smollar J. *Adolescent relations with mothers, fathers and friends.* Chicago: University of Chicago Press, 1985.
45. Kurdek LA, Fine MA. Family acceptance and family control as predictors of adjustment in young adolescents: linear, curvilinear or interactive effects? *Child Dev* 1994; 65: 1137–1146.
46. Smetana JG, Asquith P. Adolescents' and parents' conceptions of parental authority and personal autonomy. *Child Dev* 1994; 65: 1147–1162.
47. Hundleby JD, Mercer GW. Family and friends as social environments and their relationship to

young adolescents use of alcohol, tobacco and marijuana. *J Marriage Family* 1987; 49: 151–164.

48. Wills TA, Vaughan R. Social support and substance abuse in early adolescence. *J Pediatr Psychol* 1989; 14: 321–339.

49. Baumrind D. Current practices of parental authority. *Dev Psychol* 1971; 4 (Monograph 1): 1–103.

50. Baumrind D. The influence of parenting style on adolescent competence and substance abuse. *J Early Adolescence* 1991; 11: 56–95.

51. Conger JJ. *Adolescence: generation under pressure.* New York: Harper and Rowe, 1979.

52. Santrock JW. *Adolescence: an introduction.* Dubuque, IA: William C. Brown, 1984.

53. Erikson EH. *Dimensions of a new identity.* New York: Norton, 1974.

54. Hartup WW. Peer relations. *In:* Hetherington EM, Ed. *Handbook of Child Psychology: socialization, personality and social development.* Vol. 4, 4th ed. New York: Wiley, 1983: 103–196.

55. Brown BB, Mounts N, Lamborn SD, Steinberg L. Parenting practices and peer group affiliation in adolescence. *Child Dev* 1993; 64: 467–482.

56. Dunphy DE. The social structure of urban adolescent peer groups. *In:* Collins JK, ed. *Studies of the Australian adolescent.* Melbourne: Cassell, 1975.

57. Lerner RM, Karabenick SA, Stuart J. Relations among physical attractiveness, body attitudes and self-concept in male and female college students. *J Psychol* 1973; 85: 119–129.

58. Lerner RM, Karabenick SA. Physical attractiveness, body attitudes and self-concept in late adolescence. *J Youth Adolescence* 1974; 13: 307–317.

59. Schuster CS, Ashburn SS. *The process of human development.* 2nd ed. Boston: Little, Brown, 1986.

60. Collins J, Harper JF. *The adolescent boy.* Sydney: Cassell, 1978.

61. Bennett D. Sexual concerns of adolescent boys. *Patient Management* 1980; July: 105–106.

62. Storz N, Greene W. Body weight, body image and perception of fad diets in adolescent girls. *J Nutrition Educ* 1983; 15: 15–19.

63. Eisele J, Hertsgaard D, Light HK. Factors relating to eating disorders in young adolescent girls. *Adolescence* 1986; 21: 283–290.

64. Page R. Indicators of psychosocial distress among adolescent females who perceive themselves as fat. *Child Study J* 1991; 21: 203–212.

65. Taylor MJ, Cooper TL. Body size overestimation and depression. *Br J Med Psychol* 1986; 25: 153–154.

66. Davies E, Furnham A. Body satisfaction in adolescent girls. *Br J Med Psychol* 1986; 59: 279–287.

67. Newman BM, Newman PR. *Development through life.* 5th ed. Pacific Grove, CA: Brooks/Cole, 1991.

68. Felice ME, Friedman SB. Behavioral considerations in the health care of adolescents. *Pediatr Clin North Am* 1982; 29: 399–412.

69. Simmons RG, Blyth DA, Van Cleave E, Bush D. Entry into early adolescence: the impact of school structure, puberty and dating on self-esteem. *Am Sociological Rev* 1979; 44: 948–967.

70. Mussen PH, Jones MC. Self conceptions, motivations and interpersonal attitudes of late and early maturing boys. *Child Dev* 1957; 28: 243–256.

71. Harper JF, Collins JK. The effects of early or late maturation on the prestige of the adolescent girl. *In:* Collins JK, ed. *Studies of the Australian adolescent.* Melbourne: Cassell, 1975.

72. Peterson AC. Adolescent development. *Annual Rev Psychol* 1988; 39: 583–608.

73. Jones MC, Mussen PH. Self conceptions, motivations and interpersonal attitudes of early and late maturing girls. *Child Dev* 1958; 29: 491–501.

74. Johnson-Soderberg S. The development of a child's concept of death. *Oncology Nursing Forum* 1981; 8: 23–26.

75. Koocher GP. Children's conceptions of death. *In:* Bibace R, Walsh ME, eds. *Children's conceptions of health, illness and bodily functions.* San Francisco: Jossey-Bass, 1981.

76. Krause DM. Children's concepts of death. *In:* Martinson IM, ed. *Home care for the dying child: professional and family perspective.* New York: Appleton-Century-Crofts, 1976.

77. Elkind D. *The hurried child.* Reading, Mass.: Addison-Wesley, 1981.

78. Bibace R, Walsh ME. Children's conceptions of illness. *In:* Bibace R, Walsh ME, eds. *Children's conceptions of health, illness and bodily functions.* San Francisco: Jossey-Bass, 1981.

79. Wilkinson SR. *The child's world of illness: the development of health and illness behaviour.* Cambridge: Cambridge University Press, 1988.

80. Harbord MG, Cross DG, Botica F, Martin AJ. Children's understanding of cystic fibrosis. *Aust Paediatr J* 1987; 23: 241–244.

81. Gaffney A, Dunne EA. Developmental aspects of children's definitions of pain. *Pain* 1986; 26: 105–117.

82. Harbeck C, Peterson L. Elephants dancing in my head: a developmental approach to children's concepts of specific pains. *Child Dev* 1992; 63: 138–149.

83. Favaloro R, Touzel B. A comparison of adolescents' and nurses' postoperative pain ratings and perceptions. *Pediatr Nursing* 1990; 16: 414–416, 424.

84. Mussen PH, Conger JJ, Kagan J, Huston AE. *Child development and personality.* 7th ed. New York: Harper & Rowe, 1990.

85. Hornick JP, Doran L, Crawford SH. Premarital contraceptive usage among male and female adolescents. *Family Coordinator* 1979; 28: 181–190.

86. Frydenberg E, Lewis R. Adolescent coping: the different ways in which boys and girls cope. *J Adolescence* 1991; 14: 119–133.

87. Dusek JB, Flaherty JF. *The development of self concept during the adolescent years.* Monographs of the Society for Research in Child Development, 46 (4) Serial No. 191, 1981.

ALTERATIONS TO HEALTH IN INFANCY, CHILDHOOD AND ADOLESCENCE

Maintaining a standard of clinical excellence in practice, striving to meet the complexity of needs of the child with altered health and to provide appropriate and ongoing support for the family are critical aspects of the paediatric nurse's role. Part Two contains contributions from nursing specialists in which standards of practice and practice ideals are clearly explicated.

The contributions have been invited from expert nurse clinicians from various paediatric centres who are highly experienced in the care of infants, children and adolescents with altered health needs in acute hospital and community settings. Their sections explore nursing responsibilities in the provision of care, reflect the high level of specialisation that currently exists in paediatric nursing practice, and emphasise the influence of contemporary health-related issues on children's care.

Part Two addresses congenital and acquired health problems in children, from infancy to adolescence. The chapters in Part Two include discussion on the care of the infant, child and adolescent with inflammation and infection (Chapter 5), an alteration to structure (Chapter 6) and altered cellular function (Chapter 7). The content in these chapters has been organised according to a range of disturbances in the regulation of physiological functioning: oxygenation and acid-base balance; blood volume, pressure and flow; neuromuscular function; musculo-skeletal and integumentary function, gastro-intestinal function; genitourinary function; haematopoietic and immunological function and sensory function.

Chapter 8 describes the care of the infant, child and adolescent with health needs in the community. It details the nursing care of children requiring home ventilation and discusses sudden infant death syndrome and feeding problems in infancy. Discussion is also included on genetic and chromosomal abnormalities in children, with particular emphasis on the support required by families.

Chapter 9 discusses the psychological care of the infant, child and adolescent with an illness. This chapter addresses the implications of professional nursing practice in long-term illness and hospitalisation, stress, grief and bereavement, and the role and responsibilities of the paediatric nurse in supporting children and their families during times of critical stress. Chapter 9 also examines the issues surrounding abuse of children and the assessment, care and support of abused children and their families.

Chapter 5

Care of the Infant, Child and Adolescent with Inflammation and Infection

Tonsillectomy and Adenoidectomy

Lynne Brodie

The combined procedure of tonsillectomy and adenoidectomy has received considerable scrutiny in recent years, both in the media and in medical literature. Much of the controversy arises from the fact that traditionally the operation has been performed as a combined procedure, despite widespread agreement among otolarnygologists about the differing indications for each of these surgical procedures.[1-3] There has also been debate concerning the frequency of such operations. There is a trend in Australia and many other countries, for more precise criteria to be applied to the selection of patients for surgery. Beckenham defines the indications for both operations.[4]

INDICATIONS

Tonsillectomy

Recurrent infection.
3 to 4 attacks over 2 years.
6 attacks in 1 year.
Obstruction.
Obstructive sleep apnoea with cyanosis (urgent surgery).
Obstructive sleep picture.
Neoplasm.

Adenoidectomy

Chronic postnasal obstruction confirmed by lateral airway x-ray.
Recurrent attacks of acute otitis media, particularly if otitis media with effusion does not persist between attacks.
Infective postnasal discharge.

Preoperative nursing assessment

Tonsillectomy and/or adenoidectomy are performed as elective operations and the child is generally assessed in the surgeon's rooms or at an outpatient clinic before admission to hospital. At the time of admission the surgeon may have ordered pathology tests such as haemoglobin and clotting studies. Many paediatric centres have high-dependency units and children who are at risk of developing complications in the acute postoperative phase may have a bed reserved so that they can be more closely monitored. This need is determined by the surgeon and anaesthetist. Children with obstructive indications for tonsillectomy are particularly at risk and sleep studies or overnight oximetry may be ordered to determine the severity of obstruction.

The first priority of preoperative nursing assessment is to record baseline observations and document the child's general condition. The anaesthetist and registrar should be notified of any concerns. Surgery is usually rescheduled if the child is febrile or unwell as there is an increased risk of complications.

During the nursing admission, explanations should be given to the child and parents concerning the need for an adequate fluid intake postoperatively. The child should be told that medication will be given regularly to ease the sore throat. The nurse should determine the child's level of understanding of the operation and attempt to allay any fears or unrealistic expectations. Loose teeth need to be recorded on the preoperative checklist.

Postoperative nursing management

General principle: Close monitoring for airway patency as oedema and excessive secretions may cause obstructive problems.

Nursing action: Rate and quality of respirations should be recorded at a minimum of every 30 minutes for the 1st 4 hours and if satisfactory, hourly for 24 hours. Oximetry may be ordered.

General principle: Close monitoring for bleeding in the 1st 24 hours postoperatively.

Nursing action: Report excessive swallowing as this may indicate bleeding. Record pulse at least every 30 minutes for the 1st 4 hours and then hourly if stable. Note type and amount of emesis and report excessive vomiting or presence of fresh blood. It is not uncommon for children to vomit old blood and mucous in the early postoperative period. Antiemetics may be ordered if vomiting is excessive.

General principle: Adequate pain relief.

Nursing action: Analgesia is given as ordered. Paracetamol or codeine are most commonly recommended. Aspirin is not used as it prolongs clotting time. Narcotics are used at the discretion of the surgeon. Narcotics may have been given intraoperatively.

General principle: Ensure adequate fluid intake to maintain hydration and promote healing.

Nursing action: Monitor rate of IV fluids and encourage clear fluids as tolerated. Grade slowly to a light diet. Soft foods may be preferred.

General principle: Promote oral hygiene.

Nursing action: Gentle mouth washes can be given but the child should not gargle as this may cause bleeding.

The child should be encouraged to rest for the first 24 hours and parents are encouraged to stay with their child and participate in the care. If the child is febrile, antibiotics may be ordered before discharge. The length of hospital stay varies, but tonsillectomy usually requires only a short stay of 1 to 2 days.

Reactionary haemorrhage may occur in the acute postoperative period. Early signs include excessive swallowing of secretions and elevation in pulse and respiratory rates. The child may vomit fresh blood. In the event of reactionary haemorrhage, the nurse should elevate the child's head and notify the surgeon or registrar immediately. Ice packs applied to the neck may be recommended to try to control the bleeding, but in most cases arrangements will be made to return the child to the operating theatre. The child should be closely monitored with respirations, pulse and blood pressure recorded every 15 minutes.[5]

Instructions for parents on discharge

Parents should be taught about the risk of secondary bleeding. The risk is highest at 5 to 7 days postoperatively, when the slough begins to separate. If any bleeding or high temperatures occur, parents should seek urgent medical advice. The child may also complain of earache. This occurs in approximately 50% of patients and is caused by otalgia referred from the tonsillar bed. If parents are concerned they should again seek medical advice.

Parents should also be advised about suitable analgesia such as paracetamol, diet and the need to ensure adequate fluid intake. Spicy foods are not recommended. Quiet activity should be encouraged during the 1st week after discharge and contact with ill children avoided. The child can usually return to school after a week to 10 days. Follow-up appointments are generally arranged for 2 to 3 weeks after discharge.[5]

Nursing care following adenoidectomy

Adenoidectomy is increasingly being performed as a day stay procedure in paediatric centres, unless the child has obstructive symptoms. Generally the child experiences minimal pain and paracetamol provides sufficient analgesia. There are rarely problems with encouraging oral intake and intravenous fluids are seldom indicated. As for tonsillectomy, the child should be closely monitored in the early postoperative period for evidence of respiratory difficulty or bleeding. Postoperative instructions are the same as for tonsillectomy.

REFERENCES

1. Rosenfeld RM, Gree RP. Tonsillectomy and adenoidectomy: changing trends. *Ann Otol Rhinol Laryngol* 1990; 99: 187–191.
2. Norinkavich KM, Howie G, Cariofiles P. Quality improvement study of day surgery for tonsillectomy and adenoidectomy patients. *Pediatr Nursing* 1995; 21: 341–344.
3. Colman BH. *Diseases of the nose, throat and ear and head and neck.* Edinburgh: Churchill Livingstone, 1992: 95–102.
4. Beckenham EJ. Tonsils and adenoids. *Mod Med Aust* 1990; 33: (3) 84–87.
5. Nursing guidelines for care of children following tonsillectomy. *Royal Alexandra Hospital for Children Camperdown nursing policy and procedure manual.* Sydney: The Hospital, 1991.

Disturbances in Oxygenation and Acid-based Balance
Helen Sharp

Lower Respiratory Tract Infection

Five per cent of acute respiratory infections in children involve the trachea and lower respiratory tract.[1] Severe infections are more prevalent in the first 3 to 4 years of life, although the highest incidence of serious respiratory disease occurs in infants under 12 months of age.[1,2] Various factors contribute to the increased incidence of respiratory dysfunction in this age group. Not only do infants have a smaller airway and greater resistance to air flow, their normal oxygen consumption is approximately 3 times per kilogram body weight greater than an adult's.[1,3] Any obstruction or dysfunction in the bronchi, bronchioles or alveoli can lead to ventilation/perfusion inequality which will result in reduction of the oxygen delivered to the bloodstream. The amount of oxygen combining with haemoglobin may be insufficient for normal cellular respiration, resulting in interruption of homeostasis and death of cells through oxygen deprivation.

Nursing assessment

A complete respiratory assessment is undertaken and the child is carefully observed for the degree of respiratory dysfunction. Cyanosis, difficulty with breathing, chest recession, respiratory noises such as grunting or wheezing, and fatigue are symptoms that should be noted. Irritability and restlessness may be important indications of impaired gaseous exchange. The child is examined for signs of a 'barrel chest' caused by hyperinflation of the lungs, and clubbing of the fingers and toes, which may indicate chronic hypoxaemia. A set of observations including pulse, temperature and respiration is important to provide baseline data from which to monitor the progress of the dysfunction. In addition to recording the rate and depth of respiration, respiratory effort and rhythm should also be noted. Oxygen saturation should be assessed by pulse oximetry, transcutaneous oxygen monitor, or blood gas levels whenever impairment of gaseous exchange leading to hypoxaemia is present or suspected. The nurse also needs to assess the degree and appearance of mucus production, and if possible obtain a specimen for pathology.

Chest pain, which may be present, is very difficult to assess in infants and very young children. Changes in pulse and respiratory rate, restlessness, crying, irritability or loss of appetite may suggest that the infant is in pain. Older children can verbalise the degree of pain and its location, especially with the aid of a pain chart.[4]

In obtaining the nursing history, the nurse asks questions to ascertain when the symptoms were first noticed and if they are more evident at certain times of the day. The sound of the cough, whether it is productive or non-productive and its frequency are important to determine the method of nursing intervention. For example, a child with the whooping sound associated with pertussis will need to be nursed in isolation while a child with a frequent, productive cough may be more comfortable nursed upright in bed.

Further, the nurse in obtaining a nursing history from the primary caregivers and/or child, ascertains the child's eating habits, weight gain or loss and any past history of respiratory illness in the child or family. Recent exposure of the child to infectious micro-organisms, any increase in environmental irritants and the child's current immunisation status also need to be recorded. If the child or family have travelled, especially overseas, in the past weeks this should be included in the nursing history, as it may help to identify any unusual organisms.

The nurse should question whether the child has been frequently exposed to an environment in which the primary caregivers or others smoke, and whether the child, if old enough, also smokes. The occurrence of pneumonia and bronchitis, especially during the first year of life, is more than doubled in children if both primary caregivers smoke, and increased by 50% when 1 primary caregiver smokes.[1] Research has shown that wheezing attacks after an acute episode of bronchiolitis are increased in children whose primary caregivers smoke.[5]

Implementation of care

The role of the nurse in the care of a child with lower respiratory tract infection is mainly supportive, and includes helping the child maintain respiratory function, conserve energy and remain comfortable. The child is observed for signs of hypoxaemia as demonstrated by tachycardia, tachypnoea, restlessness, cyanosis and low blood gas levels. Oxygen administration is required in children with impaired gas exchange. Various delivery devices, such as face mask, nasal prongs, oxydome or other specialised equipment may be used. The rate of oxygen provided will depend on the level of oxygen saturation, which is monitored continuously by means of a pulse oximeter, or transcutaneous oxygen monitor. Rest is encouraged in these children to conserve oxygen demand and reduce respiratory effort, thereby lowering the risk of respiratory fatigue.

Oximeter and probe.

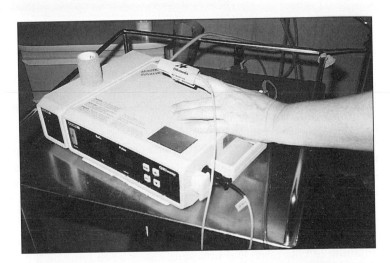

Placement of oximeter and probe on infant.

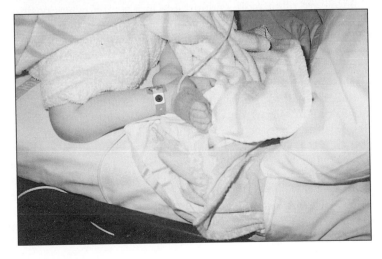

Child with chest recession and hyperinflation.

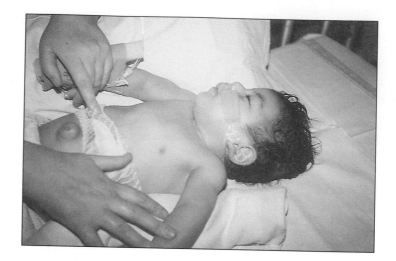

The infant or child should be observed for increasing signs of ineffective breathing patterns, including marked chest recession and retraction, the use of accessory muscles, asymmetry of movement of the chest and alteration in the depth, rate and rhythm of breathing. Infants, especially, should be observed for signs of tiring from the effort of breathing as they may need mechanical ventilation. Suctioning of the nasopharyngeal area to remove thick secretions may be necessary in the infant and young child to enable them to breathe more freely. Older children may need encouragement with productive coughing and nasal clearance. Chest physiotherapy may be ordered to clear accumulated mucus from the lower respiratory passages. Vital signs need to be assessed as frequently as every 30 to 60 minutes during the acute stages of the illness to provide data on which to base the continued treatment of the child's condition.

Positioning is important to the comfort of children with lower respiratory tract dysfunction. Infants often find breathing easier when lying on a flat surface, whereas older children are often more comfortable in a semi-Fowlers position.

Fluid intake is encouraged to prevent a fluid volume deficit. Approximately two-thirds of the child's daily insensible fluid loss occurs via the respiratory tract. This loss is increased by the accelerated breathing rate associated with respiratory infections. An adequate fluid intake also prevents the mucus from becoming too dry and thick to expectorate. Fever may be present, further increasing the body's fluid requirements. If the child is too ill to drink, intravenous therapy is required. Careful clinical assessment and monitoring of output are vitally important to complete evaluation of a child's hydration status. Diversionary activities for these children should be of a sedentary nature to conserve energy. If the child requires supplemental oxygen, all care is taken to eliminate flammable objects and friction toys. Respiratory illness can often cause anxiety in the primary caregivers and child, therefore a quiet, calm environment will assist them to relax. The primary caregivers and child should be given adequate opportunity to ask questions and voice any fears they may have. Children admitted with acute respiratory dysfunction frequently have had no preparation for hospital, therefore the nurse needs to show understanding, and help facilitate the child's adaptation to the new environment.

ACUTE INFECTIONS

Bronchiolitis

Bronchiolitis is a viral infection resulting in an inflammatory obstruction of the bronchioles. It develops in infants up to 2 years of age, with a peak incidence between 1 and 6 months of age, and is more commonly found in boys. In many areas including the south-eastern states of Australia, there is an increased incidence during the coldest months of the year with approximately 1% of affected infants being admitted to hospital.[1,3,5]

The illness characteristically begins with a 2 to 3 day history of upper respiratory tract infection and harsh cough. Affected infants develop a low-grade fever, increasing dyspnoea, tachypnoea, wheezing and difficulty with feeding. In the moderate to severely ill infant the chest becomes 'barrel shaped' due to hyperinflation. Intercostal and subcostal retraction and tracheal tug may also be present. Typically, the course of the disease is 7 to 10 days.[1,3,6]

Respiratory synctial virus is the predominant organism isolated, but occasionally other viruses such as rhinovirus and parainfluenza virus are responsible.[1,3,5] The virus colonises the bronchiolar mucosa causing necrosis of ciliated epithelial cells. Oedema, mucus and debris predispose the bronchioles to blockage. The infant can breathe in but has difficulty exhaling. Hyperinflation of the lungs is a characteristic feature and thus air is trapped in the alveoli, causing inadequate gas exchange and often leading to hypoxaemia and occasionally hypercapnia.[1,3] Diagnosis is based on observation, chest x-ray and immunofluorescent techniques on nasopharyngeal aspirate.

Nursing management

Infants with bronchiolitis are nursed in isolation until the results are obtained from the immunofluorescence of a sample of nasopharyngeal aspirate. The sample is collected by passing a polythene catheter via the nares into the nasopharynx.[5] If these results are positive for respiratory synctial virus, the infant remains in isolation to prevent the spread of infection.[3] Hand washing is of particular importance as the mode of transfer is thought to be by fomite or from hand to hand.[1,3] Oxygen is administered to correct the hypoxaemia which has resulted from impaired gas exchange. The infant is nursed in an oxydome, head box or tent to maintain an optimum concentration of humidified oxygen while the nurse carries out continual clinical assessment.[1,3] All observations and nursing interventions are planned so that interruptions to rest are minimised and unnecessary handling is reduced. Coordination is required as these activities increase oxygen consumption and tire the infant. Oxygen saturations are monitored by pulse oximetry, a non-invasive method of measuring, with oxygen delivery regulated to maintain oxygen saturation above 95%.[1,7] Once the infant's condition improves, oxygen may be delivered by nasal prongs at a maximum rate of 2 L/min and subsequently reduced as the oxygen saturation improves. The infant is observed frequently for signs of increasing distress, including nasal flaring, tracheal tug, intercostal and subcostal retraction, wheezing and cyanosis. Elevating the head of the bed may decrease pressure on the diaphragm and ease the work of breathing. Many of these infants are more comfortable in the prone position. Occasionally, nasopharyngeal suctioning will be required to clear the nasal passages.[3] One to 2% of infants admitted to hospital with bronchiolitis will require assisted ventilation as a result of respiratory fatigue.[1,3,6] Adequate oral hydration may be difficult as the infant becomes physically tired from the increased respiratory effort. Dehydration may occur from increased insensible loss and reduced oral intake. Some infants maintain an adequate intake with smaller, more frequent feeds, others may require intravenous therapy until the respiratory rate is reduced. Once intravenous therapy has corrected any dehydration, the fluid is subsequently administered at 50% maintenance to reduce the risk of fluid overload.[1,3] Antibiotics are not as a rule used in bronchiolitis,[1,3,6] but recently ribavarin, an antiviral agent, has been found to be effective against the respiratory synctial virus.[7] Currently, treatment with this drug is very controversial and only recommended for those who are severely ill or immunocompromised.[8,9] The child is nursed in isolation and the ribavarin is administered by small particle aerosol generator into a head box or tent.[1,10]

Primary caregivers will often need support as they watch their child struggling to breathe. Minimal handling, intravenous and oxygen therapy all contribute to the primary caregiver's feelings of helplessness.[3]

Bronchitis

Bronchitis commonly results from an acute viral respiratory tract infection, causing transient inflammation of the trachea and large bronchi. The primary clinical finding for the first 1 to 2 days is usually a dry cough which later becomes productive, and persists for 1 to 2 weeks. Fever may be present and retrosternal discomfort may be a problem in older children. The child may develop a few coarse crackles and low-pitched wheezes. When symptoms persist a secondary bacterial infection may be present. In a small percentage of children, bronchitis may be severe and associated with alteration to homeostasis. Bronchitis is most frequently caused by rhinovirus, although respiratory synctial virus, influenza, parainfluenza, adenovirus and coxsackie virus have also been isolated. In addition, bronchitis commonly accompanies measles and pertussis.[1,11] Diagnosis is based on sputum collection, viral titres, chest x-ray and the findings of clinical assessment.

Nursing management

Nursing management aims primarily to maximise rest and provide an adequate fluid intake to prevent a fluid volume deficit. Antibiotics are used if a secondary bacterial infection is suspected.[11] Cough mixtures are not recommended as there is no evidence that 'expectorant mixtures' have any useful pharmacological action and cough suppressant mixtures are usually contraindicated in any child with a productive cough. A mixture of honey and lemon juice in warm water may be given for soothing relief.[1,12]

Pneumonia

Pneumonia is an acute inflammation of the alveoli which results in lobar consolidation or an inflammatory infiltration of the interstitial tissue, depending on the causative organism. Often there is an associated inflammatory exudate in the smaller bronchi and bronchioles.[1,13] This illness is a common cause of hospital admissions in infancy and early childhood; it is relatively less frequent in older children.[12]

In children under the age of 4 years, pneumonia is mainly caused by viral infections, the most important agent being the respiratory synctial virus. Influenza, parainfluenza and adenovirus may also be responsible.[1,2,9,11,14] Pneumococcal pneumonia is the primary cause of bacterial pneumonia in infants and very young children, with a peak incidence occurring early in the 2nd year of life.[1,9,15] Older children, especially between the ages of 5 and 15 years, more commonly develop *Mycoplasma pneumonae* pneumonia.[1,9,12,16] The most severe form of pneumonia is caused by *Staphylococcus aureus*, and results in early and extensive pleural effusion and empyema leading to development of pneumatocoeles.[1,9] Beta haemolytic streptococcus and *Haemophylus influenzae* have also been isolated as important causative agents of pneumonia in children,[6,14] while *Pneumocystis carinii* is a leading cause of pneumonia in immunocompromised children.[9]

Symptoms vary greatly depending on the age of the child and the causative agent. Infants and young children often present with non-specific signs such as fever, lethargy, loss of appetite, stiffness of the neck and abdominal pain. In very young infants the only indication of pneumonia may be a rapid sleeping respiratory rate, and in neonates the only indication may be apnoeic episodes, lethargy or loss of interest in feeding.[9] Tachypnoea, respiratory distress, grunting respiration, cyanosis, fever, localised rales and abnormal breath sounds are usually present in children with extensive pneumonia.[9,12,17] Cough may or may not be present. Viral pneumonia frequently has a more gradual onset and less systemic toxicity than bacterial infection, although some adenoviruses can cause a very acute disease, with rapid onset and severe systemic symptoms.[1,6]

Diagnosis is primarily confirmed from the clinical assessment and chest x-ray, but blood may be taken for culture if bacterial infection is suspected. When pleural fluid is present, pleural aspiration may be attempted for culture and antibiotic sensitivity. Nasopharyngeal aspirate, throat swab, stool and urine may be collected for viral studies.[1,2,9,15]

Nursing management

Oxygen is administered via nasal prongs or face mask to improve gaseous exchange and maintain oxygen saturation above 95%. Continuous monitoring is achieved by pulse oximeter or transcutaneous oxygen probes and regular blood gas analysis. The child is observed frequently for signs of increased fever and respiratory distress. Pyrexia can be treated as required with antipyretics and cooling measures such as fanning. Intravenous therapy is frequently required to prevent a fluid volume deficit related to the child's loss of interest in food and fluid. Antibiotic therapy is usually ordered for any child who is moderately or severely ill with pneumonia, as bacterial infection cannot, as a rule, be excluded. Ampicillin, penicillin and flucloxacillin are generally used depending on which bacteria are considered the most likely cause of infection.[2,6,12] Erythromycin is the treatment of choice for *Mycoplasma pneumonae*, while bactrim is used for *Pneumocystis carinii*.[11,12]

Aspiration pneumonia

Subacute and chronic lung disease are often associated with inhalation of food, particularly milk, and other foreign substances into the lower respiratory tract. Milk when inhaled causes an acute inflammatory reaction in the peripheral airways and alveoli. The alveoli are filled with exudate, including large foamy vacuolated macrophages, containing globules of milk. Within a few days the reaction becomes granulomatous and may progress to fibrosis after some weeks. Repeated aspiration leads to chronic interstitial pneumonia, and secondary bacterial infection may occur.[1] Inhalation of large quantities of milk causes serious homeostatic disturbances including high fever, respiratory distress and cyanosis.[1] Sugar solutions, including 5% dextrose, can also cause acute pulmonary oedema and inflammatory changes in the airway and alveoli.[1]

Reflux of gastric contents is the most frequent cause of aspiration pneumonia, although disorders of swallowing and sucking are also common. Rarely, a fine communicating passage develops between the oesophagus and respiratory tract.[1] Cough, fever, tachypnoea, and rattling or wheezy breathing are the common symptoms. On auscultation, wheezes and fine or coarse crackles can be detected, especially posteriorly. Some infants have a 'barrel chest' because of air trapping.[1]

Diagnosis is based on clinical assessment and chest x-ray as well as observation of the infant or child while feeding. The child is clinically examined for structural abnormalities of the mouth, tongue, jaw and palate. The neurological state is assessed to determine the level of motor function and whether there is evidence of cranial nerve palsy, myopathy, or other neurological lesion.[1] Radiological examination of the swallowing mechanism is undertaken using thin barium to determine the degree of spilling into the airway. Prolonged monitoring of lower oesophageal pH to determine the level of gastric acid reflux is often considered to be of more value than barium studies. A milk scan, using radioactive labelled milk and nuclear scanning, can also aid in diagnosis. An endoscopy may be undertaken to look for evidence of oesophagitis or an abnormal anatomical connection between the oesophagus and trachea as an indication of reflux. Additionally, as an aid to diagnosis, tracheal aspirate is examined for fat filled macrophages and free fat globules.[1,18,19]

Nursing management

Care of the child with aspiration pneumonia will be influenced by the cause of the aspiration. If gastro-oesophageal reflux is diagnosed, the child will need to be positioned carefully when lying, and most of these children will benefit by having the head of the bed elevated. Milk feeds thickened with cornflour or carob bean gum are frequently ordered, and care should be taken when winding these infants.[1,18,20] Some infants and children may require medication to aid in reducing the incidence of reflux.[18,21] If reflux is severe, transpyloric feeds may be implemented, until surgical intervention in the form of Nissen fundoplication or gastrostomy is performed.[1,18]

Children with impaired swallowing or sucking reflexes can often be helped with oral stimulation before feeds, and external manipulation of the tongue and jaw. Special feeding methods are successful with some of these children and include placing the food well

Child with gastrostomy tube for feeding.

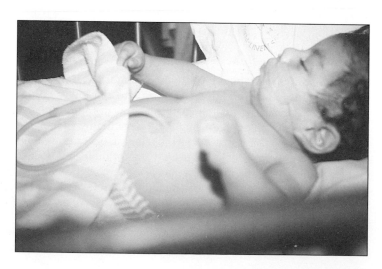

back in the child's mouth and using specially designed cups. The speech pathologist is often involved in developing special techniques, and primary caregivers can be taught these skills to enable them to care more fully for their child. The family's potential for growth will thus be enhanced, as improved knowledge and methods of caring will lead to effective coping skills.[13]

REFERENCES

1. Phelan P, Landau L, Olinsky A. *Respiratory illness in children*. 3rd ed. Oxford: Blackwell Publications, 1990.
2. Stansfield S. Acute respiratory infections in the developing world: strategies for prevention, treatment and control. *Pediatr Infect Dis J* 1987; 6: 622–629.
3. Simkins R. The crises of bronchiolitis. *Am J Nursing* 1981; 81: 514–516.
4. Wong DL. Pain assessment in children. *International Paediatric Nursing Down Under Conference Notes*. Balgowlah: The Medicine Group, 1990: 78–92.
5. Welliver R, Wong D, Sun M, McCarthy N. Parainfluenza virus bronchiolitis. *Am J Dis Childh* 1986; 140: 34–40.
6. Kilham H, ed. *The Children's Hospital Handbook*. Sydney: Alkan Press, 1993.
7. Herzog K, Dunn S, Langham M, Marmon L. Association of parainfluenza virus type 3 infection with allograft rejection in a liver transplant recipient. *Pediatr Infect Dis J* 1989; 8: 534–535.
8. Steele R. Antiviral agents for respiratory infections. *Pediatr Infect Dis J* 1988; 7: 457–461.
9. Peter G. The child with pneumonia: diagnostic and therapeutic considerations. *Pediatric Infect Dis J* 1988; 7: 453–456.
10. Department of Pharmacy, The Hospital for Sick Children. Ribavarin inhalation therapy, policies and drug information sheet for nurses. Toronto: The Hospital, 1990.
11. Gooch M. Bronchitis and pneumonia in ambulatory patients. *Pediatr Infect Dis J* 1987; 6: 137–140.
12. Pinney M. Pneumonia. *Am J Nursing* 1981; 81: 517–518.
13. Mott SR, James SR, Sperhac AM. Nursing care of children and families. Menlo Park: Addison-Wesley, 1990.

PERTUSSIS

Pertussis or whooping cough is a serious, sometimes fatal, bacterial infection of the respiratory tract caused by the Gram-negative bacillus *Bordetella pertussis*.[1-5] The bacilli attach to and multiply in the ciliated epithelial cells, leading to marked decrease in cilial activity and eventually death and sloughing of the cells. The mucosa lining the trachea, bronchi and bronchioles becomes oedematous, and mildly inflamed. Thick tenacious mucus is produced and accumulates in the respiratory tract.[1,4,6-8] *Bordetella pertussis* is endemic in most countries of the world and epidemics occur approximately every 3 to 4 years.[1,4,6,8,9] In Australia, these epidemics tend to occur in summer and last approximately 4 to 5 months.[10,11] The illness is so highly contagious that approximately 70% of unimmunised children will develop pertussis, most of them by their 5th birthday.[4,9] Newborns and infants under 3 months of age are most at risk of severe infection as maternal antibodies to pertussis are not transferred across the placenta.[3,4,12,13] Since the introduction of pertussis vaccination, there has been a dramatic decrease in the incidence of the disease, especially in the 1 to 9 year old age group.[1,3,4,14] There has, however, been an increase in the number of cases reported in children under 1 year and those over 15 years of age.[1,9,15] Transmission of the bacteria is by close contact with respiratory droplets or as a result of handling contaminated articles.[1-3,5] Unimmunised toddlers and school-age children, particularly siblings of an infected child, are the most common source of infection.[4,8,16] There is, however, reason to believe that a growing number of adults are also transmitting the disease.[4,8,14,17] This increase in adults contracting the illness may in part be due to the fact that they were not immunised as children or that their immunity is waning. Another contributing factor is the recent realisation that the illness occurs in adults and consequent increase in diagnosis.[8,12,13,17]

The incubation period lasts from 7 to 20 days, and is followed by symptoms resembling a mild upper respiratory tract infection. This stage is often referred to as the catarrhal or coryzal period. A non-specific irritating cough, transient fever, rhinorrhoea and sneezing may be present.[1-5,18] Within 2 weeks of this initial stage, the cough becomes paroxysmal or spasmodic. The child produces a series of staccato coughs with little or no effective inspiration between each in an effort to remove the thick, tenacious secretion. Following the coughing episode there is a deep inspiration which produces the characteristic whoop as air is inhaled forcefully through vocal cords and glottis that may be partly blocked by secretions or spasm.[1,2,5,8,14] Vomiting frequently occurs after the coughing episode, most likely as a result of secretions collecting in the pharynx.[1,2,8,14] Feeding, another person's cough, disturbances in the environment, suction, or attempted examination of the pharynx may all contribute to the initiation of a paroxysm.[1,8] Each paroxysm may appear to be life threatening to observers and is likely to result in significant hypoxia, especially in young infants.[1,8] At the height of the illness, the child may experience 20 or more paroxysms in 24 hours.[1,8] Frequent periods of cyanosis may occur in the young child as a result of the paroxysms.[2,8,12,13] Most complications and deaths from pertussis occur during this stage.[1] The paroxysmal stage lasts from 1 to 4 weeks, although if severe may last for 6 months or more before resolving, and minor exacerbations may occur with subsequent intercurrent respiratory infections.[1,3,8] The child is considered contagious from 1 week before to approximately 3 weeks after the onset of paroxysms of coughing. The coryzal stage is considered to be the most contagious period.[1,2,18] Diagnosis of pertussis is largely overlooked during this stage unless there is known contact with an infected individual.[3,12] Older children and adults, in addition to the typical syndrome, may display a milder atypical disease which is manifested by a persistent cough associated with lingering tracheobronchitis. The symptoms sometimes persist for weeks and complications may also occur.[1,8,19,20] Many young infants under 6 months of age, and especially those under 3 months of age, do not exhibit the characteristic inspiratory whoop, making it difficult in this group to diagnose the illness.[1,3,12,14] Apnoea as a result of the infection is also a problem in the very young infant and may lead to death.[3,12,21] Hypoxia and secondary pneumonia may also lead to death in this age group.[3]

Complications may occur very occasionally and include secondary bacterial infection leading to pneumonia and bronchopneumonia.[1,4,8] Otitis media is a more frequent infectious complication of the acute disease, especially in infants.[1,8] Severe central nervous system disturbances are rare and occur most commonly in infants as a result of hypoxia or anoxia during the paroxysmal stage.[1,8] Signs and symptoms may include persistent seizures, hemiplegia, paraplegia, ataxia, aphasia, blindness, deafness and decerebrate rigidity.[1] Children who experience central nervous system involvement as a result of pertussis frequently develop permanent sequelae or illness leading to death.[1] The prolonged and forceful expiratory efforts during pertussis paroxysms may lead to hemorrhagic events such as epistaxis, petechiae, and subdural haematoma. Increased pressure may also cause umbilical or inguinal hernias and pneumothorax.[1,8] Uncertainty exists over the length of the immune period after contracting pertussis, as it was thought to be lifelong, but recent research casts doubt on this.[1,3]

Nursing assessment

A nursing history should be completed to identify when the symptoms were first noticed and to determine the frequency and severity of paroxysms. The history should include any loss of appetite, vomiting, disturbed sleeping habits, irritability or anxiousness in the child. Recording the child's immunisation status is also important.[2,7] The child is observed for signs of respiratory distress, such as tachypnoea, nasal flaring, chest recession, tracheal tug, dyspnoea, apnoea and cyanosis. In addition, the hydration status and degree of exhaustion of the child is assessed.[22] The primary caregivers are asked about their concerns, such as fear for the life of child, and fear of brain and lung damage, to determine the level of education required.[22]

Diagnosis is primarily based on observation and is unmistakable in most cases when the typical whooping sound is present.[1,8] Marked leukocytosis and lymphocytosis is evident in blood samples.[1,8,13] Nasopharyngeal specimens, obtained with calcium alginate swabs rather than cotton swabs, may be taken and directly plated onto selective media such as fresh Bordet-Genou medium or Regan-Lowe culture plates.[1,7,16,20]

Nasal secretions may also be collected for immunofluorescence and antibody detection.[15,20] Once the diagnosis is established, it must be reported to the health authorities in all states of Australia.[11]

Implementation of care

Older children are usually cared for at home unless they become extremely cyanosed with the paroxysms or their hydration and nutrition is compromised by vomiting.[2,4,5] Young infants should be hospitalised until it is clear that paroxysmal episodes, apnoea, cyanosis and feeding problems can be safely managed at home.[1,2,4] Once hospitalised, the child will need close observation or monitoring and should be nursed in the lateral position with the head of the cot slightly elevated.[5,8] During coughing episodes the infant should be positioned upright with the nurse supporting the neck or chin.[5] The duration, and a description of the cough should be recorded along with the colour of the child during paroxysms and any bradycardic episodes that may occur. Pulse oximetry is useful to determine the degree of oxygen desaturation.[5] Temperature, pulse and respiratory rate should also be recorded at frequent intervals as tachypnoea and significant fever may indicate secondary bacterial infection.[1] The area in which the child is nursed should be well lit to enable the nurse to make accurate observations.[5] Oral or nasopharyngeal suctioning is contraindicated unless the mucus is causing severe obstruction. The equipment, however, should be readily available.[5,8] Vomiting often follows coughing spasms and may lead to problems with nutrition, hydration, aspiration and weight loss.[2,8,21] Smaller, more frequent feeds or meals are usually well tolerated although some children may require intravenous therapy during the acute period. The child should be weighed daily and an accurate intake and output chart recorded.[5] Strict handwashing is necessary to prevent the spread of infection.[5] Prevention of serious hypoxia is another important consideration, and in hospitalised children oxygen is routinely administered during coughing spasms. Equipment such as bag and mask should be available in case ventilatory assistance is required.[4,8,13,21] In infants with frequent apnoeic episodes, mechanical ventilation may be necessary.[4,13,21]

Antibiotic therapy with erythromycin is frequently given over 10 to 14 days to shorten the period of communicability. The course of the disease, however, is not shortened nor is the severity lessened by the antibiotic.[1-3,5,8] Erythromycin is also given to any contacts of the infected person to prevent or reduce the effects of subsequent pertussis infection.[3,7,8,18] Strict respiratory isolation should be observed for 5 days after starting erythromycin therapy.[1,13] Children who are not receiving antibiotic cover are isolated for 3 weeks after the onset of the paroxysms.[1] Siblings should be excluded from visiting unless they are receiving prophylactic treatment.[5] The affected child should be excluded from school for 2 weeks or until fully recovered.[5,18]

Nursing management is also aimed at educating the primary caregivers so that they understand the cause and normal course of pertussis. Education in such things as maintenance of airway, nutrition and fluid intake and treatment of symptoms enables the primary caregivers to be more confident in the care of their child at home.[2,8]

Prevention

The pertussis vaccine used in most countries of the world today is a whole cell vaccine consisting of a suspension of killed *Bordetella pertussis* bacilli.[3,12] It has been highly effective in reducing the incidence of disease and death due to pertussis.[3,8,23] Substantial epidemics have occurred in countries when the vaccine has been withdrawn due to its possible link with increased encephalopathy.[1,3] In most countries, the pertussis vaccine is given in conjunction with diphtheria and tetanus toxoids. Primary immunisation is carried out with 3 doses of triple antigen at 2 months, 4 months and 6 months, and a booster at 18 months of age.[1,3,6,23] Vaccination for pertussis is not recommended after the child's 7th birthday, as reactions are alleged to increase significantly in older individuals.[1,8,12] Whole cell pertussis vaccines, although generally considered safe, are associated with a variety of adverse reactions including local erythema, swelling and tenderness, fever and other mild systemic events such as drowsiness, irritability and anorexia.[3-5,23] More severe side effects to the vaccine, which occur occasionally, include febrile convulsions and hypotonic–hyporesponsive state. This disorder occurs between 1 and 12 hours after immunisation. Initial symptoms include fever and irritability. The child then becomes pale, limp and unresponsive. Respirations become shallow and cyanosis is frequently present. The duration may be as short as a few minutes or it can persist for days. No adverse long-term effects have been reported.[1,3,8,23] Rarely, central nervous system disorders may occur after vaccination. The estimated rate of occurrence of permanent neurological sequelae that may possibly be related to pertussis immunisation is estimated to be 1 in 310 000 or greater, which is considerably lower than the rate for the actual disease.[1,3,4,8] Paracetamol should be given after immunisation with triple antigen to reduce the risk of fever, especially in children with a family history of seizure or other central nervous disorders.[1,23] Contraindications for pertussis vaccination include the following.

1. A hypersensitive reaction to a previous dose.
2. Fever in excess of 40.5°C up to 48 hours after immunisation.
3. A hypotonic–hyporesponsive episode.
4. Persistent, inconsolable crying which lasts 3 hours or more after immunisation.
5. Convulsions which occur within 3 days of immunisation.
6. Encephalopathy occurring within 7 days of immunisation.[1,4]

Recently, interest has been shown in the development of a new generation of acellular pertussis vaccine. This interest has been stimulated in large part by continued dissatisfaction with the efficacy and safety of traditional whole cell vaccines.[6] New acellular vaccines, which are currently in use in Japan and undergoing trials in the United States, appear to be as effective as whole cell vaccine and cause fewer reactions. It is believed that these acellular vaccines will be of use for booster immunisation in older children and adults. The duration of immunity, safety and effectiveness of the booster administration, however, is as yet unknown.[1,6,8,12,16,23] There is currently a need for booster doses as present-day pertussis vaccines confer only partial and relatively transient protection, which begins to wane after approximately 3 years.[5,12]

REFERENCES

1. Cherry JD, Brunell PA, Golden GS, Karzon DT. Report of the Task Force on Pertussis and Pertussis Immunisation 1988. *Pediatrics* 1988; 81 (Suppl): 939–984.
2. Mott SR, James SR, Sperhac AM. *Nursing care of children and families.* 2nd ed. Menlo Park: Addison-Wesley, 1990.
3. National Health and Medical Research Council. *The Australian immunisation handbook.* 5th Ed. Canberra: AGPS, 1994.
4. Phelan P, Landau L, Olinsky A. *Respiratory illness in children.* 3rd ed. Oxford: Blackwell Publications, 1990.
5. Policy and Procedure Committee. *Staff information — pertussis.* Camperdown: The Children's Hospital, 1990.
6. Fine PE, Clarkson JA. Reflections on the efficacy of pertussis vaccines. *Rev Infect Dis* 1987; 9: 866–881.
7. Long SS, Welkon CJ, Clark JL. Widespread silent transmission of pertussis in families: antibody correlates of infection and symptomatology. *J Infect Dis* 1990; 161: 480–486.
8. Mortimer EA. Pertussis (whooping cough). *In:* Krugman S, Katz SL, Gershon AA, Wilfert CM, eds. *Infectious diseases of children.* 9th ed. St Louis: Mosby Year Book, 1992.
9. Binkin NJ, Salmaso S, Tozzi AE, Scuderi G, Greco D. Epidemiology of pertussis in a developed country with low vaccination coverage: the Italian experience. *Pediatr Infect Dis J* 1992; 11: 653–661.
10. Ashwell M. Pertussis outbreak in Western Australia. *Communicable Diseases Intelligence* 1993; 17: 378–379.
11. Condon R, Ashwell M, Rouse I, Roberts M, Sprague D, eds. Pertussis outbreaks in Western Australia from 1 January 1986 to 31 December 1990. *Communicable Diseases Intelligence* 1992; 16: 494–497.
12. Bass JW, Stephenson SR. The return of pertussis. *Pediatr Infect Dis J* 1987; 6: 141–144.
13. Isaacs D, ed. Nosocomial whooping cough. *Communicable Diseases Intelligence* 1992; 16: 530–531.
14. Herceg A, Mead C, Passaris I, Gordon A. *Bordetella pertussis* in an ACT school: outbreak investigation and vaccine efficacy study. *Communicable Diseases Intelligence* 1993; 17: 284–286.
15. Uren E. Pertussis at Royal Children's Hospital, Melbourne, 1988 to 1991. *Communicable Diseases Intelligence* 1992; 16: 498–499.
16. Onorato IM, Wassilak SG, Meade B. Efficacy of whole-cell pertussis vaccine in preschool children in the United States. *JAMA* 1992; 267: 2745–2749.
17. Mortimer EA. Pertussis and its prevention: a family affair. *J Infect Dis* 1990; 161: 473–479.
18. Kilham H, ed. *The Children's Hospital Handbook.* Sydney: Alken Press, 1993.
19. Editorial. Pertussis: adults, infants and herds. *Lancet* 1992; 339: 526–527.
20. Mertsola J, Kuronen T, Turunen A, Viljanen MK, Ruuskanen O. Diagnosis of pertussis. *J Infection* 1984; 8: 149–156.

21. Gillis J, Grattan-Smith T, Kilham H. Artificial ventilation in severe pertussis. *Arch Dis Childh* 1988; 63: 364–367.
22. Mark A, Granstrom M. Impact of pertussis on the afflicted child and family. *Pediatr Infect Dis J* 1992; 11: 554–557.
23. Recommendations of the Immunisation Practices Advisory Committee. Pertussis vaccination: acellular pertussis vaccine for reinforcing and booster use — supplementary ACIP statement. *Morbidity Mortality Weekly Report* 1992; 41 (No. RR-1): 1–10.

TUBERCULOSIS

Tuberculosis is an infectious disease which through vaccination programs and improved living standards has been controlled although not eradicated.[1] It is prevalent world wide and after a period of decline the incidence is again increasing. Outbreaks in developed countries are occurring, in particular among homeless people, migrants from areas with a high prevalence of tuberculosis and people with acquired immunodeficiency syndrome or human immunodeficiency virus infection.[2-7] In Australia, however, tuberculosis has become comparatively rare and the number of notified new cases has remained fairly constant over the last 5 years.[8] The disease remains a problem in high-risk groups such as Aborigines, and immigrants to Australia from South-east Asia, Central and South America, Africa and the Pacific Islands.[5,8-10]

The organism responsible for tuberculosis is *Mycobacterium tuberculosis*, or rarely *Mycobacterium bovis* bacilli and other atypical mycobacteria.[3,10] Tubercle bacilli are spore forming and have the capacity to remain viable and virulent for extended periods inside or outside the host, provided they are kept in the dark. Death of the bacillus occurs through exposure to ultraviolet rays such as sunlight, or boiling for 1 minute.[1,3,11] Many people infected by mycobacterium tuberculosis do not acquire clinical disease. In these people the presence of antibodies to the organism can be detected.[1,3] Chronic illness, malnutrition, chronic fatigue, any acute illness, or alteration in metabolism or immunity will increase the person's susceptibility to tuberculosis.[1] Infants and young children are very susceptible to the disease, as are young adolescents.[1,3,11-13] Tuberculosis is usually acquired in the home environment before the disease is diagnosed in the primary case.[2,13-16] Initially, the mycobacteria invade the tissue at the site of entry, which is usually the middle or lower lobes of the lungs. The bacilli multiply in this area over a period of 3 weeks to form a small inflammatory lesion.[1,3] Immediately after invading the lung, the bacilli enter the lymphatic system and are transported to the nearest group of lymph nodes, where they proceed to produce inflammatory lesions.[1,3] The degree of inflammatory response at these sites is determined by the number of invading bacilli.[3] Within 3 to 12 weeks of the initial infection, a cellular or humeral immune response is detectable by a skin test.[1,3,11] The immune response causes changes in the lesion and the lesion may even dissolve or disappear. Some phagocytosis of the tubercle bacilli may occur as a result of non-specific cellular resistance, and produces suppuration as well as necrosis in the central section of the lesion. At the same time, bacilli continue to multiply at the edge of the lesion.[3]

This lesion too may spontaneously resolve, or mycobacterium-specific lymphocytes and antibodies may stimulate a fibroblastic reaction at the edge of the lesion. As a result, the lesion becomes encapsulated by fibroblasts and collagen fibres to form a non-caseating granuloma. Finally, hyalinisation and calcification of the lesion occurs.[1,3,12] Viable tubercle bacilli may persist for years in the calcified lesions, especially those in the regional lymph nodes, with the potential for reactivation during periods of decreased host resistance.[1,3] Calcified lesions may be permanent or may begin to be reabsorbed within 3 to 5 years after the initial infection.[12]

Uncomplicated primary infection is usually symptomless and is the most common form of tuberculosis found in infants and young children.[1,3,4,9,11,17] Many primary lesions heal without any evidence of ill health, although in hindsight an infant or child may have shown signs of fretfulness and failure to gain weight in previous weeks.[10] Some children may develop symptoms of a hypersensitivity reaction, including pyrexia, erythema nodosum or phlyctenular conjunctivitis between 6 and 12 weeks after the onset of the infection.[10,12] A cough which lasts for more than two weeks may be present. The cough is at first non-productive and may progress to a mucopurulent cough with occasional blood-streaked secretions.[1,15] Infants and young children may also develop hilar lymph node pressure due to the increased size or the lymph glands may perforate and discharge their contents into the small soft bronchi. This pressure or erosion can result in segmental or lobar collapse and consolidation in the lung, which may resolve without requiring surgery. Resolution is usually a slow process over a period of 4 to 6 months and may occasionally take longer.[10]

An additional complication is the haematogenous dissemination of bacilli resulting in a subclinical bacteraemia and the production of inflammatory lesions throughout the body which may lead to miliary tuberculosis.[1,10,16] This form of tuberculosis is manifested by the acute onset of fever. The child looks extremely ill. Symptoms and signs of local disease may not be evident. Breathlessness, cyanosis, enlarged liver, spleen and lymph nodes, symptoms of meningeal irritation and drowsiness may be present.[1,10] The position and the degree of inflammation of the systemic lesions depends on the number of bacilli which are disseminated and the length of time it takes the host to produce an immune response.[3] Most complications of tuberculosis occur during the 1st year after the onset of the disease and follow on from haematogenous dissemination.[1,3] Tuberculous meningitis is the most severe and is a particular risk in children less than 5 years of age. If it is diagnosed early and chemotherapy is commenced immediately, tuberculous meningitis can almost always be cured.[1,10,18]

After the 1st year, complications are relatively uncommon until adolescence, when the adult form of tuberculosis may develop. This occurs more frequently in girls than boys.[1] The most common site of reactivation is in the lesions of the upper lobes or at the apex of the lower lobes in the lungs.[9] These lesions may also cause obstruction of the bronchus. Air inspiration is less hindered than expiration, causing air entrapment.[1] An additional complication in recent years is the emergence of multiresistant strains of *Mycobacterium tuberculosis* which pose problems for clinical management.[2,5,7,10]

Tuberculosis is usually transmitted by airborne microdroplets, each containing a viable tubercle bacilli, which are expelled from the respiratory tract of a person with active pulmonary tuberculosis.[10] Every time the infected person coughs, sneezes, sings, laughs, shouts or talks, virulent tubercle bacilli are released into the air.[3,10,11] The droplets, which must be small enough to pass the bronchial mucosal defences, are then inhaled into the alveoli of the host lung.[3,10,11] Household contacts, particularly young children, are extremely susceptible to inhaling the infected droplets. Any adult, adolescent or older child who has active pulmonary tuberculosis is an infection risk.[3] The person remains infectious until the sputum and gastric secretions are negative for tubercle bacilli. Some people remain intermittently contagious for years, even though there are demonstrable areas of calcification indicating that at least partial healing has occurred.[1,3,11] Children with non-progressive pulmonary tuberculosis are not usually considered to be contagious.[1] Non-pulmonary disease is also as a rule non-infectious.[10]

Nursing assessment

The nursing history should include any previous positive skin test or BCG (Bacillus Calmette Guerin) vaccination and any immunosuppression or chronic disease in the child. Any history of exposure to tuberculosis in family members is also recorded. A background of contact with an adult or older child who has tuberculosis should lead immediately to the child being tested.[1] The primary caregivers are asked whether the child has displayed any weight loss, anorexia, generalised weakness or fatigue. Low-grade fever with chills and night sweats, although common only in patients with advanced disease, may be present and if so are included in the history.[1,10,15] The nurse determines whether the child has been coughing, how long the cough has been present and whether it is productive or non-productive. The child is observed for signs of tachycardia, fever and pain or difficulty on breathing. The current nutrition and hydration status are also noted.[3,11] Questions should be asked and the child examined to exclude tuberculosis in other organs or systems.[10]

Diagnosis is based on sputum cultures, which are normally positive for mycobacteria within 2 to 3 weeks of active disease. In young children sputum is difficult to obtain.[15] Tuberculosis is often confirmed in this younger age group through culture of gastric contents collected by gastric lavage or nasogastric aspiration. The gastric specimens are collected over 3 consecutive days, preferably first thing in the morning before breakfast.[1,10] Tubercle bacilli are frequently found in gastric contents from children with tuberculosis because they swallow sputum rather than expectorate it.[1,4,11,15,18] The tubercle bacilli stains positive for acid fastness with the Ziehl-Neelson test and appears as a brilliant red, slender rod under microscopy.[1,3,10,15,16]

Skin testing for hypersensitivity with an intradermal injection of tuberculin purified protein derivative (PPD) such as the Mantoux test is carried out in children suspected of mycobacterial infection. The test is normally read within 48 to 72 hours.[3,9,13,15,18] A positive reaction often indicates a past natural infection, but it may also indicate a past BCG vaccination.[10,17] Increase in skin reaction above 10 mm in diameter or above 15 mm when there is a BCG scar indicates recent infection.[1,3,4,10,15,17] Chest x-ray is also used for diagnostic purposes, although it is often negative for primary tuberculosis in children.[10,15] Computed tomography scanning is often more diagnostically accurate.[15,16] Bronchoscopy, bronchial washing and tissue culture may be employed to obtain a positive result for mycobacterium tuberculosis.[1,3,15] When pleural effusion is present as a result of suspected tuberculosis, pleural needle biopsy may be carried out and is normally positive for tuberculous granulomas.[3,19] Tuberculosis is a notifiable disease and once the diagnosis is made, should be notified to the relevant state health department.[10]

Implementation of care

Medication is the first line of treatment with isoniazid and rifampicin being considered the essential and most effective drugs used in anti-tuberculosis therapy. These drugs are frequently combined with other drugs such as ethambutol, pyrazinamide and streptomycin.[2-4,10,11,6] Isoniazid and rifampicin are administered throughout the 6 months of treatment with supplemental pyrazinamide being given as well for at least 2 months. Ethambutol is rarely used in children. If a further drug is required, streptomycin is the drug of choice.

Occasionally, isoniazid and rifampicin will be continued for a period of 9 to 12 months.[10] Corticosteroids may be added if tuberculous meningitis is present.[10]

Once the illness and drug therapy have been stabilised, most children can be cared for at home with regular outpatient visits.[3] The child should be monitored for compliance with drug therapy, side effects and response.[3,5,10] Drug reactions such as skin rash, peripheral neuropathy, nausea, jaundice and dizziness will require immediate attention.[3,10] Monthly sputum checks are carried out until the sputum is negative for mycobacteria.[10] Temperature, pulse and respiration are checked on a regular basis to monitor any change which may indicate a complication of primary tuberculosis. Isolation of the child should be observed until antimicrobial therapy is successfully initiated. As a rule, 2 to 3 weeks provides sufficient antimicrobial cover to prevent sputum-positive patients from spreading tuberculosis to others. The close contacts of the child are examined and tested to identify persons with active disease and other people who may be at risk of infection.[1,3,10,11,17]

Primary caregivers are educated in how to care for the child at home, including correct disposal of tissues, hanging clothes and bed linen in the sun to dry, sterilisation of eating utensils by boiling or prolonged heat and using good handwashing techniques and hygiene.[3,10,11] Education is also given on the need for good nutrition and fluid intake.[1,3,11] The primary caregivers should also be aware that the child will need adequate rest and protection from other people with infections, as any acute infection or alteration in physiology, immunity or metabolism will expose the child to increasing risk of complications.[1,11] Repeated education and reassurance of the child and family is necessary to ensure the compliance, which is essential for continued care.[10]

Prevention

Isoniazid therapy is given for 1 year to recent converters and close household contacts of persons with active pulmonary tuberculosis.[1-3,10,11] At the completion of this 12-month period, a repeat chest x-ray and skin test are carried out.[10] Neonates delivered to mothers with active pulmonary tuberculosis should be offered prophylactic isoniazid until the mother's sputum is culture-negative. The infant should then be tested to ascertain that there is no infection. If found to be negative, the neonate is given a BCG vaccination unless parental permission is withheld.[10] BCG vaccination is also given to children and infants who are at high risk for contact with active cases and who are skin test negative and not immunosuppressed. Immunosuppressed children are most susceptible to death from rapidly progressive infection.[9,11,14]

The BCG vaccine is made from a live attenuated strain of *Mycobacterium bovis*.[10] It is administered by injecting 0.1 mL of vaccine intradermally. In infants the dose should be reduced to 0.05 mL. Skin testing is carried out 6 to 8 weeks later to evaluate the success of the vaccine in conferring immunity. Contraindications to vaccination include acute illness, septic skin conditions and immunodeficiency or malignant disease involving bone marrow or lymphoid systems. Children receiving corticosteroids, immunosuppressive drugs or irradiation and skin test positive people should also not receive the vaccine.[9,10] A past positive skin test or BCG vaccination does not always confer lifelong immunity.[9]

REFERENCES

1. Kendig EL, Chernik V. *Disorders of the respiratory tract in children.* 5th ed. Philadelphia: WB Saunders, 1990.

2. Clinical Briefs. Tuberculosis update. *Am Family Physician* 1992; 46 (Suppl): 100S–102S.
3. Grimes DE, Grimes RM, Hamelink M. *Infectious diseases*. St. Louis: Mosby Year Book, 1991.
4. Khouri YF, Mastrucci MT, Hutto C, Mitchell CD, Scott GB. Mycobacterium tuberculosis in children with human immunodeficiency virus type 1 infection. *Pediatr Infect Dis J* 1992; 11: 950–955.
5. Pang SC, Clayton AS, Harrison RH. Culture-positive tuberculosis in Western Australia. *Aust N J Med* 1992; 22: 109–113.
6. Rieder HL. Misbehaviour of a dying epidemic: a call for less speculation and better surveillance. *Tubercle Lung Disease* 1992; 73: 181–182.
7. Watson JM. Tuberculosis in Britain today. *BMJ* 1993; 306: 221–222.
8. Cheah D. Tuberculosis notification rates, Australia, 1991. *Communicable Diseases Intelligence* 1992; 16: 398–400.
9. National Health and Medical Research Council. *The Australian immunisation procedures*. 5th ed. Canberra: AGPS, 1994.
10. Patel A, Streeton J. *Tuberculosis in Australia and New Zealand into the 1990's*. Canberra: AGPS, 1990.
11. Mott SR, James SR, Sperhac AM. *Nursing care of children and families*. 2nd ed. Menlo Park: Addison-Wesley, 1990.
12. Behrman RE, Kliegman RM, Nelson WE, Vaughan VC, eds. *Nelson textbook of pediatrics*. 14th ed. Philadelphia: WB Saunders, 1992.
13. Schutze GE, Rice TD, Starke JR. Routine tuberculin screening of children during hospitalisation. *Pediatr Infect Dis J* 1993; 12: 29–32.
14. Citron KM. BCG vaccination against tuberculosis: international perspectives. *BMJ* 1993; 306: 222–223.
15. Migliori GB, Borghesi A, Rossanigo P, Adriko C, Neri M, Santini S, et al. Proposal of an improved score method for the diagnosis of pulmonary tuberculosis in childhood in developing countries. *Tubercle Lung Disease* 1992; 73: 145–149.
16. The Children's Hospital Camperdown. Extrapulmonary tuberculosis. *Monthly Infectious Diseases Report* 1991; 23 (Sept.): 1–7.
17. Veen J. Microepidemics of tuberculosis: the stone in the pond principle. *Tubercle Lung Disease* 1992; 73: 73–76.
18. Berman S, Kibel MA, Fourie PB, Strebel PM. Childhood tuberculosis and tuberculous meningitis: high incidence rates in the Western Cape of South Africa. *Tubercle Lung Disease* 1992; 73: 349–355.
19. The Children's Hospital Camperdown. Pleural effusion. *Monthly Infectious Diseases Report* 1992; 29 (March): 1–2.

Disturbances in Blood Volume, Pressure and Flow

Carmel McQuellin

Inflammatory Diseases of the Heart

The inflammatory diseases of the heart (rheumatic and non-rheumatic) occurring in children are uncommon, yet important from a nursing perspective. The following discussion briefly reviews the inflammatory and infective processes affecting the heart namely, infective endocarditis, myocarditis, pericarditis, Kawasaki syndrome and acute rheumatic fever. These processes cause varying degrees of debilitation to the infant or child because of the myocardial dysfunction that develops.

INFECTIVE ENDOCARDITIS

Infective endocarditis (IE) is a potentially life-threatening inflammation of the endocardium, heart valves and the endothelial lining of the vasculature.[1] The susceptibility to IE of infants and children with structural heart defects is well documented. Recent research links immunodeficiency with congenital heart disease in 25% of children.[1-4] The risk of IE is increased after cardiac surgery, especially where prosthetic material has been implanted, for example with valve replacements and grafts, and following invasive cardiac procedures.

Nursing assessment

Children present with fever and generalised symptoms of malaise, headache, muscular tenderness and joint pain. Petechial lesions are common and may result from microemboli. Embolisation of vegetations from the left heart into the central nervous system may result in significant debilitation with renal emboli causing haematuria and renal impairment, whereas emboli from the right heart may result in pulmonary embolus.[2,5]

Pathophysiology

Recently, with increased use of invasive monitoring in the neonatal period an increased incidence of IE has been reported in critically ill newborn infants without associated structural heart defects.[6,7] Invasive monitoring catheters cause damage to the endothelium on which the bacteria can develop and grow.

The factors responsible for the development of IE include bacteraemia in combination with the shunting of blood across a defect at an intracardiac or extracardiac level. The jet lesion which results causes turbulence in the blood flow and damage to the endocardium or the endothelial lining of the heart or great vessel.[1,2] Platelets and fibrin adhere to the damaged surface and enmesh to form a thrombus which harbours the organism in its fibres.[1,6] The organisms become encased in a fibrin mass, form vegetations on valve leaflets and may invade the myocardium, destroying the tissue. The vegetations are protected by a fibrin barrier that resists phagocytic leucocytes and antimicrobial preparations.[1,8]

Alpha haemolytic streptococcus is the most common organism causing IE in children, with a 41% incidence. This organism is responsible for the subacute symptoms and an insidious onset. The organisms responsible for severe and acute illness are *Staphlococcus aureus* (affecting 25% of neonates and children), *Streptococcus pneumonia* and beta haemolytic streptococcus.[1,6]

Treatment

Diagnosis is confirmed by positive blood cultures and visualisation of the vegetations on two-dimensional echocardiography. Therapeutic intervention requires the administration of parenteral bacteriocidal preparations for a period of 4 to 6 weeks. Long-term antibiotic regimens necessitate administration via central venous access, using a strict aseptic technique.[5]

Surgical intervention is indicated in children with worsening cardiac failure due to valvular involvement and in those who suffer from embolic events.[1] The outcome is dependent on the micro-organism, the drug sensitivity and the possibility of surgical clearance of the offending tissue. There is a mortality rate of up to 40% for children contracting IE from *Staphlococcus aureus*.[4]

Implications for nursing

Heightened awareness of the mechanisms responsible for the inflammation and infection are essential. The psychosocial effects of prolonged hospitalisation and regular treatment regimens hold major implications for nursing care. Due to the risk of bacteraemia associated with dental procedures or surgery, children with structural heart disease are given prophylactic antibiotic cover to reduce the risks of systemic infection and to minimise IE.[5,9] From an educational viewpoint, nurses fulfil an important role in reassuring and advising parents of the children's need for prophylactic antibiotic cover at times of increased bacteraemic risk.

MYOCARDITIS

Myocarditis is an inflammatory disease affecting the heart muscle. It may present in children as an acute, subacute or chronic illness.[10] Viruses are the common causative agents of myocarditis, dominated by the coxsackie virus, influenza, rubella and the ECHO viruses. Less commonly, the inflammation may result from bacterial, rickettsial, spirochaetal or protozoal infections.[11] Rheumatic myocarditis is discussed separately.

Nursing assessment

The diverse clinical presentation of children with viral myocarditis makes definitive diagnosis difficult, as the effects upon the heart may be masked by the viral effects upon other body systems. Various factors determine the degree of myocardial involvement and include the nature of the viral agent, the age and sex of the child, the immune response of the child and the host-genetic interaction. A fetus who contracts viral myocarditis *in utero* presents with congestive cardiomyopathy within days of birth. In contrast, the older infant or child may present with a history of generalised viral symptoms over a period of several days. Exclusion of myocarditis is warranted when signs of cardiac involvement are detected. These signs include an increase in heart rate, gallop rhythm, tachypnoea and dyspnoea associated with other signs of cardiac failure. Children who present with an acute onset of myocarditis experience severe respiratory distress and exhibit the clinical signs of shock. Of the children who recover from the acute illness, a significant number may develop congestive cardiomyopathy.[8,11,12]

Treatment and nursing implications

Supportive measures are the only options available to care for children with acute viral myocarditis. Support may include the use of anti-arrhythmic preparations to control dysrhythmias, diuretics, inotropes and vasodilator preparations for support of myocardial function and ventilation when cardiorespiratory compromise is evident. Extreme caution is essential in the nursing assessment of these children as sudden cardiovascular collapse is a characteristic feature of the illness.[5,10,11]

Bed rest is essential during the acute phase of illness, as research indicates that exercise results in an overwhelming increase in virulence and proliferation of the coxsackie virus. The use of immunosuppressive agents for the treatment of viral myocarditis is not without controversy, although the literature indicates the use of steroids and azathioprine have improved the outcome in selected patients.[11]

PERICARDITIS

Pericarditis is a potentially life-threatening condition due to inflammation of the parietal and visceral pericardium. Commonly, pericarditis is attributed to bacterial or viral infections. Several other causes have been documented, such as collagen diseases like rheumatoid arthritis, rheumatic fever, uraemia and radiation therapy of mediastinal masses.[2,9,11]

Nursing assessment and intervention

Children present with a history of upper respiratory tract infection, low-grade fever and chest pain. On clinical examination, a pericardial friction rub is often detected. When the pericardial fluid is purulent the children appear toxic, have a high fever and are often dyspnoeic.[2,9] The diagnosis is confirmed by two-dimensional echocardiography.

Pathophysiology

Inflammation and infection of the pericardium imposes significant haemodynamic consequences as a result of either pericardial fluid accumulation or the fibrosis of pericardium causing restrictive pericarditis. When fluid accumulates rapidly in the pericardium the intra-pericardial pressure is increased. This impedes the diastolic filling of the ventricles, resulting in decreased cardiac output, and constitutes cardiac tamponade. In contrast, when pericardial fluid accumulates slowly, the 'intact' myocardium accommodates the increase in pericardial pressure and the pericardium stretches to accommodate the fluid accumulation. The cardiac output in this circumstance remains essentially unaltered.[2,11]

During cardiac tamponade, the body initially compensates by increasing the heart rate to maintain cardiac output. The venous pressure increases to augment ventricular filling and initiates a potent sympathetic nervous system response by stimulating vasomotor tone which increases vasoconstriction and reverses any hypotension.[2,11] Once tamponade is diagnosed and confirmed by echocardiography, it has to be relieved urgently. The reader is referred to the discussion on cardiac tamponade included in Chapter 11.

Treatment and nursing implications

The treatment of choice for purulent pericarditis is intravenous antibiotics and surgical drainage of the pericardium, undertaken through the creation of a pericardial window, and insertion of a pleural drain.[8] High doses of antibiotics are generally required for 4 to 6 weeks. The treatment of viral pericarditis in children is supportive. Bed rest is imposed and anti-inflammatory preparations are administered with additional analgesic medication required for relief of the chest pain. Use of steroids is controversial, with reports indicating rebound effects once treatment is withdrawn.[11]

KAWASAKI DISEASE
(Mucocutaneous lymph node syndrome)

Kawasaki disease is an acute inflammatory process of unknown aetiology which causes a vasculitis in many of the body systems, including the cardiovascular system.

Nursing assessment

Kawasaki disease usually affects young children and presents as a generalised febrile illness with persistently high fever of at least 5 days' duration.[2,11,13] The children have associated skin rashes, cervical lymphadenopathy, conjunctival changes, skin changes of the hands and feet and redness of the oral mucosa.[9,11,14]

Pathophysiology

There are a number of cardiovascular problems associated with Kawasaki disease. Aneurisms develop in the coronary arteries in up to 25% of children, which may lead to scarring, calcification and coronary artery insufficiency, dilatation and hypertrophy of the heart, acute myocardial infarction and unexpected collapse.[2,9,11,13]

Treatment

Treatment is supportive, requiring the use of anti-inflammatory agents (usually aspirin) and anti-thrombotic preparations.[11] The intravenous administration of gammaglobulin remains controversial, with disagreement over its efficiency in reducing the incidence of coronary artery lesions.[13]

ACUTE RHEUMATIC FEVER

Acute rheumatic fever (ARF) is considered the most common cause of acquired heart disease in children between the ages of 6 and 15 years. Currently, a resurgence of the disease, not confined to developing countries, is being experienced.[1]

Group A streptococcus is the agent responsible for the development of pharyngitis. In susceptible children there is a dormant period of several weeks, following which symptoms of inflammation develop affecting various organ systems including the heart, brain, joints and skin. The subsequent damage is a result of an immune response to the streptococcus.[15,16]

Nursing assessment

The clinical presentation of these children is varied and may include any or all of the following symptoms, making definitive diagnosis elusive. Arthritis is the most common symptom occurring in up to 70% of the children and is associated with fever and tachycardia. Carditis, macular skin rashes, Sydenham's chorea and arthralgia are also frequently seen.[15,16]

Pathophysiology

The inflammatory process affects connective or collagen tissue, explaining the clinical findings of rheumatic carditis. All the cardiac valves may become involved although mitral valve involvement is the most frequent complication associated with ARF, pulmonary valve involvement being quite rare. The early phase of the endocarditis causes valvular insufficiency with persistent inflammation resulting in valvular fibrosis and calcification.[15]

Treatment and nursing implications

Treatment consists of penicillin for eradication of the causative organism followed by penicillin prophylaxis for extended periods of time, generally over many years. When there is valvular involvement, prophylaxis continues until adulthood and throughout life in susceptible populations.[16]

Salicylates are administered as the treatment of choice due to their anti-inflammatory properties, but steroids are administered when the salicylates fail to control the carditis. Bed rest is encouraged for the duration of the acute inflammatory process and may be required for a period ranging from weeks to several months. Anti-failure medication may also be required and strict attention is paid to the diet to minimise the sodium intake.[16]

Outcome following acute rheumatic fever

The long-term outcome depends on the degree of cardiac involvement at the time of presentation and the effectiveness in preventing recurrence.[15,16] Of the clinical effects outlined, only the carditis is associated with long-term sequelae. The arthritis dissipates within days to weeks of the illness and the chorea subsides within several months causing no neurological deficit.[16]

Eradication of ARF remains a primary health care issue, reliant upon self-reporting of streptococcal throat infections. Primary prevention must be the goal of care with educational programs conducted to inform the general public of the devastating effects that can occur from an essentially preventable disease process.

An increased involvement of nursing personnel in primary health care programs that are aimed at control and eventual eradication of ARF is essential. Heightened awareness of the aetiology of the disease, the mode of spread and the risk factors are required in the fight for elimination of this disease.

The inflammatory and infective problems which affect the myocardium of infants and children cause cardiac failure, often resulting in severe deterioration of the clinical status. For a detailed discussion of the nursing assessment and management principles surrounding cardiac failure in infancy and childhood the reader is referred to Chapter 11.

REFERENCES

1. Kaplan EL, Shulman ST. Endocarditis. *In:* Adams FH, Emmanoulides GC, Riemenschneider TA, eds. *Moss' heart disease in infants, children and adolescents.* 4th ed. Baltimore: Williams and Wilkins, 1989: 718–730.
2. Park Myung K. *Pediatric cardiology for practitioners.* 2nd ed. Chicago: Year Book Medical, 1988: 226–237.
3. Radford DJ, Thong YH. The association between immunodeficiency and congenital heart disease. *Pediatric Cardiology* 1988; 9: 103–108.
4. Sholler GF, Hawker RE, Celermajer JM. Infective endocarditis in childhood. *Paediatric Cardiology* 1986; 6: 183–186.
5. Hazinski MF. Cardiovascular disorders. *In:* Hazinski MF, ed. *Nursing care of the critically ill child.* 2nd ed. St Louis: Mosby, 1992: 117–394.
6. Millard DD, Shulman ST. The changing spectrum of neonatal endocarditis. *Clinics Perinatology* 1988; 15: 587–608.
7. Snider AR. Two-dimensional and doppler echocardiographic valuation of heart disease in the neonate and fetus. *Clinics Perinatology* 1988; 15: 523–564.
8. Cantor RM. Cardiac infections in infancy and childhood. *Topics Emergency Med* 1990; 12: 30–41.

9. Flynn PA, Engle MA, Ehlers KH. Cardiac issues in the pediatric emergency room. *Pediatric Clinics North Am* 1992; 39: 955–983.

10. Bonadio WA, Losek JD. Infants with myocarditis presenting with severe respiratory distress and shock. *Pediatric Emergency Care* 1987; 3: 110–113.

11. Noren GR, Staley NA, Kaplan EL. Nonrheumatic inflammatory diseases. *In:* Adam FH, Emmanoulides GC, Riemenschneider TA, eds. *Moss' heart disease in infants, children and adolescents.* 4th ed. Baltimore: Williams and Wilkins, 1989: 730–748.

12. Werner NP. Congestive heart failure: pathophysiology and management throughout infancy. *J Perinatal Neonatal Nursing* 1993; 7: 59–76.

13. Newburger JW, Sanders SP, Burns JC, Parness IA, Beiser AS, Colan SD. Left ventricular contractility and function in Kawasaki syndrome. *Circulation* 1989; 79: 1237–1246.

14. Baker A. Acquired heart disease in infants and children. *Crit Care Nursing Clin North Am* 1994; 6 (1): 175–186.

15. Ayoub EM. Acute rheumatic fever. *In:* Adams FH, Emmanoulides GC, Riemenschneider TA, eds. *Moss' heart disease in infants, children and adolescents.* 4th ed. Baltimore: Williams and Wilkins, 1989: 692–704.

16. Park Myung K. Acute rheumatic fever. *In:* Park Myung K. *Pediatric cardiology for practitioners.* 2nd ed. Chicago: Year Book Medical, 1988: 238–244.

Disturbances in Neurological Function

Angela M Jones

Inflammatory Brain Disease

Meningitis is inflammation of the meninges, the protective coverings of the brain and spinal cord. In cases of bacterial meningitis, the causative agent is a bacterial pathogen. Aseptic meningitis, also known as viral, non-bacterial or non-purulent meningitis, refers to an inflammatory process without evidence of a bacterial pathogen in the cerebrospinal fluid.[1]

BACTERIAL MENINGITIS

The incidence of bacterial meningitis is greatest during childhood. Approximately two-thirds of cases occur in children under 15 years of age and, of these, 80% occur in the first 5 years of life.[2] Neonates and children between 6 and 12 months of age are at the greatest risk for bacterial meningitis. Bacterial meningitis remains a serious threat to life in the paediatric population.[3] Early diagnosis and intervention are essential if significant morbidity and mortality are to be avoided.

The most common pathogens found in children with bacterial meningitis are:

Children under 1 month of age

- Group B streptococcus
- *Escherichia coli*
- *Listeria monocytogenes.*

Children over 3 months of age

- *Haemophilus influenza* type B
- *Neisseria meningitidis*
- *Streptococcus pneumoniae.*

Group B streptococcus accounts for most cases of bacterial meningitis in infants during the newborn period. The organism is acquired through contact with the mother's genital tract or bowel flora or from the hands of hospital personnel in the nursery. Children between 1 and 3 months of age are in a 'transitional stage'. They may be infected by organisms commonly found both in newborns and in children beyond 3 months of age. Beyond the newborn period, the incidence of bacterial meningitis is highest in the 3 to 8 month old period, and remains high until 2 years of age. The incidence declines after 2 years of age.

Pathophysiology

Direct extension of a bacterial infection in a site adjacent to the meninges such as the ear, sinuses or mastoids is responsible for only a small percentage of cases of bacterial meningitis.[4] The causative agent usually enters the central nervous system by way of the systemic circulation. Access via the cranial and peripheral nerves is also possible.

The development of bacterial meningitis usually follows 4 steps.[5]

1. Infection of the upper respiratory tract.
2. Invasion of the blood by the pathogen.
3. Seeding of the meninges by the blood-borne organism.
4. Inflammation of the meninges and the brain.

Other causes of meningitis include penetrating injuries, skull fracture, ventriculostomy catheters, cerebral abscess, encephalitis and neurosurgical procedures.

In cases of bacterial infection, formation of an exudate and an increase in the white blood cell count account for the cloudy appearance of the CSF. Inflammation of the meninges alters the permeability of the blood–brain barrier, leading to the development of cerebral oedema.[5] Hydrocephalus may be caused by aqueduct stenosis, meningeal scarring or obstruction of the arachnoid villi. Petechial haemorrhage leads to cerebral ischaemia and permanent neurological deficit. If hydrocephalus and cerebral oedema are present they will markedly increase the child's intracranial pressure.

Clinical presentation

The clinical presentation of meningitis frequently follows 1 of 2 patterns. In the 1st, the course is insidious with symptoms progressing over 1 to several days. The child may have a recent history of a non-specific febrile illness. In the 2nd pattern, symptoms of acute meningitis develop rapidly within a few hours. Cerebral oedema may be severe and cause herniation, brainstem compression and death in some children.

Signs and symptoms of bacterial meningitis are as follows.

Infants

- Fever
- Pallor
- Vomiting

- Lethargy
- Irritability
- Poor feeding/sucking
- Inability of parents to calm child
- Full or tense fontanelle
- Seizures
- Toxic or septic appearance
- Poor muscle tone.

Children over 3 years

- Headache
- Fever
- Neck stiffness
- Vomiting
- Delirium
- Impaired consciousness.

Meningitis may also cause pain and inflammation of the spinal nerves and their roots. The child may manifest the following signs of meningeal irritation.

- Nuchal rigidity — the child immobilises the neck and resists flexion of the neck.
- Kernig's sign — the child is placed in the supine position, the hip is flexed at a 90° angle, extension of the leg at the knee causes back pain.
- Brudzinski's sign — the child is placed in the supine position, passive flexion of the neck causes involuntary flexion of the hips and knees.

These signs are rarely seen in an infant. In many instances, the signs of meningitis may be non-specific, especially in neonates and infants. In a paediatric population, it may be difficult to distinguish between the signs and symptoms of meningitis and an uncomplicated febrile illness.

Diagnosis

A diagnosis of meningitis is confirmed by lumbar puncture. Lumbar puncture is contraindicated in the presence of raised intracranial pressure with cerebral herniation, a significant change in level of consciousness or focal neurological deficit. The signs of cerebral herniation may include a change in pupil size, a bulging fontanelle and irregular breathing. In this instance, blood and urine cultures are taken.

Nursing care

Aggressive antibiotic therapy is begun as soon as a diagnosis of bacterial meningitis is reached. In some cases the child's condition mandates that antibiotics be given in the absence of a lumbar puncture. The mainstay of current antimicrobial therapy in cases of bacterial meningitis in Australia is the 3rd generation cephalosporins. These drugs are broad-spectrum and cover the 3 most common causes of meningitis. Therapy continues until the results of CSF culture are known.

Supportive therapies consist of fluid replacement and anticonvulsant therapy when indicated. The use of high-dose steroids, such as intravenous dexamethasone, remains controversial.

Table 5.1 Comparison of cerebrospinal fluid analysis in aseptic and bacterial meningitis

Cerebrospinal fluid	Aseptic meningitis	Bacterial meningitis
Cerebrospinal	Aseptic meningitis	Bacterial meningitis
Pressure	Normal or slightly elevated	Elevated
Leucocytes ($\times 10^6$/ml) (Normal < 5)	< 10–100s	1000s
Protein (g/L) (Normal < 0.4)	Normal to slightly increased	Increased
Glucose (mmol/L) (Normal ≥ 2.5 or ≥ 50% blood level)	Normal	Decreased
Appearance	Clear	Cloudy

The child's neurological observations are carefully monitored along with the anterior fontanelle and head circumference in infants. An alteration in level of consciousness may indicate increasing intracranial pressure. The child is nursed in a quiet, dim environment and allowed to assume a position of comfort. Many children are especially sensitive to bright lights and noise during the acute phase of the disease. Minimal handling is employed to reduce agitation and increase comfort.

The child is observed for any signs of seizure activity. Cot sides and padding are used to ensure the child's safety in the event of a seizure. Oxygen and suction should be available at the bedside at all times. The child's fluid intake and urine output are monitored carefully. Fluids may be restricted in the presence of cerebral oedema. The intravenous infusion should be closely observed for signs of infiltration as many antibiotics are irritating to veins.

Upon discharge, the child's parents or primary caregivers should be advised to contact their doctor or return to the hospital if there is any change in the child's condition. This applies especially to children discharged from an emergency centre with a febrile illness. Changes in the child's behaviour and feeding patterns may be indicative of deterioration. Parents of children with meningitis due to haemophilus B bacteria should observe other siblings closely. They should seek medical advice immediately should these children become unwell.

ASEPTIC MENINGITIS AND ENCEPHALITIS

Aseptic meningitis may be caused by a number of non-bacterial agents. In children, these generally include but are not limited to arboviruses and enteroviruses. Aseptic meningitis and encephalitis may be associated with other diseases such as measles, mumps and herpes. In most cases of aseptic meningitis, the offending agent is not identified in the CSF in spite of extensive laboratory investigations. Enteroviruses are suspected to cause almost 80% of known cases. The time of year may be a consideration as some viral agents show a seasonal prevalence.

The onset of aseptic meningitis may be abrupt or gradual. The child may present with headache, fever, gastrointestinal disturbances and signs of meningeal irritation. The symptoms usually subside over 7 to 10 days without any residual effects. Treatment of aseptic meningitis is symptomatic. Antibiotic therapy may be instigated until a diagnosis of bacterial meningitis is ruled out.

Encephalitis is defined as an inflammatory process of the brain; however, many children with this disorder also have evidence of meningeal involvement.[6] Many of the organisms found in aseptic meningitis are also responsible for encephalitis. The course of the disease, however, is usually acute and the consequences may be devastating for the child and family. Death or recovery with permanent neurological deficit are possibilities.

The child may present with a focal neurological deficit, such as a hemiparesis. Language deficits, ataxia and sensory disturbances may also occur. The clinical presentation varies according to the area of the brain invaded by the offending agent.The cardinal feature of encephalitis is an alteration in the child's level of consciousness or behaviour.[2] This may be accompanied by neck stiffness.

Treatment consists of supportive measures. Cases of herpes simplex encephalitis may be treated with the drug acyclovir.

REYE'S SYNDROME

Reye's syndrome is characterised by toxic encephalopathy with hepatic dysfunction. Typically, the child has a recent history of viral illness a few days before the onset of signs and symptoms of encephalopathy.[7] The child presents with protracted vomiting, fever, impaired liver function, lethargy and agitation, which rapidly proceed to coma.[8] Intracranial pressure increases due to the presence of cerebral oedema.

Characteristically, the liver is fatty and enlarged. Laboratory tests reveal an elevated serum ammonia level due to a reduction in the enzymes which convert ammonia to urea. Transaminase levels are also elevated. The CSF may have a reduced glucose content but is otherwise normal.[2]

Early diagnosis and aggressive therapy are essential in preventing serious sequelae from Reye's Syndrome.[9] Whilst the exact aetiology of the condition is unknown, it often develops following infection with the influenza or varicella virus. In recent years an association between aspirin administration and Reye's syndrome has also been suggested.[10] Families should be educated about over-the-counter products which may contain aspirin. These products should be avoided in children with influenza-like symptoms.

REFERENCES

1. Benchot R. Aseptic meningitis in children. *Adv Clin Care* 1991; 6 (3): 7–12.
2. Robinson MJ, Gilbert GL. Meningitis and encephalitis in infancy and childhood. *In:* Robinson MJ, Roberton DM, eds. *Practical paediatrics* 3rd ed. Melbourne: Churchill Livingstone, 1994: 291–299.
3. Vulcan BM. Acute bacterial meningitis in infancy and childhood. *Critical Care Nurse* 1987; 7 (5): 53–65.
4. Sinkinson CA, Egherman WP, eds. Bacterial meningitis in children: a diagnostic dilemma. *CME-TV Study Guide* 1991; 2:6, 1–17.
5. Feigin RD, McCracken GH, Klein JO. Diagnosis and management of meningitis. *Pediatr Infect Dis J* 1992; 11: 785–814.
6. Ho DD, Hirsch MS. Acute viral encephalitis. *Med Clin North Am* 1985; 69: 415–429.
7. Hall SM. Reye's syndrome and aspirin: a review. *Br J Clin Practice* 1990; Symposium Supplement, 70: 4–11.

8. Breningstall GN. Diseases of ammonia metabolism. *In:* Swaiman K, ed. *Pediatric neurology. Principles and practice.* 4th ed. St Louis: Mosby, 1994: 1233–1242.
9. Wong DL. *Whaley and Wong's nursing care of infants and children.* 5th ed. St Louis: Mosby, 1995: 1423.
10. Barrett MJ, Hurwitz ES, Schonberger LB, Rogers MF. Changing epidemiology of Reye syndrome in the United States. *Pediatrics* 1986; 79: 598–602.

Disturbances in Musculoskeletal and Integumentary Function

Arthritis

Isobel Taylor

ACUTE SUPPURATIVE ARTHRITIS

Also known as septic arthritis, in children the usual infecting organism is *staphylococcus aureus*, although *streptococcal* infection is probably the next most common. Occasionally *Pneumococcus, Haemophilus influenzae* or *Escherichia coli* are responsible. Children with sickle-cell anaemia are prone to salmonella infection.

Infection reaches the joint as a sequel to penetrating joint injury or from local spread through adjacent infected bone (osteomyelitis). Haematogenous spread from a distant septic focus, e.g., abscesses of the skin or teeth or middle ear infection, may be identified, but often no reason is found for the onset of joint infection. In the neonate the spread may be from an infected umbilical cord.

The child presents with high fever, tachycardia and marked muscle spasm accompanied by pain at the affected joint, which is held very still, usually in a position of flexion. Suppuration inside the joint capsule raises the temperature and pressure within the joint with very destructive effects on articular cartilage. Treatment to decompress the joint and control the infection is a matter of urgency. Under anaesthesia, the joint is aspirated or opened and drained and the pus sent to pathology for culture and sensitivity studies. Parenteral antibiotic therapy is begun before waiting for the laboratory results. Penicillin is the drug of choice since the infection is most likely to be due to staphylococci.

The child needs pain relief with appropriate analgesics and careful support and protection of the joint. Padded splints or traction control muscle spasm and maintain the joint in a good position. The nurse should realise that the child will resent movement at the joint, which induces muscle spasm, and should handle the limb gently if the child has to be moved.

Once the acute symptoms are relieved, the child's general condition is satisfactory (e.g., afebrile) and the joint is no longer painful, and warm, gentle, progressive joint movements are encouraged to restore function. Gradual weight-bearing is allowed in the absence of any flare up of the infection. If the joint is badly damaged it may need to be kept splinted in as functional a position as possible while ankylosis (fusion) occurs. In such children future arthroplasty may be required.

TUBERCULOUS ARTHRITIS

Bones or joints are affected in about 5% of patients with tuberculosis (TB). The spine and the large synovial joints seem to be more commonly affected in children infected with tuberculous bacilli.[1] There may be a history of recent contact with tuberculosis. The child complains of a painful joint and the parent may report attacks of lassitude and weight loss. Investigations towards a diagnosis include the Mantoux or Heaf test and synovial biopsy.

Treatment consists of a prolonged course of combined antituberculous drugs. These include rifampicin, isoniazid, streptomycin and ethambutol or pyrazinamide for 8 weeks. The first 2 drugs are continued for a further 6 months. Ethambutol and streptomycin are more toxic and are used for short term treatment.

Bed rest and splinting of the limb to protect the joint from further damage until the symptoms subside is the usual regimen. Gradual, restricted activity is encouraged over the next 4 to 6 months until the joint changes seen on x-ray resolve. As in acute suppurative arthritis, if there is significant joint destruction splintage and rest will be prolonged to prevent the fusion of the joint in a bad position.

The parents and child will need reassurance and information about tuberculosis infection. Immediate family members and people in close contact with the child can be screened for TB to trace the source of infection or detect spread. The child and parents may need advice about the roles of optimum nutrition, healthy lifestyle and immunisation in improving immunity against the effects of tuberculosis infection.

REFERENCE

1. Apley AG, Solomon L. *Apley's system of orthopaedics and fractures*. 7th ed. London: Butterworth Heinemann, 1993.

Dermatomyositis

Robyn Pedersen

Dermatomyositis is an inflammatory disease of the skin and muscles, the cause of which is obscure. Whenever a child with this condition is admitted to hospital or seen in the community, nursing intervention is assessed on an individual basis as the disease has a wide range of severity.

Nursing assessment

In dermatomyositis there is a skin rash, muscle weakness and misery.[1] The age of presentation varies, and one-fifth of patients are less than 15 years of age. Most children with dermatomyositis will be admitted to hospital for a muscle biopsy, electromyography and a blood test for estimation of creatine kinase levels. Creatine kinase is an enzyme produced during muscle breakdown.

Pathophysiology

Significant complications of this disease include subcutaneous calcification, joint contractures (which can be severe) and vasculitis. All of these complications are more frequent in children than adults. The duration of the disease can extend from months to years. The disease can follow a monophasic course but, in protracted cases, relapses often occur.

Management

Nursing care depends on the severity of symptoms and whether contractures are present. Along with medication (steroids and/or immunosuppressants) physiotherapy is absolutely necessary to maintain joint mobility. Treatment extends over a long period and the nurse will need to encourage the child to maintain physiotherapy as the exercises can be quite painful.

In severe cases, a child may be admitted to hospital in order to have intensive physiotherapy. In the case of protracted illness, the stress on a growing child or adolescent is such that episodes of psychological or psychosomatic symptoms are common. It is important for the nurse to be aware of this possibility in children with a long-term illness and to initiate the most appropriate intervention. Death can result if the disease is not treated.

REFERENCE

1. Dubowitz V. *A colour atlas of muscle disorders in childhood.* London: Wolfe Medical Publications, 1989.

Disturbance in Gastrointestinal Function

Viral Hepatitis

Jennifer Backhouse and Lean Tan

Viral hepatitis is inflammation of the liver caused by immunologically distinct viruses: hepatitis A (HAV); hepatitis B (HBV); hepatitis C (HCV); hepatitis D (HDV); and hepatitis E (HEV). The clinical, epidemiological and immunological features of these five forms of viral hepatitis may be similar or different.[1,2]

Hepatitis may also occur during the course of disease caused by cytomegalovirus, Epstein-Barr virus, herpes simplex virus, varicella-zoster virus, adenovirus, enterovirus, rubella virus, arboviruses and drugs and alcohol.[2,3]

AETIOLOGY AND EPIDEMIOLOGY

Hepatitis A

Hepatitis A has also been known as infectious hepatitis, endemic jaundice and acute catarrhal jaundice. The fulminant form of the disease is called yellow atrophy of the

Table 5.2 Clinical and epidemiologic features of viral hepatitis[1,3,15,17]

Features	Hepatitis A	Hepatitis B	Hepatitis C	Hepatitis D	Hepatitis E
Virus	HAV	HBV	HCV	HDV	HEV
Incubation period	15–50 days	50–180 days	30–195 days	21–90 days	14–63 days
Average	28–30 days	60–90 days	155 days		
Period of communicability and sequelae	It can survive on objects and surfaces for several weeks and in natural water for up to 100 days. Virus in blood and faeces 2 to 3 weeks before onset of jaundice.	Variable. Varies in blood (probably in stool). During late incubation period and acute stage of disease. May persist in carriers and at least 1 week before onset of jaundice. The infection period is about 1 month before jaundice occurs to about 1–3 months after jaundice occurs. Some people may carry the virus for life.	The person will be infectious a few weeks before evidence of infection from a blood test. Some will continue to be infectious for an indefinite period leading to chronic hepatitis.	Cirrhosis and complications of portal hypertension occur more often and progress more rapidly.	The hepatitus E virus is apparently very labile. During epidemics it has been mild or inapparent in children and common in adolescents and young adults.
Type of onset	Usually acute	Usually insidious	Usually insidious	Usually acute	Usually acute
Specific signs	Symptoms more common in adults than children.	More insidious compared to hepatitis A. Rash is common, arthralgia, pruritus	Arthralgia may be present.	In general hepatitis D infection is a more severe disease.	Same as hepatitis A.

Mode of transmission	Usually oral (faecal) Food or water borne	Usually parenteral Perinatal	Usually parenteral	Usually parenteral	Usually oral (faecal). Water borne in developing countries.
Prognosis	Relatively benign disease, occasionally may be prolonged but complete recovery with no evidence of fatal fulminant hepatitis A	Most patients recover completely. Risk of chronic infection is extremely variable. May be low in young healthy adults and very high in young infants born to HBsAg carrier mother.			Hepatitis E is a relatively benign disease that does not progress to chronic hepatitis. However, it is a highly fatal disease in pregnant women.
Mortality	0.1% to 0.2%	0.5% to 2.0% in uncomplicated cases; may be higher in complicated cases.	1% to 2% in uncomplicated cases	2% to 20%	20% in pregnant women; 1% to 2% in general population.

liver.[1] One attack of hepatitis A provides life-long protection from hepatitis A only.[3] The highest incidence of hepatitis A is in children under 15 years of age.[4]

Hepatitis B

Hepatitis B is the most significant liver disease in the world,[5] with an estimated 300 million chronic carriers.[6] Hepatitis B is also known as serum hepatitis, homologous serum jaundice, transfusion jaundice, syringe jaundice and post-vaccinal jaundice.[7] A high prevalence of seromarkers of hepatitis B virus infection has been reported in Australian Aborigines.[8] Significant migration of people from highly endemic areas has added to the overall reservoir of infection in the Australian community.[1,9,10] Hepatitis B virus is the most common and most important cause of neonatal hepatitis infection.[7] To date, perinatal transmission of hepatitis A virus, hepatitis C virus, hepatitis D virus and hepatitis E virus has not been well documented.

Hepatitis C

Hepatitis C virus is the major causative agent in parenterally transmitted non-A, non-B (NANB) hepatitis, the most common serious consequence of blood transfusion.[1,7,11–13] The current incidence of post-transfusion hepatitis appears to be less than 1% and perhaps under 0.5%.[4] Hepatitis C is transmitted by parenteral routes. The exact risk of perinatal transmission is unknown, but would appear to be much less than that of hepatitis B virus.[11,14] Mother-to-infant (vertical) transmission appears to be uncommon (less than 10%), but is much higher if there is coinfection with HIV.[4,11]

Hepatitis D

Although the clinical manifestations and course of hepatitis D are similar to those of acute or chronic hepatitis B, it is a more severe disease.[7] Hepatitis D virus is defective in that it requires hepatitis B virus for its transmission.[7] Perinatal infection by hepatitis D virus is rare.[7]

Hepatitis E

Hepatitis E, previously called enterically transmitted NANB (ET-NANB) is distributed mainly in India, China, Mexico and North Africa. The clinical manifestations and course of hepatitis E are essentially the same as hepatitis A, except for several striking differences.[1,4,7] During various epidemics, the disease has been rare in children and common in adolescents and young adults[1] with high mortality among pregnant women.

Hepatitis F

There is the possibility of another parenteral non-A, non-B agent (hepatitis F and more) as reported by Fox and Sharp.[15]

SIGNS AND SYMPTOMS

Hepatitis A

Feeling unwell, tiredness, aches and pains, fever, nausea and vomiting, lack of appetite, abdominal discomfort, darkening of urine, pale stools followed by jaundice, yellowing of eyeballs and skin within a few days.[3]

Hepatitis B

May be frequently symptomless. Loss of appetite, nausea, vomiting, abdominal distension, fever, tiredness, often jaundice, yellowing of eyes and skin, darkening of urine and pale stools.[16]

Hepatitis C

Tiredness, mild abdominal discomfort and nausea. About 50% of people with hepatitis C will develop chronic hepatitis and some with chronic hepatitis will develop cirrhosis of the liver and/or liver cancer.[17]

Hepatitis D

The signs and symptoms resemble chronic or acute hepatitis B. In general hepatitis D infection is a more severe disease.[1]

Hepatitis E

The signs and symptoms are the same as hepatitis A.

TREATMENT

There is no specific treatment for children who are infected with hepatitis A, B, C or D virus. Management of patients with acute hepatitis involves decisions about: (i) the duration of bed rest; (ii) the choice of a diet; and (iii) the value of various non-specific drugs. Diet and return to activity usually are gauged by the child's desire.[1,18]

Corticosteroids and antiviral agents are not recommended for the treatment of acute hepatitis. Corticosteroids or other immunosuppressive forms of therapy are not indicated in chronic persistent hepatitis.[1]

Hepatitis A

The child is to be kept away from school and other children for 7 days from the first sign of jaundice. It is not necessary to keep contacts at home. Family contacts may need vaccination.[9]

Hepatitis B

It is not necessary to keep the child at home, but some children are too sick to go out. Contacts should see their family doctor for immunisation advice.[15] Hepatitis B is more commonly recognised in adults than children, and is therefore not normally a problem in child care facilities, but awareness of the potential hazards and precautions must be ensured among the staff.

Hepatitis C

One of the most important issues surrounding hepatitis C virus infection is the risk that individuals with this form of disease will eventually develop significant morbidity and mortality from the disease. Interferon (α-IFN) is the only agent shown by controlled trials to be effective, although the optimal dose and duration of treatment are still unclear.[14]

Consideration is to be given to significant side effects and high costs and also uncertain and indolent natural history of the disease. Relapse rates are 50% to 60%. Only 20% to 25% of all patients treated will have a sustained response to 6 months' treatment.[19] Side effects of treatment include transient flu-like symptoms. More chronic side effects include lethargy, loss of well-being and mild weight loss, depression, leucopenia, thrombocytopenia, alopecia and mouth ulcers and skin lesions.[17]

Hepatitis D

The effect of various antiviral and immunomodulatory agents has been evaluated for the treatment of chronic hepatitis B, C and D infections. Corticosteroid therapy is not recommended as it has not been beneficial in treating chronic hepatitis D.[1,18] A controlled trial of α-IFN revealed transient improvements. Cessation of α-IFN therapy was followed by a return of viral replication and liver disease.[20]

Hepatitis E

There is currently no vaccine for hepatitis E.

PREVENTION

Vaccines are available for the control of hepatitis A and B.[1] Hepatitis C vaccine is being developed. Immune globulins are important tools for preventing infection and disease before or after exposure to hepatitis viruses.[1]

Hepatitis A

Faecal–oral spread of hepatitis A virus may occur in households, day care centres and schools. Travellers and young children may be exposed to poor hygiene conditions in developing countries.[1,18]

Procedures designed to prevent faecal–oral spread of HAV include thorough handwashing, sterilisation of food utensils, fly abatement and exclusion of potentially infectious food handlers. Prophylactic value of immunoglobulins is greatest (80% to 90%) when given early in the incubation period and declines thereafter.[1] It is likely that inactivated HAV vaccines will replace immunoglobulins for pre-exposure vaccination.[1]

Hepatitis B

Vaccination is recommended for recipients of certain blood products including those with clotting disorders who are at an increased risk of HBV infection.[21,22] Donor blood should be tested routinely for HBsAg and anti-HBC. Several studies have confirmed the efficacy of combined passive and active immunisation. It is recommended for all infants whose mothers are HBsAg positive.[21–23] Breastfeeding should not be discouraged because hepatitis B immune globulin and hepatitis B vaccine are very effective in preventing neonatal hepatitis B infection.[1,8,21]

The vaccines that are currently used in Australia are Engerix-B and H-B-VaxII.[24]

Engerix-B

Engerix-B provides active immunisation against hepatitis B virus infection in persons who are at substantial risk and have been shown to be susceptible to HBV. The vaccine can be administered at any age from birth onward. Enerix-B should be injected into the deltoid muscle of bigger children and the anterolateral thigh of neonates and infants with a small deltoid muscle. Exceptionally, the vaccine may be given subcutaneously in patients with severe bleeding tendencies (e.g., haemophiliacs). It must not be given intravenously. Primary vaccination in adults and children consists of three intramuscular doses of vaccine, the 2nd dose being given a month after the 1st, and the 3rd dose at 6 months. For children over 10 years of age, a vaccine dose of 20 µg is recommended, and for neonates and children under 10 years, a dose of 10 µg.

Engerix-B should not be administered to patients with severe febrile infections. Patients who develop symptoms suggestive of hypersensitivity after injection should not receive further doses.

H-B-VaxII

The immunisation regimen consists of 3 doses, the 2nd dose being given a month after the 1st, and the 3rd dose 6 months after the 1st. The mode of injection and recommended sites are similar to those of Engerix-B. For adolescents (11 to 19 years), the doses are 5 µg each, and for infants and children up to 10 years, are 2.5 µg.

For infants born to HBsAg positive mothers, the 1st dose (5 µg) of H-B-VaxII may be given at birth at the same time as hepatitis B immune globulin, but should be given in the opposite anterolateral thigh to ensure absorption of the vaccine. Alternatively, H-B-VaxII may be given within the first 7 days of exposure. The 2nd and 3rd doses may be given at 1 and 6 months respectively after the 1st dose.

Patients who develop symptoms suggestive of hypersensitivity after an injection should not receive further doses. Caution should be exercised in administering H-B-VaxII to patients with severely compromised cardiopulmonary status or in those in whom a febrile or systemic reaction could pose a significant risk.[24]

Hepatitis C

The risk of perinatal transmission appears to be very low[19] and no data is yet available on prevention of possible perinatal or neonatal transmission.[19] Before blood banks in Australia began testing for HCV, there was the risk of acquiring hepatitis from a blood transmission.[2] Watson reported that HCV was responsible for 90% of post-transfusion hepatitis, although the risk is relatively low in Australia.[10,18] Due to its long incubation period until the antibody test becomes positive, there remains a small definite risk of acquiring HCV.[11] No vaccine is yet available against hepatitis C.

Hepatitis D

HDV perinatal infection is rare.[1] Hepatitis B vaccination provides a means for preventing hepatitis D.

Hepatitis E

There is no vaccine for hepatitis E prevention to date.

REFERENCES

1. Krugman S, Katz SL, Gershon AA, Wilfert CM. *Infectious diseases of children*. 9th ed. St Louis: Mosby, 1992.

2. Becton Dickinson. What is hepatitis? *The B-D Initiative* 1993; 2 (3): 2.
3. New South Wales Health Department. *Hepatitis A — Fact Sheet.* Sydney; 1991.
4. McIntosh EDG. Report with recommendations. International Symposium on Viral Hepatitis and Liver Disease. (The 8th Triennial Congress) Tokyo, 1993.
5. Treadwell TL, Keeffe EB, Lake J, Read A, Friedman LS, Goldman IS, et al. Immunogenicity of two recombinant hepatitis B vaccines in older individuals. *Am J Med* 1993; 95: 584–588.
6. Lau JYN, Wright TL. Molecular virology and pathogenesis of hepatitis B. *Lancet* 1993; 342: 1335–1344.
7. Krugman S. Viral hepatitis: A, B, C, D and E infection. *Pediatrics Rev* 1992; 13: 203–212.
8. Campbell DH, Sargent W, Plant AJ. The prevalence of markers of infection with hepatitis B virus in a mixed-race Australian community. *Med J Aust* 1989; 150: 489–492.
9. Campbell DH, Plant AJ, Sargent JW, Mock PA, Barrett ER, Archer KH. Hepatitis B infection of children in a mixed-race community in Western New South Wales. *Med J Aust* 1991; 154: 253–256.
10. Burgess MA, McIntosh EDG, Allars HM, Kenrick KG. Hepatitis B in urban Australian school-children. *Med J Aust* 1993; 159: 315–319.
11. Watson C. Hepatitis C infection in Australia. *Mod Med Aust* 1991; July: 18–31.
12. Alter HJ, Purcell RH, Shih JW, Melpolder JC, Houghton M, Choo Q, Kuo G. Detection of antibody to hepatitis C virus in prospectively followed transfusion recipients with acute and chronic Non-A, Non-B hepatitis. *N Engl J Med* 1989; 321: 1494–1510.
13. Fairley CK, Leslie DE, Nicholson S, Gust ID. Epidemiology and hepatitis C virus in Victoria. *Med J Aust* 1990; 153: 271–273.
14. Nowicki MJ, Balistreri WF. The hepatitis C virus: identification, epidemiology and clinical controversies. *J Pediatr Gastroenterol Nutr* 1995; 20: 248–274.
15. Fox R, Sharp D. The A to F of viral hepatitis. *Lancet* 1990; 336: 1158–1160.
16. New South Wales Health. *Hepatitis B.* State Health Publication (HPA) 92–59, 1992.
17. New South Wales Health. *Hepatitis C.* State Health Publication (HPA) 92–72, 1992.
18. Krugman S. Viral hepatitis: A, B, C, D and E — prevention. *Pediatr Rev* 1992; 13: 245–247.
19. Watson C. Recent advances in hepatology. *Fellowship Affairs* 1991; June: 15–16.
20. Rizetto M, Rosina F, Saracco G. Treatment of chronic delta hepatitis with alpha 2 recombinant interferon. *J Hepatol* 1986; 3: S229–233.
21. Centres for Disease Control. Protection against viral hepatitis: recommendations of the Immunisation Practices Advisory Committee (ACIP). *Morb Mort Weekly Rev* 1990; 39: RR-2, 1–26.
22. Centres for Disease Control. Hepatitis B virus: a comprehensive strategy for eliminating transmission in the United States through universal childhood vaccination. Recommendations of the Immunisation Practices Advisory Committee. *Morb Mort Weekly Rev* 1991; 40: 1–25.
23. Reznik RB. A hepatitis B vaccination programme for inner metropolitan Sydney neonates. *Med J Aust* 1991; 155: 153–156.
24. Badewitz-Dodd LH. *1993 Mims Annual.* 17th ed. Sydney: Australia Print Group, 1993.

Gastroenteritis

John Leach

Gastroenteritis is a condition which occurs throughout the lifespan, affecting infants through to adults. The effect on the adult can be mild and self-limiting; on a child or infant, however, the effect of gastroenteritis can be devastating. According to Branski et al.,[1] viral gastroenteritis is a major cause of morbidity among infants and young children around the world. De Silva states that acute gastroenteritis causes between 5 and 10 million deaths per year in children in developing countries.[2]

Gastroenteritis has 3 main causative agents: viral, bacteria and protozoa. Other causes, such as ingestion of toxins, drugs, food allergies and even enzyme deficiencies are uncommon, but can produce gastroenteritis.

De Silva states that the published studies of diarrhoeal disease have only succeeded in detecting bacterial or parasitic agents in 20% to 40% of cases.[2] He concludes, therefore, that viruses 'must play an important role in this condition'.

While as adults we tend to shrug off gastroenteritis as a 'not too serious disease', as nurses we should realise the serious effect it can have on our paediatric patients.

Nursing assessment

The child usually presents with a history of diarrhoea, vomiting or both. It is important that the nurse takes a thorough history, noting:

- length of illness
- approximate amount of vomiting
- appearance of vomitus
- number of wet nappies
- oral intake since onset of illness
- number of bowel actions the child has passed
- description of stool, noting blood and mucus.

The overall appearance of the child is one of the most important features. A child who is alert, thirsty and irritable will be in better shape than a child who is lethargic, has sunken fontanelles and eyes, and a history of poor urinary output.

Bacterial gastroenteritis

Common causative agents are: *Salmonella; Escherichia coli; Shigella; Campylobacter;* and *Yersinia*.

The stools are usually very offensive and often contain blood and pus. Children usually complain of urgency and frequency in the passing of stools and may only pass a small amount of fluid each time they go to the toilet. Antibiotics are sometimes prescribed to treat this form of gastroenteritis, but this is a controversial issue and will be discussed later in this section.

Viral gastroenteritis

This is the most common form of gastroenteritis. Causative agents include: rotavirus; adenovirus; and small round virus.

The stools are often less offensive than those of bacterial gastroenteritis and do not contain blood. The appearance is usually watery and loose and the colour can range from brown through to green. It can take up to 5 days to isolate the causative agent.

Protozoal gastroenteritis

Common causative agents include *Giardia* and *Cryptosporidium*.

These stools can be explosive, foul smelling and watery. There may be abdominal pain and weight loss.

DEHYDRATION

The infant or child who is admitted to hospital with gastroenteritis should be assessed for dehydration and intravenous therapy commenced, if appropriate.

When assessing the child for dehydration the nurse should look for the following signs.

- Mild dehydration is indicated by a decrease in urine output and an increase in thirst.
- Moderate dehydration is indicated by sunken fontanelles in infants, sunken eyes, lethargy, poor urine output, dry mucus membranes.
- Severe dehydration is indicated by a notable lack of skin tone, apathy, coldness, sweatiness, no urine output.

The nurse should arrange for the following procedures to be instigated.

- Venous blood should be taken for electrolytes, urea and creatinine.
- An intravenous line should be inserted and fluids commenced.
- Oral rehydration should be commenced if the child is able to tolerate oral fluids.

FLUID REPLACEMENT THERAPY

Intravenous therapy is considered the first line fluid replacement therapy for children who present with dehydration and gastroenteritis. Serum electrolyte levels will determine the type and amount of fluid therapy to treat dehydration.

Hypernatremia and hyponatremia are 2 features of dehydration which need to be considered when selecting intravenous replacement therapy.

Hypernatremia dehydration occurs when there is more fluid lost than electrolytes. This form of dehydration is the most serious because of the risk of serious neurological complications. Kilham recommends that rehydration should be a slow process using a half normal saline (0.45% sodium chloride) and 2.5% dextrose solution over 36 to 48 hours to prevent the risk of convulsions, cerebral damage and death associated with this condition.[3] This form of dehydration is usually uncommon but because of the potential complications should be closely monitored.

Hyponatremia is the most common form of dehydration associated with gastroenteritis. The fluid of choice is, again, half normal saline (0.45% sodium chloride) and 2.5% dextrose, but will need to be infused at a greater rate than for hypernatremic dehydration.

For the infant or child who presents with a short history of vomiting and diarrhoea with no clinical signs of dehydration, the following treatment is recommended.

Breast fed infants

- Breast feeds should continue.
- Supplement feeds of clear fluids should commence.
- Stop all solids until vomiting ceases.

Formula fed infants

- Cease milk formulas and solids.
- Offer clear fluids at approximately 100–140 mL/kg/day.
- Return to milk and solids when vomiting ceases.

Table 5.3 A suggested rehydration schedule[3]

Age	mL/kg/day
Newborn	60–90
Day 2	90–120
Day 3 to 9 months	120–140
9 to 12 months	120
1 to 2 years	90–100
2 to 4 years	70–80
4 to 8 years	60–70
8 to 12 years	50–60

Table 5.4 Recommended electrolyte requirements[5]

Electrolyte	Composition
Sodium	50–90 mmols/L
Potassium	20 mmols/L
Chloride	40–80 mmols/L
Citrate	10 mmols/L
Glucose	2%

Children over 12 months

- Cease milk and solids.
- Offer clear fluids at approximately 90—100 mL/kg/day.
- Return to milk and solids when vomiting ceases.

It is important to reintroduce an oral intake within 24 hours to prevent further breakdown of body protein and fat stores. Even if diarrhoea continues, a diet should be commenced.

Once the child shows signs of improvement after commencing clear fluids, a return to normal feeds and diet should begin. For mild dehydration this should be within the first 24 hours. For moderate to severe dehydration it may take as long as 48 hours. A suggested rehydration schedule is listed in **Table 5.3**.

There are many commercial oral rehydration preparations available for the treatment of gastroenteritis. The glucose and electrolyte content of these preparations need to be taken into account and should be similar to that listed in **Table 5.4**.

There are many schools of thought as to how regrading of normal milk feeds should commence. It is thought best for milk feeds to begin at half-strength and grade up to full strength after 2 or 3 feeds. Half-strength feeds are comprised of milk and water in equal proportions. The milk product should be the milk that the child was receiving prior to admission to hospital.

LACTOSE INTOLERANCE

A small percentage of patients recovering from gastroenteritis will develop lactose intolerance after recommencing milk feeds. According to Thompson,[6] a disaccharide intolerance can develop secondary to a number of conditions, including enteritis. The most susceptible of these enzymes is lactase. Lactase activity is very sensitive to injury, being the first disaccharidase to decrease in production, and the last to recover.

This secondary complication will be manifested in the form of persistent loose stools immediately after the milk feed. The stool may be yellow in colour but extremely loose, and the amount of stool will be large in comparison to the usual bowel action.

The presence of reducing sugars in the stool can be determined by pathology test or by the Clinitest tablet method. A fresh specimen is required for either procedure. The Clinitest tablet method is carried out on the ward by the nurse. Five drops of stool are collected in a test tube with ten drops of water. The Clinitest tablet is placed in the mixture and the test tube is gently shaken. A positive result, (i.e., an abnormal result) is one where the indicator on the colour chart is greater than 0.5%.

The management of this complication is to give a lactose-free formula such as Delact or Digestelact. According to The Gut Foundation,[5] once the child is established on a lactose-free formula, it should be continued for approximately 4 weeks before a gradual change back to the regular formula is begun.

One suggested approach to the reintroduction of formula feeds is to introduce one feed a day of the formula while maintaining the diet of lactose-free milk. Formula feeds can be increased by one feed a day until the child is off lactose-free milk. Should watery stools recommence during this regrading phase, then the milk formula should cease and lactose-free milk continue until a further trial in 2 to 4 weeks. While the child is having lactose-free milk, a lactose-free diet should also be maintained.

DRUG THERAPY IN GASTROENTERITIS

According to Wyeth and Kamath,[7] antiemetics and anti-diarrhoeals commonly prescribed for children with gastroenteritis, in the majority of cases, can be unwarranted and may even be harmful to the patient. A survey of 100 general practitioners on the use of drug therapy in patients with gastroenterits was conducted by Wyeth and Kamath. The results of the survey revealed:

- 81% prescribed anti-diarrhoeals
- 33% prescribed anti-emetics
- 12% prescribed antibiotics.

The authors concluded that the use of drug therapy should be limited to specific circumstance, such as bacteremia or bacteria-isolated gastroenteritis.

NURSING MANAGEMENT

Diagnosis: Fluid volume deficit related to increased loss of fluid and dietary intake.

Management: Accurate recording of all intake and output. It is important to determine stool fluid loss and urinary output. Disposable nappies should not be used because they can mask the distinction between stool and urine loss. Oral fluids should be introduced as soon as possible.

Fever usually accompanies gastroenteritis and should therefore be monitored closely. Pulse and respirations can also indicate the well-being of the child. A slow thready pulse is indicative of dehydration which could lead to shock in the most severe cases.

Diagnosis: Alteration in nutrition, less than body requirements related to diarrhoea, vomiting and decreased dietary intake.

Management: Bare weigh daily to determine loss in weight and possible further dehydration. The child should be weighed on the same scales each day and approximately at the same time of the day. Bare weight is preferred, but older children should have their privacy maintained and could therefore be weighed in their undergarments. Once there has been definite improvement in the child's condition, a light diet should be introduced.

Diagnosis: Potential for infection related to presence of infective organisms.

Management: Handwashing is the most effective means of reducing the spread of gastroenteritis. Jewellery should be removed before attending the patient and the hands thoroughly washed before and after entering the room. The use of gowns is a controversial issue and provides the staff with little protection from vomiting and diarrhoea.

Diagnosis: Alteration in bowel elimination related to frequent loose stools and identification of infective organism.

Management: Handwashing is of particular importance when collecting specimens from nappies and placing them into containers. Two stool specimens should be collected for pathology. At least 5 mL is required for each specimen. The stools are collected for: 1) microscopy, culture and sensitivity plus cysts, ova and parasites; and 2) virology. The stools should be sent to pathology as soon as they are collected. This should be, however, when pathology services are available.

Emotional support

Parents can become very distressed by the sight of their sick infant or child. Feelings of guilt can be experienced if the parent feels that they have kept their children at home too long before bringing them to the hospital or medical centre.

The nurse has a responsibility to provide emotional support for the parent as well as the patient. Parents' anxieties can be alleviated by involving them in as much of the child's care as possible. They should be encouraged to stay with the child for the duration of the illness if this is possible. Parents should be encouraged to talk about their fears and these should be put into perspective by the nurse where possible. Parents should be educated on the signs of gastroenteritis and the severity of the disease. During the acute phase parents can support their child by offering feeds at a predetermined rate set by the nurse or medical officer. The nurse should be made aware of all nappy changes so that stools can be examined and the urinary output assessed and recorded.

The parents can play an important and extremely beneficial role in the recovery phase of a child with gastroenteritis. Their input should be encouraged for their own well-being and, more importantly, the well-being of their child.

Standard isolation practices

Most hospitalised patients with gastroenteritis are nursed in standard isolation. Isolation may be achieved through the use of isolation/infectious disease wards or single rooms and the use of gowns and other barrier techniques. While this practice has been in place in the major teaching hospitals for many years, the principle of isolation is both controversial and costly.

Gastroenteritis can be spread from person to person through direct or indirect contact. Therefore, the spread of gastroenteritis can be enhanced by nurses, medical officers, physiotherapists, play therapists and parents. In the acute care setting a patient can be visited by a great array of people interested in the disease process of the condition, as well as nursing personnel and sundry other people involved in the care of the child.

The simple act of handwashing can prevent the spread of gastroenteritis between patients nursed in a general paediatric ward. The enforcing of a handwashing policy is by no means an easy accomplishment for nursing staff to convey to patients and visitors. In emergency situations, handwashing may be of little significance to a patient in crisis.

As a barrier, the use of gowns and gloves can be expensive and may not aid a decrease in cross-infection. Their use does little to protect the clothes of health workers and can add a psychological barrier to the child and parent.

Cross-infection can be hazardous to the patient and can cause hardship to the patient and family by causing a longer hospital stay which is, in turn, costly to the institution. Whether the use of standard isolation continues or whether the practice is deemed outdated and costly, becomes a matter of choice for all institutions.

Psychological effects of isolation

Infants and children nursed in isolation should still be allowed as much interaction and stimulation as the nurse is able to offer. While infants may require less than older children, they still require appropriate toys and colour stimulation. Bright mobiles and interaction during nappy changes and feeding should be an integral part of nursing care.

Toddlers need greater attention by nursing staff when they are confined to isolation. Toys may not be enough to distract them from the psychological effect of being isolated from other children. If the institution has a volunteer service, such people can be of extreme importance in providing the toddler with a one-to-one interaction and aiding in a speedy recovery.

Children can understand the reasons for isolation when they are explained to them in simple, easy to understand language. However, children still need diversionary therapy when they are isolated. Television, books and toys can be used with great effect.

None of these diversionary tactics are substitutes for human contact. Parents should be encouraged to stay with the child for as long as possible. Relatives can also be of use when the parents have other siblings at home to care for.

Follow-up

Most children will not need to be followed up after discharge. However, they should routinely see their early childhood nurse or local medical officer to make sure that they are gaining weight and to confirm that their stools are returning to normal.

The nurse plays an important role in educating parents on foods their child should receive after discharge. Most importantly, fatty foods including fried cooked meats and full-strength juices should be avoided until normal bowel actions have returned.

REFERENCES

1. Branski D, Dinari G, Rozen P, Walker-Smith J. *Paediatric gastroenterology: aspects of immunology and infections.* Vol. 13. New York: Karger, 1986.

2. de Silva L. Viruses and gastroenteritis. *In:* Procopis P, Kewley G, eds. *Current paediatric practice.* Sydney: Harcourt Brace Jovanovich, 1991.
3. Kilham H, ed. *The Children's Hospital handbook.* Sydney: Aiken Press, 1993.
4. Anderson C, Burke V, Gracey M. *Paediatric gastroenterology.* 2nd ed. Melbourne: Blackwell Scientific, 1987.
5. Barnes G, Bishop R, Cameron D, Davidson G, Kamath R, Sheperd R. *Diarrhoea in children.* Randwick: The Gut Foundation, The Prince Of Wales Hospital, 1987.
6. Thompson S. Infant feeding. *In:* Procopis P, Kewley G, eds. *Current paediatric practice.* Sydney: Harcourt Brace Jovanovich, 1991.
7. Wyeth B, Kamath R. Outpatient and home management of acute gastroenteritis. *In:* Procopis P, Kewley G, eds. *Current paediatric practice.* Sydney: Harcourt Brace Jovanovich, 1991.

Appendicitis

Trish Comerford and Margaret Yates

Appendicitis is inflammation of the vermiform appendix. Obstruction of the lumen of the appendix by a faecalith (hardened faeces) is the most common cause of inflammation.

Appendicitis is the most common reason for abdominal surgery during childhood. The incidence is most frequent in adolescents between the ages of 15 and 24 years.[1] Appendicitis is less common under the age of 3 years.[2]

NURSING ASSESSMENT

The child will walk into the unit with a stoop, presenting with a history of periumbilical pain which eventually localises to the right lower quadrant. Fever and vomiting and either constipation or diarrhoea will be present. The child will have a rigid abdomen with reduced bowel sounds and rebound tenderness on physical examination. The most significant indication of appendicitis is a change in the child's behaviour. Young children assume a tense, still posture while lying on their side with the knees flexed. The older child will manifest the same signs and symptoms and will describe their pain and how sick they feel.[3]

If peritonitis ensues, the child will experience sudden relief of pain which is followed by an increase and change in the character of the pain from being localised and colicky to a dull, diffuse pain. This is accompanied by progressive abdominal distension, rigidity and guarding, tachycardia, rapid shallow respirations (because of the non-use of abdominal muscles to breathe) and pallor. The behavioural indications will be agitation and apprehension.

During any physical examination, reassure and comfort the child while their painful abdomen is being touched. Any clinical assessment of the child, or movement such as experienced during transfer for organ imaging, must be carried out with an awareness that the child is suffering severe pain. Nurses act as the first-line patient advocate and will protect the child from any pain being imposed unnecessarily.

INVESTIGATIONS

A rectal examination may be performed to rule out other possible conditions. It has been suggested that this procedure contributes little to the diagnosis of appendicitis.[1] The white blood cell count is usually elevated. Diagnostic imaging may demonstrate the presence of a faecalith.

The signs and symptoms manifest in the child will usually confirm the diagnosis without further investigation.[3]

THE CHILD UNDERGOING APPENDICECTOMY

Preoperative nursing care

The preoperative phase is rapid and urgent for the child and family. Preparation for transfer to the operating suite is carried out as quickly as possible. This leaves the nurse little time to explain clearly all the routine preoperative procedures.

Postoperative nursing care

The postoperative care is consistent with the care of the child undergoing abdominal surgery. The child having had a ruptured appendix will be acutely ill after surgery and not inclined to be active or mobile after return to the unit. The hospital stay for this child may be prolonged in comparison to the child with a non-ruptured appendix. It is essential to keep the child and parents well informed as to the length of recovery time.

Incentive spirometry may be necessary in conjunction with deep breathing and coughing exercises to prevent respiratory complications.

Positioning the child in high Fowler's position is thought to assist in the prevention of abscess formation. There is, however, no substantial evidence to support the effectiveness of this position or the necessity to nurse the child this way. The nurse should therefore encourage the child to assume whatever position is most comfortable.

Intravenous antibiotics are usually commenced intraoperatively. When administering antibiotics the child is observed for a local or generalised allergic response.

Any child may develop the complication of postoperative paralytic ileus or diarrhoea from an irritated colon. Abscess formation in extreme cases will be demonstrated by pleuritic and shoulder tip pain. During the convalescent period the child may exhibit signs and symptoms suggestive of an intra-abdominal abscess. These will include vomiting, abdominal pain, diarrhoea, fever, tachycardia and shoulder tip pain. Many of these signs and symptoms are non-specific, but shoulder tip pain suggests a subphrenic collection.

REFERENCES

1. Shandling B. *In:* Walker, Durie, Hamilton, Walker-Smith, Watkins. *Paediatric gastrointestinal disease. Pathophysiology, Diagnosis, Management.* Vol. 1. Toronto: BC Decker, 1991.
2. Hutson JM, Beasley SW. *The surgical examination of children.* Oxford: Heinemann Medical Books, 1988.
3. Wong DL. *Whaley and Wong's nursing care of infants and children* 5th ed. Toronto: Mosby, 1995.

Crohn's Disease

Trish Comerford and Margaret Yates

Crohn's disease is seen predominantly in adolescent patients. On assessment, the patient may be pale, miserable, thin, with muscle wasting and evidence of growth failure and delayed puberty.

The adolescent and parents will relate a history of a loss of energy and lethargy, an inability to participate in sports previously played and pain during and after meals. Additional signs observed by the nurse and symptoms described by the adolescent will depend on which areas of the gastrointestinal tract are affected. In the upper gastrointestinal tract, anorexia, nausea, vomiting, stomatitis, dyspepsia, dysphagia and malnutrition, evidenced by wasting, are common. If the colon is the affected area, diarrhoea with associated abdominal cramping, urgency to defaecate, perianal tissue damage, fistula and/or abscess and rectal bleeding are likely. Growth retardation with retarded height velocity and, in the older child, delayed puberty and secondary sex changes are features of Crohn's disease.[1]

Extra-intestinal manifestations may include erythema nodosum, pyoderma gangrenosum, iritis, conjunctivitis, ankylosing spondylitis, arthritis and jaundice caused by inflammation and scarring in the bile ducts of the liver.[2]

PATHOPHYSIOLOGY

Crohn's disease is a chronic inflammatory process which can affect any segment of the gastrointestinal (GI) tract. This includes any area from mouth to anus. The inflammation affects all layers of the intestinal wall (transmural) in discrete regions, as distinct from ulcerative colitis which involves a continuous segment of bowel.[1] The terminal ileum, colon and anus are the most commonly affected areas of gut in the majority of children or adolescents with Crohn's disease. The involvement of the small bowel accounts for the specific nutritional deficit which is characteristic of the illness. The colon is involved with the small bowel and is seldom involved in isolation. Involvement or oral, oesophageal and gastric segments are rare without bowel involvement.

INVESTIGATIONS

Nutritional assay

1. Measurement of height, estimation of growth velocity, determination of percentile position and assessment of pubertal development.
2. Full blood count, serum iron, protein and albumin estimations.

Organ imaging

1. Barium enema study of small bowel.
2. Barium enema or colonoscopy.
3. Upper GI endoscopy.
4. Stool cultures to eliminate bacterial infection, which can mimic the disease.
5. Sigmoidoscopy.

There is no diagnostic test which will give a differential diagnosis. The combined results of the above investigations serve to support a clinical diagnosis.

MEDICAL TREATMENT

The main focus of medical intervention is to control bowel inflammation, associated symptoms and the subsequent affect on the child's growth and development. Optimum management is achieved through a combination of pharmacological agents, nutritional support and relevant surgical intervention.[1]

Pharmacologic therapy

Corticosteroids will arrest the acute phase of the disease and effect a remission. These drugs are used in response to symptoms, but are not effective in preventing the onset of symptoms. The additional benefits of the anti-inflammatory action include the stimulation of appetite and improvement of the child's sense of well-being through the drug's direct action on the appropriate brain centres. Steroids are administered cautiously to offset the potential side effect of growth retardation. This is best achieved by administering the drug on alternate days if possible. The desired effects of steroids are the suppression of intestinal inflammation and the associated symptoms of pain, fever, anorexia, weakness, fatigue, abdominal tenderness and bleeding from inflamed tissue. Steroids are also used to suppress extraintestinal disturbances such as iritis, conjunctivitis, erythema nodosum and arthritis.[2]

Sulfasalazine is used for its anti-inflammatory effect during the chronic phase of the disease. This drug has been shown to be useful in patients with Crohn's colitis and ileocolitis, but is of no benefit to patients with small bowel disease alone. It has not been shown to be effective in maintaining remission, regardless of where the disease is located. It is unclear why sulfasalazine is therapeutic. Its advantages are considered by some researchers to be the inhibition of the release of harmful chemicals known as inflammatory mediators into the intestine. The drug also improves the transport of sodium and water in the colon which may have an antidiarrheal effect.[2] Side effects of sulfasalazine include headache, nausea, vomiting or bloody diarrhoea.

Metronidazole is used in paediatric patients as an adjunct to steroids and/or sulfasalazine. Metronidazole is useful as an antibacterial agent in those patients with small intestine bacterial overgrowth or perianal disease such as fissures, fistulas and abscesses.[1]

If metronidazole is used over long periods, the child may develop numbness in the feet and lower legs and heightened sensitivity to the cold. This can be distressing for the child, but both side effects will abate if the drug is withdrawn.

The use of non-steroidal anti-inflammatory drugs such as Ketorolac is becoming increasingly common practice for pain management. Ketorolac is a potent analgesic and moderate anti-inflammatory agent. Clinical studies indicate that in single dose trials, the efficacy and tolerability of the drug is greater than that of morphine or pethidine. The initial findings from trials also indicate fewer adverse effects than with the two commonly used narcotics.[3]

Nutritional support

The goal of nutritional therapy is to recover metabolic homeostasis, promote catch-up growth and enable progression to puberty. A low residue diet is indicated to avoid potential intestinal obstruction in those children with a segment of narrowed lumen. Foods which are difficult to digest such as raw or dried foods, raw vegetables, bran, whole grains, nuts or seeds should be avoided. Some children may experience lactose intolerance. Since dairy foods are an important source of dietary calcium, protein and calories, possible lactose intolerance should be investigated before restricting dairy food intake. In some instances, diet supplements such as Ensure Plus are encouraged to provide a balanced range of nutrients. Such supplements are low residue and free from the potential bowel irritants, lactose and gluten.

Total parenteral nutrition is administered to provide nutritional supplementation by sustaining additional energy and protein intake. It also may help bring the disease under control or into remission by facilitating bowel rest and improving nutritional status. Bowel rest alone has not been proven to have a significant therapeutic value.[1]

Nocturnal nasogastric feeding is implemented for those patients who are unable to increase their nutritional intake voluntarily. Elemental formula, for example, Vivonex is delivered where malabsorption is significant, if there is evidence of bowel stricture or where disease activity has not been arrested by previous medical therapy.[1]

Surgery

Surgery may be indicated when the child does not respond to medication and nutritional regimens or when complications develop. Local resection and temporary ileostomy will be considered for patients not responding to treatment. Indications for resection include intestinal perforation, uncontrolled GI bleeding, fistula formation and fixed intestinal obstruction.

There is no conclusive surgical solution to Crohn's disease. Many patients who undergo bowel resection will experience relapse regardless of long periods of remission. In the event that a patient requires repeated resections, short bowel syndrome may ensue.

NURSING INTERVENTIONS

Nursing care of the child with Crohn's disease parallels the care of the child with ulcerative colitis as well as other chronic illnesses. Nursing care is central to the multidisciplinary team approach necessary for the ongoing care of these children. Care is planned and managed over time, in accordance with the chronicity of the disease and episodes of relapse. The effectiveness of care is reliant on the degree of understanding and participation in self-management the child and family are prepared to undertake both at home and in hospital and the family's capacity to cope with chronic illness. Affiliation with The Australian Crohn's and Colitis Association Inc. (ACCA) support group will benefit the child and family in learning how to live with a life-long disease. This will be particularly beneficial when compliance to treatment regimens and lifestyle adjustments become difficult to cope with, particularly for the adolescent patient who will often resent having a condition which sets them apart from their peers.

Adolescence is a time when taking control and becoming independent is something to which the young person looks forward and represents the threshold of adulthood and self-determination. Episodes of acute exacerbation with pain, diarrhoea, fatigue and other symptoms requiring hospitalisation will impinge upon the adolescent's sense of self. This form of chronic disease serves as a disruption to life and isolation from their friends and peers. At times professional counselling may be necessary for the child and the whole family. It should be reinforced that there are certain steps which the adolescent can take to assert control over their life. For example, determining times with the medication regimen, choosing foods which are suitable and avoiding foods which exacerbate symptoms can enhance a sense of autonomy. Maintaining treatment and adhering to nutritional recommendations can be difficult for adolescents with the large variety of fast foods available. These foods may prove difficult to digest and equally as difficult to resist under peer pressure. Encouraging adolescents to participate in discussion about their hospital care with medical, nursing and allied health care staff will also enhance their sense of being in control.

Nursing care is also determined in accordance with the reason for admission to hospital. In the event that the child is admitted for conservative treatment such as nutritional support, the child's needs assessment will include total parenteral nutrition or enteral feeding management and pain management. Abdominal pain is the most common symptom described by children.[4] Careful pain control is fundamental to patient care, therefore involvement with the pain management team will greatly assist in the comprehensive assessment of pain and the initiation of appropriate analgesia. Continuous narcotic infusion, patient-controlled analgesia infusion or the use of a non-steroidal anti-inflammatory agent will be chosen. The nursing care will include ongoing assessment of pain relief and patient comfort.

Admission for surgical intervention requires careful physical and psychological preparation to help the patient and family deal with the fear of surgery and the likely outcome of a conventional ostomy (see nursing care of the child undergoing abdominal surgery). Involvement by the stomal therapy nurse is imperative and should begin in the very early preoperative stage. If the child is to have a stoma as a result of surgery, the stomal therapy nurse will teach the child and the family about what to expect, including all aspects of ostomy care both in hospital and after discharge. The community nurse should be notified for continuing care once the child is discharged. Apart from the physical requirements, ostomy management includes the psychological aspects of altered body image and subsequent low self-esteem. A stomal therapist is best placed to arrange contact with a carefully chosen peer with Crohn's disease who is also an ostomate. Relating to another child will help through the realisation that there are other children in the same situation.

Aspects of physical care coordinated by the stomal therapist include skin protection, stoma observation, appliance selection and application and containment of stoma output. Crohn's disease causes considerable disruption and requires adjustment to an altered life style for both the child and the family. Caring for these families requires great sensitivity, patience and support. The establishment of a trusting relationship is necessary in order to encourage the child and the family to express their fears, feelings and frustrations about living with the disease. Hospitalisation becomes a natural part of their way of life. Nursing staff too, can become an integral part of their life.

ACKNOWLEDGMENT

Mrs Marie Hiscock, Clinical Nurse Consultant, Stomal Therapy, John Hunter Hospital.

REFERENCES

1. Jackson W, Grand R. Crohn's disease. *In:* Walker WA, Durie PR, Hamilton JR, Walker-Smith JA, Watkins JB. *Pathophysiology, management and diagnosis. Paediatric gastrointestinal disorders.* Vol. 1. Toronto: BC Becker, 1991.

2. Brandt LJ, Steiner-Grossman P. *Treating IBD. A patient's guide to the medical and surgical management of inflammatory bowel disease.* New York: Raven Press, 1989.
3. Buckey MT, Brogden RN. Ketorolac: a review of its pharmacodynamic and pharmacokinetic properties, and therapeutic potential. *Drugs* 1990; 39: 87–109.
4. Hanauer SB, Kirsner JB, Kirschner BS, Colwell JC. *Inflammatory bowel disease. A guide for patients and their families.* New York: Raven Press, 1985: 145.

Ulcerative Colitis

Trish Comerford and Margaret Yates

The child with ulcerative colitis will present with a history of growth retardation related to gastrointestinal dysfunction. The child may have anorexia, nutritional and caloric depletion from chronic colon dysfunction and increased metabolic demands from extensive inflammation, and seriously impaired growth velocity and secondary sexual development.

Children may be subjected to frequent admissions to hospital for correction of anaemia and malnutrition. The number of admissions to hospital may well reflect not only the severity of the illness, but also the capacity for the child and family to manage at home.

The child with an acute exacerbation of ulcerative colitis will present as thin, pale, anorexic, dehydrated, febrile, small for age, with severe abdominal pain and frequent urgent diarrhoea. Nausea and vomiting may also be presenting features.

The nursing assessment will consider:

1. The context of current hospitalisation and the severity of the present acute episode.
2. The ongoing support of the child and family, particularly in regard to the child's nutritional needs and compliance to medication.
3. Children requiring drug therapy with sulphasalazine and corticosteroids require diligent encouragement to comply. The side effects of both drugs mimic the signs and symptoms of the disease and include growth retardation, premature closure of the epiphyses in prepubertal children and increased susceptibility to infection (e.g., stomatitis) from long-term steroid therapy. Bloody diarrhoea, abdominal pain, fever, anorexia, nausea and vomiting are side effects of sulfasalazine.[1] It is, therefore, very difficult for the child and the family to believe in the benefits of drug therapy.

PATHOPHYSIOLOGY

Ulcerative colitis is distinguished by chronic extensive inflammation of the mucosa and submucosa of the distal colon and rectum. The inflammation extends the length of the colon with varying degrees of ulceration, abscess formation, haemorrhage, oedema and patchy granulations. The absorption of nutrients and fluid and electrolyte status is seriously compromised because of the extensive damage to the mucosa.

The extensive inflammation increases bowel motility and causes diarrhoea, urgency with incontinence, tenesmus (the urge to pass a stool with little or no faeces in the rectum) and an urge to pass stools during the night. Stools will contain pus (leucocytes), blood and mucous and have a loose, watery consistency.

Children with ulcerative colitis run a great risk of developing cancer of the colon in later life. The duration and severity of the illness increases the risk.[2]

AETIOLOGY

The aetiology remains unknown. No infectious agent has been identified, although the lesions resemble changes seen in infectious colitis. An autoimmune or immunologic defect has been postulated with no definitive data to support the theory.

No evidence supports psychosomatic aetiology. Emotional and sociological factors, however, may influence the presentation and course of the illness. Ulcerative colitis affects individuals between 10 and 19 years of age and is seen in males and females equally. There is a higher incidence of the illness where there is a family history.[3]

INVESTIGATIONS

The diagnosis is based on the clinical presentation and history, radiological findings, macroscopic appearance of the mucosa and histology.

Laboratory pathology

A fresh stool specimen is collected to exclude infectious agents such as *Campylobacter*, *Shigella*, *Salmonella*, *Esherichia coli* and *Yersinia*. A stool should also be investigated for the presence of blood, leucocytes, ova and parasites.[3]

Radiology

Abdominal and chest x-rays are taken to determine the degree of colonic distension and are useful in diagnosing obstruction from stricture. Barium enema is rarely used diagnostically. Gastrointestinal series and small bowel follow-through with fluoroscopic study of the terminal ileum will indicate small bowel involvement.

Endoscopy

Sigmoid and/or colonoscopy with mucosal biopsy will provide the most definitive of diagnostic information. Colonoscopy is contraindicated in toxic megacolon because of the potential to perforate the bowel and induce haemorrhage. Toxic megacolon as a complication of ulcerative colitis is very rare in the paediatric patient.[3]

MEDICAL TREATMENT

The goal of treatment is to control the symptoms and prevent relapses. Children with mild cases are managed at home on bed rest, a low residue diet and with sulfasalazine which is introduced gradually.

Moderately ill children who have systemic disturbance, are hospitalised for observation and evaluation for complications. Treatment includes bed rest, a low residue diet and corticosteroids. Sulfasalzine may be used as an adjunct to the steroids. If the child is hypoalbuminaemic and anaemic, blood transfusion may enhance recovery. In the event the child fails to respond to this regimen, enteral resting and hyperalimentation is implemented.

Where severe disease is present, profuse bloody diarrhoea, weight loss, fever, abdominal tenderness and distension, anaemia and hypoalbuminaemia constitute loss of homeostasis. This amounts to a medical emergency requiring hospital admission and aggressive intervention to correct dehydration and electrolyte disturbance.[3] Where children respond poorly to medical treatment, surgical intervention becomes necessary. An elective temporary colostomy may be performed to rest the colon. Because ulcerative colitis is confined to the colon colectomy, performed in extreme cases, eliminates the disease.[1] See nursing care of the child undergoing abdominal surgery.

NURSING MANAGEMENT

Dehydration related to profuse diarrhoea

1. Assess and document frequency, volume and consistency of stools and urine.
2. Maintain a strict fluid balance record. A urinary output of 1–2 mL/kg/hour is a guide to adequate hydration.
3. Administer intravenous fluids in accordance with weight and age.
4. Assess the mucous membranes for moisture, colour, presence of secretions and moistness of tongue.
5. Assess skin colour, whether pale or flushed; temperature and skin turgor.
6. Offer small amounts of clear fluids or ice to suck.

Nutrition depletion related to bowel dysfunction

1. Encourage the child with a low residue diet which is age appropriate. Invite the child to choose food which they like to eat, taking into account the child's anorexia.
2. Document the dietary intake.
3. If the oral intake is inadequate, administer nasogastric dietary supplements as ordered.
4. When total parenteral nutrition is used, administer accordingly via a central venous access.

Growth failure related to malnutrition

1. Measure the child's height and weight regularly. Document these growth parameters on a height-weight growth chart.
2. Explain to the child and family that growth retardation is related to impaired nutrient absorption. Include in discussions an explanation regarding delayed secondary sexual development.
3. Confirm with the child and family that growth and development recommences once the disease is controlled.

Disruption to family lifestyle related to chronic illness

1. Assist the child and parents to devise a nutrition plan in consultation with the dietitian. The plan should include high caloric foods. Meals should be coordinated with the times medications are taken. This plan should be flexible enough for use during hospitalisation and practical for home management.
2. Encourage the child and family to vent their thoughts and feelings about episodes of exacerbation and the consequent disturbance to daily home life.
3. Keep the child and family informed at all times about investigations, treatment and progress.
4. In the event the child is to undergo bowel surgery, stress the positive aspects such as growth acceleration, permanent recovery, relief from bowel dysfunction and the capacity to live a 'normal' life.

5. Arrange for long-term consultation and discussion with social workers and appropriate community-based support networks which will assist the family to maintain close contact with relatives and friends.
6. Encourage the child to mix with other children while hospitalised.

REFERENCES

1. Wong D. *Whaley and Wong's nursing care of infants and children* 5th ed. St Louis: Mosby, 1995.
2. Mott SR, James SR, Sperhac AM. *Nursing care of children and families.* 2nd ed. Redwood City: Addison-Wesley, 1990.
3. Jackson W, Grand R. Ulcerative colitis. *In:* Walker WA, Durie PR, Hamilton JR, Walker-Smith JA, Watkins JB. *Paediatric gastrointestinal disorders. Pathophysiology, management and diagnosis.* Vol. 1. Toronto: Becker, 1991.

Disturbances in Genitourinary Function

Jill Farquhar

Urinary Tract Infection

Infection of the urinary tract is one of the most common childhood infections. Early detection and investigation is important so that children with structural abnormalities of the urinary tract can be identified and treatment to prevent renal damage can begin.

A urinary tract infection occurs when bacteria enter the urinary tract. Infections are mostly caused by gut flora. These organisms colonise the perineum and enter the urinary tract via the urethra. *Escherichia coli* is the most common invading organism, although coagulose-negative *Staphylococcus*, *Klebsiella* and *Proteus* are often isolated.[1] *Proteus* often colonises the foreskin in uncircumcised boys and commonly causes infection.

The presence of greater than 10^5 organisms per millilitre of a single species in a midstream urine culture is defined as a urinary tract infection.[2] Urinary tract infection is generally associated with pyuria.

Lower urinary tract infections are most common in adolescents and symptoms include haematuria, frequency, pain and foul-smelling urine.

Infections of the upper urinary tract involve the kidney and renal pelvis (pyelonephritis). Pyelonephritis is usually caused by an ascending infection originating in the bladder and causes infants and children to be very unwell. The children present with high fevers, loin pain, lethargy and associated lower urinary tract symptoms. Severe sepsis may occur if treatment is delayed, particularly in the neonate.

Outside the neonatal age group, urinary tract infections are far more common in girls because of their shorter urethra and the potential for infection from the perineum.

CAUSES

There are several predisposing factors to urinary tract infection in children.

The major risk is urinary stasis, which can be caused by obstruction to urine flow by structural defects of the kidney and urinary tract such as pelvo-ureteric junction obstruction, vesico-ureteral obstruction or posterior urethral valves. Vesico-ureteric reflux is a functional abnormality that causes urinary stasis and infection and is the most common structural abnormality of the urinary tract predisposing children to urinary tract infection.

Bladder catheterisation places the urinary tract at risk of infection.

NURSING ASSESSMENT

Children present with varying signs and symptoms of urinary tract infection depending on where the infection is located in the urinary tract and the age of the child. Children under 2 years of age usually present with failure to thrive, feeding problems, vomiting, diarrhoea, fever, offensive-smelling urine, periods of screaming and irritability.

Because the symptoms are so variable in infants, urinary tract infection may be overlooked and go untreated, which may result in scarring of the kidneys and irreversible damage.

A urine culture is an important investigation for any infant presenting with fever of unknown origin.

The initial nursing assessment of the child should include a history of the child's voiding patterns and careful documentation of any alterations such as poor urinary stream, painful urination, frequent urination, offensive-smelling urine or abnormally coloured urine. Older children may complain of loin pain, abdominal pain, dysuria, frequency, offensive-smelling urine, urgency and vomiting. Enuresis and daytime wetting may recur in children who were toilet trained before the infection.

A clean specimen of urine should be collected and a full ward urinalysis attended.

Blood pressure should be recorded carefully as well as temperature, pulse and respirations.

Weight should be recorded and compared to previous weights as an assessment of hydration and nutritional status.

NURSING MANAGEMENT

Urine specimen collection

When a child presents with a suspected urinary tract infection it is a nursing responsibility to collect a clean and, if possible, midstream specimen of urine for culture of invading organisms so that the appropriate antibiotic therapy can be instigated.

While this procedure appears to be a simple task to perform, too often urine specimens are contaminated by organisms from the perineal area in girls and the foreskin in boys. This can be avoided in most cases if sufficient care is taken when the urine is collected. The method used to collect the urine specimen varies according to the age of the child. It is difficult to collect a midstream specimen from an infant, but it may be possible to collect a specimen from a boy if the nappy is removed and there is sufficient time to wait until he voids. While this is not very practical in a busy paediatric ward, a well informed mother of a child with frequent urinary tract infections can be taught to do this.

Paediatric urine specimen collection bags are available and it may be necessary to use them to collect the urine.[3] The genitalia and entire nappy area should be cleansed with mild unperfumed soap and water, and then dried thoroughly before applying the bag. Care should be taken to thoroughly cleanse the folds of the labia in girls. Uncircumcised boys should have the foreskin cleaned and then pulled back gently to clean the glans. The foreskin may not be freely retractable in newborns and should not be forced. The bag should be applied carefully to prevent leakage and positioned as far away from the anal area as possible to avoid contamination of the urine by faeces. A nappy is placed loosely on the infant to prevent the bag being pulled off if they are kicking. Check the infant regularly and remove the bag immediately urine has been passed. The bag should not be folded or creased. Remove the bag slowly and gently to prevent skin irritation. Bags are not used on infants with nappy rash.

If the child is toilet trained, a midstream sample may be collected after a thorough explanation using simple terms which the child will be able to understand. The child may be more cooperative if parents assist with the collection.

Urine samples should be sent to the laboratory for culture immediately because bacteria will multiply at room temperature. If this is not possible, the urine must be refrigerated at 4°C.

Suprapubic bladder aspiration is another method of obtaining a urine specimen. This method is used when attempts to obtain a clean bag specimen have been unsuccessful. With the baby lying on his back, the skin between the umbilicus and symphysis pubis is cleansed. A 23 gauge sterile needle is introduced midline through the skin about 1 to 2 cm above the symphysis pubis.[4] Once the needle is in the bladder, urine is gently aspirated into a sterile syringe. When the needle has been removed a clean gauze swab is placed over the hole and gentle pressure is applied for a few minutes.

Bladder aspiration should not be attempted immediately after the baby has voided or if the bladder is not palpable.

Urethral catheterisation is occasionally performed to collect a sterile urine specimen.

Urine analysis

Urinalysis should be performed to check for the presence of red blood cells, protein, white blood cells and urinary pH. The urine becomes more alkaline when it is infected.

Blood pressure

Blood pressure must be recorded on children with urinary tract infections because blood pressure may be elevated if renal damage is present. The blood pressure recording is also a useful observation for assessment of the child's hydration status.

Fluid intake and hydration

Children with urinary tract infections have a fluid volume deficit because of a temporary reduction in renal concentrating capacity caused by the infection. Other factors which have the potential to lead to a deficit are fluid losses through the skin related to high fever and reduced intake due to malaise and abdominal pain.

An accurate record of fluid intake and output should be kept to assist in the assessment of kidney function. Intravenous fluids are administered to infants and children who are particularly unwell and who are not taking adequate oral fluids.

The child should be encouraged to increase his or her oral fluid intake in order to dilute the infected urine. It may be possible to increase the oral fluid intake of children who are reluctant to drink by tempting them with icy poles or jellies.

Pain when passing urine

The child with a urinary tract infection may experience pain when passing urine because of inflammation of the bladder mucosa. Dysuria has the potential to cause urine retention if the child is reluctant to pass urine because of the pain. Sitting the child in a warm bath may relax the child and provide some relief.

Hygiene

Education of the child and parents regarding hygiene may help to prevent further urinary tract infection. The importance of only wiping the perineal area from front to back to avoid contamination of the urethra with faeces should be stressed.

Infants should have nappies changed regularly and the nappy area cleaned at changes. It is also important that the perineal area is wiped from the front to back.

Parents should be advised to discourage incorrect potty position. Some girls sit forward on their potty with the knees together, this allows bacteria to be forced into the vagina and from there it may be transferred into the urethra.[5]

Highly perfumed soaps and bathing with bubble bath irritate the urethra and interfere with normal defence mechanisms. Parents should be advised against using these products.

Parent education

Parents and children are taught to recognise the signs of urinary tract infection and the importance of early intervention to prevent renal damage should the infection recur.

The importance of completing a full course of antibiotics, even if the child appears to be recovered before completion of the course, must be stressed.

INVESTIGATIONS

Urinary tract infection is usually diagnosed on the symptoms and on the result of the urine culture. It will take approximately one day to obtain the results of the culture, and a further day to obtain full organism sensitivities. White cells will be present in infected urine, and therefore the number of white blood cells which can be seen on microscopy is useful in making a diagnosis.

Boys of any age and girls under 6 require investigation of the urinary tract when they initially present.[5]

Renal ultrasound

This is usually the first investigation performed and is a very popular diagnostic investigation because it is not invasive.[6] Ultrasound of the kidneys yields information on pelvicalyceal dilatation, ureteric dilatation, renal size and gross renal scarring.

Micturating cystogram

This test is useful in diagnosing ureteric reflux. A urinary catheter is inserted and a contrast medium is then administered via the catheter into the bladder. X-rays are taken before and during voiding. Reflux may occur while the bladder is filling, however, in some cases can only be seen when the child voids.[7] To prevent infection by infective organisms at the time of catheterisation, antibiotic coverage is administered for two days before the cystogram, continuing for two days thereafter.

Radionuclide scanning

A radioactive compound is administered intravenously prior to scanning the kidneys. Either 99mTc-DMSA or 99mTc-DTPA are the compounds used in this test.[8] Renal scars and tumours show up on the scan as areas differing in density from the rest of the kidney.[7] Renal function and obstructions can be assessed using radionuclide scanning techniques.

Intravenous pyelogram

This investigation is used very occasionally in centres which do not have other facilities. It is, however, a poor study in infants because of their immature renal function.

A contrast medium is injected intravenously and the atoms of iodine in it make the kidneys radio-opaque.[7] X-rays are taken immediately and then at intervals for 20 to 40 minutes after the injection. This investigation provides good anatomical detail of the kidney and urinary tract in older children.

Unlike radionuclide scanning, there is a risk of allergic reaction to the contrast medium used in this test. When compared to radionuclide scanning, the radiation exposure is much higher in intravenous pyelogram.

MEDICAL INTERVENTION

Both blood and urine cultures are collected from children with an upper urinary tract infection.

Broad-spectrum antibiotic therapy is commenced after a urine sample has been obtained. Oral therapy is chosen unless the child is particularly unwell. If a child is acutely unwell they will be given intravenous antibiotics.

The duration of antibiotic therapy is fairly controversial. Some physicians suggest long-term prophylactic therapy for children with vesicoureteric reflux to prevent reinfection.[6]

Obstructive lesions are usually treated surgically.

A repeat urine culture should be obtained 1 to 2 weeks after commencing antibiotic therapy. In the child who is not responding to treatment, however, cultures are repeated in 2 to 3 days. Initial symptoms clear in 2 to 3 days.

REFERENCES

1. Bailey RR. *In:* Whitworth JA, Lawrence JR, eds. *Textbook of renal disease.* Melbourne: Churchill Livingstone, 1987.
2. Hicklin M. Urinary tract infection in children, *Paediatric Nursing* 1993; 5 (10): 24–27.
3. Taylor C. *Handbook of renal investigations in children.* London: Wright, 1989.
4. Behrmann RE, Vaughan VC. *Nelson. Textbook of pediatrics.* Philadelphia: WB Saunders, 1987.
5. O'Brien WM, Gibbons DM. *Am Family Physician* 1988; 38: 101–112.
6. Brooks D, ed. *Urinary tract infection.* Lancaster: MTP Press, 1987.
7. Uldall R. *Renal nursing.* 3rd ed. Boston: Blackwell Scientific, 1988.
8. Shaffer A. Infections and inflammation of the genitourinary tract. *In:* Walsh, Relick, Stamen, Vaughan. *Campbells urology.* 6th ed. Philadelphia: WB Saunders, 1992.

Glomerulonephritis

Glomerulonephritis is an inflammation of the glomerulus caused by an immunological reaction. It may be either an acute, reversible process or chronic and progressive, leading to irreversible renal failure. There are several types of glomerulonephritis, which are classified as either a primary disease or a secondary characteristic of an underlying disease.

ACUTE POST-STREPTOCOCCAL GLOMERULONEPHRITIS

Pathophysiology

Acute post streptococcal glomerulonephritis is an acute inflammatory process of presumed immunological origin affecting the filtration surface of the glomeruli.

Following exposure to beta haemolytic streptococci, a reaction develops and antigen–antibody complexes form which become trapped in the glomeruli. The complement system is activated and the inflammatory process that follows causes increased vascular permeability, endothelial swelling, fibrin formation and platelet aggregation resulting in congestion and increased pressure in the glomeruli.[1]

The glomerular lesions cause glomerular filtration to be reduced with protein and red blood cells leaking out of the glomerulus and into the tubules.

Presentation

The child shows evidence of the disease about 10 days after the onset of a streptococcal infection. The infection is usually of the throat, upper respiratory tract or skin. It generally affects children between the ages of 2 and 12 years, and is twice as common in boys. The child and the parents may not always outline a history of infection.

Children usually present with a history of dark, bloodstained urine, and oedema, but in some children the haematuria is microscopic. The oedema and proteinuria are rarely as severe as that seen in the children with nephrotic syndrome. The amount of protein in the urine is usually between 30 to 100 mg/L and 1 g/L.[2] Some children have a mild form of the disease and present with haematuria only.

Other clinical features the children display are oliguria, fluid overload and hypertension. Diminished renal function may cause hyperkalaemia, acidosis, raised serum urea, creatinine, phosphate, and uric acid levels, as well as sodium and water retention.

Nursing assessment

The nurse responsible for the initial assessment of the child should obtain a sample of urine for testing and inspection. Ask the child and parents about any changes in the child's elimination pattern such as abnormal colour of urine or obvious blood staining, reduction in urine output or in the number of wet nappies.

A bare weight must be obtained and compared to a recent weight if available. Weight gain indicates fluid retention. The child is observed for signs of oedema, such as swelling around the eyes and face; the ankles and sacral area may also appear oedematous.

An accurate blood pressure recording is an important nursing assessment; ask the child if he or she has a headache. Hypertension accompanied by a headache indicates cerebral oedema and requires medical intervention.

Medical intervention

Penicillin is usually the most appropriate antibiotic therapy. Pharmacological treatment varies according to the degree of fluid overload, hypertension and renal impairment. Hypertension is most often caused by fluid retention and may be treated with Frusemide or Spironolactone. If diuretic therapy is ineffective then an antihypertensive agent such as Nifedipine will be administered.

Investigations

Blood samples

Blood is collected for urea, electrolytes and creatinine levels to assess if the child has acute renal impairment.

Immunological investigations aid in the diagnosis of acute post-streptococcal glomerulonephritis. Anti-streptococcal antibody levels are elevated (ASOT, Anti DNase B). Serum complement levels (C3) are low.[3]

Urine

The urine should be tested using a dipstick, checking for the presence of blood and protein. A urinometer will determine specific gravity, which may be raised due to increased solute load in children with a reduced urine output.

Additionally, a spot urine sample (about 20 mL collected in a clean container) may be required for microscopic analysis of red blood cells, white cells and casts.

A 24-hour urine collection is sometimes required to quantify the amount of protein contained in the urine.

Throat swab

A throat swab or a swab of skin lesions is useful in choosing the antibiotic therapy.

Nursing management

Altered body fluid status

Children with glomerulonephritis may have an intravascular fluid volume excess which is related to an impairment in the kidney's filtration mechanism. This complication introduces the potential for hypertension, hypertensive encephalopathy and pulmonary oedema. Nursing care should therefore be planned around prevention and recognition of the complications of fluid overload, so that appropriate intervention may be implemented.

The following observations and interventions will prevent further fluid retention and help to maintain blood pressure within normal limits.

Daily bare **weight** on the same set of scales is a most important tool in assessment of body fluid status. Weight gain may require intervention strategies such as fluid restriction, diuretic therapy or antihypertensive medication. The child's physician should be notified of significant weight gain (500 g or more) immediately, so that medical treatment can be initiated.

Depending on the presence and degree of hypertension, **blood pressure** should be recorded every 2 to 4 hours, with an appropriate-sized blood pressure cuff. Ensure that the internal bladder of the cuff completely encircles the arm and covers 75% of the upper arm.

All children with glomerulonephritis should have their blood pressure recorded at least twice daily, regardless of whether they are hypertensive at their initial presentation. Hypertension may not present until later in the course of the disease and therefore could be missed.

Normal and acceptable blood pressure levels are related to the age and size of the child. Guidelines for acceptable upper and lower limits of blood pressure recordings should be discussed with the child's physician. Hypertension must be reported to medical staff promptly so that antihypertensive medication may be ordered and administered if necessary. Abnormal readings should be confirmed by a second person to avoid unnecessary administration of antihypertensives because of errors in blood pressure readings.

Fluid balance — All fluid intake and output must be recorded carefully.

Children will require a **fluid restriction** if they have hypertension or their urine output is reduced. The fluid restriction must include all oral and intravenous fluids and any fluid given with medications.

This intervention may cause a great deal of distress to the child and the parents because the child will feel thirsty. The thirst is due to an increased solute level in the blood caused by the reduced filtration capacity of the diseased kidney. Importantly, the reason for introducing and adhering to the fluid restriction should be explained to them.

The child requires supervision at any time that there may be temptation and access to fluid, including when cleaning teeth and when in the bathroom.

Sodium restriction — A no-added-salt diet and avoidance of foods excessively high in sodium should be introduced for children with fluid retention and hypertension. Common examples of foods that are high in sodium are Vegemite, tomato sauce and potato crisps.

Abnormal urine content

Children with glomerulonephritis have abnormal urinary excretion of blood and protein, which is related to inflammation of the glomeruli and impaired glomerular filtration. Nursing interventions make it possible to monitor the disease progression so that appropriate treatment may be implemented.

All urine voided should be tested for the presence of blood, protein, specific gravity and pH. Twenty to 30 mL of the first urine voided each day should be saved in a container. This observation is useful in assessing the degree of macroscopic haematuria present and also acts as a guide to effectiveness of the child's treatment.

Disease progress and outcome

In most cases there is a full recovery within 4 weeks. Oliguria rarely persists beyond 2 to 7 days, and the haematuria usually becomes microscopic within 10 to 14 days, disappearing in the following 2 weeks. Microscopic haematuria may persist for many months.

HENOCH SCHONLEIN PURPURA

Henoch Schonlein purpura is a disease that is characterised by a systemic vasculitis of the small blood vessels. The blood vessels of the skin, joints, gastrointestinal tract and kidneys are affected.

The cause of this disease is thought to be an allergic reaction to food, drugs, insect bites or infective agents.[2]

Children between the ages of 2 and 8 years are most commonly affected, however adults do occasionally develop this disease. Boys are affected about twice as often as girls.[2]

The child usually presents with a low-grade fever and feels quite lethargic and unwell, with loss of appetite common. Some children are noted to have had an upper respiratory tract infection a few weeks before presentation, while others may report a recent allergic reaction to a particular food, drug or an insect bite.[4]

All children develop a characteristic purpuric rash, mainly affecting the lower limbs, ankles, buttocks and arms. The face and trunk are not usually affected by the rash. Additional to the rash, children may have some or all of the following symptoms of the disease.

Gastrointestinal system

Two-thirds of children with Henoch Schonlein purpura present with abdominal pain, vomiting and diarrhoea,[5] with a small number of children having malaena or haematemesis. These problems are caused by the occurrence of petechiae throughout the gut.

Arthralgia

Swelling, inflammation and pain occurs in all joints in the majority of children.

Nervous system

A small number of children have neurological symptoms such as irritability and head-ache, with reports of cerebral haemorrhages in a small number of children.[5]

Renal involvement

The kidneys are affected by Henoch Schonlein purpura in approximately 10% to 40% of children. Of the children with renal involvement, approximately 80% have microscopic haematuria only, with fewer showing clinical symptoms of acute nephritis such as haematuria, proteinuria and hypertension. A small number of children develop nephrotic syndrome and reduced renal function.

Medical management

Non-steroidal anti-inflammatory agents are administered to treat the arthritis and abdominal pain, but steroids may help severe abdominal pain. Steroids and cytotoxic agents are given if the child has significant renal involvement, such as nephrotic syndrome with or without reduced renal function.

The child with Henoch Schonlein purpura may relapse, especially during the 6 months following the onset of the disease. Most children make a complete recovery, but those with nephritis require regular follow-up every 3 to 6 months. A small number of children develop hypertension or chronic renal failure and end-stage renal failure in the 5 to 10 years following the onset of the disease.

Nursing care

Nursing care of children with Henoch Schonlein purpura varies according to the system affected by the disease. Not all children display all of the symptoms.

All children who present with a diagnosis of Henoch Schonlein purpura should have their blood pressure, weight and urinalysis recorded daily so that renal involvement is detected early. Refer to guidelines for nursing care of children with glomerulonephritis, arthritis and gastrointestinal disorders.

IgA NEPHROPATHY

A common cause of glomerulonephritis in children and adults is IgA nephropathy. Characteristically, children develop macroscopic haematuria when they have an upper respiratory tract infection. Other children may be found incidentally to have microscopic haematuria or haematuria and proteinuria. The diagnosis is confirmed from the finding of deposits of immunoglobulin A in glomeruli on renal biopsy. Some children will progress to end-stage renal failure.

CHRONIC GLOMERULONEPHRITIS

Glomerulonephritis may be chronic and lead to progressive destruction of renal tissue and end-stage renal failure. Chronic glomerulonephritis occurs less frequently in children than in adults. Only 25% of adult patients with nephrotic syndrome have the acute, minimal change type of nephrotic syndrome, compared with 90% in young children.[6]

OTHER TYPES OF GLOMERULONEPHRITIS

Other types of chronic glomerulonephritis are mesangiocapillary glomerulonephritis, rapidly progressive glomerulonephritis, membranous glomerulonephritis, hereditary nephritis, and systemic lupus erythematosis nephritis.

Glomerulonephritis may present with microscopic or macroscopic haematuria, proteinuria, proteinuria and haematuria, acute nephritis, nephrotic syndrome, acute or chronic renal failure.

REFERENCES

1. Davison AM. *A synopsis of renal diseases.* Bristol: John Wright & Sons, 1981.
2. Behrmann RE, Kleyman R. Nelson essentials of pediatrics. Philadelphia: WB Saunders, 1990.
3. Whitworth JA, Lawrence JR. *Textbook of renal diseases.* Melbourne: Churchill Livingstone, 1987
4. Oliver C. Triage decisions. A 4 year old with petechial rash. *Emergency Nurses Assoc* 1994; 20: 164.
5. Lynch M, Potter M. Henoch Schonlein purpura: a case study. *Pediatric Nursing* 1990; 16: 561–566.
6. Cameron S. *Kidney disease. The facts.* Toronto: Oxford University Press, 1981.

Nephrotic Syndrome

The nephrotic syndrome is not a distinct disease. It is a term used to describe a clinical picture caused by an abnormality of the glomerular basement membrane such that it becomes more permeable to protein, particularly albumin, a relatively small molecule.

Characteristics of the nephrotic syndrome are as follows.

- Heavy proteinuria (3–5 g/day in adults; or > 3 g/1.73 m^2/day in children).
- Hypoproteinaemia and hypoalbuminaemia (Serum albumin < 25 g/L).
- Hyperlipidaemia.
- Oedema.
- Hypovolaemia is present early in the disease and then plasma volume normalises.
- Decreased urine output.

PATHOPHYSIOLOGY

Proteinuria

Large amounts of protein leak out through the glomerular basement membrane into the tubules and are excreted in the urine, resulting in serum protein levels becoming severely reduced.

Protein is a colloid which exerts an osmotic pressure to keep fluid inside the body's intravascular compartment. A reduction in osmotic pressure allows fluid to escape out of the intravascular compartment and into the interstitium and third spaces resulting in oedema and hypovolaemia.

Ascites

Fluid may collect in the child's abdominal cavity and become infected. Pneumococcal peritonitis is not an uncommon complication of the nephrotic syndrome.

Susceptibility to infection

The child with nephrotic syndrome has an increased susceptibility to infection due to the loss of molecules known as opsonins which are lost with albumin. Opsonins are required to process encapsulated organisms such as *Pneumococcus* and *Haemophilis*. Infections may be fatal to the child with nephrotic syndrome, particularly those children who require large doses of immunosuppressive medications to treat the disease.

Lipid abnormalities

Hypercholesterolaemia and hyperlipidaemia are also features of the nephrotic syndrome. The exact cause of these raised levels is not known. It is known that the liver attempts to compensate for protein loss by rapid protein synthesis and may inadvertently manufacture cholesterol and lipids.[1]

MINIMAL CHANGE NEPHROTIC SYNDROME

The most common cause of the nephrotic syndrome in children is minimal change glomerulonephritis, the cause of which is not known.[2] Characteristically, the glomeruli obtained on renal biopsy appear normal on light microscopy.

Onset of minimal change nephrotic syndrome occurs between the ages of 2 and 7 years and is reportedly more common in boys.[3]

INVESTIGATIONS

Blood analysis

Blood is tested for urea, electrolytes and creatinine. Urea and creatinine are usually normal in minimal change glomerulonephritis. Serum albumin levels are reduced.

Urine analysis

Urine is examined for protein and red blood cells. It is unusual for macroscopic haematuria to occur, but about one-third of children have microscopic haematuria.

Renal biopsy

Renal biopsy is only performed in children who do not respond to steroid treatment or who have hypertension, macroscopic haematuria or reduced renal function.

NURSING MANAGEMENT

Assessment

Nursing assessment is similar to that for the child with glomerulonephritis.

The oedema of the nephrotic syndrome is more severe than that seen in glomerulonephritis and results in the child's entire body having a swollen appearance. The oedema is particularly noticeable in the face and around the eyes. Oedema settles with gravity, causing the eyelids to appear especially puffy in the mornings. Some children can not open their eyes when they wake, particularly if they have been lying flat to sleep. Boys often have scrotal oedema and girls have labial oedema which worsen throughout the day as children walk around.

Urine output is decreased and urine may have a frothy appearance due to the presence of large amounts of protein and lipids.

Temperature, pulse and respirations must be recorded. Blood pressure should be recorded at the initial nursing assessment and should continue to be observed every 4 hours, although it is unusual for children with minimal change nephrotic syndrome to have hypertension.

Intervention

Children with nephrotic syndrome have an altered body fluid status related to an accumulation of excess fluid in the interstitial and third spaces. Additionally, there is depletion of fluid in the intravascular compartment caused by the alteration to kidney function.

Observations are directed towards assessment of the child's current fluid status so that further fluid accumulation can be prevented.

Skin Care

There is a potential for impaired skin integrity as a result of oedema inhibiting blood flow to the tissues, causing poor cellular nutrition.[4] Reduced activity and poor nutrition also place the child at increased risk for tissue damage. The skin must be kept clean and dry to prevent skin breakdown and infection.

Check that clothing is not too tight and that the elasticised waist of pyjama pants does not create too much pressure on the oedematous skin.

Bathe eyes frequently if they are swollen.

Table 5.5 Nursing observations of children with nephrotic syndrome

Observation:	Weigh daily before breakfast, on the same set of scales each time.
Rationale:	For accurate assessment of the child's body fluid status. Body fluid status fluctuates according to the degree of oedema.
Observation:	Record blood pressure every 4 hours. Ensure that the blood pressure cuff covers 75% of the child's upper arm.
Rationale:	Blood pressure recording is a useful assessment of the child's fluid status. Intravascular fluid retention is indicated by hypertension, and intravascular fluid depletion is indicated by hypotension.
Observation:	Twice daily girth measurements. Ensure the measurements are accurate by marking the child's abdomen with a pen and placing the tape measure around the marked area each time.
Rationale:	The presence of ascites is indicated by an increased girth measurement.
Observation:	Accurate recording of fluid intake and output.
Rationale:	To assess the progression of the disease and to assess the child's fluid status and fluid replacement requirements.
Observation:	Perform a dipstick urinalysis for blood and protein daily.
Rationale:	To assess the progression of the disease.

Activity

Bed rest is not encouraged since children with nephrotic syndrome have hypercoagulation tendencies, and is only necessary if the child is extremely oedematous or hypertensive.[5] Hypertension is uncommon in children with minimal change nephrotic syndrome, however, they are quite often lethargic and limit activity because of the increased fluid load.

Frequent pressure area care and change of position is important in those children spending a lot of time in bed.

Scrotal support

Scrotal support may be required to make boys with severe scrotal oedema more comfortable. Adhesive urine collection bags should not be used on children with genital oedema.

Nutrition

Nutritional status is often impaired because children have an oedematous gut, causing them to be anorexic and to vomit. Lethargy contributes to the child's lack of interest in food, and heavy proteinuria also affects the child's state of nutrition. Providing adequate nutrition is a challenge for caregivers. Children should be encouraged to eat nutritious, high protein meals, snacks and milkshakes. Favourite foods should be provided if possible.

Children should not be disturbed to perform nursing care while they are eating.

Restriction of fluid and salt intake is sometimes indicated if fluid retention is severe enough to cause hypertension.[6]

Prevention of infection

Children with nephrotic syndrome have an increased susceptibility to infection related to the loss of gammaglobulins, opsonins and immunosuppressive therapy. As a result, peritonitis, septicaemia, cellulitis and pneumonia may occur. The following strategies are implemented when planning nursing care to assist in the prevention of infection.

- The child and family are informed of the increased risk of infection. They should be advised to avoid contact with persons suffering infectious diseases, e.g., chickenpox, measles, colds and influenza.
- Temperature is recorded every 4 hours and even low-grade fevers reported to the attending physician because prednisolone masks fevers.
- Abdominal pain should always be investigated immediately because it could indicate peritonitis.
- Intravenous cannula sites are inspected regularly and the cannula removed immediately if the entry site appears inflamed.
- It is important to wash hands before attending nursing care to avoid cross-infection.

Medications

Administer medications (e.g., steroids and diuretics), and intravenous albumin as ordered. Children quite often refuse to take prednisolone because of its bitter taste. A lot of patience and explanation about the importance of the drug is necessary to encourage children to take this medication. Steroids must be given with food to avoid gastric ulceration.

Altered body image

There is a potential for non-compliance with medication after discharge from hospital related to concern about steroids affecting the child's appearance. Side effects such as obesity and moon facies understandably cause considerable distress to both the child and parents.

Education and counselling to promote acceptance and understanding of the disease should begin at an early stage in the child's disease. A well informed family is more likely to comply with the medication regimen.

The child and family should be allowed to express their anxieties, but the importance of following medication orders must be stressed.

MEDICAL INTERVENTION

The goal of treatment is to reduce urinary protein loss, restore the intravascular fluid volume and eliminate oedema.

Medical treatment usually begins with administration of oral prednisolone. Daily steroid therapy continues for 4 to 6 weeks. Most children go into remission, losing their proteinuria completely within 2 to 3 weeks. Prednisolone is then given in reducing doses, on alternate days to prevent side effects. Steroids usually continue for several months to reduce the likelihood of relapse. If there is no response to prednisolone therapy, or the child has frequent relapses of the disease, an immunosuppressant such as cyclophosphamide or cyclosporine may be used.[7]

When oedema is excessive and the child feels uncomfortable, intravenous albumin may be given. Albumin infusions raise the intravascular oncotic pressure and drag fluid back into the intravascular space. An intravenous diuretic is also given to remove excess fluid from the body. The diuretic should be given before the administration of the albumin to establish a urine output before restoring the intravascular fluid volume. This treatment will provide only temporary relief from the discomfort and complications of oedema and fluid retention.

PROGRESSION AND OUTCOME OF THE DISEASE

A successful outcome of nursing and medical intervention is indicated by an increase in serum albumin and protein, reduction of excess fluid in the extravascular compartments and increased intravascular fluid. Nurses are able to assess the efficiency of interventions clinically by observing a decrease in the child's weight and degree of oedema, decreased abdominal girth measurement, a reduction in the amount of protein in the urine and the observation of normal blood pressure.

Minimal change nephrotic syndrome quite often follows a course of remission and relapse and in most cases resolves by adolescence.

FOCAL SEGMENTAL GLOMERULONEPHRITIS

Children presenting with this type of nephrotic syndrome may be mistakenly diagnosed as having minimal change glomerulonephritis. In its early stages the disease only affects the glomeruli at the corticomedullary junction and if a diagnostic renal biopsy is performed the diseased glomeruli may be missed.

Characteristically, these children present with nephrotic syndrome resembling minimal change glomerulonephritis but have a poor response to steroid therapy.[8] The disease is progressive and destroys the kidney, resulting in end-stage renal failure, with the disease recurring in transplant kidneys.

Other causes of nephrotic syndrome which present as a primary disease process are mesangial capillary glomerulonephritis, membranoproliferative glomerulonephritis and membranous glomerulopathy.

Nephrotic syndrome may also present as a secondary characteristic of an underlying disease such as post-streptococcal glomerulonephritis, Henoch Schonlein purpura and systemic lupus erythematosis.

REFERENCES

1. Uldall R. *Renal nursing.* 3rd ed. Boston: Blackwell Scientific, 1988.
2. Brodehl J. Conventional treatment for idiopathic nephrotic syndrome in children. *Clinical Nephrology* 1991; 35 Suppl. 1: S8–S15.
3. Behrmann RE, Kleyman R. *Nelson essentials of pediatrics.* Philadelphia: WB Saunders, 1990.
4. Carpenito LJ. *Nursing diagnosis. Application to practice.* 5th ed. Philadelphia: JB Lippincott, 1993.
5. Johnson DL. Nephrotic syndrome: a nursing care plan based on current pathophysiologic concepts. *Heart and Lung* 1989; 18: 88–93.
6. Wong DL, Whaley LF. *Clinical manual of pediatric nursing.* St Louis: CV Mosby, 1990.
7. Niaudet P, Broyer M, Habib R. Treatment of nephrotic syndrome with cyclosporin A in children. *Clinical Nephrology* 1991; 1: 530–534.
8. Mallick NP. Epidemiology and natural course of idiopathic nephrotic syndrome. *Clinical Nephrology* 1991; 35 suppl. 1: S3–S7.

Disturbances in Immunological Function

Juvenile Rheumatoid Arthritis

Isobel Taylor

Juvenile rheumatoid arthritis (JRA) is synonymous with juvenile chronic arthritis (JCA) and Still's disease. George Still was a registrar (in the 19th Century) at St Thomas's Hospital, London, where he documented case descriptions of children with inflammatory arthritis which clearly differentiated the disease process from rheumatic fever.

Juvenile rheumatoid arthritis is a disease of low prevalance (affecting 1 in 1000) characterised by chronic inflammation of one or more joints and lasting a minimum of 6 weeks in children under 16 years of age. JRA differs from adult-onset rheumatoid arthritis by its tendency toward spontaneous remission (70% of affected children will achieve permanent remission by adulthood). Joint pain in childhood is a common occurrence and, since the presentation and course of JRA is so variable, joint pain or tenderness alone are insufficient for a diagnosis of JRA. The diagnostic process may take time until all other causes of arthritis can be excluded and a pattern of symptoms and signs characteristic of JRA becomes evident.

A classification system of types and subtypes has been developed under the auspices of the International League Against Rheumatism (ILAR) to aid the diagnostic process and to improve the management of the condition.[1]

CHARACTERISTICS OF JRA TYPES

Type 1: Pauciarticular JRA

This is the most common type, representing 50% of all children presenting with JRA. It is more common in girls. There are the following 3 subtypes within this group.

1. Girls with circulating antinuclear antibodies (ANA) who are at risk of developing the serious inflammatory eye disease of iridocyclitis.
2. Older boys who are Human Leucocyte Antigen (HLA) B27 positive and who are at risk of development of ankylosing spondylitis.
3. Children who are neither ANA or HLA B27 positive but have involvement of the large joints such as the knees.

The involvement of the temperomandibular joints may be a feature of all 3 subtypes.

Type 2: Polyarticular JRA

This type is represented in 25% to 30% of children with JRA and again is more common in girls. It is characterised by involvement of 5 or more joints. There are 2 subtypes within this group.

1. Those children who have circulating rheumatoid factor (RF), that is, an antibody with antiglobulin activity (usually IgM anti-IgG). These children are at risk of developing progressive, erosive, nodular disease persisting throughout adult life.

2. No RF but chronic arthritis most often in knees, ankles, wrists, elbows, metacarpal phalangeal (MCP) joints and proximal interphalangeal (PIP) joints.

Type 3: Systemic JRA

This type accounts for 20% to 30% of JRA presentations and occurs equally in boys and girls. It is characterised by the onset in younger children of polyarthritis accompanied by fever, an evanescent rash, pericarditis and pleuritis.

ASSESSMENT

A systematic approach to the nursing assessment and management includes physical assessment as well as an appraisal of the impact of the disease on the child and the family. This will allow the nurse to plan the most effective type of problem-solving care to meet the identified needs of that particular child and family. An assessment tool is needed which incorporates a functional assessment report and an arthritis impact measurement scale adapted to the age of the child and which takes into account the social and cultural environment of the child and family.

NURSING MANAGEMENT

An appropriate clinical nursing focus in the management of children and families affected by JRA is that which encompasses the nursing competencies suggested by Benner's domains of nursing practice.[2]

The helping role

Providing comfort measures and preserving personhood in the face of pain and extreme breakdown.

Interpreting kinds of pain and selecting appropriate strategies for pain management and control.

Providing emotional and informational support to patients' families.

Maximising the patient's participation and control in his or her own management.

The teaching-coaching function

Timing: capturing a patient's readiness to learn.

Assisting patients and families to integrate the implications of the illness and recovery into their lifestyles.

Eliciting and understanding the patient's interpretation of their illness.

The diagnostic and monitoring function

Anticipating problems.

Understanding the particular demands and experiences of the illness: and anticipating patient care needs.

Assessing the patient's potential for wellness and for responding to various treatment strategies.

Administering and monitoring therapeutic interventions and regimens

Administering medications accurately and safely: monitoring untoward effects.

Combating the hazards of immobility: ambulating and exercising patients to maximise mobility and rehabilitation.

Planning the care

An effective management approach to the child and family who have to learn to cope with a chronic illness, the aetiology of which is uncertain and for which there is as yet no cure is a *patient problem model*.[3] Frequently occurring problems of children with rheumatic diseases can be assembled into 4 distinct groups.

1. alterations in comfort;
2. functional alterations;
3. adaptational alterations; and
4. physical alterations.

Each group contains a cluster of specific alterations which relate to each other and interact with alterations in other groups. Identification of problems using this schema facilitates the formulation of nursing diagnoses and the development of a management plan.

Alterations in comfort

Pain, stiffness, fatigue and sleep pattern disturbance are common problems experienced by children with JRA. The pain may be due to inflammation and muscle spasm or poor positioning and overuse of the joint. Sometimes stiffness is perceived as pain. Fatigue may be due to the disease process, anaemia, anxiety and inadequate sleep. Careful observation of the child to identify the factors contributing to the comfort alterations will enable the nurse to choose the most effective management options.

Interventions: Basic comfort measures include changing position, checking the fit of splints and the tightness of bandages and adjusting as necessary. The use of bed cradle and foot board relieves pressure and supports the lower limbs while the child is in bed. Local measures include the use of hot or cold packs. A gentle range of motion exercises, massage and traction are some mechanical options that help relieve muscle spasm. The correct timing of the prescribed analgesic and anti-inflammatory medications is important to maintain therapeutic blood levels of the drugs. The joint stiffness is most marked in the morning, and a late evening and early morning dose of the anti-inflammatory drug is indicated. To protect the gastric mucosa, these doses are given with a snack and a milk drink.

Functional alterations

Changes in mobility and a change in the activities of daily living are related to pain, stiffness and muscle weakness. It is difficult to build muscle strength without stressing inflamed joints. A child who has reached independence in personal hygiene and dressing and whose social life revolves around physical pursuits may now need the kind of assistance he or she required at an earlier developmental stage. Many children react to this with a degree of anger, anxiety and depression. It is important that nurses and parents avoid the trap of taking over completely the child's daily living skills. It may be quicker and seem kinder to do everything for the child, but it is vital that the child continues to

Table 5.6 Investigations used in JRA

Diagnostic tests

Blood tests
Antinuclear antibodies
Antibodies to DNA
Tests for immunoglobulins
Blood concentrations of complement (C3, C4, C5)
Tests for rheumatoid factor
Tissue typing for HLA B27

Tests useful for monitoring the course of the disease and treatment

Synovial fluid analysis
X-rays
Bone scan
Haemoglobin, haematocrit and reticulocyte count
White blood cell count
Platelet count
Erythrocyte sedimentation rate
Liver function tests
Urinalysis

---

do as much as possible. The correct use of appropriate assistive devices will protect joints during activities of daily living.

The child's natural response to joint pain will be to assume a position of comfort and stay still. The assumed position is usually one of flexion and will result in flexion contractures if the position is not corrected. The concept of the risk to the child of flexion contracture resulting from assuming non-functional positions for long periods, e.g., lying curled up in bed or on a couch watching TV, must be grasped by the parent and child and guarded against at all costs. Hips and knees are vulnerable, as is the cervical spine. Good posture during sitting, lying, standing and walking should be demonstrated to the parents and the child and strategies such as regular short periods of prone lying and the use of adjustable desk and chair heights should be encouraged.

Adaptational alterations

Change in self-esteem and limitations in insight are problems that may be missed unless careful assessment and observation are done. It should be recognised that a child's and indeed the family's self-esteem may be threatened or changed by JRA. The child and family will need patient teaching and coaching to help them understand the disease process and how they can take control and gain mastery over their own lives. It is worthwhile for the nurse to establish good communication with the child and family. Open communication will allow the airing of any problems and difficulties within the family, so that these may be addressed and appropriate referrals made. The siblings of children with chronic illnesses sometimes suffer from a perceived lack of attention from the parents and guilt feelings because they may experience strong resentment or negative feelings towards the ill child.

While the aetiology of this disease remains unclear, recent research has increasingly focussed on immunogenetic aspects, and this is reflected in the type of laboratory tests undertaken (**Table 5.6**).

tre
thi
me

C

In
be
se
pe
si
di
m
a
v
a

P

T
c
v
c
f
l
l

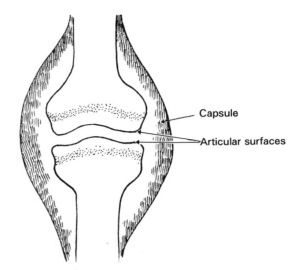

Figure 5.1 Normal synovial joint.

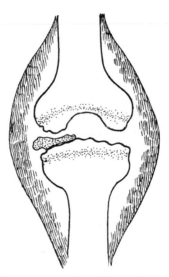

Figure 5.2 Destructive changes to the articular surfaces of the synovial joint due to inflammatory reactions in the synovium.

The synovium lining the joint undergoes inflammatory changes, thickens and becomes destructive to the articular cartilage and soft tissues (**Figures 5.1 and 5.2**). It is hypothesised that an autoimmune response results from a trigger factor such as a virus in a genetically susceptible individual and the immune system targets certain of the body's own cells as foreign cells and sets up the inflammatory reaction.

Chicken Pox

Jennifer Backhouse

Chicken pox is a common, generally benign contagious disease caused by the varicella zoster virus, a member of the herpes virus group. It predominantly affects young children aged 4 to 10 years, but can occur well into adolescence and adulthood.[1–3] After contracting chicken pox a person is immune to reinfection. Except in some instances, immunity is life-long.[1,2] Man is the only source of infection, which is by either person-to-person contact, or droplet infection. However, airborne transmission has been documented.[1,2] The virus gains entry at the conjunctivae and/or mucosa of the upper respiratory tract. It then multiplies in regional lymph nodes.[1,2] The virus is highly communicable for 1 to 2 days before the onset of the rash, and can be contagious for 5 days after,[1–4] or until the lesions are all crusted.[2,3] The incubation period is usually 14 to 16 days, but some cases occur as early as 11 days and as late as 21 days.[2–4]

The disease is characterised by a generalised pruritic vesicular rash, with a mild fever and few systemic symptoms (headache, malaise and anorexia).[2,3,5] The skin lesions, which tend to erupt in crops, usually begin on the neck or the trunk and spread to the face, scalp, mucous membranes and extremities. These first appear as small, flat, red blotches that progress to raised vesicles. The vesicles contain fluid which contains the varicella virus. As the lesion progresses the fluid is absorbed and a scab is formed. The scab is first adherent, then later becomes detached, leaving a shallow pink depression which eventually becomes white without scar formation etching. Prematurely removed scabs or secondarily infected lesions may cause scarring.

Complications from chicken pox can vary from mild to severe or even fatal.[1,2,4,6] The most common is bacterial superinfection; others are thrombocytopenia, arthritis, hepatitis, encephalitis or meningitis, glomerulonephritis and Reyes syndrome.

Encephalitis occurs in less than 1 in every 1000 cases of varicella. Encephalitis can have cerebellar involvement or affect the central nervous system. Cerebellar involvement with ataxia is more common in varicella than in measles encephalitis and this usually has a good prognosis. The symptoms of central nervous system involvement usually develop between the 3rd and 8th days after the rash appears. The signs are those of meningoencephalo-myelitis: fever, headache, stiff neck, change in sensorium and occasionally convulsions, stupor, coma and paralysis. This has a more guarded prognosis.[2,6]

A study in New Mexico found the incidence of Reye syndrome to be 2.5 per 1000 cases. Symptoms usually develop within a few days to several weeks. The condition is almost self-limiting and requires no specific therapy. Until then it was not realised that the liver can be involved in uncomplicated varicella.[2]

Varicella of the newborn infant can occur if the mother has been exposed to the disease shortly before delivery. Maternal varicella usually occurs 5 to 10 days before delivery. Congenital varicella syndrome is extremely rare, but may develop after maternal varicella in the 1st or early 2nd trimester of pregnancy. The malformations can be limb atrophy, cicatricial skin lesions, central nervous system and eye manifestations.[1,2,7]

Immunocompromised patients have a high risk of serious varicella infection. The best-studied group in this category is the leukaemia or lymphoma patient. The complications are pneumonia, hepatitis and encephalitis, which can be fatal to these patients.[8–11] The duration of the vesicular eruption can be a week or longer in immunocompromised patients.[10,12,13]

Varicella-Zoster immune globulin (VZIG) should be given to the following susceptible individuals at high risk.

- Immunocompromised children.
- Newborn infants of mothers who had varicella within 5 days before delivery or within 48 hours after delivery.
- Sick or unstable infants whose mothers lack a prior history of chicken pox.

The patient should receive VZIG within 96 hours of exposure, but preferably before 72 hours.[1] Those patients who receive VZIG should remain in isolation until 28 days after exposure.

Most children will not require hospitalisation as the illness can be managed at home. The child may need antipyretics (no aspirin because of the relationship of Reyes syndrome). Baths with local applications of calamine lotion or antipruritic ointment help to control the itching. Fingernails should be kept short and clean to minimise scratching of the vesicles, which may then develop secondary skin infection.[1,2]

The child who is hospitalised will need to be isolated until lesions are all crusted, and treated as above with antipyretics, baths and calamine lotion. An antiviral such as Acyclovir may be given, usually by intravenous infusion.

REFERENCES

1. Committee on Infectious Diseases. *Report of the Committee on Infectious Diseases.* 21st ed. Illinois: American Academy of Pediatrics, 1988.
2. Krugman S, Katz SL, Gershon AA, Wilfert CM. *Infectious diseases of children.* 9th ed. St Louis: Mosby, 1992.
3. Mott SR, James SR, Sperhac AM. *Nursing care of children and families.* 2nd ed. Menlo Park: Addison-Wesley, 1990.
4. Plotkin SA. Varicella vaccine: a point of decision. *Pediatrics* 1986; 78: 703–707.
5. Department of Health, NSW. Some infectious diseases of children. *Symptoms and signs: exclusion from school.* Sydney: The Department, 1992.
6. Krywanio ML. Varicella encephalitis. *J Neurosci Nursing* 1991; 23: 363–368.
7. Grose C. Variation on a theme by Fenner. The pathogenesis of chicken pox. *Pediatrics* 1981; 68: 735–737.
8. Arbeter AM, Granowetter L, Starr SE, Lange B, Wimmer R, Plotkin SA. Immunization of children with acute lymphoblastic leukemia with live attenuated varicella vaccine without complete suspension of chemotherapy. *Pediatrics* 1990; 85: 338–344.
9. Brunell PA, Taylor A, Wiedeman J, Greiser CF, Frierson L, Lydick E. Risk of herpes zoster in children with leukemia. Varicella vaccine compared with history of chicken pox. *Pediatrics* 1985; 77: 53–56.
10. Feldman S, Lott L. Varicella in children with cancer: impact of antiviral therapy and prophylaxis. *Pediatrics* 1987; 80: 465–472.
11. Gershon AA, Steinberg SP, The Varicella Vaccine Collaborative Study Group of the National Institute of Allergy and Infectious Diseases. Persistence of immunity to varicella in children with leukemia immunized with live attenuated varicella vaccine. *N Engl J Med* 1989; 320: 892–897.
12. Prebud SR. Varicella: complications and costs. *Pediatrics* 1986; 78: 723–735.
13. Stevens M. *Resource manual, oncology unit.* Sydney: RAHC, 1992.

Measles

Helen Sharp

Measles is a highly contagious, acute febrile illness caused by the morbilli virus of the paramyxovirus family.[1-4] It is transmitted by direct contact with respiratory droplet spray from coughing or sneezing, or by small infected droplets which remain suspended in air for considerable periods of time.[1,2,5,6] In young children, the measles virus may also be spread from one person to the next when the child handles infected nasal secretions before touching his or her own nose.[1] The virus is highly communicable for 1 to 2 days before the onset of symptoms, with infectivity peaking during the late prodrome and lasting until 3 to 4 days after the appearance of the rash.[1-4,7,8] Clinically, it is a cyclic, epidemic disease, which with the introduction of live measles vaccine has become less frequent and more isolated in developed countries.[1-4,9] Live vaccination has also altered the age distribution of susceptible people, leading to a rise in the number of older children and adults contracting the disease. As a result a greater percentage of young women of childbearing age are at risk of gestational measles and the possible teratogenic effects on the unborn child.[10-15] Approximately 95% of children infected with the measles virus will manifest some symptoms. These range from the very mild modified measles which appears in the partially immune person, to the more serious form in which high fever, generalised rash and cerebral involvement occurs.[1,3,16] Immunocompromised children, and those under 2 years of age are at greatest risk for severe infection and mortality from the disease.[17-21]

The illness typically presents with fever, cough, coryza, conjunctivitis and malaise, after an 8 to 12 day incubation period.[5-8,10] These symptoms increase in severity over the next 4 days with the fever reaching 39.5°C to 40.5°C. During this period the buccal mucosa becomes reddened and small bluish white spots, called Koplik spots, appear on its surface. Approximately 48 hours later a maculopapular rash appears on the body. The rash, which begins behind the ears and on the forehead at the hair line, progresses distally, coalescing as new areas become affected. It begins to clear 3 to 5 days later, turning a coppery colour as it fades. Desquamation frequently occurs while the discoloured areas heal. With the appearance of the rash the cough loosens up, and the conjunctivitis and nasal symptoms gradually subside. The fever usually peaks around the 2nd to 3rd day of the rash, then subsides over the next 24 to 48 hours.[1-3,18] After recovering from the infection the child will normally have a life-long immunity.[2,3]

Complications resulting from measles infection occur in approximately 1 in 15 people and can vary from mild to severe, or even fatal.[1,3,10,15,17] The complications mainly involve the respiratory or nervous systems, although occasionally disorders such as thrombocytopenic purpura and hepatitis have been reported.[1,3] Viral bronchitis, bronchiolitis and pneumonia are frequently present, while approximately 15% of laryngotracheobronchitis cases may be related to measles, especially during the prodromal stage.[1,8] Pneumonia and bronchopneumonia may occur as a result of secondary bacterial infections caused by the common respiratory pathogens, and are the most likely cause of death.[2,4,8,15] In infants and young children, otitis media is frequently present.[1,3,4,17]

Encephalitis may also occur as a complication of measles infection. When present, it is usually evident within 8 days from the onset of the illness, although occasionally it may develop during the prodromal stage.[4,13,15,20,22] A small number of children and adolescents will develop subacute sclerosing panencephalitis, which is a rare degenerative central nervous system disease due to a persistent measles viral infection. Subacute sclerosing panencephalitis has an incubation period of 5 to 7 years, with a greater risk in children who acquire measles at an early age. There is at present no cure, and death usually occurs within 6 to 9 months of onset.[1-3,8] Fortunately, since the introduction of routine vaccination this disorder has been virtually eradicated.[14,17]

NURSING ASSESSMENT

Most commonly, the typical appearance of the bleary-eyed, miserable, febrile, coughing child with a developing blotchy, maculopapular rash will alert the nurse to the diagnosis of measles.[3] A nursing history is obtained to establish when the symptoms were first noticed and whether the child has been in contact with another confirmed case of measles.[12] Baseline observations of temperature, pulse and respirations are recorded to establish the degree of fever and respiratory distress. The child or parents are asked whether there have been any signs of neurological involvement such as headaches, convulsions, lethargy or irritability.[13,20,22] The child's mouth should be examined for the presence of Koplik spots,[3,18] and the child observed for signs of photophobia. When necessary, the diagnosis can be confirmed by serology[1,3,22,23] or viral isolation in tissue culture.[2,6,18,24] Once measles is diagnosed it should be notified to the health authorities, in all States of Australia.[11,14,17]

IMPLEMENTATION OF CARE

Most children will not require hospitalisation, as the illness can be managed quite satisfactorily at home. If, however, the child develops increasing respiratory distress, unresponsive croup, persisting tachypnoea, unexplained drowsiness or convulsions, marked toxicity, persisting hyperpyrexia, or the recurrence of significant fever, hospital admission may be necessary.[3,22] Once in hospital, the child will need to be nursed in respiratory isolation until approximately 4 days after the onset of the rash, to prevent the spread of infection.[2,8]

The child should be observed for any change in respiratory or neurological status and any increase in temperature. Bed rest and quiet activity is advisable while the child is febrile, to conserve energy. Bright lights are best avoided if photophobia is present. Antipyretics such as paracetamol may be required to control the fever, while antibiotics may be prescribed for secondary bacterial infections. Fluid intake is encouraged to prevent a fluid volume deficit, especially when fever is present, and a soft diet should be offered as tolerated.[1,3,8,18] The child should be excluded from school for 5 days after the appearance of the rash, or until fully recovered.[7,10]

PREVENTION

Measles is a preventable illness which has been greatly reduced in incidence since the introduction of the vaccine.[1,3,4] The measles vaccine is a live attenuated vaccine produced in chicken embryos and may safely be used before and after exposure.[1-4] This vaccine should be stored at temperatures between 2°C and 8°C, used within 1 hour of reconstitution and should be protected from light. Failure to do this can result in inactivation of the virus.[2,4,25] Ideally, it is given as a single subcutaneous dose, either alone or in combination with the mumps and rubella vaccine.[2,4,12,25] There has, however, been some suggestion that 2 doses should be given due to reported outbreaks of measles in vaccinated children who have failed to seroconvert.[1,4,15,22]

The vaccine is safe and effective, and can be used in children who are suffering from mild fever or who are human immunodeficiency virus positive.[2,4,5,21] It should not, however, be used in children who are suffering from defective cell-mediated immunity such as leukaemia or lymphoma and those receiving immunosuppressive therapy. These children can be given normal human immunoglobulin within 6 days of exposure to the virus.[1,3,6,7,18] Children who have received treatment with gammaglobulin should not be given the vaccine for 3 months after cessation of the treatment.[2–4,18,25] No adverse reactions have been reported in children who have been given the vaccine when already immune.[4,10,16,25] Side effects occur rarely and usually consist of fever or irritability with or without a rash. Very rarely a more serious reaction may present.[1,3,4,25]

While the vaccine can be given to any age group, the recommended age for routine immunisation is between 12 and 15 months,[2,7,9,22,26] as children under 12 months of age usually have acquired their mothers' antibodies to the illness.[4,20,26] In developing countries and communities at risk, however, routine immunisation is carried out at 9 months and again at 15 to 18 months.[4,9,20,26] During an outbreak of measles, the spread of infection can be contained by immunising susceptible children within 72 hours of contact with an infected person.[4,10,26]

REFERENCES

1.   Cherry DJ. Measles. *In:* Feigin RD, Cherry JD, eds. *Textbook of pediatric infectious diseases.* 3rd ed. Philadelphia: WB Saunders, 1993.
2.   Committee on Infectious Diseases. *Report of The Committee on Infectious Diseases.* 21st ed. Elk Grove Village, Ill: American Academy of Pediatrics, 1988: 277–289.
3.   Kennedy DH. Measles. *The Practitioner* 1990; 234: 895–900.
4.   National Health and Medical Research Council. *The Australian immunisation procedures handbook.* 5th ed. Canberra: AGPS, 1994.
5.   Farizo KM, Ster-Green PA, Simpson DM, Markowitz LE. Pediatric emergency room visits: a risk factor for acquiring measles. *Pediatrics* 1991; 87: 74–79.
6.   Rivera ME, Mason WH, Ross LA, Wright HT. Nosocomial measles infection in a pediatric hospital during a community-wide epidemic. *J Pediatrics* 1991; 119; 183–186.
7.   Kilham H, ed. *The Children's Hospital handbook.* Sydney: Alken Press, 1993.
8.   Nelson JD. *Current therapy in pediatric infectious disease — 2.* Toronto: BC Decker, 1988: 256–258.
9.   Levy MH, Bridges-Webb C. Just one shot is not enough — measles control and eradication. *Med J Aust* 1990; 152: 489–491.
10.   Cheah D, Scott R, Passaris I. Measles outbreak in Canberra. *Communicable Diseases Intelligence* 1992; 16: 114–117.
11.   Communicable Diseases Intelligence Laboratory Reporting Scheme. Measles — CDI Laboratory Reporting Schemes and National Notifiable Diseases Data. *Communicable Diseases Intelligence* 1991; 15: 313–315.
12.   Hutchins SS, Escolan J, Markowitz LE, Hawkins C, Kimber A, Morgan RA, Preblud SR, Orenstein WA. Measles outbreak among unvaccinated preschool-aged children: opportunities missed by health care providers to administer measles vaccine. *Pediatrics* 1989; 83: 369–374.
13.   Morbidity and Mortality Report, Centers For Disease Control, Atlanta. Current trends measles — United States, 1987. *Arch Dermatol* 1988; 124: 1627–1628.

14. Nolan T. Measles — eradication or procrastination. *Med J Aust* 1990; 152: 449–450.
15. Weinstein P, Carrangis J. Measles resurgence in South Australia. *Communicable Diseases Intelligence* 1991; 15: 312.
16. Conway SP, Phillips RR. Morbidity in whooping cough and measles. *Arch Dis Childh* 1989; 64: 1442–1445.
17. Christopher PJ. Measles campaign: $11 million saved in New South Wales. *Med J Aust* 1989; 151: 485–486.
18. Gershon AA. Childhood exanthema. *In:* Kass EH, Platt R, eds. *Current therapy in infectious disease — 3.* Toronto: BC Decker, 1990: 68–69.
19. Jeffs DA, Wenzel WA. Birthday card reminders to increase measles immunization rates. *Med J Aust* 1989; 151: 723.
20. Kakakios AM, Burgess MA, Bransby RD, Quinn AA, Allars HM. Optimal age for measles and mumps vaccination in Australia. *Med J Aust* 1990; 152: 472–474.
21. Sension MG, Quinn TC, Markowitz LE, Linnan MJ, Francis HL, Nzilambi N, Duma MN, Ryder RW. Measles in hospitalized African children with human immunodeficiency virus. *Am J Dis Childh* 1988; 142: 1271–1272.
22. Morbidity and Mortality Weekly Report. Measles — United States, first 26 weeks, 1989. *JAMA* 1990; 263: 497–498, 501.
23. Brennan R, Gokel G, Maloney M. Tennant Creek measles outbreak February–March 1992. *Communicable Diseases Intelligence* 1992; 16: 271–272.
24. Schepetiuk S, Norton R. Measles diagnosis by viral culture. *Communicable Diseases Intelligence* 1992; 16: 383–384.
25. Editorial. Measles/mumps/rubella vaccine. *Lancet* 1988; 2: 860.
26. Isaacs D, ed. Measles in New South Wales. *Communicable Diseases Intelligence* 1991; 15: 208–209.

Mumps

Helen Sharp

Mumps or parotitis is an acute illness caused by a strain of the paramyxovirus, which is readily transferred by direct contact with an infectious carrier. The virus enters the host via the nose or mouth and settles in the salivary glands or upper respiratory mucosa where it proliferates, causing viraemia and generalised illness.[1-4] The incubation period is most commonly 16 to 18 days following contact with an infected person, although cases have been reported anywhere between 12 and 25 days after exposure.[1,2,4,5] Once the child is infected the period of communicability normally lasts 1 to 2 days before the onset of parotid swelling and 5 days afterwards. In some children, however, the period of communicability may last as long as 7 days before the onset of symptoms and 9 days after swelling.[1,2,5,6] Until recently, the illness predominantly affected young children between the ages of 5 and 9 years.[1,2,4,7,8] While this age group is still affected, there has been an increase in the number of children between 10 and 19 years contracting the disease since the introduction of vaccination for mumps. This shift is related to the absence of, or inadequate vaccination of the older age group. Over all however, there has been a decline in the incidence of mumps since the introduction of live vaccine.[2,3,7,9,10]

The illness is usually characterised by painful swelling of the parotid glands, which may be unilateral or bilateral, and causes discomfort rather than tenderness.[1-5,11] One-third of mumps infections fail to produce clinically apparent swelling.[1,2,5] Symptoms progress in severity over 1 to 3 days, remain virtually the same for an equal length of time, then gradually subside over the next week.[1,5] In the acute stage, a subcutaneous gelatinous infiltration may be present over the affected gland, extending down to the clavicular area.[4] Anorexia is a common complaint, whereas fever may or may not be present.[1,4] Meningitis is a frequent complication of mumps, although it is usually a short, self-limiting disorder lasting 2 to 4 days.[1,2,4,8,12] Meningoencephalitis is a rare postinfectious complication which may produce focal neurological symptoms and even death.[4,7] Other rare complications include arthritis, pancreatitis, renal involvement, thyroiditis, oopharitis and mastitis as well as hearing impairment, which may be severe, and is usually unilateral.[1,2,4,5,7,8,12,13] Orchitis is a common complication after puberty, but may occur as early as 3 years of age.[1,2,4,7,8,12] There is no documented evidence that mumps infection in pregnancy leads to congenital deformities of the foetus.[2,7]

NURSING ASSESSMENT

The child is assessed to determine the degree of swelling and discomfort around the ears. The amount of pain experienced behind the ear when the child is chewing or swallowing should also be assessed.[14] A set of baseline observations is recorded to determine the degree of fever, if any, and the child is observed for any signs of dehydration. A nursing history is obtained to establish when the symptoms were first noticed and whether there has been any contact with a known case of mumps. The child or parents should also be asked whether there have been any signs of neurological involvement such as headaches, increased drowsiness or irritability. Boys should have their scrotal area checked for signs of swelling. If a definite diagnosis is required the mumps virus can be isolated from throat swabs, or in tissue cultures innoculated with throat washings, urine or spinal fluid.[1–4] Serological studies will also confirm the presence of the mumps virus.[3,4,13,15]

IMPLEMENTATION OF CARE

Nursing management is mainly supportive, with symptomatic treatment as required.[1,2,5] Analgesics such as paracetamol may be used to relieve pain and fever.[1,5,11] A fluid volume deficit may be prevented by adequate hydration while a soft diet will reduce the discomfort caused by chewing. Sour foods such as citrus fruits, highly seasoned foods, or other mucous membrane irritants such as peppermint should be avoided as they aggravate the pain by encouraging rapid salivary flow.[1,5,11] A scrotal sling may be required if there is marked swelling in this area, to relieve the discomfort caused by the weight and size of the scrotal sac.[14]

Hospitalisation for mumps is rarely necessary unless the child has developed severe manifestations or is immunocompromised. In these circumstances the child should be isolated until the swelling has subsided or other distinct signs of the illness have cleared. This usually occurs by the 9th day after the onset of swelling.[2,4,5] An audiology test after mumps is recommended, to determine whether there is any hearing loss.[13] School-age children should be kept at home until fully recovered.[6]

PREVENTION

To reduce the incidence of mumps, the live virus, which has been grown in chick embryo cell cultures, should be given routinely to children between the ages of 12 and 15 months.[6,8,12] Children suffering from minor illness, with or without low-grade fever, may quite safely be vaccinated. There is no increased risk of reaction if an individual is vaccinated during the incubation period of mumps, or if already immune.[2,7,8] The live virus, however, should not be given within 3 months of administration of immunoglobulin or blood transfusion as the passively acquired antibody may neutralise the vaccine virus.[2,7,8] The vaccine is administered in a single subcutaneous injection according to the manufacturer's directions, either alone or in combination with the measles and rubella vaccines.[1,2,4–8] Vaccination has been found to be approximately 95% effective in preventing mumps infection, especially when given between 12 and 15 months of age.[1–5,7,12] There are virtually no side effects, and those which have been recorded, such as allergic reactions including rash, purpura and pruritis, are uncommon, mild and brief.[1,2,4,7,8,13]

REFERENCES

1. Brunell PA. Mumps. *In:* Feigin RD, Cherry JD, eds. *Textbook of pediatric infectious diseases* 3rd ed. Philadelphia: WB Saunders, 1993.
2. Committee on Infectious Diseases. *Report of the Committee on Infectious Diseases.* 21st ed. Elk Grove Village, Ill: American Academy of Paediatrics, 1988.
3. Hersh BS, Fine PE, Kent K, Cochi SL, Kahn LH, Zell ER, Hays PL, Wood CL. Mumps outbreak in a highly vaccinated population. *J Pediatr* 1991; 119: 187–193.
4. Mott SR, James SR, Sperhac AM. *Nursing care of children and families* 2nd ed. Menlo Park, CA: Addison-Wesley, 1990.
5. Marcy SM. Infection of the salivary glands. *In:* Nelson JD, ed. *Current therapy in pediatric infectious disease — 2* Toronto: BC Decker, 1988.
6. Kilham H, ed. *The Children's Hospital handbook* Sydney: Alken Press, 1993.
7. Immunisation Practices Advisory Committee. Mumps prevention. *Morbidity and Mortality Weekly Report* 1989; 38: 388–400.
8. National Health and Medical Research Council. *The Australian immunisation procedures handbook.* 5th ed. Canberra: AGPS, 1994.
9. Centers for Disease Control. Leads from the MMWR — Mumps — United States, 1985–1988. *JAMA* 1989; 261: 1702, 1707–1708.
10. Davis J. Cases of mumps following previous vaccinations. *Am J Dis Childh* 1988; 142. 1022.
11. Dudley JP. Infection of the mouth, salivary glands, and neck spaces. *In:* Kass EH, Platt R, eds. *Current therapy in infectious disease — 3.* Toronto: BC Decker, 1990.
12. Kakakios AM, Burgess MA, Bransby RD, Quinn AA, Allars HM. Optimal age for measles and mumps vaccination in Australia. *Med J Aust* 1990; 152: 472–474.
13. Kayan A, Bellman H. Bilateral sensorineural hearing loss due to mumps. *Br J Clin Pract* 1990; 44: 757–759.
14. Pachman DJ. Cases of mumps following previous vaccinations [letter]. *Am J Dis Childh* 1988; 142: 1022.
15. Smith H. Mumps. *Practitioner* 1990; 234: 903–904.

Disturbances in Integumentary Function

Helen Sharp

Impairment in Skin Integrity

The skin, which covers the entire surface of the body, acts as a protective barrier, holding in moisture and preventing harmful bacteria and ultraviolet rays from damaging the underlying tissues. It also plays an important role in the maintenance of normal body temperature, storage of chemicals, synthesis of vitamin D and excretion of wastes. Any damage to the skin results in alteration of homeostasis, and increased susceptibility to infection.[1]

Nursing assessment

Obtaining a nursing history of the child's condition is an important aid to planning care. After introduction to the child and primary caregivers, the nurse asks questions to ascertain whether there have been any recent changes in lifestyle that may have predisposed the child to the skin problems. These include the use of different soaps, shampoos or skin products. New animals, recent travel or the move to a different house can also be associated with some skin conditions. The nurse also needs to inquire about any history of allergies or skin problems affecting the child or other members of the family.

The nursing history should identify any symptoms prior to admission; when and where the eruptions were first noticed; whether the lesions have undergone any changes; the way in which they have spread; and whether itch or pain is present. Through careful observation the nurse can detect the size, colour, distribution, form, number and type of lesions; whether the lesions are dry, moist, scaly, greasy, smooth or rough, and whether there is any associated exudation. While obtaining the history the nurse can also ask questions which aid in understanding how the child and family are coping with the condition.

Implementation of care

Pruritis is often present when there is altered skin integrity. It can be localised or generalised in nature and is usually worse in the evening and at night, as there is less distraction for the child.[2,3] The goal of care in nursing these children is to prevent exacerbation of the skin condition and reduce itching. The nurse can explain the importance of not scratching to the older child, and encourage children to participate in their own care. The younger child can have mittens applied and the areas of pruritis covered to discourage scratching.[4] Fingernails should be kept short and clean to prevent secondary infection and exacerbation of the skin condition.[4] The child should be encouraged to avoid the type of clothing or activity which would cause overheating. Any allergens and irritants such as wool, sand, perfumes and soap should also be avoided.[5,6] The provision of diversional activities will aid in distracting the child from the itch. Additionally, antihistamines, topical corticosteroids, soothing creams or dressings may be ordered to alleviate the problem.

Alteration in comfort related to pain is sometimes associated with skin conditions, especially those caused by infection. Care is aimed at reducing or alleviating pain. Providing diversional activities for the young child and relaxation therapy for the older child can reduce their perception of pain.[7,8] Sometimes, elevation of the affected area may help. Analgesics should be administered if the pain is severe.

Alteration in self-image often needs to be addressed when skin integrity is impaired, as many of these conditions are very noticeable and cause people to stare at or avoid the child. At times the child and family have difficulty in accepting the condition, especially when it can be treated but not cured. Encouraging the child and the primary caregivers to discuss the disorder, as well as helping them to accept the diagnosis and treatment, are important aspects of the nursing role. Acceptance of the child is important and can be achieved through free communication and the open demonstration of affection. Alteration in fluid and nutritional requirements is another important consideration. Skin conditions may cause fever, or fluid loss from lesions. In some diseases both may be present. Dehydration occurs if there is an associated reduction in fluid intake. Exudation from lesions can also result in a depletion of protein, leading to poor wound healing. Nursing care therefore, should include education for and encouragement of a good fluid intake and a well balanced diet.

Normal motor development needs to be promoted by the provision of age-appropriate activities, relative to the child's tolerance and physical mobility. Appropriate participation in their own care can often aid normal development in children as well as providing diversional activity. This is especially important when scratching and pruritis are present.

Maintaining optimal conditions such as keeping the skin clean and free of urine, faeces, and other irritants aids healing, promotes healthy skin and prevents infection. Exposing the skin to artificial ultraviolet light, or sunlight for short periods can also aid healing in certain conditions, such as psoriasis.[4,6]

Inflammation

ATOPIC DERMATITIS

Atopic dermatitis is characteristically a disease of childhood, in which 75% of children will show the first signs by 6 months of age, although 50% are relatively free of the active disease by puberty.[2,9] The disease can occur as an acute weeping dermatitis or as a chronic condition in which the skin becomes lichenified or thickened. There is often a family history of asthma, allergic rhinitis, or atopic dermatitis,[10] and only very rarely is

Table 5.7 Comparison of characteristic features of atopic dermatitis in different age groups

Infancy	Young children	Older children
75% show first signs by the age of 6 months.		50% relatively free by puberty.
Lesions mainly on face, trunk and limbs.	Lesions on extensor surface of limbs, especially the legs.	Lesions in the limb flexures.

Atopic dermatitis of the face.

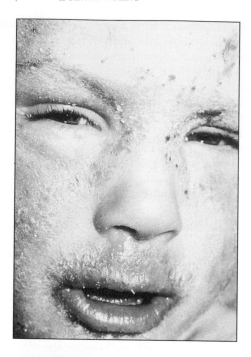

Atopic dermatitis of the face.

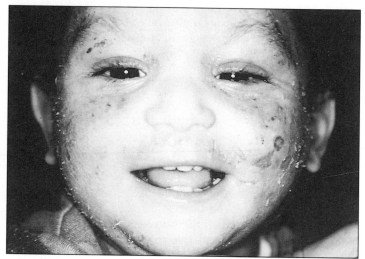

it related to food allergies.[4,6] The skin is very dry and itchy, with a low irritation threshold.[2,9] In infancy, the lesions most commonly occur on the face, although they may also be found on the trunk and limbs. Young children usually have lesions on the extensor surfaces of limbs, especially the legs, whereas lesions are found in the limb flexures in older children.[2,9,11]

Nursing management of atopic dermatitis includes the use of dispersible oils in the bath, emollient creams such as glycerine 10% in sorbolene applied all over the body at

Atopic dermatitis on lower limbs showing thickened skin.

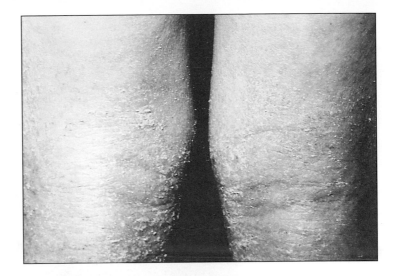

Application of cream before wet dressing.

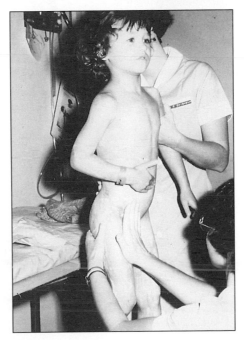

least twice a day. Severe manifestations may also require the application of topical corticosteroids.[2,6,9] Wet dressings may be applied 3 times a day if there is widespread disruption to the skin integrity. Wet dressings increase the hydration of the skin, enhance the penetration of the corticosteroid, reduce the itch and help prevent scratching. The dressings consist of pieces of clean old linen soaked in warm water which are wrapped around the affected areas, once the creams have been applied. Bandages are used to hold the linen in place. This treatment usually results in significant improvement within 3 to 4 days.[9] Antihistamines are frequently ordered to allay itching, especially at night.[4,9]

Wet dressing to body.

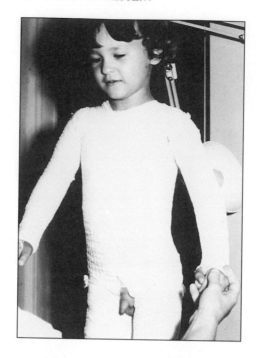

Wet dressing to face.

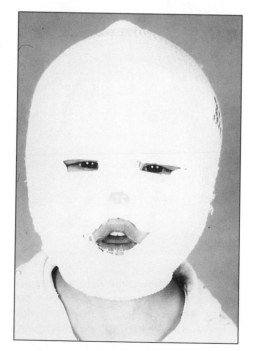

Seborrhoeic dermatitis.

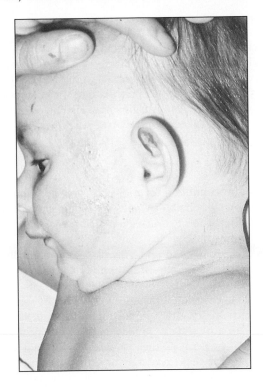

Children with atopic dermatitis are particularly susceptible to secondary infections, especially from *Staphylococcus aureus* and herpes simplex virus. Any infected lesion should be swabbed and the specimen sent for culture and antibiotic sensitivity. While the lesions are infected it is advisable to nurse the child in isolation to prevent the spread of the organism. If the infection is bacterial, oral antibiotics are administered.[2,5]

Ensuring that the child (if old enough) and the primary caregivers understand the condition is an important aspect of the nursing management of children with atopic dermatitis. The child and family will require continued encouragement, understanding and education in the treatment of the skin disorder.

SEBORRHOEIC DERMATITIS

Seborrhoeic dermatitis is a condition which occurs either in the 1st year of life, or after puberty.[12] The characteristic appearance is a background erythema and a greasy yellow scale.[13] It is a non-itchy condition mainly found on the scalp, in the nasolabial folds, on the eyebrows, behind and inside the ears, and in the axilla and groin.[4,5]

Nursing management is directed at removing the scale, treating the condition and any secondary infection. The most common method of treatment is to apply a weak corticosteroid preparation to the affected areas on the face and body. The scalp can usually be cleared by applying a preparation containing sulphur and salicylic acid at night and washing it out in the morning. Thick scale can be softened by applying warm olive oil or paraffin before the cream.[4,5]

CONTACT DERMATITIS

In children, contact dermatitis is usually caused by plants such as the Rhus tree or poison ivy. It appears as streaks of very acute, often blistering dermatitis accompanied by severe pruritis.[12] Nursing management is primarily aimed at making the child more comfortable, either through the application of strong fluorinated corticosteroids to the rash or oral administration of corticosteroids. Antipruritics may also be ordered and in some children wet dressings may be required (see atopic dermatitis).[12]

PSORIASIS

Acute guttate psoriasis, the childhood form of psoriasis, commonly presents as an acute eruption of tiny papules or very small plaques on the surface of the skin. This eruption is often preceded by a sore throat. Psoriasis can also present in the adult form with large erythematous plaques and a thick silvery scale, mainly on the scalp, elbows, knees and buttocks. The lesions are widespread and may also extend to the face.[4-6,14] Creams are applied to restore skin integrity. Preparations containing tar are the treatment of choice.[4] Corticosteroid creams are often used for infants, however, as tar preparations tend to cause skin irritation in this age group. In children who are not sensitive to tar preparations guttate psoriasis can be treated with 4% liquor picis carbonis and 4% salicylic acid in an aqueous cream base twice a day, with half-strength preparations on face and flexures.[5] The treatment is usually long term as the condition is difficult to control.

The nurse should be aware that there may be a disturbance in self-concept related to body image as psoriasis can be very unattractive. Both the child and family may need a lot of support and encouragement to enable them to cope with the condition and treatment.

Infection

Alteration in the integrity of the skin can be caused by a variety of mechanisms including invasion of wounds or infection of hair follicles by micro-organisms. Evidence of local infection includes pain, redness, heat, oedema and sometimes enlarged lymph nodes. Malaise and fever may develop later if the infection is not treated.[3]

IMPETIGO

Impetigo occurs primarily in preschool and early school-age children, usually through direct contact. The most common causative agent is *Staphylococcus aureus*. Occasionally it may be caused by group A beta haemolytic streptococcus or a combination of both of these bacteria.[15] Impetigo is often superimposed on other skin conditions, including atopic dermatitis.[6] There are two forms of impetigo:

1. Bullous impetigo, which is always caused by *Staphylococcus aureus* and starts as a blister, developing on previously normal skin. The blisters increase in size and number and rupture to produce superficial erosions with a peripheral brown crust.

Bullous impetigo.

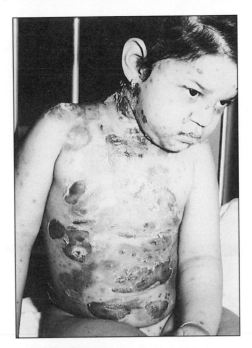

Bullous impetigo.

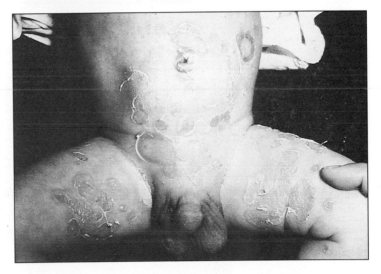

2. Non-bullous impetigo consists of small pustules surrounded by erythema. The pustules rupture to produce an exudate which forms a thick, honey-coloured crust.

In both conditions, the lesions are neither itchy nor painful, and are found mainly on the forearm and lower leg. However, lesions may also group around the mouth and nose.[6,15]

The child should be isolated and barrier nursing instituted. Handwashing is especially important to prevent the spread of infection. Saline baths are used to cleanse the skin, remove crusts and promote healing. Oral antibiotics are used to treat the infection. Topical

Staphylococcal scalded skin syndrome.

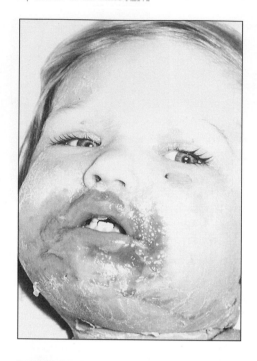

Staphylococcal scalded skin syndrome.

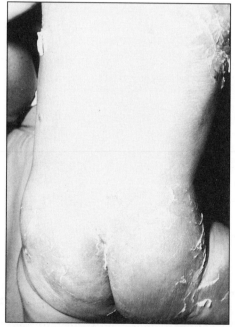

mupirocin may be used occasionally.[4,15,16] The child should be encouraged to avoid handling the lesions and to participate in self-care.

Glomerulonephritis is a rare complication of Group A beta haemolytic streptococcus. If the organism is isolated in samples taken from the lesions, the child must be screened by regular urinalysis over an 8-week period.[5] Evidence of glomerulonephritis will include haematuria, an increase in urine specific gravity, oliguria and mild generalised oedema.[3]

STAPHYLOCOCCAL SCALDED SKIN SYNDROME

This condition is caused by the toxin of *Staphylococcus aureus* entering the bloodstream from an infection in the eye, nose, throat or a wound,[17] resulting in the skin splitting high in the epidermis. Initially, the child develops a fever and macular erythema, and within approximately 48 hours large flaccid blisters develop. Skin disruptions begin on the face, especially around the mouth and eyes, spread to flexural areas and progress to involve the rest of the body. The skin then sheets off and the erosions become dry and crusted. Extreme tenderness of the skin is usually present. The mucosa is unaffected and fluid loss from the lesions is minimal. Complete recovery is normally achieved in 10 to 12 days.[6,15,18,19]

Swabs are taken from the eye, nose, throat or wound for culture and antibiotic sensitivity when the child is first admitted. The blisters themselves are sterile.[6,17,19]

Children with this condition are nursed naked on a non-stick material such as melanin, and handled as little as possible to lessen the potential for trauma and pain. Oral antibiotics and adequate oral or intramuscular analgaesia are given. Bath oils and emollients can be used to restore skin integrity once the initial tenderness has passed.[15,19]

Mobiles, television or other visual stimuli help divert the child's attention away from the condition, and they should be nursed where they can see the nursing staff and others as much as possible. Nurses, primary caregivers, or others should spend time talking and reading to the child, especially during the acute phase when physical mobility is impaired.

FURUNCLES

Furuncles or boils are cutaneous abscesses caused by virulent *Staphylococcus* strains which start as firm, tender, red raised spots on the skin, and develop into fluid-filled lumps. They commonly occur in areas of increased friction and sweating such as the neck, groin, waistline and axilla. Occasionally these abscesses need surgical intervention for drainage of pus.[6,15] Pain relief is achieved through positioning the child and giving adequate analgaesia. Swabs are taken from the lesions for culture and sensitivity to determine the most appropriate antibiotic.

CELLULITIS

Cellulitis is an infection involving the subcutis as well as the dermis of the skin and is usually caused by a beta haemolytic streptococcus, although *Haemophilus influenza* may also cause this condition. The lesions are erythematous, swollen, warm, painful and sometimes have a bluish or purple hue. The most common sites in young children are the face and perianal area. The infection may appear on intact skin or following trauma.[4,6,15] Cultures are obtained from the nose, throat and blood before antibiotic therapy is begun. The nursing management includes attention to pain relief. Intravenous antibiotics are administered to treat the infection and restore skin integrity.

CANDIDA ALBICANS

Candida albicans is a fungal infection which is commonly associated with napkin dermatitis in infants. It may also occur as a secondary infection in psoriasis. Napkin dermatitis is treated with a mild antifungal cream, such as cotrimoxazole, often combined with a weak corticosteroid. The cream is applied sparingly 3 times a day.[4,12]

TINEA

Tinea is an infection caused by dermatophyte fungi and occurs on all areas of the skin, including the hair and nails. The characteristic appearance is an area of erythema studded with papules or pustules in a circular formation. The centre tends to be clear with a superficial scale. Between the toes it mainly appears as maceration with a thick white scale. Nail tinea causes a white discolouration and crumbling of the nail plate with an accumulation of debris beneath the nail. Scalp tinea varies from a mild erythema and a fine dandruff-like scale to a pustular carbuncle-like lesion. Localised or patchy alopecia is present with all the hairs breaking at the same length. Tinea is diagnosed by scraping hairs or scales onto a slide, and examining the specimen microscopically.[4,5,20] Topical antifungals may be used on small localised lesions, while griseofulvin is the treatment of choice for long-standing or severe cutaneous tinea, and all hair and nail tinea. A 3-month course is generally used, but nail tinea may require longer treatment.[4,5,20]

Infestation

SCABIES

Scabies is transmitted by physical contact. The mites burrow into the skin, particularly between the fingers, the ulnar border of the hand, around the wrist and elbows, the anterior axillary fold, the nipples and the penis. In infants the palms and soles may be affected. The burrows are rarely seen although papules, pustules, wheals and bullae may be present. The primary eruption is usually followed by a secondary eruption of multiple, very pruritic papules, which appear mainly on the abdomen, thighs and buttocks.[4,5,21]

Diagnosis is by microscopic slide examination of specially prepared skin scrapings,[21,22] or by rubbing ink or black felt pen over the area of suspected burrows. The ink is then removed with an alcohol swab leaving the burrows outlined.[5,6]

If hospitalised, the child is isolated until the skin has been treated, to prevent the spread of infection. To minimise the risk of reinfestation, it is essential for the child, family members and other close contacts to be treated simultaneously with 1% gamma benzene hexachloride. The cream is applied to all external surfaces, avoiding the face. In older children and adults, the preparation is left on the skin for a period of 12 hours.[4,21] Children under 12 months of age have the cream applied for 6 hours at a time as their skin is more sensitive. The cream is then removed by washing with mild soap and water.[22] This application is repeated the next day, and subsequently on the same 2 days of the following week. Sulphur or crotamiton creams, though less effective, may be ordered for premature or ill infants, as their skin is extremely sensitive.[5,21] Recent studies have

Table 5.8 Treatment of scabies

Premature and ill infants	Young children	Older children
Sulphur or crotamiton cream is used due to extreme skin sensitivity.	Gamma benzene hexachloride 1% applied to all areas of the body omitting head. Leave on for 6 hours.	Gamma benzene hexachloride 1% applied to all areas of the body omitting head. Leave on for 12 hours.

compared Permethrin 5% and gamma benzene hexachloride in the treatment of scabies. Permethrin 5% was found to have improved therapeutic results and fewer side effects.[22,23]

Bed linen and clothing are washed in the normal manner, then left unused for a week as the mite cannot survive away from the host for more than 4 days.[5,22]

PEDICULOSIS

Pediculous or head lice are commonly found among school-age children and occasionally epidemics occur. Intense pruritis of the scalp is often the first symptom. The adult louse attaches her eggs to the hair shafts. They are small, translucent, white, oval-shaped eggs which are very difficult to remove. These eggs may be found in most areas of the scalp hair although the nape of the neck is the commonest site of infestation. Adult lice are transferred by direct contact or by sharing combs, hats and other personal articles.[4,21] Restoration of skin integrity includes the use of a pediculocidal shampoo such as gamma benzene hexachloride. As this is not guaranteed to kill all the eggs, the hair should be fine tooth combed, and the treatment repeated in 7 to 10 days. Clothing should be laundered in hot water, and combs and brushes soaked in pediculocide.[21]

Fleas, bedbugs, mosquitoes, bees and wasps are other organisms which can cause local urticaria and pruritis. In a small percentage of susceptible children, bees and wasps can cause a hypersensitive reaction, sometimes leading to anaphylaxis and requiring immediate intensive care.[24]

REFERENCES

1. Tortora GJ, Anagnostakos NP. *Principles of anatomy and physiology.* 7th ed. New York: Harper and Row, 1993.
2. Krowchuk DP. Practical aspects of the diagnosis and management of atopic dermatitis. *Pediatr Ann* 1987; 16: 57–67.
3. Mott SR, James SR, Sperhac AM. *Nursing care of children and families.* 2nd ed. Menlo Park, CA: Addison-Wesley, 1990.
4. Verbov J. *Essential paediatric dermatology* Bristol: Clinical Press, 1988.
5. Rogers M. Skin disorders commonly encountered in children. Student Information Sheet. Camperdown: The Children's Hospital, 1990.
6. Schachner LA, Hansen RC, eds. *Pediatric dermatology* Vols. 1 & 2. New York: Churchill Livingstone, 1988.
7. Beyer J, Bournaki M. Assessment and management of postoperative pain in children. *Pediatrician* 1989; 16: 30–38.
8. Kuttner L, Bowman M, Teasdale M. Psychological treatment of distress, pain and anxiety for young children with cancer. *J Dev Behav Pediatr* 1988; 9: 374–382.
9. Rogers M. Atopic dermatitis. *Cur Ther* 1987; June: 115–124.

10. Burks AW, Mallory SB, Williams LW, Shirrell MA. Atopic dermatitis: clinical relevance of food hypersensitivity reactions *J Pediatr* 1988; 113: 447–451.
11. Broadbent JB, Sampson HA. Food hypersensitivity and atopic dermatitis. *Pediatr Clin North Am* 1988; 35: 1115–1125.
12. Rogers M. Childhood forms of dermatitis. *Mod Med Aust* 1985; August: 21–23.
13. Faergemann J. Treatment of seborrhoeic dermatitis of the scalp with ketaconazole shampoo. *Acta Derm Venereol* 1990; 70: 171–172.
14. Honig PJ. Guttate psoriasis associated with perianal streptococcal disease. *J Pediatr* 1988; 113: 1037–1039.
15. Rogers M. Bacterial skin infections in children. *Mod Med Aust* 1990; March: 26–32.
16. McLinn S. Topical mupirocin vs systemic erythromycin treatment for pyoderma. *Pediatr Infect Dis J* 1988; 7: 785–790.
17. Murono K, Fujita K, Yoshioka H. Microbiologic characteristics of exfoliative toxin producing *Staphylococcus aureus*. *Pediatr Infect Dis J* 1988; 7: 313–315.
18. Hoeger PH, Elsner P. Staphylococcal scalded skin syndrome: transmission of exfoliation-producing *Staphylococcus aureus* by an asymptomatic carrier. *Pediatr Infect Dis J* 1988; 7: 340–342.
19. Hurwitz S. The skin and systemic disease in children. Chicago: Year Book Medical, 1985.
20. Frieden IJ. Diagnosis and management of tinea capitis. *Pediatr Ann* 1987; 16: 39–48.
21. Lane AT. Scabies and head lice. *Pediatr Ann* 1987; 16: 51–55.
22. Haustein U, Hlawa B. Treatment of scabies with permethrin versus lindane and benzyl benzoate. *Acta Derm Venereol* (Stockholm) 1989; 69: 348–351.
23. Schultz M, Gomez M, Hansen R, Mills J, Menter A, Rodgers H, et al. Comparative study of 5% permethrin cream and 1% lindane lotion for the treatment of scabies. *Arch Dermatol* 1990; 126: 167–170.
24. Berhman R, Vaughan V. *Nelson's textbook of pediatrics.* 14th ed. Philadelphia: WB Saunders, 1992.

Disturbances in Sensory Function

Inflammation and Infection of the Eye

Julie Bleasdale and Jill Molan

Fear of the unknown will be the biggest hurdle for paediatric eye patients. Most parents will want to be able to take part in their child's care and should be encouraged to do so. Some parents will feel afraid and unsure and will need extra support and encouragement.

Probably the most common eye problems are those of infection and inflammation. A most important part of the nursing role in caring for children with these conditions is that of parent education, especially on aspects relating to hygiene, eye assessment and instillation of the appropriate treatment. Inflammation and infections of the eye and surrounding tissues in children can be divided into 2 groups: those which affect the external parts of the eye and are relatively superficial (lid infections); and those which are of a more serious nature and may not only be sight threatening but life threatening cellulitis and other disorders.

Table 5.9 Distinguishing features of conjunctivitis of bacterial, viral and allergic aetiology

Feature	Bacterial	Viral	Allergy
Lid oedema	yes	yes	yes — may be severe
Red eyes (Conjunctival injection)	yes	yes	yes
Discharge	yes	maybe — scant	yes — stringy mucopurulent and watery exudate
Photophobia	yes	yes	yes
Itchiness	yes	irritating	yes — severe
Pupil reaction	normal	normal	normal
Contagious	yes	yes	no
Duration	5–7 days	varies 2 days to 4 weeks	varies after removal of irritant

LID INFECTIONS

Blepharitis

Blepharitis is a chronic inflammation characterised by redness and scaling of the skin at the eyelid margins.

Use cotton buds dipped in baby shampoo to remove the crusts with a gentle scrubbing motion on the lid margins. Then cleanse away shampoo with saline and gently massage antibiotic ointment onto the clean lid margins using cotton buds.

Hordeolum (stye)

Hordeolum (stye) is an acute staphylococcal infection of the Zeis gland at the base of an eyelash. The abscess usually 'points' outwards and resolves spontaneously.

Warm compresses will relieve discomfort and promote resolution. Instillation of an antibiotic ointment may be necessary.

Chalazion

Chalazion is a chronic inflammation of a meibomian gland on the inside of the lid. Oral and topical antibiotics may help resolution. The chalazion may require incision and drainage if it is large and not resolving. A general anaesthetic is usually required for this procedure in children.

Conjunctivitis

Conjunctivitis is the most common cause of bilateral red eyes. The common causes of inflammation of the conjunctiva are bacterial, viral or allergic. (**See Table 5.9.**)

Recurrent conjunctivitis could be caused by a retained foreign body underneath the upper lid. It may be necessary to evert the upper lid to observe and remove the foreign body. (**See Figure 5.3.**)

Educate the caregiver and child with regard to hygiene measures to prevent cross-infection in the family. Separate towels and face cloth are used by the child. Parents are

Table 5.10 Distinguishing features of preseptal cellulitis and orbital cellulitis

Feature	Preseptal	Orbital
Lid swelling with redness	yes	yes
Ocular motility	full range	restricted
Pain	slight	severe
Visual acuity	normal	may be impaired
Proptosis (protruding eyeball)	no	yes

taught about handwashing and the correct technique for installation of drops. Eye toilets relieve itching and discomfort. Sunglasses or a darkened room may alleviate photophobia.

Dacrocystitis

Dacrocystitis is an inflammation of the nasolacrimal duct. Sometimes an acute infection can occur which needs systemic antibiotics. Incision and drainage may be required.

CELLULITIS

Cellulitis of the orbit is an acute, purulent inflammation of the tissue of the orbit. It is usually unilateral. The child has a fever and general malaise and requires hospitalisation and intravenous antibiotic treatment. There are two types of cellulitis — preseptal and orbital. Preseptal cellulitis is the more common form of cellulitis in children, and is usually milder than orbital cellulitis, which may be both sight threatening and life threatening. The two types are differentiated in **Table 5.10**. Both types of cellulitis can be caused by infection from neighbouring structures, usually sinuses, a penetrating injury or following surgery.

The complications which can arise include meningitis, optic nerve atrophy which leads to visual impairment and cavernous sinus thrombosis, a rare but life-threatening complication.

Nursing care involves pain relief, eye toilets and cool compresses, fluid balance and nutritional maintenance, intravenous cannula care and vital signs. Medical treatment will include intravenous antibiotic therapy and topical antibiotic drops or ointment. Most children have a speedy recovery once antibiotic treatment has begun.

OTHER DISORDERS

Other significant ocular infections and inflammations include herpes simplex virus, an infection of the cornea; gonococcal or chlamydial conjunctivitis of the newborn; uveitis, a sterile intraocular inflammation often associated with juvenile arthritis; and endophthalmitis, a severe intraocular infection.

Ophthalmic Nursing Procedures

Julie Bleasdale and Jill Molan

INFANTS

Infants will not cooperate with attempts to carry out an ophthalmic procedure. It is important to provide explanation and reassurance to the caregivers and to seek their assistance. The simplest technique is to wrap the baby firmly in a bunny rug, remembering to tuck its hands away, and ask the caregiver to hold the infant's head.

TODDLERS

It is usually best to have one person restrain the toddler firmly while another carries out the procedure. If the caregiver is to learn to do the procedure, (e.g., eye toilet or installation of drops) it may be useful for the nurse to be the restraint person. After the procedure has been demonstrated the caregiver can practise under supervision.

GENERAL PRINCIPLES

- Remember that both child and caregiver will be experiencing fear of the unknown until they are familiar with the procedure.
- Prepare all equipment beforehand in order to minimise the time required with the child.
- Make procedures as comfortable and painless as possible.
- Be prepared for the child to scream and cry during the procedure. If the procedure is done quickly and confidently the child will settle more readily after the procedure.
- Learn to assess the eye mainly by looking rather than touching.
- Eye ointment may be instilled while the child is asleep, if it is impossible when the child is awake.
- When it is essential that the examination is accurate, for example, measuring intraocular pressure, an examination under general anaesthesia will be necessary.

EYE EXAMINATION AND OBSERVATIONS

The aim of these procedures is to detect abnormalities or complications following surgery or trauma and monitor effectiveness of treatment.

- The eyes should be examined following cleansing and before instillation of drops or ointment.
- An examination torch should be used for accurate assessment.
- The eye is examined systematically from 'outside in'.
- Note any discharge on the eye pad or lashes.
- Always look at the patient's face as a whole to determine facial symmetry and note any obvious palsy, ptosis, proptosis, allergy or trauma.

Table 5.11 Eye examination and observations

Structure	Normal	Abnormal
Lids	Symmetrical Clean	Ptosis (drooping lid) Irregularity/lesions, lacerations, swelling, bruising, redness, itching, crusting
Conjunctiva	Translucent, flat White sclera is visible beneath conjunctiva	Injected Bloodshot Chemosis (swelling which looks like a bubble or blister. In extreme cases the swelling may protrude between lids.) Haemorrhage, lacerations
Cornea	Bright, clear Smooth surface	Scarring and opacities Haziness (can indicate corneal pathology. If associated with eye pain, irritability and watery eye may indicate raised intraocular pressure.) Foreign body, rust ring, abscess
Anterior Chamber	Clear, bright Deep	Hyphaema (blood, note level) Hypopyon (pus, note level, may indicate infection or non-infective inflammation) Check depth (deep or shallow)
Pupil and Iris	Variable size (pupils should be round and central). Reacts to light right = left	Dilated, constricted, irregular shape (oval, keyhole, tear drop)

EYE CARE

Because the eye is very delicate and sensitive, the caregivers should be extremely gentle with their hands and manner. The eye is small and there is not much room to manoeuvre around when performing nursing procedures. The principles of asepsis apply as for any other aseptic technique. The following points relate specifically to eye care.

- Always have the child's head tilted backwards and supported. The patient can be lying or sitting with head supported. This is important for patient comfort.
- Forceps are never used when performing eye care. Forceps may cause trauma.
- Fingernails should be clean and short. Direct hand contact is necessary for the eye care procedures.
- Clean the unaffected eye first. This helps prevent cross-infection.
- Hands are supported on the patient's face. If the patient suddenly moves, hands will move as well, preventing touch with the eye.
- Do not apply pressure to the globe of the eye. Pressure on the globe is not only painful, it can increase intraocular pressure and may produce wound dehiscence.
- If the eye is discharging pus it is not covered. A pad is a perfect medium for bacterial growth.

EYE TOILET AND DRESSING TECHNIQUE

- Explain the procedure to the child and parents.
- Wash hands.

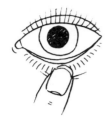
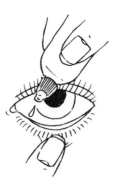

1. Wash hands.
2. Uncap bottle.
3. Pull lower eyelid gently down with your finger to form a pocket.
4. Look up.
5. Instil drop into the pocket you've formed. Avoid contact between drop bottle tip and hands or eye.
6. After instillation gently close eye.

Figure 5.3 Instillation of eye drops.

- Prepare equipment.
- Position the child. Older children may be encouraged to remove their eye pad and participate in the procedure, which helps to decrease their anxiety and gain their cooperation. If eye drops need to be instilled, the child should be instructed to lie down.
- Wash hands.
- Moisten swab with saline and gently clean the eye from the inner canthus to the outer using the swab once. Discard the swab and repeat until the eye is clean, paying particular attention to the lashes.
- Assess the eye, noting any discharge or abnormalities.
- Instil drops or ointment if ordered.
- Apply eye pad if necessary.
- Discard equipment and wash hands.
- Sign the prescription/medication chart.

INSTILLATION OF EYE DROPS AND OINTMENT

- Wash hands.
- Position the child. If the child's cooperation can be gained, ask him or her to look up and gently pull down on the lower lid. If cooperation is not possible, place the thumb and first finger gently on the upper and lower lids, close to the lashes and carefully pull the lids apart, being sure not to apply any pressure to the globe of the eye.

Drops

- Squeeze a drop inside the lower lid. *Do not* touch the eye, lids or lashes with the nozzle.

Ointment

- Hold the tube parallel to the eye, pointing toward the nose. Squeeze about 0.5 cm of ointment into the lower lid pouch. *Do not* touch the eye, lids or lashes with the nozzle.
- Release the lids, allow the child to blink, and wipe away excess, but do not allow the child to rub his or her eyes.

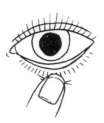
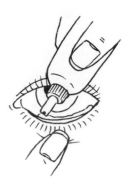

1. Wash hands.
2. Uncap tube.
3. Pull lower eyelid gently down with your finger to form a pocket.
4. Look up.
5. Apply a small strip of ointment into the pocket you've formed. Avoid contact between tube and hands or eye.
6. After instillation gently close eye.

Figure 5.4 Instillation of ointment.

Step 1   Step 2   Step 3

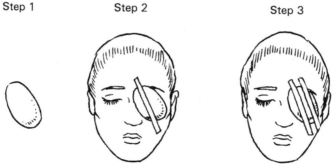

Figure 5.5 Applying a light pad.

- If drops and ointment are ordered, instil drops first. When instilling a number of eye medications, the drops are instilled in the following order, to allow maximum absorption. 1. Mydriatics (dilating) /miotics (constricting) 2. Antibiotics 3. Anti-inflammatories (steroids). Wait 1 to 2 minutes after each drop for absorption of the drug to take place in the eye. Ointment is instilled last of all.

APPLYING A PAD

A light pad

A light pad may be used to lightly cover and protect the eye after surgery or when a penetrating injury is suspected.

- Position the child comfortably.
- Ask the child to close both eyes and keep them closed.
- Maintain sterility of the underside of the eye pad, apply about 10 cm of tape along one side. Pick up the pad using tape, apply gently, sticking tape on forehead and cheek. Apply a second strip of tape to the other side of the pad.
- Ensure the eye is closed underneath the pad or a corneal abrasion may result.

Step 1   Step 2   Step 3

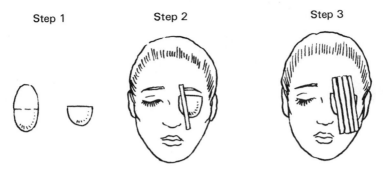

Figure 5.6 Applying a firm pad.

Step 1   Step 2

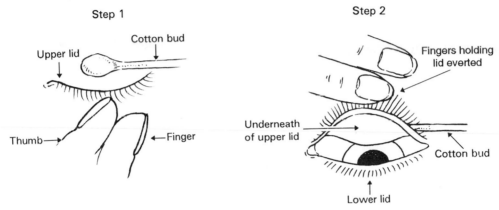

Figure 5.7 Everting the upper lid.

A firm pad

A firm pad may be used to cover the eye and apply gentle pressure to keep the lids closed after removal of a corneal foreign body and/or corneal abrasion. Follow the same procedure as for application of a light pad, only double the pad by folding it in half. Apply the straight edge under the child's eyebrow. Apply several pieces of tape over the pad to ensure gentle but firm pressure over the globe. Try to overlap tape on forehead and cheek to reduce the amount of skin involved.

EVERTING A LID

This is never attempted if there is any reason to suspect a penetrating eye injury.

- A cotton bud is needed.
- Ask the patient to look down and not close the eye. The chin is slightly up.
- Gently but securely grasp the upper lashes between the thumb and index finger.
- Place the cotton bud about 1.5 cm above lid margin in the lid crease. (This is the upper border of the tarsal plate.)
- Gently lift the lashes, maintaining firm pressure with the cotton bud.
- The lid should 'flip over'.

- The patient should continue to look down while the lid is everted or it will not be possible to keep lid everted.
- To return lid, release lashes and ask the patient to blink.

BIBLIOGRAPHY

Pavan-Langston D. *Manual of ocular diagnosis and therapy.* 4th ed. Boston: Little, Brown & Company, 1995.

Stollery R. *Ophthalmic nursing.* 2nd ed. Oxford: Blackwell Science, 1996.

Vaughan D, Asbury T, Riordan-Eva P. *General ophthalmology.* 14th ed. East Norwalk: Appleton & Lang, 1995.

Otitis Media

Lynne Brodie

CLASSIFICATION

Otitis media refers to a condition involving inflammation of the mucosal lining of the middle ear and associated structures. There are a number of different forms of otitis media described in the medical literature.[1-3] Inflammation may be acute or chronic. The fluid that collects in the middle ear and mastoid process may be purulent (suppurative) or serous (non-suppurative or secretory). Infection can enter the middle ear cavity externally via a perforated tympanic membrane or internally from the nasopharynx via the eustachian tube. Infection via the bloodstream has also been described, but the most common route in children with intact tympanic membranes is the eustachian tubes.[4]

INCIDENCE AND AETIOLOGY

Studies consistently confirm the frequent nature of otitis media. It is seen in children of all ages, but particularly in those under 2 years. A recent study from Finland reported a relatively low risk for otitis media during the first 6 months of life. The risk was found to increase rapidly after this, with the greatest risk occurring at 12 months then, decreasing during the 2nd year.[5]

Many factors have been implicated as contributing to otitis media. These include a high incidence of respiratory infections in children, a less competent, more compliant eustachian tube which may predispose to obstruction, increased risk of regurgitation of milk and secretions via the eustachian tubes during feeding, middle ear congestion during teething and active growth of lymphoid tissue obstructing the eustachian tubes. There is an increased incidence in children with cleft palate, probably due to dysfunction of the muscles involved in swallowing. Skull fractures and surgical trauma may also involve eustachian tube damage which may interfere with the normal mucociliary clearance mechanism.[4]

CLINICAL PRESENTATION AND MANAGEMENT OF ACUTE OTITIS MEDIA

Most children with acute otitis media are treated by their general practitioner or pediatrician. The typical history is that the child has been unwell with an upper respiratory tract infection. Infants may show generalised symptoms such as crying, fever, rhinorrhea, feeding problems, disturbed sleep patterns, and general irritability. Older infants may pull the affected ear or roll and bang their head. Children who are old enough to verbalise, may complain of earache or decreased hearing. Pain may be intense as fluid accumulates, causing pressure on the tympanic membrane, but is generally relieved spontaneously if the membrane ruptures.[6]

Examination will reveal changes in the appearance of the membrane depending on the stage at presentation and type of inflammation. In suppurative otitis media the drum typically appears very inflamed and bulging. No light reflex is seen. There may also be mastoid tenderness as the mucosa is continuous from the eardrum to the mastoid.[7]

If the child has serous otitis media, pain is unlikely to be severe and often the only symptom is hearing loss reported by older children. Examination of the drum will reveal a variety of appearances from dull red through to amber or grey depending on whether the accumulated fluid is bloodstained or serous.[8]

NURSING MANAGEMENT

If the child has been admitted to hospital for treatment during an acute episode, a course of intravenous antibiotics is typically ordered. Unless the tympanic membrane has ruptured, the child is likely to be in pain and analgesics should be given as prescribed. Antipyretics are given to help reduce body temperature, which is often very high. A tepid sponge may also be indicated.

Oral intake is encouraged although the child may refuse food due to referred pain during chewing. Adequate hydration can generally be maintained by offering frequent small amounts of fluids.

Any discharge should be noted and reported. The outer ear and pinna can be gently cleaned using wool swabs soaked in normal saline. Progress will be monitored by the specialist and generally the child can be discharged on appropriate oral antibiotics once the acute symptoms have settled. Recurring episodes are not uncommon and in some cases the specialist will recommend insertion of ventilating tubes or grommets.

MYRINGOTOMY AND INSERTION OF GROMMETS

This combined procedure is a very common one in paediatric hospitals and is usually performed on a day-stay basis. Myringotomy alone may be performed to allow drainage of fluid from the middle ear. Ventilating tubes (grommets) may be inserted to prevent closure of the myringotomy. Postoperative recovery is generally unremarkable and the child may be discharged as soon as observations are satisfactory and oral fluids are tolerated.

Parents need specific instructions on discharge. The child's ears should be kept dry until the tubes are removed or fall out. A variety of commercial earplugs is available to protect the ears during bathing and hairwashing or more simple measures such as silicon putty, blue tac or cotton balls coated with vaseline can be used. Earplugs and a bathing cap are recommended for swimming. No attempt should be made to clean the ears. Advice should be sought if there is any persistent discharge, raised temperature or earache.[9]

REFERENCES

1. Bluestone CD, Klein JD. Otitis media, atelectasis and eustachian tube dysfunction. *In:* Bluestone CD, Stool SE. *Pediatric otolaryngology.* Vol 1. Philadelphia: Saunders, 1990: 321.
2. Curotto JH. Acute otitis media. *Mod Med Aust* 1990; 33 (5): 25–30.
3. Bordley JE, Brookhouser PE, Tucker GF. *Ear nose and throat disorders in children.* New York: Raven Press, 1986: 65–97.
4. Ransome J. Acute suppurative otitis media and acute mastoiditis. *Scott-Browne otolaryngology.* London: Butterworth, 1987: 177.
5. Alho O, Koivu M, Sorri M, Rantakallio P. The occurrence of acute otitis media in infants. A life-table analysis. *Int J Pediatr Otorhinolaryngol* 1991; 21: 7–14.
6. Colman BH. *Disease of the nose, throat and ear and head and neck.* Edinburgh: Churchill Livingstone, 1992: 223–229.
7. Maw AR. Otitis media with effusion (glue ear). *Scott-Browne's otolaryngology.* London: Butterworth, 1987: 164–165.
8. Bluestone CD. Modern management of otitis media. *Pediatr Clin North Am* 1989; 36: 1371–1387.
9. Royal Alexandra Hospital for Children. Nursing guidelines for children following insertion of grommets (tubes). *Nursing policy and procedure manual.* Sydney: RAHC, 1991: 06.08.

Mastoiditis

Lynne Brodie

This condition may range from acute inflammation of the mastoid air cells, to severe infection involving underlying tissue and bony destruction. Symptoms include localised pain and tenderness, discharge, swelling (which may cause protrusion of the ear), fever and in rare cases, facial paralysis which indicates that the infection has spread to the facial nerve.[1]

Treatment involves a course of intravenous antibiotics, pain relief and close monitoring for complications such as facial nerve paresis or meningism. The child may be irritable, febrile and anorexic and the nurse should ensure fluid intake is satisfactory. A soft diet may be preferred initially to avoid referred pain during chewing. In some cases, surgery is indicated to drain accumulated pus and prevent further bony destruction.

After surgery, the child generally has a pack in the affected ear and a soft occlusive dressing. The incision line lies posterior to the ear and a drain may be *in situ.* This is generally removed after a few days. Dressings should be checked and changed regularly and the area kept clean and dry. The sutures and ear pack are removed approximately 10 days after surgery. Follow-up hearing tests may be arranged to check for permanent damage.[2]

REFERENCES

1. Ransome J. Acute suppurative otitis media and acute mastoiditis. *Scott-Browne's otolaryngology.* London: Butterworth, 1987: 185–192.
2. Royal Alexandra Hospital for Children. Nursing guidelines for children following mastoidectomy. *Nursing policy and procedure manual.* Sydney: RAHC, 1991: 06–07.

Chapter 6

Care of the Infant, Child and Adolescent with Alteration to Structure

Disturbances in Blood Volume, Pressure and Flow

Carmel McQuellin

Congenital Heart Disease

Congenital heart disease (CHD) is the most common form of congenital abnormality, affecting 0.8% of births.[1] Understanding intracardiac haemodynamics enables the clinical signs associated with the various anomalies to be anticipated. When used in conjunction with information obtained from a comprehensive nursing assessment, the nurse's ability to problem solve, make critical decisions and plan nursing care appropriate for the child's needs is enhanced.

Clinical assessment combined with non-invasive ultrasound imaging provides extremely accurate diagnosis of the defects, eliminating the need for urgent cardiac catheterisation and angiographic assessment in the majority of critically ill newborn infants.[2] The following classification of acyanotic and cyanotic congenital heart disease includes the common defects and highlights the nursing assessment. The pathophysiology and treatment modalities for infants and children are also included. A number of more complex and rare lesions are not included in this discussion. Other authors have comprehensively discussed various congenital cardiac defects.[3-10] See Chapter 11 for nursing assessment and management of infants and children with myocardial dysfunction and the perioperative nursing care for children with structural heart problems.

Acyanotic Congenital Heart Disease

INCREASED PULMONARY BLOOD FLOW

The acyanotic cardiac defects that are associated with a left-to-right shunt and an increase in pulmonary blood flow (PBF) may precipitate cardiac failure in infancy, failure

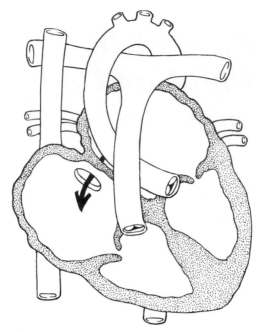

Figure 6.1 Diagrammatic representation of atrial septal defect (Ostium Secundum ASD).

to thrive, and ultimately lead to pulmonary vascular disease and severe respiratory infections which may progress to pneumonia. Increased PBF imposes an additional haemodynamic load on the left heart as a left-to-right shunt directs an additional volume of oxygenated blood from the systemic circulation to the right heart. Additional volume load increases the work of the right heart, the lungs and, therefore, the left ventricle. Factors that control the degree of shunting include:

- size of the defect
- pressure gradient across the defect
- resistance to blood flow beyond the defect
- compliance of the right ventricle.[11]

Atrial septal defects (ASD)

These are common lesions occurring in 7% to 9% of children with CHD, with twice as many females as males affected.[12,13] The ostium secundum ASD is the most common (occurring in 70% of cases) and is generally situated in the region of the fossa ovalis. Less common lesions include the ostium primum ASD (partial atrioventricular canal defect) and sinus venosus ASD.[12–14] (**Figure 6.1.**)

Nursing assessment

Most infants with an ASD are asymptomatic; however, a large left-to-right shunt can result in fatigue and dyspnoea and the development of cardiac failure during infancy, especially when associated with other anomalies.[15,16] (See: Nursing Assessment of Infants with Cardiac Failure, Chapter 11).

Pathophysiology

The degree of left-to-right shunt occurring across the defect determines the added load placed on the right atrium, right ventricle and pulmonary circulation.[13] The inherent non-compliance of the right ventricle during the neonatal period restricts the degree of left-to-right shunting across the defect. As the compliance of the right ventricle improves with age, the magnitude of the shunt and the pulmonary blood flow increases. An ASD which remains uncorrected will usually lead to increased pulmonary vascular resistance and, when associated with supraventricular arrhythmias, right heart failure.[13]

Treatment modalities

Surgery to close a defect should be scheduled even when the child is asymptomatic and before the child begins school (between 4 to 5 years of age). When cardiac failure is a problem in early infancy and a child does not respond to medication for control of cardiac failure, surgery may be scheduled at an earlier time. Outcome following surgery with an ostium secundum ASD is excellent with minimal morbidity and almost no mortality.[15] Following closure of an ostium primum ASD, the child is more susceptible to atrial and junctional rhythm disturbances, usually transient in nature and a consequence of surgical trauma. These children will, however, require long-term follow-up because of associated deformity of the mitral valve (See Chapter 11, Perioperative nursing assessment and management).

Ventricular septal defects

Ventricular septal defects (VSD) are the most common cardiac lesions, occurring in 20% of children with CHD. The birth incidence for VSD is 1.5 to 2.5 per 1000 as an isolated lesion. VSDs also form a complex of cardiac anomalies, such as tetralogy of Fallot and truncus arteriosus.[8,11,15,17,18]

VSDs are classified according to anatomical position of the defect on the ventricular septum.

- Perimembranous VSDs lie in the region of the membranous septum near the tricuspid and aortic valves, and are the most common (75% to 80% of VSDs).
- Supracristal septal defects lie immediately beneath the pulmonary valve (5% to 7% of lesions).
- Isolated inlet septal defects lie posteriorly and inferiorly to the membranous septum (5% to 8% of VSDs).
- Muscular septal defects (10% of VSDs) may occur as an isolated lesion or a component part of a complex cardiac anomaly with multiple defects.[11,17] (**See Figure 6.2.**)

Nursing assessment

The infant or child with a small VSD is generally asymptomatic. The only sign may be a systolic murmur and thrill detected at routine screening. Spontaneous closure of a small defect may occur within the 1st 2 years in 60% of children.[11] An infant with a moderate to large VSD will present in cardiac failure, resulting from the increased left-to-right shunt which develops across the defect as the pulmonary vascular resistance decreases. The increased blood volume causes an overload of the left heart precipitating cardiac failure. Initially, infants display fatigue on exertion when feeding and crying, increased

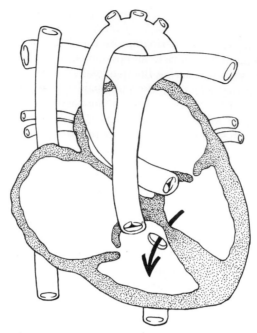

Figure 6.2 Diagrammatic representation of ventricular septal defect.

irritability and excessive sweating and have a history of feeding difficulties, and failure to thrive. They may present with an asymmetrical appearance of their chest wall — precordial bulge. The asymmetry of the chest develops in response to the cardiomegaly imposed by the cardiac failure. A systolic thrill indicative of intracardiac shunting of blood may be detected. Chapter 11 provides nursing assessment and management principles for the infant or child with cardiac failure.

Cardiac catheterisations are not routinely undertaken in children with small, isolated VSDs, as echocardiographic assessment provides the information for highly accurate diagnosis. In children with a moderate to large VSD, catheterisation is undertaken to:

- evaluate the size of the left to right shunt
- estimate pulmonary vascular resistance
- locate the position of the defect/s.[11]

Pathophysiology

Haemodynamically, blood shunting left to right across the VSD is dependent upon the size of the defect, the resistance to blood flow determined by the systemic and pulmonary vascular resistance and the pressure gradient across the defect.[11] The resistance offered by the pulmonary vasculature is of extreme importance in an infant with a left-to-right shunt. At birth, the increased pulmonary vascular resistance (PVR) drops markedly with the transition from the fetal to the postnatal circulation reaching a near adult level by 4 to 6 weeks of age.[19] The PVR drops due to changes within the vessel walls, whereby the muscularity in the medial layer of the arteriolar network is reduced.[20] Thus the small, narrow lumen of the fetal pulmonary arteries alter to become the wide lumen seen in the older infant. Once the PVR decreases, the pulmonary blood flow concomitantly increases.

It is the increase in the left-to-right shunt that results in volume overload of the left heart. The left ventricle subsequently dilates and hypertrophies in a compensatory response to the imposed volume load. These effects are additional to the stimulation which occurs to both the neuroendocrine and sympathetic nervous systems which evokes the other common clinical signs seen in cardiac failure.[11] The decrease in the PVR which occurs between 4 and 6 weeks of age explains the characteristic presentation of cardiac failure in infants with a large VSD at that age.

Treatment modalities

Small VSDs in children with normal pulmonary artery pressure warrant regular clinical assessment and an echocardiograph to determine the degree of left-to-right shunt. These children are at risk of endocarditis and therefore require prophylactic antibiotic cover at times of high risk, for example dental or oral, genitourinary and gastrointestinal surgery.[11]

In infants with moderate to large VSDs, control of cardiac failure may require diuretic regimens in addition to digoxin. When infants remain unresponsive to this therapy, systemic vasodilators, for example, captopril, may be effective.[11] These infants are at significant risk of severe pulmonary infection which may be life threatening. When medical therapy fails to control the cardiac failure, primary surgical repair is undertaken at an early stage.[21] (See Chapter 11, Nursing assessment and management principles of cardiac failure in infancy and perioperative considerations of care.)

Outcomes

The outcome in children with small defects is excellent, as most defects close spontaneously and there is a normal life expectancy when risks of endocarditis are eliminated.[18] Infants with moderate-sized defects will require anti-failure medication if symptomatic. The period of greatest risk is between 1 to 6 months of age. Only 15% to 20% of these infants will have persistent, moderately large shunts beyond infancy. Such defects should be electively closed between 3 to 5 years of age, beyond which time further spontaneous reduction in size is not expected. Infants with a large left-to-right shunt pose the most difficult problem due to the development of cardiac failure, their increased incidence of pulmonary infections and the risk of developing increased pulmonary vascular resistance. These infants generally require primary surgical closure of the defect within the first 6 months of life.[11]

Patent ductus arteriosus

Patent ductus arteriosus (PDA) has an incidence of approximately 1:2000 births, accounting for approximately 5% to 10% of CHD. There is a 2:1 female to male ratio.[18,22,23]

Perinatal considerations

The ductus arteriosus is a large vascular channel that exists within the foetus which diverts blood from the high resistance of the pulmonary circulation to the descending aorta during intrauterine life (**Figure 6.3**). Ductal patency *in utero* is maintained by endogenous prostaglandins which act to relax ductal smooth muscle.[19] The gestational age of the baby determines the responsiveness of the ductus to endogenous prostaglandins.[24-27]

Before delivery, the fetus has high serum levels of prostaglandin, particularly prostaglandin E_2 (PGE_2). Prostaglandins are locally synthesised and act locally within the

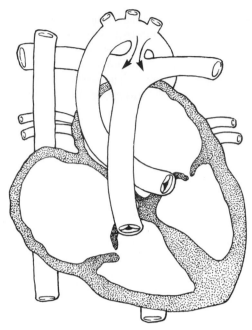

Figure 6.3 Diagrammatic representation of patent ductus arteriosus.

ductus arteriosus, placenta, umbilical vessels, pulmonary artery and aorta.[27] The catabolic pathway of prostaglandin occurs via the lungs.[25] *In utero*, only 7% of the cardiac
output of the fetus perfuses the fetal lung to produce a trivial pulmonary blood flow.[28] As
the lungs of the fetus during intrauterine life are essentially non-functional the PGE_2 is
not metabolised and thus the high serum levels of prostaglandin are explained.

Functional closure of the ductus arteriosus occurs due to the following:

- An increase in oxygen tension of the blood occurring with initiation of extrauterine
  respiration, which stimulates constriction of ductal smooth muscle.[27–29]
- Elimination of the endogenous prostaglandin supply resulting from neonatal respiration and removal of the placenta.[25]
- The release of vasoactive substances, for example, bradykinin and endogenous
  catecholamines.[25,29]

Nursing assessment

Infants with a large PDA: The term infant of 4 to 6 weeks of age presenting in cardiac
failure demonstrates poor feeding and slow weight gain, irritability, tachycardia, tachypnoea
and diaphoresis. On clinical assessment, the nurse will note bounding peripheral pulses
characteristic of rapid aortic run-off, a wide pulse pressure and an overactive precordium,
with a continuous systolic thrill detected at the upper left sternal border.[4,18,22,23] Pulmonary rales may be heard within the base of the lung with systemic venous engorgement
evidenced by liver enlargement. (Refer to subsection on nursing assessment and management of infants with cardiac failure included in Chapter 11.)

Infants with a moderate PDA: Infants with an isolated PDA of moderate size will not
present until several months of age, and will have subtle clinical signs. Weight gain is

generally adequate although the infants are often below the average percentiles for mass and length. A history of upper respiratory tract infection is common and there may be a problem with the infant experiencing exertional dyspnoea.[4,18,22,27]

Infants and Children with a Small PDA: The infant or child with a small PDA is asymptomatic and has no significant alteration to the haemodynamic state, displaying essentially normal growth and development patterns.[18,22,27]

Pathophysiology

The detection of the clinical signs of cardiac failure in an infant with a PDA is determined by the degree of left-to-right shunt across the ductus. Before delivery, the pulmonary vascular resistance (PVR) is extremely high due to the marked proliferation of the medial muscle layer in the pulmonary arterioles, which develops from approximately 38 weeks of gestation.[30] Following birth, PVR drops dramatically and reaches near adult levels by about 4 to 6 weeks of age. The proliferation of smooth muscle tissue protects against the high pulmonary blood flow in the first weeks of life.

Age is an important factor in infants presenting with the clinical signs of cardiac failure attributed to a large PDA. There are two characteristic ages of presentation. Once the PVR drops significantly below the level of the systemic vascular resistance, there is progressive left-to-right shunting of blood across the ductus, from the aorta to the pulmonary artery.[2,30,31] The volume overload results in pulmonary plethora, an increase in pulmonary venous return and left heart enlargement. Unless relieved, left ventricular failure and pulmonary hypertension will develop.[23,30]

In contrast, the preterm infant does not have the same development of the medial smooth muscle layer of the pulmonary arterioles. The younger the gestational age of the infant and the lower the weight, the more significant the haemodynamic effects.[22,27] Consequently, a large left-to-right shunt at ductal level can precipitate severe cardiac failure with development of pulmonary hypertension at a very early age.[29,32] The relative incidence of PDA in infants of 26 to 30 weeks' gestation is 77%, 50% at 31 to 32 weeks gestation and 27% at 35 to 36 weeks. Birth weight of less than 1000 g carries an associated incidence of PDA in 83% of infants, but only 40% of the last group are significantly affected haemodynamically.[22]

Treatment modalities

Pharmacological manipulation of the ductus is commonly indicated to either effect ductal closure in the preterm infant or ensure patency in newborns with ductal-dependent congenital cardiac lesions.

The preterm infant with persistent patency of the ductus arteriosus will require fluid restriction with or without diuretics, as these infants cannot tolerate intravascular volume overload. Anaemia must also be corrected as it potentiates the cardiac failure.[29,30]

Pharmacological treatment of the cardiac failure with digoxin presents special problems for preterm babies because of the:

- increased amounts of connective tissue and water within the myocardium which decrease the distensibility of the left ventricle;
- increased risks of arrhythmia and subendocardial ischaemia;
- increased potential for toxicity because of a prolongation of the half-life of digoxin (57 hours in the preterm infant compared with 35 hours in the term infant). This is attributed to liver and kidney immaturity.[30]

Indomethacin is the current pharmacologic agent used to constrict the ductus in the preterm infant with a large left-to-right shunt.[25,27,29,30,32-34] Its use is advocated in the preterm infant weighing less than 1500 g and has been very effective in closing the ductus in extremely low birthweight infants of less than 1000 g in weight.[25,29,32]

Heyman maintains that pulmonary vascular disease in the preterm infant may be established within a few days of life, only requiring a moderate degree of left-to-right shunt at ductal level to produce the change.[29] The link between respiratory distress syndrome in the preterm infant and continued patency of the ductus arteriosus is well substantiated. Studies have shown a reduced incidence of ventilator dependency and bronchopulmonary dysplasia in infants receiving early intervention with indomethacin.[29,30,32,33]

Implications for nursing practice

From a nursing perspective, astute assessment of the infants to detect evidence of a significant ductus arteriosus will facilitate prompt intervention. Following indomethacin treatment, complete closure or significant constriction of the ductus occurs in 50% to 75% of infants.[29,30] Up to 25% of infants may later regain their shunt;[34] however, they may respond to a further course of indomethacin.[27,29] It is important to note there is a difference in the half-life of indomethacin in infants less than 32 weeks' gestation due to their delayed metabolism of the drug. Lower doses of the drug are therefore being used.[30] The side effects of indomethacin may restrict this form of therapy for a small number of infants. Though transient in nature, the side effects documented with its use include renal dysfunction and inhibition of platelet function. Indomethacin is contraindicated in infants with necrotising enterocolitis, shock and any dysfunctional state which may potentiate further complications.[25,27,29,30,34]

Special considerations

It is now possible to achieve non-surgical, though invasive, PDA closure using plugs or a modified Rashkind PDA occlusion device. The procedure gaining rapid and wide acceptance uses a double umbrella device of polyurethane foam discs mounted on surgical steel struts. The device is inserted in a folded configuration into a femoral vein via a percutaneous approach.[23,35-38] The device is positioned in the ductus and as the sheath that controls the device is withdrawn, one set of arms is allowed to open on to the aortic side and the second set of arms opens on the pulmonary side. Technical modifications of the device, together with adequate premedication and anaesthesia, have enhanced the rate of success which approaches 100%.[35,37] With rapid technological achievement, the early development of suitable delivery systems appropriate for use in the preterm infant is foreseen.[38]

Surgical closure: ligation of the ductus arteriosus

The asymptomatic infant in whom spontaneous closure of the PDA does not occur, will require elective surgery to ligate the duct to prevent the risk of bacterial endocarditis. The operative mortality associated with ligation is negligible. Long term, the children progress normally with full life expectancy unless pulmonary vascular disease becomes established before surgery. Without the surgery, infants with a large PDA who live to adulthood, develop pulmonary vascular disease and right ventricular failure.[22]

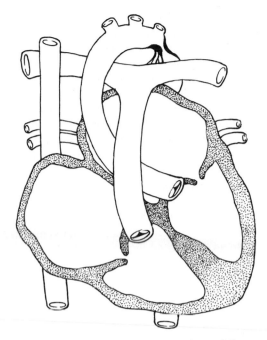

Figure 6.4 Diagrammatic representation of coarctation of the aorta.

There are special considerations for the preterm infant with a significant PDA. Most units advocate an attempt at medical closure of the PDA in an infant, and surgery if this is unsuccessful. Importantly, reports indicate an association with necrotising enterocolitis (NEC) in infants with a large PDA. This is attributed to the reduction in cardiac output and the resultant organ hypoperfusion which ultimately produces gut ischaemia.[22] Recent research undertaken on infants of less than 1000 g with haemodynamically significant PDAs indicates that an aggressive surgical ligation program reduces the incidence of NEC from 30% to 8%, questioning whether 'prophylactic' surgical ligation might be indicated.[30] Refer to subsection on perioperative nursing assessment and management principles included in Chapter 11.

NORMAL PULMONARY BLOOD FLOW

Coarctation of the aorta

Coarctation of the aorta accounts for 5% to 8% of CHD, with a ratio of 2:1 males to females being affected.[40–44] It is an anomaly where the distal aortic arch or the proximal descending aorta become narrowed, causing varying degrees of obstruction to the systemic blood flow. **See Figure 6.4**.

Nursing assessment

The newborn infant with coarctation of the aorta: Newborn infants presenting during the first weeks of life with coarctation of the aorta are often critically ill. The time of clinical presentation of these newborns is variable, from a few days of life to several weeks of age. This is partly explained by ductal patency, which facilitates the adequate flow of blood to the lower extremities and trunk. As the ductus arteriosus closes, the perfusion to the lower half of the body diminishes rapidly.

Astute nursing assessment of these infants will enable subtle early signs of heart failure to be detected and the initiation of treatment, thus avoiding decompensation to a critical state. These infants are unsettled, increasingly irritable and unable to feed, tachycardic, tachypnoeic and diaphoretic. On examination the femoral pulses are impalpable. It is essential to obtain differential blood pressure recording between limbs. Oliguria would be present due to minimal renal perfusion and venous engorgement would be reflected by the enlargement of the infant's liver. Hypertension in the upper extremities is seen if there is no associated large VSD.

When heart failure is severe hypertension is masked and, left untreated, the infant can develop cardiovascular and respiratory collapse. Approximately 10% of infants with coarctation will develop cardiac failure. Two-thirds of these have associated cardiac defects, for example, patent ductus arteriosus, ventricular septal defects, aortic or mitral stenosis.[43] Infants who have an associated VSD or PDA are predisposed to develop heart failure at a very early stage. Refer to subsection on nursing assessment and management of cardiac failure in infancy included in Chapter 11.

The older child with coarctation of the aorta: Asymptomatic children with coarctation of the aorta will generally remain so until early adolescence.[42] Clinically, there is a marked discrepancy between the arterial pulses of the upper and lower limbs with the children displaying hypertension in the upper extremities.[40]

Often in the older child extensive collateral circulation develops between the proximal aorta and the region distal to the coarcted segment.[40,41] The collateral supply enhances the perfusion to the trunk and lower extremities and rib notching develops, a phenomenon seen in children and adolescents who have an extensive collateral network.[40,42,44,45] The collateral vessels may cause erosion of the ribs, most commonly at the level of the 3rd and 7th ribs.[43]

Without surgery, the mean survival for patients with coarctation of the aorta is 35 years.[43] The complications that develop relate to systemic hypertension, cardiac failure, cerebrovascular accidents, aortic aneurisms and endocarditis.

Pathophysiology

The obstruction to systemic blood flow that occurs in children with coarctation of the aorta results from 2 different mechanisms. A proliferation of fibrous tissue develops in the wall of the aortic arch adjacent to the origin of the left subclavian artery.[43] It is thought that an extension of ductal smooth muscle tissue into the arch constricts as the ductus arteriosus closes.[41] Hypoplastic development of the aortic arch is the 2nd mechanism responsible for varying degrees of obstruction to systemic blood flow, which may vary from minimal in nature to near complete obstruction.

Haemodynamically, the degree of mechanical obstruction will determine pressure gradients, the level of hypertension experienced by the infant or child and ultimately the ability or inability of the infant or child to compensate effectively. Pressure gradients do not develop across the constricted segments of arch until the aortic lumen is 50% occluded.[42,43] It is postulated that the level of hypertension the infants and children experience results from carotid baroreceptor sensitivity and the renin–angiotensin mechanisms.[43] If there is a major associated VSD, significant systemic hypertension does not occur.

Classification of coarctation of the aorta

Coarctation of the aorta is classified according to the specific site of aortic arch narrowing. The preductal form of coarctation occurs proximal to the site of the ductus arteriosus. Haemodynamically, systemic blood flow in the newborn infant is maintained via the ductus arteriosus while the PVR remains elevated. With the circulatory changes that occur at birth and the marked decrease in PVR of the neonatal period, the shunting of blood from right to left across the ductus arteriosus will cease.[19] The left ventricular pressure will subsequently rise secondary to pressure overload of the ventricle, which ultimately fails unless relieved. In the periductal form of coarctation, the aortic obstruction occurs at the level of the ductus arteriosus, while in the postductal coarctation, the obstruction is situated distal to the ductus.

Perioperative considerations

Urgent intervention to support the newborn infant with severe coarctation of the aorta or aortic arch interruption is imperative as these infants are at risk of total cardiovascular and respiratory collapse.

The importance of the nursing role cannot be overemphasised in the care of the critically ill newborn in heart failure. The nursing assessment performed at the time of presentation is a continuing process. These infants require immediate intervention to relieve the obstruction to systemic blood flow. Urgent stabilisation is effected through the use of prostaglandin infusions, ventilation, correction of acidosis, relief of cardiac failure and correction of hypoglycaemia.[45]

A prostaglandin E_1 infusion will dilate the ductus arteriosus and re-establish perfusion to the lower extremities.[46] Support of the infant's compromised cardiorespiratory condition through reversal of the acidotic and hypoxic state will be enhanced through intubation and ventilation. Diuretics are used to reduce the preload of the heart and inotropes to improve the contractile state of the myocardium.[47] Postoperatively, vasodilators may be used to reduce afterload and allow recovery of the stressed myocardium. A combination of digoxin and diuretic therapy may be effective in controlling the cardiac failure (Refer to the discussion on management principles of myocardial failure in Chapter 11). In the critically ill newborn, dopamine in low doses will have the desired beta effects on the myocardium and vasculature by reducing the afterload and improving renal perfusion. Re-establishing the infant's fluid and electrolyte state and ensuring adequate glucose levels in the infant who would have depleted glycogen stores in response to the stress state will further promote cardiovascular and neuroendocrine homeostasis.

Surgical intervention and outcome

Following initial control of the infant's cardiac failure, the method of surgical relief remains controversial. The technique favoured for the newborn infant with severe coarctation is the subclavian flap aortoplasty.[40,42] This technique decreases the risk of aortic recoarctation following surgery.[48] The subclavian artery maintains normal growth and is used to patch the narrowed segment of aorta. Alternatively, resection of the coarctation and an end-to-end anastomosis is used in some newborn infants and in the older child.[48] Less commonly, a patch graft aortoplasty may be performed, although it carries an incidence of postoperative aortic aneurisms.[49]

Postoperative mortality rates from subclavian flap repair of coarctation in the newborn period are 2% to 10%.[42] These statistics have improved with the aggressive pharmacological and interventional support manoeuvres now used which resolve cardiac failure in the preoperative period.[48] Infants who have associated intracardiac defects have a markedly increased operative mortality, many requiring simultaneous pulmonary artery banding. Gestational age and weight also influence the outcome in the neonatal group.[40] The reader is referred to the subsection on perioperative nursing assessment and management included in Chapter 11.

Interventional catheterisation

Controversy surrounds balloon angioplasty and dilatation of the aortic coarctation as opposed to the surgical approach. Most centres avoid balloon dilatation in infants with a primary coarctation due to the poor results from unsatisfactory relief of pressure gradients and the risks of complication. The procedure is associated with intimal and medial tears of the aortic wall and hence, there are increased risks of aneurism formation. The procedure does, however, have growing support and is deemed suitable for children with postoperative recoarctation of the aorta.[35,36,50,51] Scar tissue develops in these children and provides the support necessary for the vessel wall, offering low risk and an effective rate of success at close to 90%.[50]

Postoperative considerations

The major problems the infants and children experience during the postoperative period relates to hypertension and collateral vessel development from the aorta.[49] Hypertension may require pharmacological intervention to minimise the risks of postoperative haemorrhage.[42] Continuous infusion of sodium nitroprusside or other vasodilators may be required and can then be followed by oral antihypertensive preparations if necessary.

A postcoarctectomy syndrome can develop, particularly in older children several days after surgical repair. The children experience severe abdominal cramps and distension and in severe forms a paralytic ileus, fever, melena, acidosis and leucocytosis develop. The syndrome is attributed to a mesenteric arteritis resulting from the change in pressure and flow patterns to the gut following the repair.[40,45]

Aortic arch interruption

Aortic arch interruption (AAI) is a rare anomaly with an estimated incidence of 0.003 per 1000 births,[42] where there is complete discontinuity of the aortic arch. A fibrous cord may connect the 2 segments of arch in a small number of infants.[42,43] The classification of aortic arch interruption is determined by the site of the lesions.

- Type A: distal to the left subclavian artery (40%).
- Type B: the left common carotid and the left subclavian artery (55%).
- Type C: the innominate artery and the left common carotid artery (5%).[42]

Aortic arch interruption is almost always associated with other anomalies, for example, ventricular septal defects, atrial septal defects or transposition of the great arteries.

Nursing assessment

The presentation of these infants is similar to those infants with severe coarctation of the aorta. They are critically ill and display all the clinical signs of cardiac failure.[42,52,53]

From a nursing perspective, these critically ill infants pose a special management problem from the time of their presentation. Their critical preoperative state demands careful nursing assessment and an ability to problem solve to prevent deterioration to an irreversible clinical state. The operative mortality for AAI has been as high as 80% to 100% in previous years, but current experience suggests a mortality as low as 10% is achievable.[42]

Pathophysiology

In newborn infants with AAI, the blood flow to the descending aorta is effected via the ductus arteriosus.[53] Irrespective of the classification of AAI, desaturated blood crosses the ductus arteriosus from right to left to perfuse the trunk and lower extremities. As the ductus closes, clinical signs of cardiac failure develop rapidly.[42,46,53]

Special perioperative considerations

The critical condition of these infants warrants urgent supportive measures and early surgical relief of the aortic obstruction. A prostaglandin infusion will maintain ductal patency and facilitate the perfusion from the right ventricle to the lower body.[12,53]

Controversy exists about the timing of corrective procedures between a primary and second stage repair. Current research advocates primary surgical repair of the aortic interruption and, whenever possible, the repair of the associated intracardiac defect with the support of cardiopulmonary bypass.[42,46,53]

Aortic stenosis

Aortic stenosis can occur at a valvular level, subvalvular or supravalvular level. Valvular aortic stenosis is the most common form occurring in 3% to 6% of all children with CHD, with a 4:1 male to female ratio. In 20% of the children it is associated with other anomalies, for example, coarctation of the aorta and VSD.[54] Subaortic stenosis occurs in 8% to 10% of children with aortic stenosis with 2:1 males to females affected. A fibromuscular membrane develops beneath the aortic valve in the outflow tract of the left ventricle.

Nursing assessment

Most of the children with aortic stenosis are asymptomatic, falling within the normal percentile boundaries for height and weight. The defect may be detected at a routine examination where auscultation of the heart reveals a cardiac murmur. In moderate to severe forms of aortic stenosis the children may exhibit fatigue, exertional dyspnoea, angina pectoris when the intramyocardial oxygen supply is reduced and syncope. In infancy, presentation may be with severe congestive cardiac failure and poor arterial pulses. With severe obstruction, sudden death can occur in up to 19% of the children due to myocardial ischaemia and ventricular arrhythmia.[54]

In borderline situations exercise testing may reveal electrocardiographic changes indicative of myocardial ischaemia. Dopler echocardiographic assessment of children with aortic stenosis assists selection of children for cardiac catheterisation and balloon aortic valvuloplasty. However, this remains a controversial procedure due principally to the risks of iatrogenic valvular incompetence.[54]

Pathophysiology

In valvular aortic stenosis the valve tissue is thickened and the leaflets are rigid with partial fusion of the valve commissures. A haemodynamically significant lesion will result in left ventricular hypertrophy and poststenotic dilatation of the ascending aorta as a pressure gradient develops between the left ventricle and the aorta. Further, a reduction in myocardial blood flow may develop from the intramyocardial compression of the coronary vessels, reducing the subendocardial blood flow.[54]

Treatment modalities

Only in severe aortic stenosis should the parents and child appreciate the need to avoid strenuous activity. However, the children will require life-long prophylaxis against infective endocarditis at times of risk, for example, when oral surgical procedures are undertaken. The operative mortality is less than 2% and is essentially confined to infancy, with the children experiencing excellent relief. It is suggested that within 15 to 20 years of the operation, up to 35% of children will require prosthetic valve replacement due to their deformed valve leaflets.[54]

Critical aortic valve stenosis in infancy

The newborn infant with critical aortic valve stenosis constitutes a medical emergency as these infants often present with intractable cardiac failure. They may develop myocardial infarction which may further result in endocardial fibroelastosis due to the reduced subendocardial oxygen availability.[54]

Nursing assessment

On examination the infants are noted to be pale, irritable, tachycardic and hypotensive. Pulmonary congestion is exhibited by tachypnoea, dyspnoea and chest recession with pulmonary rales detected at the bases. Cyanosis may also develop secondary to a ventilation — perfusion mismatch (V/Q inequality).

Treatment modalities

The treatment of choice for these infants is controversial. Whether surgical aortic valvotomy or balloon valvuloplasty is performed, the mortality rate is high and the procedure only palliative. Refer to the subsection on perioperative nursing care included in Chapter 11 for detailed discussion on the principles of postoperative nursing of these infants.

Pulmonary stenosis

Pulmonary stenosis may be valvular or subvalvular in nature, occurring in up to 30% of children with CHD. It may occur in isolation, but it is often associated with other anomalies, for example, tetralogy of Fallot or transposition of the great arteries. In valvular pulmonary stenosis, the cusps are fused, with 20% of the children having a bicuspid valve and 10% to 15% having dysplastic (thickened) leaflets.[55]

Nursing assessment

Clinically, the majority of the infants and children are asymptomatic. Dependent upon the degree of stenosis, the children may present with increasing dyspnoea, fatigue and signs of right ventricular failure. On exertion, the children may demonstrate signs of peripheral cyanosis. Those with severe pulmonary stenosis and a patent foramen ovale may develop central cyanosis due to the right-to-left shunt that can result. The symptomatic newborn who presents within days of birth has critical pulmonary valve stenosis, resulting in significant restriction to the pulmonary blood flow and right-to-left atrial shunt.

Pathophysiology

Haemodynamically, the pulmonary stenosis causes a secondary effect upon the right ventricle by increasing the ventricular pressure, leading to right ventricular hypertrophy.[55] Obvious narrowing of the infundibular area situated beneath the pulmonary valve is a characteristic feature of tetralogy of Fallot.

Treatment modalities

Balloon valvuloplasty is the treatment of choice to relieve pulmonary stenosis outside the newborn period, when surgery is required to relieve the obstruction of critical pulmonary valve stenosis. The technique involves balloon inflation of the valvular stenosis to effect relief of the gradient that exists between the pulmonary artery and the right ventricle. There is a 5% risk of complication with the procedure and a 0.5% incidence of mortality. The complications of the procedure may result in iliac vein thrombosis in 10% to 20% of the children with the development of pulmonary valve incompetence, usually haemodynamically insignificant, in a further 20%.[50]

Cyanotic CHD

The causes of cyanosis in the newborn infant are many and varied and include both structural heart defects associated with a right-to-left shunt (as in tetralogy of Fallot), and upper and lower airway problems. Commonly, the cause of cyanosis is related to respiratory dysfunction or metabolic problems as in hypoglycaemia, persistent pulmonary hypertension of the newborn, central nervous system dysfunction, shock or sepsis.[56]

The clinical presentations of the infants are variable dependent upon the types of lesions involved, and whether there is an increase or a decrease in pulmonary blood flow. The following classification will be helpful to identify the types of cardiac lesions affecting the infants and children.

PRESENTATIONS ASSOCIATED WITH CYANOSIS

Increased pulmonary blood flow

- Cyanotic congenital heart lesions resulting from admixture (mixing) of the systemic and pulmonary venous return is often associated with congestive cardiac failure. These lesions include total anomalous pulmonary venous return and truncus arteriosus. In admixture lesions an inverse relationship exists between the degree of pulmonary blood flow and the level of cyanosis in the infant.
- Cyanotic congenital heart lesions due to failure of the pulmonary venous return to reach the systemic circulation, for example, newborn infants with transposition of the great arteries.

Decreased pulmonary blood flow

- Cyanotic congenital heart lesions with an associated right-to-left shunt, for example tetralogy of Fallot, pulmonary atresia and tricuspid atresia. A right-to-left shunt signifies that some deoxygenated blood reaches the systemic circuit, having bypassed the lungs.

Obstruction to pulmonary venous return

- Cyanotic congenital heart lesions resulting from obstruction to the pulmonary venous return are associated with congestive cardiac failure (as exemplified in many newborn infants with obstructed total anomalous pulmonary venous return) and rare forms of hypoplastic left heart syndrome.

The presentations of infants with cyanotic congenital heart lesions are, however, variable and may also result from a combination of any of the factors outlined above.

THE NEWBORN INFANT WITH CYANOTIC CHD

Nursing assessment of cyanosis

The degree of cyanosis in the newborn infant is dependent upon the amount of deoxygenated haemoglobin carried in the blood.[56] Once the deoxygenated haemoglobin approaches 30 to 50 g/L, central cyanosis becomes apparent.[56,57] The presence of fetal haemoglobin in the newborn infant hampers recognition of cyanosis, thus there is the potential for these infants to become severely hypoxic before cyanosis is detected. From a nursing perspective this is a very important concept to appreciate, as measurement of PaO_2 in these infants is a more valuable and reliable aid to assessment than is the use of saturation monitoring.[56]

Differentiation of the cyanosis of cardiac from non-cardiac causes is greatly aided by the hyperoxia test.[56,57] An FiO_2 of 1.0 is administered to the infants for a short time. When the newborn infant is receiving an FiO_2 of 1.0 the PaO_2 will normally become elevated to a value in excess of 300 mmHg, whereas in the infant with a right-to-left shunt, the PaO_2 will not exceed 200 mmHg.[56] Prolonged administration of the high oxygen concentrations is to be avoided, especially in premature infants due to the risks associated with pulmonary atelectasis and retinopathy. The infants need to be well pacified as crying evokes variable responses in the intracardiac shunting that can significantly influence the PaO_2 and SaO_2 results obtained from the formal arterial blood gas analysis. The hyperoxia test is a simple, useful test, particularly in peripheral centres where paediatric diagnostic facilities are unavailable.

Principles of stabilisation

Stabilisation for the newborn infant with cyanotic CHD aims to minimise oxygen requirements and maximise cardiac output. This is achieved by providing warmth to ensure a neutral thermal environment, fluid and electrolyte homeostasis, appropriate blood glucose levels and the administration of oxygen that will help alleviate significant hypoxaemia in the baby. Further, the nurse responsible for the infant's care must be aware of the need for assisted ventilation and a continuous infusion of prostaglandin E_1 for the newborn infant with a ductal-dependent lesion until surgical intervention can be provided.[56]

COMPLICATIONS OF CYANOTIC CHD

Growth retardation is a common finding in these infants and children as is the development of polycythemia. The increase in red cell volume is a mechanism of compensation resulting from the continuous state of hypoxaemia. The red blood cell proliferation (polycythemia) is effective in the delivery of more oxygen to body tissues; however, it causes an increase in the viscosity of blood, thus increasing the workload of the heart and increasing the myocardial oxygen requirements. The increased blood viscosity leads to increased risks of a cerebrovascular accident. Further, these children have an increased susceptibility to develop infective endocarditis and cerebral abscesses, the result of septic embolisation from the venous circulation reaching the cerebral circulation through a right-to-left shunt. Coagulopathy poses a significant problem in this group of children[58] as the polycythemia reduces the plasma volume, thus decreasing the necessary clotting factors, while increased fibrinolysis and platelet dysfunction further contribute to the coagulation problem.[59]

Many infants and young children with cyanotic CHD experience hypoxic spells similar in nature and aetiology to that of tetralogy of Fallot, although loss of consciousness is not a usual feature. Severe episodes of hypoxaemia resulting from hyperdynamic obstruction to the pulmonary arterial blood flow cause devastating periods of hypoxaemia and metabolic acidosis.[58]

CARE OF CHILDREN WITH INCREASED PULMONARY BLOOD FLOW

In all forms of CHD where there is an increase in pulmonary blood flow (PBF), the infants and children are at risk of developing cardiac failure and more importantly pulmonary vascular disease. The increase in PBF is associated with an increase in the muscularity of the pulmonary arterial network which initially, may be potentially reversible. However, if the condition of increased pressures and flow persists, the lumen of the pulmonary arterioles becomes increasingly narrowed and eventually the lumen is obliterated. At this stage the pulmonary hypertension becomes irreversible. Once this pulmonary vascular disease becomes established, the operative morbidity and mortality are greatly increased and may result in an inability to operate on the infant.

Truncus arteriosus

In truncus arteriosus, one single arterial vessel arises from the heart to supply the systemic and pulmonary arterial systems. Often referred to as an admixture lesion, the truncal vessel overrides a VSD and receives the entire blood ejected from both the left and right ventricles.[57,60] The truncal valve is semilunar in nature and may be stenotic or insufficient. Truncal valve abnormalities are also associated with an increased surgical risk for the infants. (**Figure 6.5.**) There are 3 classifications of truncus arteriosus, dependent upon the site of pulmonary arterial connection with the truncal vessel. The anomaly is reported to occur in 0.7% of infants with CHD.[57]

Nursing assessment

The clinical presentation of infants is dependent upon the pulmonary blood flow and the degree of truncal valve dysplasia. The nurse will detect a mild degree of cyanosis in the newborn infant with truncus arteriosus, however, as the infant's pulmonary vascular

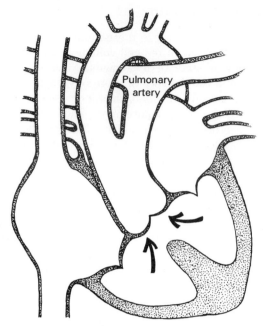

Figure 6.5 Diagrammatic representation of truncus arteriosus.

resistance decreases with increasing age, the level of cyanosis dissipates and the clinical signs of cardiac failure will be evident.[60] When the lesion is associated with truncal valve incompetence, these infants will often present in the neonatal period with severe signs of cardiac failure and respiratory embarrassment.

Pathophysiology

The pressures within the truncal vessel, pulmonary arteries and systemic arteries are equal due to the ejection of blood into the truncus from both the left and right ventricles. The volume of pulmonary blood flow is dependent upon the resistance offered by the pulmonary arteriolar network and any existent pulmonary artery stenosis.[57] The high pulmonary vascular resistance that exists at birth acts to protect the lungs from the extremely high pulmonary blood flow of the first few days of life that is associated with this defect. As soon as the pulmonary vascular resistance drops, these infants develop cardiac failure secondary to the increased pulmonary blood flow that accompanies TA.[46,57] Unless treated, the infants die of heart failure or develop obliterative pulmonary arterial disease which precludes operation. The degree of cyanosis these infants exhibit is inversely proportional to the volume of pulmonary blood flow. In the newborn, the degree of cyanosis is intensified due to the high resistance within the pulmonary circuit, but as the pulmonary vascular resistance decreases the level of cyanosis decreases. The truncal valve incompetence accentuates the volume load placed upon the left ventricle, further contributing to the myocardial dysfunction.

Treatment modalities

Current studies indicate the need for early surgical intervention in the neonatal period to support these infants and prevent the development of cardiac failure and irreversible pulmonary vascular disease. The infants will require medication to support their cardio-vascular state and relieve cardiac failure.[57] At the time of surgery, the pulmonary arterial vessels are detached from the truncal vessel and the VSD is closed, directing the blood from the left ventricle into the truncal vessel. A dacron conduit, which commonly contains a valve, or an ascending aortic allograft with valve conduit is anastomosed to the right ventricle, thus directing the systemic venous return into the pulmonary circuit.[46,61]

In the past, the treatment option in the neonate was aimed at controlling the degree of cardiac failure by performing pulmonary artery banding. In attempting to reduce the surgical risks associated with open heart surgery in these infants with severe cardiac failure, corrective surgery was often withheld for a period of several months, and the infants were supported with anti-failure medication while optimising their rest and nutritional state.[46] Results indicated an unacceptable incidence of morbidity and mortality with the delayed surgical approach. More recently, palliation has been excluded and primary surgical correction has become the treatment of choice. Statistically, the outcomes following truncus arteriosus repair are encouraging with the operative mortality currently reported between 10% and 16%.[60,62,63] When a small allograft is used to effect a repair in infants, further surgery will be required to revise the conduit which will become progressively narrow and therefore inadequate for the infant due to growth.[63]

Special considerations

These infants pose a special nursing and medical management problem following their surgery due to the risks associated with their very young age and the potentially life-threatening effects of labile pulmonary vascular resistance resulting in severe pulmonary hypertension and truncal valve incompetence.

Transposition of the great arteries

Transposition of the great arteries (TGA) is the most common CHD causing cyanosis in the newborn infant, occurring in 5% to 7% of all congenital heart defects, with a 60% to 70% male preponderance.[64] In complete TGA, the anatomical relationship of the great arteries to ventricles is transposed so that the aorta arises from the morphologic right ventricle and the pulmonary artery arises from the morphologic left ventricle. (**Figure 6.6.**)

Nursing assessment

In simple TGA (without a VSD), a patent foramen ovale and/or a PDA facilitate the bidirectional shunting of blood that sustains the life of the infant. With no treatment, 30% of infants die in the first week of life, 50% by the first month, 70% by 6 months and 90% by 1 year of age.[64]

In simple TGA, 92% of infants generally present within hours of delivery or within the first day of life.[64] The infants are generally of good size and are well at birth. However, they soon develop cyanosis which progresses in intensity over time and upon exertion and becomes worse as the ductus arteriosus starts to close. Tachycardia and dyspnoea develop with the increased hypoxaemia. The circulation remains stable with the peripheral pulses easily palpable initially. However, hypoxaemia develops very rapidly with ductal closure and without appropriate support the infants become profoundly hypoxic and are in imminent danger of complete cardiorespiratory collapse.

Nursing personnel fulfil a crucial role in detecting early clinical signs with these infants. They are totally reliant upon early evaluation of the clinical features of hypoxia

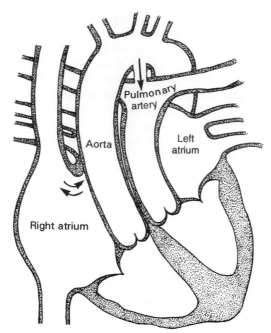

Figure 6.6 Diagrammatic representation of transposition of the great arteries.

as delay in providing therapeutic intervention may prove fatal. Extreme caution should be exercised in the care of these infants to avoid potent stimuli such as cold stress and excessive handling which may evoke an unwanted response that further exacerbates hypoxia. Infants with TGA who demonstrate early signs of cyanosis and hypoxia require the support of a prostaglandin infusion to dilate and maintain ductal patency until more definitive intervention is available.

Pathophysiology

The anatomical position of the great arteries results in the systemic venous blood returning to the right heart and being directed via the aorta back around the body, while the pulmonary venous blood returning from the lungs to the left heart, is directed via the pulmonary artery back to the lungs.[46,57,64] These 2 parallel circuits function quite independently of one another and unless adequate mixing of the 2 circulations occurs profound cyanosis, hypoxia and acidosis ensue. The defect is not compatible with life.[65,66] When a large VSD is associated with complete TGA the infants do not present as early as when the interventricular septum is intact. The VSD enables the required mixing of systemic and pulmonary blood and hence cyanosis and signs of hypoxia are not detected as early. Rather, these infants present with the clinical signs of heart failure, with mild cyanosis occurring between 2 and 6 weeks of age.[64]

Treatment modalities

Echocardiographic diagnosis has simplified the management of the critically ill newborn infant with cyanotic CHD, negating the need for cardiac catheterisation with its attendant high risks.[66,67] Following clinical and echocardiographic assessment, a balloon atrial septostomy (Rashkind procedure) can be performed to facilitate adequate mixing of the 2 circulations at atrial level, a procedure now commonly undertaken in the neonatal intensive care unit.

In this procedure, a balloon-tipped catheter is inserted via the umbilical or saphenous vein and advanced into the right atrium. The patent foramen ovale is probed and the catheter is passed into the left atrium through the patent foramen ovale. The balloon is then inflated with a saline-based solution and pulled briskly back towards the right atrium, thus tearing a hole in the atrial septum. The procedure may need to be repeated several times to effectively tear the atrial septum and enable mixing of the systemic and pulmonary circulations.[67,68] The balloon atrial septostomy is not without risks and it is essential that the nurse be aware of the various complications, anticipate potential problems and be prepared to intervene early should they arise. The complications that have been reported include cardiac tamponade, pneumopericardium,[69] arrhythmias and infection.

Until recently, balloon septostomy was the procedure of choice in neonates and provided palliation for a period of up to 6 to 9 months of age, after which the infants underwent physiological correction of their TGA following either a Mustard or Senning procedure.[64] Current trends favour the anatomical correction of the arterial switch procedure which is undertaken in the neonatal period.[66]

Arterial switch repair

The arterial switch procedure requires the division of the great vessels and their realignment with their morphologically correct ventricular chamber. Great care is necessary in relocating the coronary arteries so that myocardial function is not compromised.[46,64] This procedure is now widely accepted by most centres as the treatment of choice for most of the infants with TGA other than those with an associated left ventricular outflow tract obstruction. For infants with simple TGA, primary surgical correction is optimal in the first days of life. Balloon atrial septostomy may be avoided in these infants where ductal patency is effectively maintained with a continuous infusion of prostaglandin.[66] The timing for the arterial switch cannot be delayed beyond the first 2 to 3 weeks, as over time the left ventricle becomes increasingly unable to pump at a systemic level. The left ventricular pressure drops within the first weeks of birth in this group of infants, as pressure in the pulmonary artery undergoes its normal progressive fall.[65,66,70]

In the infants that present many weeks after birth, a 2-staged surgical procedure is advocated. In this group of babies it is considered that a pulmonary artery banding usually combined with a systemic to pulmonary artery shunt will help to increase the pressure of the left ventricle and prepare it for the arterial switch procedure. It is believed that the left ventricle can then pump against the systemic resistance.[66,71]

Atrial repair

The Mustard and Senning procedures were until recently accepted as the treatment of choice for infants with simple TGA. These procedures direct the systemic venous return to the left ventricle and the pulmonary venous return to the right ventricle, using either the infant's own atrial wall or a pericardial or dacron patch to act as the intra-atrial baffles or channels.[46,65,72]

Outcomes following surgery: physiologic versus anatomical correction

Immediate results following atrial (physiological) correction for simple TGA are good, however, late deterioration in the children's haemodynamic state is well documented. The 10-year survival following surgery is reported to be between 80% and 90% with the 20-year survival projected to be 77%.[64,65] Surgical correction for complex TGA carries a greater risk due in large part to pulmonary vascular disease and has a higher post-operative mortality with only 60% to 70% of the children surviving to 5 years.[64] The atrial reparative procedures have lost favour in recent years due to the potential for long-term complication related to right ventricular dysfunction, baffle obstruction and arrhythmia.[64–66,73,74]

Arrhythmias are important problems following atrial surgical repairs with rhythm disturbances of non-sinus aetiology occurring in 60% to 80% of the children at a 6-year follow-up.[66,75,76] Further, links have been drawn between significant arrhythmia and sudden death following the Mustard procedure, which is reported to occur in up to 9% of the children discharged from hospital.[64–66,76]

The results of the arterial switch procedure (anatomical correction) have improved steadily with current data suggesting a 5% hospital mortality.[77] The medium-term follow-up indicates no increase in sudden death or symptomatic arrhythmia, but infrequent atrial and ventricular ectopic beats have been noted in the children over time.[66,76] Although right ventricular outflow tract obstruction remains a postoperative problem, the overall outcome following the arterial switch is considered better in the long term with a reduced risk of associated complications and an excellent quality of life.[78,79]

Implications for nursing practice

The newborn infant requires special care in the recovery period following anatomic correction, with careful attention paid to maintaining cardiac output. The potential for the development of low cardiac output is significant due to the impairment of the left ventricular function in the neonate in the first 48 hours following surgery.[64,80,81] The risks of myocardial infarction or ischaemia associated with translocation of the coronary arteries with the arterial switch have to be kept in mind. These complications require close assessment for both the clinical signs of low cardiac output and electrocardiographic changes that signify infarction.

Total anomalous pulmonary venous connection

Total anomalous pulmonary venous connection (TAPVC) is an anomaly whereby all the pulmonary veins fail to connect with the left atrial chamber and are connected to the systemic venous circulation. There are several anatomic variations depending on the location of the pulmonary venous drainage, hence their classification as supracardiac, cardiac, infradiaphragmatic and mixed TAPVC, with further subdivisions between obstructed and non-obstructed.[82] The incidence of TAPVC is approximately 2% of all CHD.[57,83]

Nursing assessment

The presentation of infants with TAPVC is variable with the intracardiac haemodynamics determining the clinical features. Symptoms develop soon after birth when the right-to-left shunt at atrial level is inadequate to sustain the infant's systemic circulation. In infradiaphragmatic forms of TAPVC, an obstruction to pulmonary venous return develops.

These infants are critically ill presenting with severe cyanosis and respiratory distress with pulmonary oedema.[16,57]

When the pulmonary venous return is not obstructed and there is adequate intra-atrial communication the infants present with only a mild degree of cyanosis. When the presentation of these infants is delayed beyond the first days of life, they may appear thin and undernourished, demonstrating progressive signs of cardiac failure.[16,57]

Pathophysiology

TAPVC is an admixture lesion where all the pulmonary veins drain into a common venous vessel which returns its load, along with the systemic venous return to the right atrium. In the supracardiac TAPVC, the pulmonary venous return occurs via a vertical vein or the superior vena cava, whereas in the cardiac form it usually returns via the coronary sinus. The infradiaphragmatic form of TAPVC returns oxygenated blood via the inferior vena cava, whereas in the mixed form of the TAPVC the pulmonary veins are attached to any combination of anatomical positions.[46]

In TAPVC the pulmonary blood flow is markedly increased with the intra-atrial communication facilitating the flow of mixed blood from the right atrium to the left atrium and hence onto the systemic circulation. As the left atrium receives no direct pulmonary venous return, the systemic blood flow is dependent upon the right-to-left shunt at atrial level. In the obstructed form of TAPVC, which is usually associated with the infradiaphragmatic type, severe pulmonary hypertension with decreased pulmonary blood flow results.

Treatment modalities

Urgent corrective surgery to repair the anomaly is undertaken following echocardiographic assessment. usually within the first days of life.[46] Without surgery, the risks to the infants are extremely high with a 50% mortality at 3 months and an 80% mortality by 1 year of age.[82]

The aim of the surgery is to redirect the pulmonary venous drainage to the left atrial chamber, and close the ASD. This is accomplished well in the babies with the intracardiac and supracardiac forms of TAPVC; however, most of the infants with an infradiaphragmatic connection (due to the associated obstruction of their pulmonary veins) and those with the mixed form of TAPVC have a higher incidence of operative mortality and pose a very difficult management problem.

The overall mortality following surgery is suggested to be as low as 2 to 5%.[46] The type of anomalous connection and the presence of obstruction to the pulmonary venous flow causing pulmonary hypertension are the factors of greatest risk to the infants, often resulting in a significantly higher mortality rate.[46,82]

Hypoplastic left heart syndrome

Hypoplastic left heart syndrome (HLHS) involves a complexity of abnormalities where the left side of the heart is grossly underdeveloped. The anomalies making up the syndrome include hypoplasia of the aorta, aortic valve, left ventricle, mitral valve and left atrial chamber. A patent ductus arteriosus and foramen ovale are generally present, supporting the infants' circulation in the postnatal period.[46,84–87]. HLHS is reported to occur more commonly in male infants and in up to 9% of infants with CHD.[45,86]

Nursing assessment

These infants are generally well at birth, but may present very soon after delivery. Clinically, they show signs of tachypnoea, tachycardia and mild cyanosis. They have liver enlargement, a gallop rhythm and demonstrate a left precordial bulge. As the ductus starts to close the infant's condition deteriorates rapidly with acute and severe signs of cardiac failure, cyanosis, respiratory distress and poor perfusion. With the progression of the cardiac failure and hypoxaemia, metabolic acidosis develops and cardiovascular collapse is imminent.[46,84,86] Refer to the subsection on principles of nursing assessment and management of cardiac failure in infancy included in Chapter 11.

The nursing assessment of these infants requires early critical evaluation to detect the often subtle changes in the infants' clinical state and to effect optimal support of their failing circulation. This anomaly is the most common cause of death in the first weeks of life.[84] Research indicates 40% of the infants present within the first 2 days of life, 75% by 6 days of life and 86% by 2 weeks of age. The anomaly carries a 98% mortality rate within the first month of life.[86]

Pathophysiology

The infants with HLHS are dependent upon the ductus arteriosus and a patent foramen ovale for blood flow to the systemic circulation. Classically, these infants present within the first days of life. Their presentation may be delayed due to the combined patency of the ductus and the naturally high pulmonary vascular resistance that is characteristic in the newborn infant.[86]

As the right ventricle acts as the systemic ventricle it becomes dilated as the muscle mass hypertrophies, which further increases the myocardial oxygen requirements. Coronary artery perfusion is impeded by the structural abnormality. Myocardial fibrosis develops with ischaemic changes to the myocytes and is thought to contribute to the poor outcome in these infants.

Treatment modalities

Due to an extremely poor prognosis, some units advise against active surgical intervention for newborn infants with hypoplastic left heart syndrome. If palliation is pursued, management of these infants' critical haemodynamic state requires the use of a prostaglandin E_1 infusion to maintain ductal patency, inotropes, diuretics and ventilation to reverse the acidosis and stabilise the cardiovascular status.[86] Various treatment options have been posed to support the circulation of these infants and include cardiac transplantation and the palliative surgical procedures offered in stages known as the Norwood procedure.[62,77,84,88]

Essentially, the Norwood procedure relies on the right ventricle to pump blood to both the pulmonary and systemic circulations. The surgery is complex and carries a high operative mortality of between 53% and 91%.[46,86] A very limited number of infants reach stage 2 of the procedure and even less achieve a satisfactory result. The quality of life of the infants undergoing the Norwood-staged palliation has been questioned with the majority of infants requiring highly technical support with intensive nursing and medical care for extended periods of time. The literature abounds with technical discussion on the Norwood operation, to which the interested reader is referred.[46,84,86]

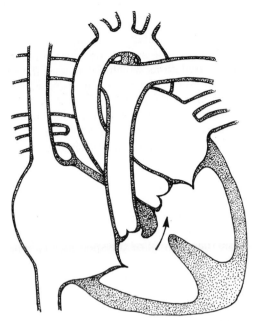

Figure 6.7 Diagrammatic representation of tetralogy of Fallot.

Tetralogy of Fallot

Tetralogy of Fallot is the most common cyanotic congenital heart defect, accounting for approximately 10% of all CHD.[58,89,90] The anomalies constituting the tetralogy include a large VSD, an overriding aorta, pulmonary stenosis (which may be valvular, supravalvular or, commonly, subvalvular in nature) and right ventricular hypertrophy.[46,57,89-92] In tetralogy, there is also malalignment of the ventricular septum and a deviated infundibular septum, which results in the VSD and the narrowing of the right ventricular outflow tract.[90] (**Figure 6.7.**)

Nursing assessment

The age of onset of symptoms is determined by the degree of right ventricular outflow tract obstruction. Most are diagnosed in infancy. Their presenting signs may include either cyanosis or a cardiac murmur or both of these signs. Tetralogy is less commonly diagnosed in the neonatal period.[89] The degree of cyanosis is variable and will increase with crying, feeding, exertion or during hot weather. Clubbing of the fingers and toes becomes apparent in infants with severe hypoxaemia after many months. Growth patterns in the children are normal initially but may become retarded over time. The squatting position is commonly assumed by children with tetralogy following exertion. This mechanism increases the systemic vascular resistance and minimises the right-to-left shunt across the VSD. Further, it decreases the volume of systemic venous return to the heart, thereby improving the oxygen saturation of the circulating blood.[90] These children require careful assessment of their hypoxaemic state. Clinical signs of heart failure are not seen in infants or children with uncomplicated tetralogy of Fallot.

Pathophysiology

The VSD in infants with tetralogy is usually large and non-restrictive in nature, causing equilibration of the ventricular pressures. It is the relative resistance to blood flow into the pulmonary and systemic circulations which determines the magnitude of the right-to-left shunt.[46,89] The more severe the right ventricular outflow obstruction, the greater the degree of shunting and level of cyanosis.[46,89,91]

Various mechanisms of compensation, which attempt to improve oxygenation, develop in the infants in response to the degree of hypoxaemia. These are exemplified by increasing polycythemia and the development of pulmonary collateral vessels.[89]

Hypercyanotic episodes

Cyanotic spells reportedly occur more frequently in the infants at a time when the systemic vascular resistance is low, for example, following sleep or feeding.[89] The episodes are sudden in onset and vary in duration and intensity. The infants may simply exhibit a greater degree of cyanosis than normal or the spell may increase in intensity such that the infant becomes increasingly restless, tachypnoeic and dyspnoeic with alteration to their level of consciousness.[90] Some spells may last minutes, others hours, with the infants left weak and lethargic and often sleeping for extended periods. They are uncommon in infants under 2 months of age.[89] The more severe spells may progress to convulsions, coma and death as a result of the profound hypoxaemia and acidosis.[57]

Hypercyanotic spells occur in various cyanotic congenital heart defects. The exact aetiology of the hypercyanotic spell in tetralogy, although unclear, is attributed to spasm of the infundibulum of the right ventricular outflow tract.[89,90] The infundibular spasms increase the degree of right-to-left shunting across the VSD, which further decreases the pulmonary blood flow. Crying exacerbates the problem. The hypoxaemia that develops leads to a state of acidosis. Both these factors contribute to further constriction of the pulmonary vasculature and worsen the cyanosis, leading to myocardial hypoxia.[57,89]

From a nursing perspective, sound appreciation of these concepts heightens the nurse's awareness of the need for early assessment and the urgent intervention required to support these infants and prevent the development of a profound state of hypoxaemia and acidosis. Parents need to be well informed regarding assessment and intervention, as these spells reportedly occur in up to 35% of the infants with tetralogy.[91]

In principle, the treatment required to reverse the spell necessitates an increase in the systemic vascular resistance to limit the right-to-left shunt, relief of the infundibular spasm, administration of oxygen and relief of the infant's pain and anxiety. The systemic vascular resistance is increased by placing the infant in the knee–chest position. The beta blocking agent propranolol relieves the spasm of the infundibular muscle, slows heart rate and promotes an increase in pulmonary blood flow.[93] Treatment of acidosis and volume expansion may be required in profoundly hypoxaemic and acidotic infants, with morphine given to relieve pain and allay anxiety.

Cyanotic spells are generally controlled with regular administration of oral propranolol until corrective or palliative surgery is undertaken. The optimal age for primary surgical correction in an infant susceptible to cyanotic episodes is 7 to 10 months of age. If the infant's anatomical features preclude correction at that time, a shunt procedure is undertaken. Special caution is observed in the nursing assessment of infants stabilised on propranolol who are scheduled for primary surgical correction. The risks of hypercyanotic episodes are increased when the medication is withdrawn 24 hours before surgery.

Treatment modalities

Primary surgical correction in early infancy is the treatment of choice practised by many centres, as it improves the long-term outcome in the children by minimising the residual haemodynamic and electrophysiologic problems previously experienced.[46,89,94] The surgical approach aims for closure of the VSD, resection of the infundibular muscle and relief of the pulmonary stenosis via a ventriculotomy or combined pulmonary artery and right atrial approach.[46,89]

The children generally recover very well after surgery, with a 2% to 5% hospital mortality following complete repair.[89,90,95,96] Most children usually require vasodilation and inotropic support in the initial recovery phase, with postoperative risks increasing with decreasing age. The infants who have required propranolol are potentially at greater risk of developing a postoperative low cardiac output state, due to residual myocardial depression from the drug.[97] Refer to the subsection on perioperative nursing care included in Chapter 11.

Dysrhythmias remain a potential problem after tetralogy repair. The majority of children are left with a right bundle branch block. A left anterior hemiblock and early atrioventricular conduction disturbances are relatively common, but the persistence of complete heart block is rare.[89,96] There is an association with exercise-induced ventricular arrhythmia in up to 25% of the children in the late postoperative period with a substantial incidence of sudden unexplained death.[89,94] Recurrent VSDs occur occasionally and require reoperation.[89] Importantly, prophylaxis for endocarditis should be continued in these children at times of greatest risk, even following surgical repair.[90]

Tricuspid atresia

Tricuspid atresia is an anomaly whereby there is complete absence of the tricuspid valve. It has an incidence of 1% to 2.9% of all CHD.[98] A system of classification is based on the associated malformations, i.e., the attachment of the great arteries and the volume of pulmonary blood flow. Type I tricuspid atresia has normally related great arteries and is the most common form, accounting for approximately 70% of infants. There may be an intact ventricular septum with pulmonary atresia (Type Ia), a small VSD and/or pulmonary stenosis (Type Ib) or a large VSD without pulmonary stenosis (Type Ic). Type Ib is the most common, accounting for up to 73% of the Type I defects.[98] (**Figure 6.8.**) In Type II the great arteries are transposed. Type IIa has pulmonary atresia, Type IIb pulmonary or subpulmonary stenosis and Type IIc, the second most common subgroup, has unrestricted pulmonary blood flow.

Nursing assessment

The complex of associated abnormalities with tricuspid atresia may, in effect, result in an increased, deceased or normal pulmonary blood flow which will determine the clinical presentation of the infants and the appropriate treatment modalities.[99]

Most infants with tricuspid atresia present early in life due to cyanosis or a cardiac murmur.[98] Central cyanosis is most often due to reduced pulmonary blood flow with tachypnoea induced by the arterial and cerebral chemoreceptors.[99] Hypoxic spells are common, occurring in up to half of the infants, resulting from a similar mechanism as that in tetralogy of Fallot.[98] When the state of hypoxaemia is attributed to closure of the ductus arteriosus, a prostaglandin E_1 infusion will dilate the duct and stabilise the infant

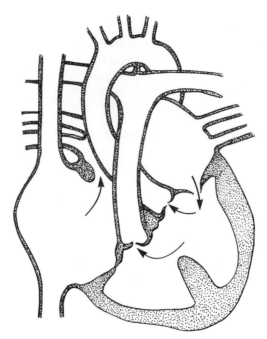

Figure 6.8 Diagrammatic representation of triscuspid atresia (Type Ib).

until a palliative shunt procedure can be undertaken.[57,99] Seven per cent of infants and children with tricuspid atresia experience life-threatening arrhythmias, with as many as 25% developing endocarditis following their palliative shunt procedures.[99,100]

Cardiac failure can develop in infants with various forms of tricuspid atresia, commonly in Type I and Type IIc. These infants have a significant increase in their pulmonary blood flow which may be severe and associated with a high mortality.[98,99] The time of their presentation can extend beyond the neonatal period. Palliation for these infants is surgical and is designed to reduce their pulmonary blood flow, for example, by pulmonary artery banding.

Pathophysiology

Tricuspid atresia Type Ib constitutes a cyanotic congenital cardiac defect with decreased pulmonary blood flow. The systemic venous return flows from the right atrium to the left atrium across an atrial septal defect. In the left atrium the deoxygenated blood mixes with the pulmonary venous return, crossing the mitral valve into the left ventricle. The majority of blood is then ejected via the aortic valve, but a small quantity crosses the ventricular septal defect to the hypoplastic right ventricle and then on into the small pulmonary arteries. The infant's pulmonary blood flow may be augmented by a patent ductus arteriosus.

Treatment modalities

When the infants present with cyanosis due to decreased pulmonary blood flow a shunt procedure, such as a Blalock Taussig or modified Blalock Taussig shunt, will augment the flow and alleviate the hypoxaemia and acidosis. When the pulmonary blood flow is excessive such that it causes cardiac failure, the infants will be treated with anti-failure medication. Most of the infants, however, will require a pulmonary artery banding in the first months of life, although the procedure remains controversial.[63,99] The Fontan procedure is recommended for children between 4 and 15 years of age with tricuspid atresia who meet the stringent criteria of having normal-sized pulmonary arteries and normal pulmonary vascular resistance and pressures.[57,99] Discussion on the principles of perioperative nursing care and a brief review of the Fontan procedure is included in Chapter 11.

Outcomes in children with tricuspid atresia

Tricuspid atresia carries a high infant mortality of 50% before 6 months of age in unoperated infants. The statistical data indicates another rise in mortality by 15 years of age attributed to congestive cardiac failure, arrhythmia and pulmonary hypertension. The Fontan procedure for tricuspid atresia currently has a 71% survival at 5 years.[99]

Conclusion

This discussion has reviewed the principles of nursing assessment and management approaches in the care of infants, children and adolescents with an alteration to cardiovascular structure. For a detailed review of the nursing assessment and management of infants and children with an alteration to their blood volume, pressure and flow dynamics and discussion on the perioperative nursing assessment and management principles, the reader is referred to the comprehensive discussion included in Chapter 11.

The high demands placed on nurses in this clinical speciality continue as neonates, young infants, children and adolescents make exacting demands because of the acute nature of their cardiac problems. The importance of the nursing contribution in meeting the established health care needs of the infants and children through the provision of a standard of clinical excellence cannot be overemphasised. Clinical assessment skills provide the foundation to nursing practice, a component fundamental to provision of quality care for the children. The primary focus of this discussion has been to highlight the importance of the nursing assessment in establishing health care needs and analysing the information obtained to determine the priorities and specific care for the infant or child and the special needs of the family.

REFERENCES

1. Oberhaensli I, Extermann P, Friedli B, Beguin F. Ultrasound screening for congenital cardiac malformations in the fetus: its importance for peri and postnatal care. *Pediatr Radiol* 1989; 19: 94–99.
2. Snider AR. Two-dimensional and doppler echocardiographic evaluation of heart disease in the neonate and fetus. *Clin Perinatal* 1988; 15: 523–564.
3. Adams FH, Emmanoulides GC, Riemenschneider TA, eds. *Moss' heart disease in infants, children and adolescents*. 4th ed. Baltimore: Williams and Wilkins, 1989.

4. Hazinski MF. Cardiovascular disorders. *In:* Hazinski MF, ed. *Nursing care of the critically ill child.* 2nd ed. St Louis: Mosby, 1992: 117–394.
5. Jordan SC, Scott O. *Heart disease in paediatrics.* 3rd ed. London: Butterworths, 1989.
6. Kirklin JW, Barratt-Boyes BG. Postoperative care. *In:* Kirklin JW, Barrat-Boyes BG. *Cardiac surgery: morphology, diagnostic criteria, natural history, techniques, results, and indications.* 2nd ed. New York: Churchill Livingstone, 1993: 195–248.
7. Liberthson RR. *Congenital heart disease: diagnosis and management in children and adults.* Boston: Little Brown, 1989.
8. Rengucci LM. Circulation; implications of abnormalities in structure and pressure. *In:* Mott SR, James SR, Sperhac AM. *Nursing care of children and families.* 2nd ed. California: Addison-Wesley, 1990: 1049–1136.
9. Sims SL. Alterations of cardiovascular function in children. *In:* McCance KL, Huether SE, eds. *Pathophysiology: the biological basis for disease in adults and children.* St Louis: Mosby, 1990: 992–1023.
10. Yacoub M, ed. *1988 Annual of cardiac surgery.* London: Gower Academic Journals, 1988.
11. Graham TP, Bender HW, Spach MS. Ventricular septal defect. *In:* Adams FH, Emmanoulides GC, Riemenschneider TA, eds. *Moss' heart disease in infants, children and adolescents.* 4th ed. Baltimore: Williams and Wilkins, 1989: 189–209.
12. Feldt RH, Porter CJ, Edwards WD, Puga FJ, Seward JB. Defects of the atrial septum and atrioventricular canal. *In:* Adams FH, Emmanoulides GC, Riemenschneider TA, eds. *Moss' heart disease in infants, children and adolescents.* 4th ed. Baltimore: Williams and Wilkins, 1989: 170–189.
13. Liberthson RR. Atrial septal defect. *In:* Liberthson RR. *Congenital heart disease: diagnosis and management in children and adults.* Boston: Little Brown, 1989: 45–60.
14. Jordan SC, Scott O. Acyanotic lesions with left to right shunts. *In:* Jordan SC, Scott O. *Heart disease in paediatrics.* 3rd ed. London: Butterworths, 1989: 71–107.
15. Kirklin JW, Barratt-Boyes BG. Atrial septal defect and partial anomalous pulmonary venous return. *In:* Kirklin JW, Barratt-Boyes BG. *Cardiac surgery: morphology, diagnostic criteria, natural history, techniques, results, and indications.* 2nd ed. New York: Churchill Livingstone, 1993: 609–644.
16. Moynihan PJ, King R. Caring for patients with increasing pulmonary blood flow. *Crit Care Nursing Clin North Am* 1989; 1: 195–213.
17. Liberthson RR. Ventricular septal defect. *In:* Liberthson RR. *Congenital heart disease: diagnosis and management in children and adults.* Boston: Little Brown, 1989; 61–74.
18. Park Myung K. Left to right shunt lesions. *In:* Park Myung K. *Pediatric cardiology for practitioners.* 2nd ed. Chicago: Year Book Medical, 1988: 125–144.
19. Heyman MA. Fetal and neonatal circulations. *In:* Adams FH, Emmanoulides GC, Riemenschneider TA, eds. *Moss' heart disease in infants and children.* 4th ed. Baltimore: Williams and Wilkins, 1989: 24–35.
20. Perloff WF. Physiology of the heart and circulation. *In:* Swedlow DB, Raphaely RC, eds. *Cardiovascular problems in pediatric critical care. Clinics in critical care medicine, 10.* New York: Churchill Livingstone, 1986: 1–85.
21. Kirklin JW, Barratt-Boyes BG. Ventricular septal defect. *In:* Kirklin JW, Barratt-Boyes BG. *Cardiac surgery: morphology, diagnostic criteria, natural history, techniques, results, and indications.* 2nd ed. New York: Churchill Livingstone, 1993: 749–824.
22. Kirklin JW, Barratt-Boyes BG. Patent ductus arteriosus. *In:* Kirklin JW, Barratt-Boyes BG. *Cardiac surgery: morphology, diagnostic criteria.* 2nd ed. New York: Churchill Livingstone, 1993: 841–859.
23. Liberthson RR. Patent ductus arteriosus. *In:* Liberthson RR. *Congenital heart disease: diagnosis and management in children and adults.* Boston: Little Brown, 1989: 75–82.
24. Bhatt V, Nahata MC. Pharmacologic management of patent ductus arteriosus. *Clin Pharmacol* 1989; 8: 17–33.

25. Clyman RI, Heyman MA. Pharmacology of the ductus arteriosus. *Pediatr Clin North Am* 1981; 28: 77–93.

26. Friedman WF, Printz MP, Skidgel RA. Prostaglandins and the ductus arteriosus. *Adv Prostaglandin Thromboxane Leukot Res* 1982; 10: 277–302.

27. Heyman MA. b). Patent ductus arteriosus. *In:* Adams FH, Emmanoulides GC, Riemenschneider TA, eds. *Moss' heart disease in infants and children.* 4th ed. Baltimore: Williams and Wilkins, 1989: 209–224.

28. Clyman RI, Heyman MA, Mauray F. Role of circulating prostaglandin E_2 in regulation of the ductus arteriosus. *Adv Prostaglandin Thromboxane Leukot Res* 1983; 12: 495–498.

29. Heyman MA. Prostaglandins and leukotrienes in the perinatal period. *Clin Perinatol* 1987; 14: 857–880.

30. Dooley KJ. Management of the premature infant with a patent ductus arteriosus. *Pediatr Clin North Am* 1984; 31: 1159–1174.

31. McNamara DG. Value and limitations of auscultation in the management of congenital heart disease. *Pediatr Clin North Am* 1990; 37: 93–113.

32. Pongiglione G, Marasini M, Silvestri G, Tuo P, Ribaldone D, Bertolini A, Garello-Cantoni L. Early treatment of patent ductus arteriosus in premature infants with severe respiratory distress syndrome. *Pediatr Cardiol* 1988; 9: 91–94.

33. Cotton RB. The relationship of symptomatic patent ductus arteriosus to respiratory distress in premature newborn infants. *Clin Perinatol* 1987; 14: 621–633.

34. Hammerman C, Zaia W, Berger W, Strokes E, Aldousany A. Prostaglandin levels: predictors of indomethacin responsiveness. *Pediatr Cardiol* 1986; 7: 61–65.

35. Roberts PJ. Caring for patients undergoing therapeutic cardiac catheterisation. *Crit Care Nursing Clin North Am* 1989; 1: 275–288.

36. Sholler G. Interventional catheterisation in paediatric cardiology. *Clinical bulletin, The Children's Hospital Sydney.* 1989; 13 (3): 1–4.

37. Monett ZJ, Roberts PJ. Patient care for interventional cardiac catheterisation. *Nursing Clin North Am* 1995; 30 (2): 335–345.

38. Callow LB. Nursing implications of interventional device placement in pediatric cardiology and pediatric cardiac surgery. *Crit Care Nursing Clin North Am* 1994; 6 (1): 133–151.

39. Cassady G, Crouse DT, Kirklin JW, Strange MJ, Joiner CH, Godoy G, et al. A randomised control trial of very early prophylactic ligation of the ductus arteriosus in babies who weighed 1000 grams or less at birth. *N Engl J Med* 1989; 320: 11–12.

40. Gersony WM. Coarctation of the aorta. *In:* Adams FH, Emmanoulides GC, Riemenschneider TA, eds. *Moss' heart disease in infants, children and adolescents.* 4th ed. Baltimore: Williams and Wilkins, 1989; 243–255.

41. Jordan SC, Scott O. Acyanotic lesions with left heart obstruction. *In:* Jordan SC, Scott O. *Heart disease in paediatrics.* 3rd ed. London: Butterworths, 1989; 108–135.

42. Kirklin JW, Barratt-Boyes BG. Coarctation of the aorta and aortic arch interruptions. *In:* Kirklin JW, Barratt-Boyes BG. *Cardiac surgery: morphology, diagnostic criteria, natural history, techniques, results and indications.* 2nd ed. New York: Churchill Livingstone, 1993: 1263–1326.

43. Liberthson RR. Coarctation of the aorta. *In:* Liberthson RR. *Congenital heart disease: diagnosis and management in children and adults.* Boston: Little Brown, 1989: 3–15.

44. Park Myung K. Obstructive lesions. *In:* Park Myung K. *Pediatric cardiology for practitioners.* 2nd ed. Chicago: Year Book Medical, 1988: 145–156.

45. Girlando RM, Belew B, Klara F. Coarctation of the aorta. *Crit Care Nurse* 1988; 8: 38–50.

46. Ilbawi MN. Current status for congenital heart diseases. *Clin Perinatol* 1989; 16: 157–176.

47. Nadas AS. Update on congenital heart disease. *Pediatr Clin North Am* 1984; 31: 153–164.

48. del Nido PJ, Williams WG, Coles JG, Trusler GA, Freedom RM. Closed heart surgery for congenital heart disease in infancy. *Clin Perinatol* 1988; 15: 681–697.

49. Schleien CL, Setzer NA, McLaughlin GE, Rogers MC. Post operative management of the

cardiac surgical patient. *In:* Rogers MC, ed. *Textbook of pediatric intensive care.* 2nd ed. Baltimore: Williams and Wilkins, 1992: 467–531.

50. Radtke W, Lock J. Balloon dilation. *Pediatr Clin North Am* 1990; 37: 193–213.
51. Rocchini AP, Kueselis D. The use of balloon angioplasty in the pediatric patient. *Pediatr Clin North Am* 1988; 31: 1293–1305.
52. Jordan SC, Scott O. Heart disease in the newborn infant. *In:* Jordan SC, Scott O. *Heart disease in paediatrics.* 3rd ed. London: Butterworths, 1989: 231–248.
53. Ruchman RN. Anomalies of the aortic arch complex. *In:* Adams FH, Emmanoulides GC, Riemenschneider TA, eds. *Moss' heart disease in infants, children and adolescents.* 4th ed. Baltimore: Williams and Wilkins, 1989: 255–273.
54. Friedman WF. Aortic stenosis. *In:* Adams FH, Emmanoulides GC, Riemenschneider TA, eds. *Moss' heart disease in infants, children and adolescents.* 4th ed. Baltimore: Williams and Wilkins, 1989: 224–243.
55. Rocchini AP, Emmanoulides GC. Pulmonary stenosis. *In:* Adams FH, Emmanoulides GC, Riemenschneider TA, eds. *Moss' heart disease in infants, children and adolescents.* 4th ed. Baltimore: Williams and Wilkins, 1989: 308–338.
56. Lees MH, King DH. Heart disease in the newborn. *In:* Adams FH, Emmanoulides GC, Riemenschneider TA, eds. *Moss' heart disease in infants, children and adolescents.* 4th ed. Baltimore: Williams and Wilkins, 1989: 842–855.
57. Driscoll DJ. Evaluation of the cyanotic newborn. *Pediatr Clin North Am* 1990; 37: 1–23.
58. Park Myung K. Cyanotic congenital heart defects. In: Park Myung K. *Pediatric cardiology for practitioners.* 2nd ed. Chicago: Year Book Medical, 1988: 157–196.
59. Moore R. Anesthesia considerations for patients undergoing palliative or reparative operations for congenital heart disease. *In:* Swedlow DB, Raphaely RC, eds. *Cardiovascular problems in pediatric critical care. Clinics in critical care medicine, vol 10*, New York: Churchill Livingstone, 1986: 169–204.
60. Mair DD, Edwards WD, Julsrud PR, Seward JB, Danielson GK. Truncus arteriosus. *In:* Adams FH, Emmanoulides GC, Riemenschneider TA, eds. *Moss' heart disease in infants, children and adolescents.* 4th ed. Baltimore: Williams and Wilkins, 1989: 504–515.
61. Kirklin JW, Barrat-Boyes BG. Truncus arteriosis. *In:* Kirklin JW, Barratt-Boyes BG. *Cardiac surgery: morphology, diagnostic criteria, natural history, techniques, results, and indications.* 2nd ed. New York: Churchill Livingstone 1993: 1131–1152.
62. Cohen DM. Surgical management of congenital heart disease in the 1990's. *Am J Dis Child* 1992; 146: 1447–1452.
63. Kirklin JW, Barratt-Boyes BG. Tricuspid atresia and the Fontan operation. *In:* Kirklin JW, Barratt-Boyes BG. *Cardiac surgery: morphology, diagnostic criteria, natural history, techniques, results, and indications.* 2nd ed. New York: Churchill Livingstone 1993: 1055–1104.
64. Paul M. Complete transposition of the great arteries. *In:* Adams FH, Emmanoulides GC, Riemenschneider TA, eds. *Moss' heart disease in infants, children and adolescents.* 4th ed. Baltimore: Williams and Wilkins, 1989: 371–423.
65. Kirklin JW, Barratt-Boyes BG. Complete transposition of the great arteries. *In:* Kirklin JW, Barratt-Boyes BG. *Cardiac surgery: morphology, diagnostic criteria, natural history, techniques, results, and indications.* 2nd ed. New York: Churchill Livingstone 1993: 1383–1468.
66. Yacoub M, Radley-Smith R. Transposition of the great arteries. *In:* Yacoub M, ed. *1988 Annual of cardiac surgery.* London: Gower Academic Journals. 1988: 37–47.
67. Kai-Chiu Lau, Che-Keung Mok, RNS Lo, M Pnig Leung, Chap-yung Yeung. Balloon atrial septostomy under two dimensional echocardiographic control. *Pediatr Cardiol* 1987; 8: 35–37.
68. Mullins CE. Therapeutic cardiac catheterisation: part 5, invasive diagnostic and therapeutic techniques. *In:* Adams FH, Emmanoulides GC, Riemenschneider TA, eds. *Moss' heart disease in infants, children and adolescents.* 4th ed. Baltimore: Williams and Wilkins, 1989: 130–167.
69. Crosson J, Ringel RE, Haney PJ, Brenner JI. Pneumopericardium as a complication of balloon atrial septostomy. *Pediatr Cardiol* 1987; 8: 135–137.

70. Jonas RA, Lang P. Open repair of cardiac defects in neonates and young infants. *Clin Perinatol* 1988; 15: 659–679.

71. Jonas RA, Giglia TM, Sanders SP, Wernousky G, Nadal-Ginard B, Mayer JE, Castaneda AR. Rapid, two stage arterial switch for TGA and intact ventricular septum beyond the neonatal period. *Circulation* 1989; 80: 203–208.

72. Blonshine SK. Transposition of the great arteries. *Assoc Operating Room Nursing J* 1989; 49: 973–987.

73. Musewe NN, Reisman J, Benson LN, Wilkes D, Levinson H, Freedom RM, Trusler GA, Canney GJ. Cardiopulmonary adaptation at rest and during exercise 10 years after Mustard atrial repair for TGA. *Circulation* 1988; 77: 1055–1061.

74. Turina MI, Siebenmann R, von Segesser L, Schonbeck M, Senning A. Late functional deterioration after atrial correction for TGA. *Circulation* 1989; 80: 162–167.

75. Denfield SW, Garson A. Sudden death in children and young adults. *Pediatr Clin North Am* 1990; 37: 215–231.

76. Martin RP, Radley-Smith R, Yacoub MH. Arrhythmias before and after anatomic correction of TGA. *J Am College Cardiol* 1987; 10: 200–204.

77. Kirklin JW, Barratt-Boyes BG. Double inlet ventricle and atretic a-v valve. *In:* Kirklin JW, Barratt-Boyes BG. *Cardiac surgery: morphology, diagnostic criteria, natural history, techniques, results, and indications.* 2nd ed. New York: Churchill Livingstone 1993: 1549–1580.

78. Gibbs JL, Qureshi SA, Martin R, Wilson N, Yacoub MH, Radley-Smith R. Neonatal anatomical correction of transposition of the great arteries: non-invasive assessment of hemodynamic function to 4 years after operation. *Br Heart J* 1988; 60: 66–68.

79. Kirklin JW, Colvin EV, McConnell ME, Bargeron LM. Complete TGA: treatment in the current era. *Pediatr Clin North Am* 1990; 37: 171–177.

80. Callow LB. A new beginning: nursing care of the infant undergoing the arterial switch operation for transposition of the great arteries. *Heart Lung* 1989; 18: 248–255.

81. Jensen CA. Nursing care of a child following an arterial switch procedure for transposition of the great arteries. *Crit Care Nurse* 1992; December: 51–57.

82. Lucas RV, Krabill KA. Anomalous venous connections, pulmonary and systemic. *In:* Adams FH, Emmanoulides GC, Riemenschneider TA, eds. *Moss' heart disease in infants, children and adolescents.* 4th ed. Baltimore: Williams and Wilkins, 1989: 580–617.

83. Hoffman JIE. Congenital heart disease: incidence and inheritance. *Pediatr Clin North Am* 1990; 37: 25–43.

84. Bailey LL, Gundry SR. Hypoplastic left heart syndrome. *Pediatr Clin North Am* 1990; 37: 137–150.

85. Panyard JL, Kaneta MK. Hypoplastic left heart syndrome: clinical manifestations and treatment. *Neonatal Network* 1988; 7 (1): 17–25.

86. Freedom RM. Hypoplastic left heart syndrome. *In:* Adams FH, Emmanoulides GC, Riemenschneider TA, eds. *Moss' heart disease in infants, children and adolescents.* 4th ed. Baltimore: Williams and Wilkins, 1989: 515–529.

87. Smith JB, Vernon Levett P. Hypoplastic left heart syndrome; treatment options. *Am J Maternal Child Nursing* 1989; 14: 180–183.

88. Johnson AB, Davis JS. Treatment options for the neonate with hypoplastic left heart syndrome. *J Perinatal Neonatal Nursing* 1991; 5: 84–92.

89. Pinsky WW, Arciniogas E. Tetralogy of Fallot. *Pediatr Clin North Am* 1990; 37: 179–192.

90. Zuberbuhler JR. Tetralogy of Fallot. *In:* Adams FH, Emmanoulides GC, Riemenschneider TA, eds. *Moss' heart disease in infants, children and adolescents.* 4th ed. Baltimore: Williams and Wilkins, 1989: 273–288.

91. Byrd LA, Bruton-Maree N. Tetralogy of Fallot. *J Am Assoc Nurse Anaesthetists* 1989; 57: 169–176.

92. Milne C. Heart disease: clinical features, tetralogy of Fallot. *Nursing Standard* 1988; 12: 28–30.

93. Flynn PA, Engle MA, Ehlers KH. Cardiac issues in the emergency room. *Pediatr Clin North Am* 1992; 39: 955–983.

94. Castaneda AR, Jonas RA. Repair of tetralogy of Fallot. *In:* Yacoub M, ed. *1988 Annual of cardiac surgery.* London: Gower Academic Journals, 1988: 26–36.

95. Kirklin JW, Barratt-Boyes BG. Ventricular septal defect and pulmonary stenosis or atresia. *In:* Kirklin JW, Barratt-Boyes BG. *Cardiac surgery: morphology, diagnostic criteria, natural history, techniques, results, and indications.* 2nd ed. New York: Churchill Livingstone 1993: 861–1012.

96. Walsh EP, Rockenmacher S, Keane JF, Hougen TJ, Lock JE, Castaneda AR. Late results in patients with tetralogy of Fallot repaired during infancy. *Circulation* 1988; 77: 1062–1067.

97. Lell WA, Reves JG, Samuelson PN. Anaesthesia for cardiovascular surgery. *In:* Kirklin JW, Barratt-Boyes BG. *Cardiac surgery: morphology, diagnostic criteria, natural history, techniques, results, and indications.* 2nd ed. New York: Churchill Livingstone 1993: 109–138.

98. Sade RM, Fyfe DA. Tricuspid atresia: current concepts in diagnosis and treatment. *Pediatr Clin North Am* 1990; 37: 151–169.

99. Rosenthal A, Dick M. Tricuspid atresia. *In:* Adams FH, Emmanoulides GC, Riemenschneider TA, eds. *Moss' heart disease in infants, children and adolescents.* 4th ed. Baltimore: Williams and Wilkins, 1989: 348–361.

100. Kulik LA. Caring for patients with lesions decreasing pulmonary blood flow. *Crit Care Nursing Clin North Am* 1989; 1: 215–229.

Disturbances in Neuromuscular Function

Laurence Dubourg

Neural Tube Defects

A neural tube defect (NTD) is a congenital anomaly of the nervous system such as anencephaly, spina bifida and cranium bifidum. The covering structures like the skin, meninges and bones can also be incomplete. The neural tube is formed towards the end of the 3rd week of embryological development and by the 11th week, the spine develops. Structural abnormalities of the nervous system appear to be related to a delay in the closure of the neural tube.

While multifactorial reasons are given to explain these anomalies, diet and genetics appear to be the most likely causes. Folic acid supplements are now recommended as a preventative measure to women planning a pregnancy. It is recommended to take folic acid orally, 12 weeks before the pregnancy and during the first 12 weeks of gestation.

INCIDENCE OF NEURAL TUBE DEFECTS

Neural tube defect incidence varies throughout the world. The highest incidence is 4 to 16 per 1000 alive births. In Victoria, Australia, the incidence has decreased to 1.59 per 1000 live births. In a family where the birth of a child with a NTD has occurred, the incidence of recurrence becomes 1 in 25 live births.[1] This justifies the follow-up of affected families to ensure proper genetic counselling. Successful counselling programs lead to effective prevention.

TYPES OF NEURAL TUBE DEFECTS

ANTENATAL PERIOD

A NTD may be diagnosed with routine ultrasonography. In addition, alpha fetoproteins positively identified at about the 16th week of gestation suggest a NTD. The decision to terminate the pregnancy may be taken. Parents require support to deal with this ethical issue and the decision must be compatible with their personal values.

If a NTD is diagnosed late in pregnancy, the infant is observed with ultrasonography. Information such as the size of the defect, the degree of hydrocephalus and the motor function below the defect are relevant to determine the appropriate type of birth. A baby with a large head, greater than 40 cm, may not permit a delivery through the narrow birth canal. A prelabour caesarean section may be recommended if the sac is large and good leg movements have been observed. The aims are to prevent rupture of the sac during delivery and avoid trauma by compression of the spinal cord, which may preserve motor function below the defect.

POSTNATAL PERIOD

In most instances, surgery is offered within hours of the delivery. If surgery is delayed, nurses must continually assess the baby to monitor the condition and support the family facing an emotional turmoil.

Preoperative assessment of the baby

Assessment of the head

Signs of raised intracranial pressure such as full or tense anterior fontanelle, 'sun setting' eyes, poor feeding or vomiting, high-pitched cry, raised blood pressure and low pulse rate are relevant signs because children may be developing progressive hydrocephalus. Head circumference measurements indicate whether the head grows within the birth percentile curve or outgrows it. A rapid growth rate, as shown in **Figure 6.12**, indicates that hydrocephalus is progressing.

Assessment of the limbs

Spontaneous movements are assessed without the baby being touched. Movement of the legs in response to touch may be reflexes. A stimulus above the lesion will lead to voluntary movements above the spinal lesion and simultaneously, the lower limbs should be observed for similar voluntary movements. A baby with strong quadriceps movements will walk as a child and possibly as an adult. To ascertain sensation in the legs, a given stimulus of the lower limbs will awaken an asleep baby.

The overall appearance of the muscles of the lower limbs indicates if the baby has been kicking during the pregnancy or if it has always been paralysed.

Assessment of the defect

The aim of the care is to prevent rupture of the protruding sac and its size affects the handling of the baby. A baby with a small and stable protruding sac can be handled more freely than a baby with a large sac. Stress on the defect must be avoided and nursing the

Table 6.1 Neural tube defects — definitions and outcome

Definition	Outcome
Anencephaly	
At birth, the baby presents with a deformed skull and brain.	Many babies are stillborn. Death may occur in hours or days. If surviving, only basic functions such as sucking, breathing and making of sounds occur.
Cranium bifidum	
A cyst protrudes through a skull defect in the midline.	
Cranial meningocele	
The cyst is filled with CSF and the brain underlying is normal.	A repair of the sac and the skull defect is necessary.
Encephalocele	
The cyst contains brain and CSF and hydrocephalus may be associated.	The surgery is complex. The aim is to repair the skull, correct hydrocephalus and preserve the brain.
Spina bifida occulta	
The skin covers underlying incomplete vertebral arches. 10% of the population has a spina bifida occulta. However, many children who have a cutaneous abnormality have an underlying defect.	This is discovered accidentally and has no consequence apart for some occasional bladder and bowel dysfunction.
Dermal sinus	
An ectodermal anomaly such as a small pit or hairy patch is apparent. This may communicate with the spinal cord and lead to infection. See Figure 6.9	The surgery consists of removing the anomaly and preventing neurological deficits such as bladder and bowel dysfunction, and lower limbs weakness.
Lipoma	
A fatty lump localised under the skin or entering the meninges leads to compression on the spinal cord.	Explorative surgery is decided upon size and intraspinal involvement. The aim is to decompress the spinal cord and to optimise the long-term neurological status.
Spina bifida cystica	
A midline sac protrudes through a spinal defect. It is commonly on the posterior lumbo sacral region but may be higher on the vertebral column. Hydrocephalus is present in 90% of the children; 70% will require treatment. Arnold Chiari malformation is commonly present.	Neurological problems present are immediately below the level of the defect. During growth and development some degree of spinal cord adhesions (tethering) may complicate the condition and lead to neurological problems.
Meningocele	
The midline sac is covered by meninges, filled with CSF and does not contain neural tissue. (See Figure 6.10)	Surgery will consist of repairing the defect and preventing infection. Neurological deficits are usually absent.

Table 6.1 (*continued*)

Definition	Outcome
Myelomeningocele The midline sac contains spinal nerve roots and/or spinal cord. 80% occur in the lumbosacral region. (See Figure 6.11)	The neurological problems are present immediately below the defect. A high defect leads to greater morbidity than a low defect. (See Table 6.2 and Figure 6.10)

[1] Lindsay KW, Bone I, Callander R. *Neurology and neurosurgery illustrated.* Edinburgh: Churchill Livingstone, 1986: 409.

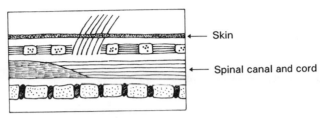

Figure 6.9 Spina bifida occulta. Incomplete fusion of the vertebral arches. A tuft of hair, a dimple or a fatty lump can be seen or palpated in the lumbo-sacral region.

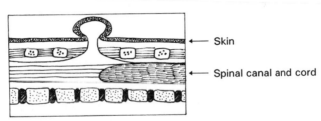

Figure 6.10 Meningocele. A sac with meninges and filled with CSF protrubes. It can be fully or partially covered by skin.

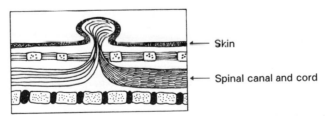

Figure 6.11 Myelomeningocele. A sac protrudes and contains meninges, CSF, cord and spinal nerves. It can be fully or partially covered by skin.

baby prone and in a flat position is usually preferred because the upright position encourages CSF to flow to the defect and may lead to increase in the sac's size. Hydrocephalus will increase the intracranial pressure, which may increase the intraspinal pressure, thus leading to sac growth. The enlargement of the defect must be reported to the medical staff.

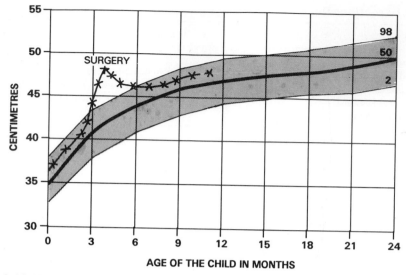

Figure 6.12 Head circumference variations showing deviations above normal limits with an infant developing hydrocephalus. Surgery is followed by a return to normal.

Monitoring of infection

The prevention of infection is the most important aspect of the nursing care. A baby with a defect not covered by skin is at risk of developing meningitis. A CSF leakage increases the risk of developing meningitis. The leak must be reported to the medical staff rapidly. To prevent contamination of a lumbosacral defect, it is essential to isolate it from urine and faeces. A surgical steridrape applied below the defect and above the nappy will protect the dressing. Parents are taught to practice a correct handwashing technique before handling their baby.

Signs such as elevated temperature, pulse, lethargy or irritability, poor feeding, arching of the neck and full anterior fontanelle must be reported as they can be signs of meningitis.

Assessment of the bladder

Nurses' observations will enable the paediatrician to make a diagnosis on the bladder function. Some of the following questions may be asked:

- Is the baby dry between wet nappies?
- Is the baby dribbling all the time?
- How often is micturition occurring?
- Is the baby's abdomen distended and hard before micturition?
- What is the volume of each micturition (nappies are weighed)?
- Is the bladder completely empty immediately after a micturition?
- What is the volume of the urine residual if present?
- What is the quality of the stream if present?
- What does a simple ward test show?
- Does the urine smell?

Assessment of the bowel

Nurses can assess bowel functioning by observing the anal tone and the movement of the pelvic floor. The bowel waste is carefully documented and problems related to constipation are discussed with the paediatrician. Glycerine suppositories may be required.

Family assessment, education and support

Parental feelings

Time is required to assess the underlying dynamics of families. Health professionals may feel they are facing a dysfunctional family while in fact the family is overwhelmed, in shock and confronting a serious crisis. Parents may experience a sense of failure. Some parents see the birth as a punishment or an unacceptable event. They may reject the baby or feel inadequate in caring for their baby. Invariably they will experience fear for the future and for the unknown they are facing.

It is important to understand how the family functions in order to provide individualised care. Conflicts between parents may have occurred very early in the pregnancy if the decision to continue the pregnancy was perceived differently. Where is the support coming from? How do both parents cope? How are decisions made within the family?

Parental knowledge

Health professionals must *explore the actual parental knowledge.*

- What did the maternity ward staff say?
- What do the parents understand about their baby's condition?
- Have parents been involved in caring for a baby with the same condition?
- Was the condition similar?

Carers must be a coordinated team and nurses ensure that consistent information is given. While medical specialists involved should optimally meet together with the family, it is common for specialists to meet individually with different family members. Information given during these multiple forums must be recorded to be shared with other medical practitioners. A primary nurse can be appointed as it often permits continuity of care, consistency of information, education and overall follow-up.

The nurse has a key role at these meetings. The nurse assists parents with the formulation of questions. In most instances, parents are overwhelmed by the circumstances or intimidated by the meeting. They have shared their concerns with the bedside carer who thus knows their concerns and needs. After the meeting, the nurse explores with the parents their understanding of the information given and reinforces information or organises further meetings to clarify issues. Anxious parents may not hear the information given, retain a small percentage of it or misunderstand it.

The mother must be included in all care issues, even if she is still in the maternity ward. She must not get 3rd hand information from her husband who may wish to protect her from unpleasant news. It is important to transfer the mother close to her baby as soon as possible and involve her in care and management decisions. Breastfeeding must be encouraged. Breast milk can be transferred between hospitals. In addition to responding to the child's needs, breast milk empowers the mother and creates a link between her and the baby. If the mother remains in the birth centre, is she kept involved in the care of her baby?

The surgical decision

The baby's health outcome, comfort and quality of life guide the decision. The surgical decision lies with the parents, guided by a team of experts: the neurosurgeon, the paediatrician, the nurse, the social worker, perhaps a religious representative, and occasionally an orthopaedic surgeon and an urologist. Parents require information on the child's intellectual development, her or his ability to move, bladder and bowel function, the medical interventions required at different ages and survival chances with and without surgery.

Health professionals will recommend surgery when the lesion is technically operable and it is anticipated that the baby will have good chances of postoperative survival with good quality of life. The surgery will occur within the first 24 hours to prevent infection and does not improve or worsen the baby's physical condition.

Hydrocephalus

Nurses must be aware that hydrocephalus occurs in approximately 90% of the children with spina bifida cystica and of those, 70% will need to be treated with a shunt. Ultrasonography of the head will confirm the dilatation of the ventricles. The ventriculoperitoneal shunt is commonly inserted when the spinal sac defect is being closed.

Nursing care following spinal defect closure

Postoperative observations

Assessment of the head, limbs, bladder and bowel continue as during the preoperative period.

Wound management

The preventative measures of the preoperative period continue after the surgery and the wound is isolated from the nappy by a sterile drape.

A CSF leakage will be reported urgently because CSF is a perfect medium for bacterial and viral growth. The neurosurgeon will want to seal the leakage immediately by adding stitches to the wound.

Handling of the baby

The neurosurgeon dictates the mobilisation of the baby, aiming at preventing wound breakdown. The preoperative size of the defect dictates the handling of the child. A small defect implies that the wound requires less skin tension to close and is less at risk of wound breakdown. The risk of wound breakdown, however, is much greater when there is a large defect which requires much skin tension.

Promoting comfort

The baby's comfort is assessed during the routine observations. Crying, restlessness and change in vital signs may be present. Pain may be related to the back wound if the cut is extended above the sensory deficit, to the head wound if the baby has had a shunt insertion and to hunger if the baby is still fasted.

Conservative management of the baby

After considerable debate, the decision to care for the baby in a conservative manner may be reached. This decision will be reviewed regularly and may be altered depending on the child's condition and parental wishes. Numerous family meetings take place to ensure that the family is informed and provided with continuous support. The aim of the nursing care is to make the baby comfortable and protected from infection. The care of the baby is a partnership between parents and health care professionals. The parents who are empowered, make the final informed decisions about the care of their baby. Parents who wish to go home with their baby will be linked to community services such as district nursing services or palliative care agencies. Medical follow-up will continue regularly.

LONG-TERM CARE ISSUES

Hydrocephalus monitoring

A neurosurgical outpatient review is required every 1 or 2 years. Shunt dysfunction is a common reason for readmission to a neurosurgical inpatient unit for a shunt revision. The problems faced can be blockage of lower or upper part of the shunt, disconnection at the valve site, displacement of the lower end and infection. Parents must know the signs and symptoms of shunt dysfunction.

Bladder care

The primary aim of bladder care is to preserve renal function and the secondary aim is to achieve continence. Renal function is preserved by preventing urinary tract infections, draining residual urine and preventing urinary reflux. Parents require education to manage their child's bladder. Each program is individualised to the child's needs and takes into account the child's age and type of bladder.

Clean intermittent catheterisation (CIC)

CIC aims to empty the bladder in a clean manner to prevent infection and promote continence. The stasis of contaminated urine in the bladder may lead to urinary infections. Continence is achieved by emptying the bladder regularly instead of letting unpredictable bladder overflow occur at random throughout the day. CIC is most effective in attaining continence if the child has a large volume, flaccid bladder. Children with small, spastic bladders will rarely be dry in between catheters.

The program consists of educating about fluid intake and frequency of catheters. A large fluid intake is suggested to help preventing infections. Young children can drink as much as they wish and wear a nappy at night. Older children needing to be dry overnight, are encouraged to drink large amounts during the day while in the evening, decreasing fluid intake helps overnight continence without needing an overnight catheter. While 4-year-old boys and 6-year-old girls have been reported to learn the technical skill of CIC, close supervision is required for overall management. The program needs to continue at school and either the district nurse or a properly trained integration aide must assist the child with the catheters during the day.

Bladder surgery

Various surgical procedures may be required to achieve continence or to prevent deterioration in renal function.

Vesicotomy is performed in infancy and consists of opening the bladder onto the skin. The aim is to let urine drain continually onto a nappy, thus primarily maintaining a low intravesical pressure, therefore preventing renal reflux and hydronephrosis and secondarily reducing residual urine and preventing infections.

Bladder augmentation increases the size of the bladder.

Artificial sphincter insertion increases resistance to urine flow through the urethra and with CIC promotes dryness.

Bladder studies

A micturating cystourethrogram (MCU) consists of filling the bladder with radio-opaque or isotopic contrast via an urethral catheter. Diagnosis of vesicourethral reflux is made if there is a back-flow of urine from the bladder into the ureters and/or the kidneys. Reflux reaching the kidneys may warrant surgical intervention while back-flow to the ureters may be controlled by CIC.

A renal ultrasound provides information on size and shape of the kidneys.

A renal isotope scan shows very accurately the renal parenchyma and may be undertaken if a MCU or a renal ultrasound detects an anomaly.

Bowel care

The aim is to prevent chronic constipation and promote continence. The principles of bowel regimen are as follows.

A morning bowel evacuation can be more successful in achieving continence because the rectum emptied in the morning is less likely to 'ooze' during the day.

Dietary manipulation, regular sitting and 'pushing' on a toilet, daily suppository, abdominal massages are the simplest types of regimen and enable most children to be clean. Passive movements of the limbs to compress the abdominal cavity may help infants to evacuate their rectum. Older children can be encouraged to bend forward on the toilet, to massage their abdomen or to blow up balloons to increase the abdominal pressure.

Stool must be formed. If it is too soft, the child may be incontinent.

In some instances, manual stimulation, manual evacuation or enemas are required to evacuate the bowels. The Willis Home Bowel Washout Programme[3] can be very successful in achieving faecal continence if other regimens fail.

High-fibre diet, stool softeners and medication increasing bowel peristalsis are often required.

Should a change in a bowel regimen be required, because the child is constipated or has soft stools, one change to one aspect of the regimen can be done at any one time. This change must be evaluated and thought through before further changes are made.

Parents and child often discover the type of food that stimulates the bowel motions, or the type of food that hardens or softens stools.

The description of the quantity of the stools must be objective rather than subjective: words like 'one table tennis ball' or 'tennis ball' or 'golf ball' will be preferred to small, medium and large. Similarly the consistency could be described using words such as pebbles, sausage, toothpaste or fluid-like. The observation can be followed by recom-

Table 6.2 Level of defect, neurological status and the child's future

Level of defect	Neurological status	Future
Cervical	Paralysis of limbs and trunk. Diaphragmatic respiration present. Neurogenic bladder and bowel.	Long-term survival is unlikely.
High thoracic	Paralysis of some intercostal muscles. Partial upper limbs problems. Lower limbs paralysis. Neurogenic bladder and bowel.	Survival to adulthood is unlikely.
Thoracic 12	Lower limbs paralysis. Neurogenic bladder and bowel.	Ambulation may be maintained using long braces and crutches. Children will use a wheelchair by adult life. Regimens to promote bladder and bowel continence are required.
Lumbar 4	Quadriceps may be present, no movement below the knees. Neurogenic bladder and bowel.	Child may walk with callipers below the knees. Regimens to promote bladder and bowel continence are required.
Below lumbar 4	A foot drop may be present. Neurogenic bladder and bowel.	Shoes to maintain feet or splints are required for the child to walk. Regimens to promote bladder and bowel continence are required.
Sacral 3	Neurogenic bladder and bowel.	Regimens to promote bladder and bowel continence are required.

mendations for the evening or the next day: 'give one additional orange juice tonight and tomorrow morning'. This is most important in the hospital environment where every shift, caregivers change. It is less an issue at home where one parent follows the child's progress and plans the care.

A child admitted to the hospital should continue the bowel care routine already established at home, or should it need to be interrupted for a surgical procedure, it must be recommenced as soon as possible.

Mobility and deformity

Mobilisation

The child's ability to mobilise is directly related to the level of the neurological lesion, the child's learning ability, understanding of instructions and motivation (**Table 6.2**). The training for walking begins by the age of 2 to 3 years with the fitting of braces and special shoes.

The physiotherapist will assist the child by optimising mobilisation, providing aids if required for ambulation, monitoring physical development and body alignment. The issue of school access is addressed to facilitate school integration. Funding for ramps and other possible aids may be requested from the city council.

Prevention of deformity

The major aim is to prevent deformity and eliminate the development of secondary problems such as abnormal spinal curves, decreased respiratory capacity, decubitus pressure sores on the sacrum or back. Maintaining symmetrical body alignment through ambulation or standing position is important. In most cases, children will need orthoses.

Orthopaedic interventions

Orthopaedic interventions may be required to correct deformities which may either cause secondary problems or impede mobility.

Back surgery may be required to stop further scoliosis, prevent further reduction of respiratory capacity, relieve back pain and decrease incidence of sacral pressure sores.

Surgery may be required to correct hip and knee flexion, deformities to allow the child to lie flat in bed and stand with orthotics support.

Feet anomalies and deformity are corrected to allow for shoes to be worn, permit the standing position and reducing the likelihood of pressure sores.

Skin care

In infancy, children may have frequent nappy rash because they are continually soiled. Later in life, common skin problems are related to pressure sores and burns. Parents and children must be educated in monitoring pressure areas such as sacrum, perineal region and feet. Pressure area care must be encouraged at least hourly when the child is sitting in the wheelchair.

Home hot water temperature must be controlled to prevent scald burns when bathing or showering, because the child's lack of sensation may prevent him or her from feeling the hot water. Parents and children are encouraged to check the temperature with the hand before bathing or showering. 'Warming the child up' in front of the heater must be discouraged because it may lead to major burns of the tissue exposed to the heater.

Sexuality

Children with spina bifida may have neurological impairment which may affect sexual functioning. The difficulties may include loss of sensation in the genitourinary area. Health care professionals need to view sexuality in a holistic manner and not as intercourse only. Parents and child require a sensitive and factual approach to the child's sexuality and that, for example, gentle touch can be pleasurable. As with all adolescents, counselling must address birth control issues. In addition, the risk related to the birth of a child with spina bifida must be raised. Information about the adolescent's physical impairment and the impact this will have on fertility, impotence and child bearing is required.

During pregnancy, difficulties with urinary drainage, prolapse of the pelvic floor and spinal column changes related to hormonal changes may occur. Most deliveries will be done by caesarean section for various reasons. Men have greater difficulties with procreation as problems which may range from impotence to retrograde ejaculation and sterility and are more complicated to overcome.

Social worker interventions

The child will require constant medical and surgical interventions which will put a strain on the family. The need for emotional support is enormous and the financial implications of caring for a child with such complex problems are great. Families must be informed about their entitlements such as disability allowances. Organisations such as the Australian Spina Bifida Association, the Program for Aids for Disabled People and Continence Aids Assistance Scheme are available. The social worker has a key role in ensuring that the child and the family are appropriately linked to up-to-date, community-based support services, and to ensure that continuity of care is provided between hospital, community services and home.

LATE NEUROLOGICAL PROBLEMS

A number of medical conditions may be responsible for late deterioration of function. Early medical intervention is required when a deterioration occurs which is reversible. A prolonged deterioration will not be correctible.

Hydromyelia

Hydromyelia (or syringomyelia or syrinx) results from high pressure CSF within the central spinal canal of the spinal cord. It can present with a variety of symptoms. Generally a slow and progressive deterioration occurs below the level of the syrinx — it can be the development of scoliosis, back pain, limb spasticity, weakness of the limbs, bladder or bowel dysfunction. The reasons for the CSF cyst or the CSF flow alteration may be related to hydrocephalus, Arnold Chiarri malformation or tethered cord. Treating the condition is likely to stop further deterioration. In the absence of a cause, a syringoperitoneal shunt may be inserted.

Arnold Chiari malformation type 2

Part of the cerebellum vermis, medulla and 4th ventricle extend through the foramen magnum, often to the mid-cervical region. The lower cranial nerves are stretched and the cervical roots run horizontally or in an upward direction.

Clinical signs

The children in difficulty from this malformation will present with neurological signs related to pressure on the lower third of their brainstem. The lower cranial nerves are stretched and problems such as squeaky voice, difficulty with swallowing or weak cough are common. Sleep apnoea is not uncommon and can be fatal. Loss of shoulder elevation, gait ataxia, decreased sensation below the neck and occipital headaches may also occur.

Treatment and nursing care

A posterior fossa decompression, which consists of removing the posterior rim of the foramen magnum and the posterior arch of the atlas, aims at increasing the space for the cerebellum tonsils, brainstem and low cranial nerves.

The postoperative nursing care is critical and consists of the following observations:

- Respiration monitoring: an apnoea monitor or an oxymeter is required for continuous monitoring of the respiration because sleep apnoea may lead to death.
- Blood pressure, pulse and temperature monitoring.
- Neurological observations are concerned with consciousness and in addition must include the assessment of the lowest cranial nerves. This involves assessing the quality

of the voice, the gag and swallowing. The voice is compared to the preoperative voice; whether it is weaker or stronger. Parents can assist with this subjective evaluation.

- Feeding will only resume if swallowing and gag reflexes are good. The swallow is assessed with a sip of water because clear water, if aspirated, is less damaging for the lungs. The gag is assessed with a tongue depressor.
- The risk of aspiration pneumonia will be decreased by positioning the child on the side to compensate for a potentially unprotected upper airway.
- Limb observations, for movements, strength and sensation, are relevant as deterioration may occur following the sudden decompression of the posterior fossa structures.
- Pain control is an important aspect of the nursing care. During surgery, the shoulder muscles have been cut to access the posterior fossa space. The child will experience pain when nodding, turning from side to side, shrugging shoulders and breathing deeply. Pain assessment includes asking the child, the parents and evaluating the child's behaviour. In addition to administering ordered analgesia, the child must be nursed to avoid stretching of the wound. Exaggerated neck flexion hurts, whether it is side to side, hyperflexion or hyperextension. The best position ensures a body alignment and a neutral head position. Pillows of different thickness are required to accommodate different-sized children. Relaxing the shoulders downward may help. Before being turned 2 hourly, children must have the procedure explained, and they must be rewarded after it.

Spinal cord tethering

During adolescence, growth is accelerated and adhesions may lead to an increase in morbidity. These adhesions occur on the site of the spinal defect repaired in infancy and the deficits can be foot drop, gait deterioration or change in bladder patterns. A spinal cord decompression or detethering is required to prevent further deterioration. This is important for walking children as they may become wheelchair bound without early surgery.

The surgery carries the risks of additional morbidity and must be explained to the family and adolescent.

Postoperative nursing care

- Pain control.
- Pressure area care every 2 hours or as required.
- Avoid wound traction when handling the child. The child is turned log rolling and if possible, a spinal turning bed is used to minimise the trauma of the turning.
- The position of the child is recommended by the neurosurgeon — it can be prone, side to side or on the back.
- Monitor vital signs for hypovolaemia, infection and the child's anxiety.
- Monitor function and sensation below the lesion — limbs, bladder and bowel.
- Recommence oral intake as tolerated, after bowel sounds have returned. Encourage a diet to prevent constipation (orange juices, high fibre diet).
- Report wound breakdown or CSF leak immediately as meningitis has devastating consequences when the child has a shunt.
- Recommence bowel care regimen on day 3 after surgery.

CONCLUSION

Children born with NTD are challenging to nursing practice at all ages of their life. Parents and children must be well informed to accept this condition, take control of the strategies and overcome problems. Tremendous support is required and they must be linked to available services and support systems. Nurses must not underestimate their responsibilities in promoting continence. Continence may be the key to the child's successful social integration while incontinence may lead to low self-esteem and social isolation.

REFERENCES

1.   Bryan, AD. Neural tube defects. *In:* Robinson MJ, Roberton DM, eds. *Practical Paediatrics.* 3rd ed. Melbourne: Churchill Livingstone, 1994: 476–481.
2.   Smith GK. Spina Bifida. *In:* Jones PG, ed. *Paediatric surgery — diagnosis and management.* 2nd ed. Oxford: Blackwell Scientific Publications, 1976: 101–112.
3.   Willis RA. Faecal incontinence — Willis Home Bowel Washout Programme. *Zeitschritt Kinderchirurgie* 1989; 44 (Suppl.1): 46–47.

Disturbances in Musculoskeletal Function

Isobel Taylor

Musculoskeletal Injuries

Accidents are a leading cause of death as well as a significant cause of residual disability among children over 1 year old. In multiply injured children, especially those with life-threatening trauma, fracture management may take a low priority until the child's condition is stable. Definitive treatment of the fracture should then be instituted as soon possible in order to ensure full restoration of function.

There are age-related differences of bone physiology that require consideration for diagnosis and management, particularly when a growth mechanism is involved (epiphyseal fractures) (**Figure 6.13**). In children the bones are still springy and incomplete, and greenstick, buckle or torus fractures are common. The greenstick fracture pattern is one of disruption of the cortex of the bone on one side only. The buckle or torus fracture pattern is one of bony deformation without fracture. Sprains and ligamentous injuries are less common in children because the young bone is weaker than the ligaments. An injury which results in a ligament tear in an adult is more likely to result in an epiphyseal fracture in a child.

CLASSIFICATION OF FRACTURES

Incomplete and epiphyseal fractures are only seen in the paediatric age group. Aside from these unique patterns, children's fractures are classified as they are in adults.

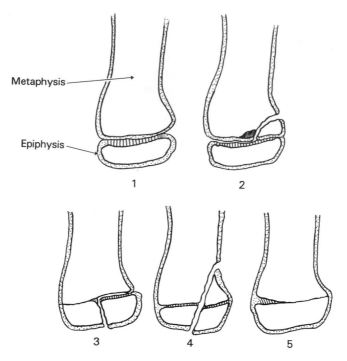

1. Complete separation of the epiphyseal plate without any fracture in the adjacent bone.
2. Separation plus fracture of the metaphysis.
3. Intra-articular fracture from the joint surface.
4. Fracture extending from the joint surface through a portion of the metaphysis.
5. A crushing force has compressed the epiphyseal plate.

Figure 6.13 Epiphyseal fractures.

For example, they are described as closed or simple fractures where the skin over the fracture site is intact and as open or compound where there is a wound over the fracture site resulting in an increased risk of contamination and infection. Complicated fractures are those where important soft tissues are damaged such as viscera, blood vessels or nerves. Further classifications are related to the anatomical location of the fracture on the bone, e.g. supracondylar, metaphyseal, subtrochanteric.

Other descriptive terminology used in the assessment of fractures relates to the radiological appearance of the fracture line, e.g., spiral, transverse, oblique, longitudinal, impacted and comminuted (**Figure 6.14**). These patterns reflect the mechanism of injury and, in the absence of an adequate history (which may be the case in an unwitnessed accident), help the hospital staff to anticipate the full extent of the injury, including any associated damage. Where there is a discrepancy between the skeletal injury pattern and the parental explanation or if there is evidence of previous unexplained injury, non-accidental injury should be suspected and referral to appropriate professionals trained to investigate and handle the situation is mandatory. Such a report is an expression of concern, not blame, and it is important for the nurse to remain an objective observer and to ask questions in a non-accusatory way.

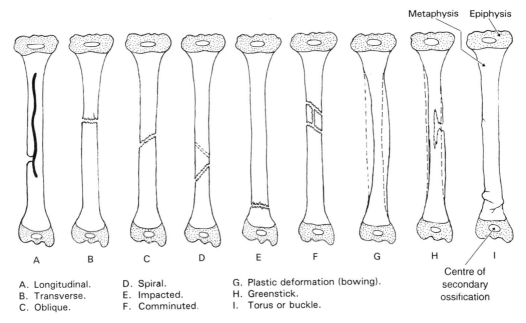

Metaphysis Epiphysis

A   B   C   D   E   F   G   H   I

Centre of
secondary
ossification

A. Longitudinal.   D. Spiral.   G. Plastic deformation (bowing).
B. Transverse.   E. Impacted.   H. Greenstick.
C. Oblique.   F. Comminuted. I. Torus or buckle.

Figure 6.14 Classification of fractures.

ASSESSMENT AND PLANNING

The principles of fracture management in children are based on recognising the unique properties of the growing skeleton in relation to aspects of anatomy, physiology and biomechanics. At the ends of the long bones the epiphyseal growth plates are active in longitudinal and diametric growth and are in various stages of ossification. This feature makes the radiological assessment and diagnosis of joint injury at the ends of bones, particularly around the elbow and ankle, more difficult. For this reason an x-ray of the opposite, uninjured side is often needed for comparison. It is important to explain the reason for the radiological examination of the uninjured side to the parents and child. The expanded use of computed tomography (CT scans), sonography and magnetic resonance (MR) imaging has greatly helped in the diagnosis of injuries to non-ossified bone where these facilities are available. Fracture through the growth plate (epiphysis) requires special assessment because of the potential for disruption to growth and subsequent deformity as the child grows. Epiphyseal fracture patterns have been classified according to the degree of damage to the growth plate and this has helped in the diagnosis and treatment of these fractures, which are unique to children (**Figure 6.13**).

FRACTURE MANAGEMENT

The principles of management of skeletal and soft tissue injury in children are essentially the same as those for adults, such as: accurate assessment to establish the mechanism of injury, early treatment aimed at restoration of form and function, prevention of complications of the injury and treatment. Fracture results in pain, deformity and loss of function and is accompanied by high levels of anxiety and distress.

The principles of management of the child must include good pain control and anxiety reducing measures. The injured limb needs to be well supported and handled very gently during the diagnostic process. The child's support person should be allowed to be present throughout any procedures. Inhalation analgesia in conjunction with parenteral narcotic administration are used during manipulation and splinting of the limb.

The aims of management of the fracture are to reduce (realign) the fracture, to immobilise or hold the reduction while healing progresses and to restore movement and function.

Reduction

Closed reduction, where the fractured bone is manipulated into alignment, is the most common method. This is achieved under light general anaesthesia or regional block. If the fracture cannot be reduced by the closed method or if it is unstable after reduction then open reduction will be performed as a surgical procedure and some form of internal fixation used.

Immobilisation

The reduced fracture is held in position by some form of splint, cast or traction until healing is secured. Children's bones heal faster than adult bone because the growing skeleton is highly active in bone replacement and remodelling. A femoral shaft fracture in a child under 12 years heals in around 8 weeks. The same fracture in a 20 year old takes almost twice as long to heal.

Since the remodelling capacity of a child's bone is greater than adults', more angulation or overriding of the fragments (bayonet apposition) after reduction can be tolerated as subsequent moulding will produce normal length and contour by the end of growth. Unreduced rotational malalignment, however, will result in deformity as the child grows and must be corrected at the time of reduction.

Restoration of function

Once the fracture is reduced and held securely the child is encouraged to move as much as possible within the limits of the immobilisation device until the fracture is healed. Most children need little encouragement to resume activities and rarely is ongoing physical therapy needed once the child and parents have been educated about activity and preservation of the fracture immobilisation. Periodic follow-up is essential until the end of the growth period to ensure that form and function are proceeding normally.

SPECIFIC FRACTURE MANAGEMENT

Fracture of the clavicle

The clavicle can be injured at birth during a traumatic delivery, but it is more commonly injured by a force transmitted to it by a fall on the outstretched hand, elbow or shoulder. Immobilisation in a figure-of-eight bandage or clavicle strap for 3 to 4 weeks is the usual treatment. Older children with displaced fractures will need closed reduction and immobilisation for 5 to 6 weeks.

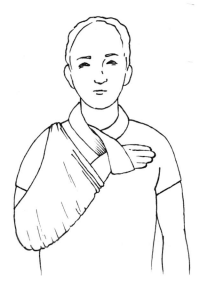

Figure 6.15 Shaft of humerus fracture. Collar and cuff with external support to the arm.

Fractures of the humerus

Fractures of the humeral neck commonly occur in adolescents from a fall on the out-stretched hand, more rarely from a direct blow or fall on the lateral shoulder. Immobil-isation with a sling is the usual treatment for minimally displaced fractures which do not need reduction. The weight of the arm tends to correct the displacement. The child is shown and encouraged to perform pendulum exercises to minimise shoulder stiffness and to regain abduction at the shoulder joint as soon as possible. Healing takes place in 3 to 6 weeks, depending on the degree of displacement.

Shaft of humerus fractures result from falls or direct blows, or may be due to indirect forces transmitted to the bone from the throwing of a ball. A fracture may occur when a child is grabbed by someone trying to prevent a fall or even by the act of pulling the child's arm forcibly in or out of a sleeve in a tight garment. After reduction the arm is immobilised with the elbow in 45° to 90° of flexion using a collar and cuff with a U-slab of plaster bandaged onto the lateral aspect of the arm (**Figure 6.15**). The loop of the U-slab is bandaged over the shoulder for more proximal fractures and over the elbow for more distal ones. The child should be asked to demonstrate active extension of the fingers to exclude radial nerve damage, since there is a possibility of this following shaft fractures of the humerus. Healing time is 4 to 6 weeks, but the U-slab may be removed and replaced after 2 weeks by a functional brace.

Supracondylar fracture of the humerus

This common fracture occurs with a fall on the outstretched hand. Usually the elbow is flexed at the moment of impact and the distal fragment displaces posteriorly. If the elbow is fully extended on impact there will be anterior displacement. The latter is a less common presentation. Undisplaced or minimally displaced supracondylar fractures are treated in a sling for 3 weeks, but more usually reduction and more secure immobilisa-tion are needed.

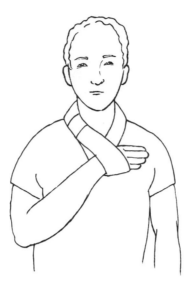

Figure 6.16 Collar and cuff immobilisation for supracondylar fracture. Adjustment can be made to increase or decrease the degree of flexion at the elbow as required.

Posteriorly displaced fractures are treated with closed reduction under anaesthesia and immobilised using a collar and cuff. The more flexion there is at the elbow, the more stable is the reduction (**Figure 6.16**). The radial pulse is assessed throughout the reduction and frequently in the post-reduction phase because occasionally the pulse is obliterated when the elbow is well flexed. In this case a less flexed position will have to be accepted and additional support using a posterior plaster slab from below the shoulder to just above the wrist will be needed. As the swelling diminishes during the next few days, the collar and cuff can be adjusted to increase the elbow flexion, provided the pulse remains palpable. The child and parents are shown and encouraged to move the wrist and fingers but the arm cannot be taken out of the cuff for 3 weeks. After that time if the check x-ray shows satisfactory alignment the child can take the hand out of the cuff for washing and dressing. The healing time is 6 to 8 weeks. Restoration of function may take months due to elbow stiffness. The child and parent are advised of this and instructed not to force elbow extension. Passive movements and carrying weights are particularly contraindicated.

An early complication of this fracture is compartment syndrome, and for this reason these children are often admitted to hospital overnight in order to assess the neurovascular status of the hand. Occasionally, if the circulation is compromised by attempted reduction and flexion, the arm will need to be placed in extended arm traction until the swelling subsides (**Figure 6.17**).

A late complication is ulnar nerve palsy due to valgus deformity as the child grows, resulting either from epiphyseal damage or inadequate reduction (**Figure 6.18**).

Fractured radius and ulna

Fracture of the neck of the radius is usually caused by a fall on the outstretched hand while the elbow is in a slightly valgus position. Sometimes the proximal ulna is also

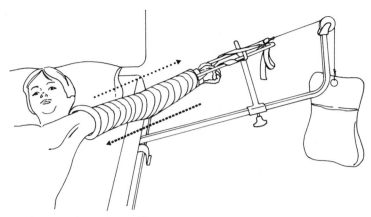

Figure 6.17 Supracondylar fracture treatment in an extended arm traction splint. This is used until the fracture is reducible without vascular compromise.[3]
(Reproduced with permission from Churchill Livingstone)

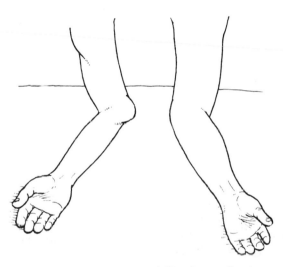

Figure 6.18 Valgus deformity of the elbow following a fracture which damaged the growth plate.[3] (Reproduced with permission from Churchill Livingstone)

fractured. After closed reduction the arm is immobilised using a posterior plaster slab with the elbow held in 90° of flexion. The slab is worn for 3 weeks and a collar and cuff for another week (**Figure 6.19**).

A fall on the hand may force the ulna backwards, dislocating the elbow. Deformity is very obvious and it is important to check for damage to blood vessels or nerves. Treatment consists of closed reduction under anaesthesia and immobilisation with a collar and cuff for 3 weeks with the elbow flexed more than 90°. Shoulder and finger exercises are encouraged from the start. After 1 week the child is shown how to gently exercise the elbow. After 3 weeks the collar and cuff are left off and gentle active elbow movements

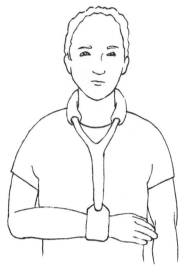

Figure 6.19 Collar and cuff immobilisation.

encouraged. As in previously mentioned injuries around the elbow, the parents and child are advised to avoid forced elbow extension.

Greenstick (incomplete) fracture of the distal radius and ulna is a common injury following a fall on the outstretched hand. The 2 bones may fracture at the same level, but more commonly the radius fractures at a higher level than the ulna.

Treatment consists of closed reduction and immobilisation in a long arm plaster cast with the elbow in 90° of flexion for 4 to 6 weeks.

Fracture of the metacarpals and phalanges

Hand injuries are usually due to direct force and are often associated with skin damage. Restoration of function is vital as fingers stiffen easily. Splintage is kept to a minimum and swelling is controlled by elevating the hand and encouraging early, repeated active movement of the fingers. The injured finger is splinted by being strapped to its neighbour so that both move as one. Healing time is 2 weeks for phalanges, 2 to 5 weeks for metacarpals.

Femoral fractures

The femur is injured in falls from heights or in traffic accidents. Treatment of shock due to blood loss is a priority in these injuries. Significant amounts of blood can be distributed along the thigh with little external evidence, and it should be kept in mind that swelling in the thigh can be due to extensive bleeding as well as fracture-related soft tissue swelling.

Fractures of the femoral shaft in infants and children under 2 years (or weighing up to 16 kg) are treated in Gallows (Bryant's) traction (**Figure 6.20**). In older children and adolescents the fracture is reduced and immobilised in skin traction, either Hamilton-Russell (for upper third or neck fractures — **Figure 6.21**) or fixed traction in a Thomas splint (for middle and lower third fractures — **Figure 6.22**), for 3 to 6 weeks. Healing

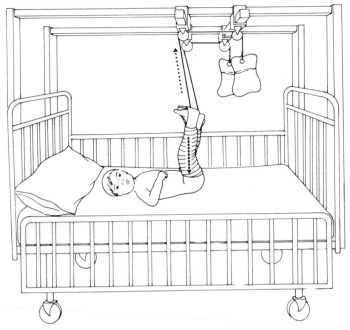

Figure 6.20 Gallows (Bryants) traction for femoral fracture immobilisation in infants weighing less than 16kg.[3] (Reproduced with permission from Churchill Livingstone)

may take up to 12 weeks in older children, in which case a cast brace is applied after 6 weeks in traction.

NURSING CARE OF CHILDREN WITH FRACTURES

An important nursing diagnosis for the child who sustains musculoskeletal trauma is the potential for neurovascular deficit related to the injury or the treatment of the injury if it involves splints, casts, traction or surgery.

A systematic approach to neurovascular assessment is essential to detect the onset of vascular or nerve impairment (**Figures 6.23, 6.24 and 6.25**).

Assessing the neurovascular status

Assess the circulation of the injured limb by noting the following:

- The colour of the skin and comparing it with the unaffected side.
- The capillary filling of the nail beds. Press on the nail to blanch the underlying tissue and watch for the return of colour when the pressure is released. The nail beds should flush with colour within 2 seconds.
- The temperature of the skin and comparing it to the unaffected side. The back of the examiner's fingers are more sensitive to temperature changes than the finger tips. Also note the presence of ice packs or fans which could influence the assessment.
- The pulse distal to the injury, and comparing the force to the unaffected side. It may be necessary to use an ultrasonic flow meter (Doppler) in infants and very young

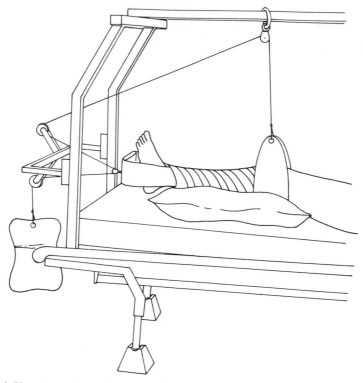

Figure 6.21 Hamilton Russell traction.[3] (Reproduced with permission from Churchill Livingstone)

children. It is helpful to mark the skin with an 'X' over the spot where a pulse is located in order to facilitate ongoing assessments.

- The amount of swelling and comparing it to the unaffected side. Also note the position of the extremity, e.g. amount of elevation. A certain amount of swelling is to be expected following an injury or surgical procedure and appropriate elevation of the limb is essential to control oedema by facilitating venous return so that the swelling itself does not become severe enough to be the cause of neurovascular impairment.
- The occurrence of increased pain when the toes or fingers are passively extended.

Assess the nerve supply by testing sensation and movement as follows:

- Touch the skin lightly and compare the child's response to the unaffected side. Test for reliability by not actually touching the child each time a response is elicited. Of course, ensure that the child cannot see whether he is being touched or not. If the child is old enough, enquire about the presence of numbness and tingling. The child may be able to relate to the sensation of the part's having 'gone to sleep' or having 'pins and needles'.
- Test both active and passive movement (see compartment syndrome below). It is important to remember that reduced movement or power may be a result of pain or fear of producing pain. Distraction techniques using toys such as finger puppets and stories might be successful in getting the unwilling child to move fingers or toes. Again compare your findings to the unaffected side.

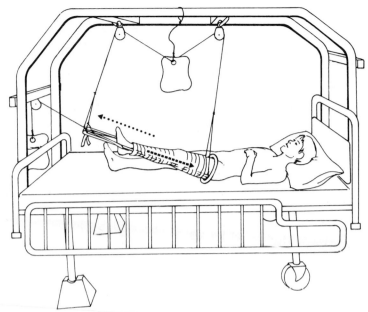

Figure 6.22 Femoral fracture management using fixed skin traction in a Thomas splint. The dotted arrow represents the traction pull exerted by the cords from the skin extensions tied to the end of the splint. The blocked arrow denotes the countertraction force transmitted along the side bars of the splint to the ring around the thigh.[3] (Reproduced with permission from Churchill Livingstone)

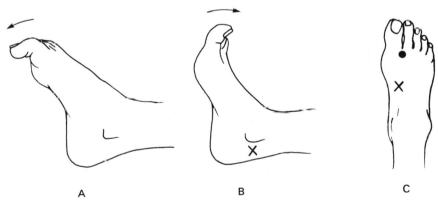

Figure 6.23 Neuromuscular assessment — testing dorsiflexion and plantar flexion. The X marks the site of the pedal pulses. The dot marks the site for testing sensation of the nerve distribution.[3]

(Reproduced with permission from Churchill Livingstone)

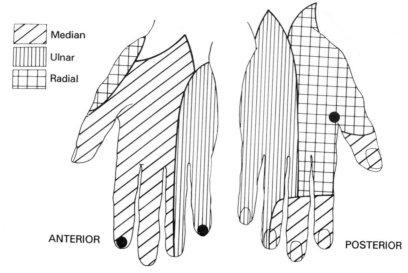

Figure 6.24 Neuromuscular assessment: the distribution of the sensory nerves of the hands. The black dots denote the site of evaluation of sensation.[3]
(Reproduced with permission from Churchill Livingstone)

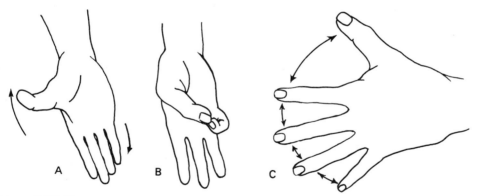

Figure 6.25 Neuromuscular assessment: testing the motor nerves in the hands. (A) radial nerve: extension of fingers. (B) median nerve: fingers and thumb opposition. (C) ulnar nerve: spreading the fingers.[3]
(Reproduced with permission from Churchill Livingstone)

The pathophysiology of neurovascular deficit can be considered in relation to impaired venous return, arterial insufficiency and compartment syndrome.

Impaired venous return occurs when venous stasis due to injury and immobility is exacerbated by an encircling cast, splint or bandage. Maintaining adequate elevation of the affected limb (higher than the heart) and encouraging the child to move fingers or toes as appropriate will help prevent venous stasis. It is essential to monitor the degree of swelling and to check the tightness of any cast, splint or bandage at each neurovascular check.

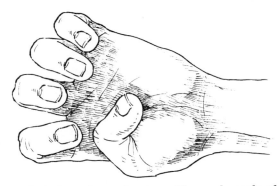

Figure 6.26 Volkmann's ischaemic contracture. The end result of unrelieved compartment pressure is this claw hand deformity.

Arterial insufficiency occurs through interruption of the blood supply in the injured limb. This may happen at the time of injury or dislocation, particularly in injuries around the elbow or knee and following fractures of the forearm and lower leg.[1] An arterial branch may be avulsed at the time of injury or the vessel may be lacerated by sharp fracture fragments or be occluded by direct pressure, thrombosis or spasm. Arterial damage is suspected if the limb is cool and pale with diminished or absent pulse. Pain can be intense until anaesthesia and paralysis signal ischaemic nerve loss. The state of the limb must be reported to the treating physician without delay so that early intervention can be undertaken to preserve function. Arteriography may be indicated to confirm the location and extent of the damage and to plan operative procedures.

Compartment syndrome occurs when swelling takes place within the tightly enclosed fascial compartments and the rising tissue pressure adversely affects the perfusion of the affected muscle groups. The two areas most at risk of this complication are the forearm, following supracondylar fractures, and the lower leg, following proximal tibial fractures. The muscles in these compartments become hypoxic and swell within the inelastic fascia. The increasing tension further compromises arterial inflow, capillary throughflow and venous outflow.[2] Even if the arterial flow is reduced, the collateral circulation may be sufficient to maintain a pulse and a seemingly adequate peripheral circulation. The presence of a pulse in this circumstance is misleading. Pain will be an indicator of ischaemia, especially when the hypoxic muscles are moved. Therefore increasing pain on passive extension of the fingers (if the arm is involved) or toes (if the leg is involved) is a reliable sign and should be included in the routine neurovascular assessment of an injured limb. If the compartment pressure is not relieved within 4 to 6 hours, ischaemic necrosis of the muscles will result in permanent contracture of the distal arm and hand. This condition is known as Volkmann's ischaemic contracture (**Figure 6.26**).

Initial management of suspected compartment syndrome is to loosen or remove any encircling tight splints, casts or bandages, leaving the limb in a neutral position. Elevation of the limb is not helpful as this further compromises arterial flow. Keeping the limb cool will reduce the metabolic needs of the compromised tissues. Treatment of an established compartment syndrome is surgical decompression by fasciotomy of the affected muscle compartments. The wound is usually left open until the swelling subsides and the limb will require meticulous care and protection until secondary closure is performed.

CARING FOR A CHILD IN A CAST

Most children with fractures do not require admission to hospital and are discharged from the accident and emergency department wearing a cast. The child, if old enough, and the parents or guardian need clear verbal and written instructions in a language they understand before the child is discharged. The instructions include: care and protection of the cast; signs and symptoms of neurovascular compromise and skin problems and what to do about them; comfort measures; and follow-up appointment dates.

Plaster of Paris is still extensively used for casts because it is easy to apply and is relatively inexpensive. It is vulnerable to wetting and soiling and may crack or crumble round the edges with active children. Fibreglass casting material is lighter, tougher and more resistant to the effects of wetting and soiling and is preferred for hip spica casts. The casted limb is kept elevated to control swelling and it is supported along the length of the cast until it is dry enough not to be indented by external pressure. When handling a wet or 'green' cast, take care to use the flat palmar surface of the hands since finger pressure can leave indentations. A sling or collar and cuff supports arm casts, and a pillow under the entire length of the cast supports the leg. The heel should be clear of the pillow and any hard surface to ensure that no flattening of the cast over the heel occurs that can lead to the development of a pressure sore on the heel under the cast. During the drying process the cast is left uncovered to allow free circulation of air to ensure even drying. A bed cradle is useful to keep the blankets off the cast. In cold weather the rest of the child should be warmly covered. With large casts the child should be turned periodically (2nd hourly) to facilitate drying of the underneath part.

Neurovascular assessment, as described above, is recorded regularly and all complaints or evidence of pain should be reported and investigated. Persisting pain after a cast is applied is a reliable sign that something is wrong. Odour and drainage seeping through the cast is a late sign of skin ulceration if the early warning signs were missed or ignored.

A window can be cut in the cast to check identified local trouble spots. The cut-out section of the cast is retained and repositioned in the gap with a bandage to avoid pressure from swelling at the window edges.

Cast application and removal can be a frightening experience for a child. To reduce the trauma, adequate age-appropriate explanation is required. Incorporating the procedure into play activities will help. A doll or teddy bear can have a cast applied and removed prior to the child's procedure. Older children can be shown pictures and allowed to see and hear the cast removing equipment in action.

The child and parent should be prepared for the appearance of the limb after cast removal. There will be some muscle wasting and the limb circumference will look smaller. The skin may look discoloured and scaly due to the build-up of sebaceous material and shed skin. The limb should be oiled and washed gently several times to gradually restore a normal appearance. Vigorous cleaning is not necessary and may traumatise the skin.

CARING FOR A CHILD IN TRACTION

Traction treatment involves the use of a pulling force to a part of the body. Essentially, this pulling force overcomes muscle spasm and shortening and, in some traction arrangements, the effects of gravity are also overcome. By controlling movement of the injured part, traction enables bone and soft tissue to heal and can be used in a variety of conditions as a method of treatment.

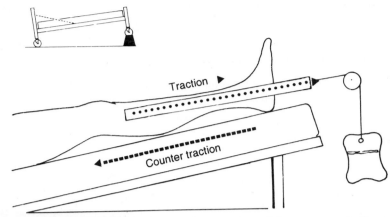

Figure 6.27 Principles of traction treatment. The dotted line represents the traction pull on the leg via skin extension. The blocked line denotes the countertraction force when the foot of the bed is elevated.[3]

(Reproduced with permission from Churchill Livingstone)

- Restoring and maintaining alignment of bone following fracture.
- Resting inflamed joints and maintaining them in a functional position.
- Gradually correcting deformities due to contracted soft tissues.
- Relieving pain due to spasm.

As well as acting on limbs, traction can be applied to the pelvis and spine.

Traction can be achieved in several ways, though certain essential principles must be observed if the traction is to have the desired effect. These principles are:

1. The grip or hold on the body must be adequate and secure.
2. Provision for countertraction must be made.
3. There must be minimal friction.
4. The line and magnitude of the pull, once correctly established, must be maintained.
5. There must be frequent checks of the apparatus and of the patient to ensure that
   a.   the traction set-up is functioning as planned,
   b.   the patient is not suffering any injury as a result of the traction treatment.

Poorly or incorrectly applied traction can cause considerable discomfort to the patient and may retard rehabilitation. It is important, therefore, that staff responsible for setting up and maintaining traction are thoroughly familiar with the principles of traction so that the mechanics of traction set-up are well understood (**Figure 6.27**).

Congenital and Acquired Abnormalities

Congenital and developmental conditions affecting the growth and function of the musculoskeletal system are treated by splinting, surgery or a combination of the two.

These modalities always require monitoring of the neurovascular assessment of the treated limbs and educating the family in the care of the child in an orthotic device.

CONGENITAL DISLOCATION OF THE HIPS (CDH)

This is a spontaneous dislocation of the hip before, during or shortly after birth. It may involve one or both hips (**Figures 6.28 and 6.29**). Bilateral dislocation occurs in two-thirds of affected babies. It is most common among first born female babies by a ratio of 6:1 and there is an increased incidence after breech deliveries. There may be a family history of CDH. The condition is looked for in the neonatal check using Ortolani and Barlow's tests (**Figure 6.30**). These diagnostic manoeuvres detect instability at the hips and a check ultrasound will confirm the clinical findings. The earlier the dislocation is reduced the better the prognosis. If untreated, walking may be delayed and the child develops a limp and waddling gait. The aim of the treatment is to use splintage to correct the dislocation and to keep the hips flexed and abducted. This position allows the femoral head to develop in conjunction with an adequate acetabulum.

The Pavlik harness is used to maintain the desired position in very young babies (**Figure 6.31**). If the hip problem is picked up later or the Pavlik device proves ineffective, a more rigid device is used. Once the harness is fitted and adjusted it must not be removed. The parents are taught how to wash the baby and apply and remove nappies without altering the straps, which maintain the leg position. The device is worn for 3 months. The baby is checked after one week and seen fortnightly thereafter to change the harness as needed. Ultrasound examination is used to periodically check the hips until 4 months, when the bones are developed enough to use x-ray. If a hip spica cast (**Figure 6.32**) is used the parents are shown how to lift, move and position the baby so that the cast is supported at all times (see caring for the child in a cast).

CONGENITAL CLUB FOOT (TALIPES EQUINO-VARUS)

One or both feet may be affected. The condition is more common in boys. The cause is essentially unknown but there may be a family history. Minor degrees of the deformity may be explained by prolonged malposition in utero. The affected foot is twisted inwards (inversion) with inward deviation of the forefoot relative to the hindfoot (adduction) and plantar flexion (equinus) (**Figure 6.33**). The foot cannot be pushed through the normal range of motion and there may be noticeable underdevelopment of the calf muscles.

Treatment

The treatment begins immediately after birth and consists of manipulation, holding the foot in the corrected position with plaster (**Figure 6.34**). The plaster is changed weekly and then fortnightly. After 3 to 4 months, if correction cannot be maintained, surgery is performed. After surgery a plaster is worn for a further 2 to 3 months. The parents should be advised that it may be necessary for the child to be fitted with orthotic shoes for a further 3 months.

Limb lengthening

Limb length discrepancy in children from congenital or acquired causes results in varying degrees of deformity and even disability in later life. The procedure of lengthening the shortened limb requires a high degree of commitment on the part of the nurse to patient

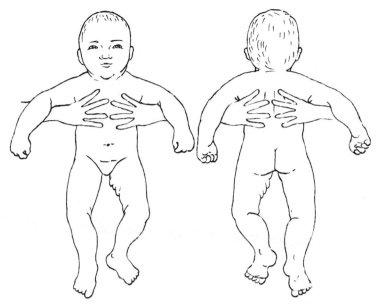

Figure 6.28 Unilateral dislocation of the left hip showing the tell-tale asymmetry of the buttock and thigh skin folds.

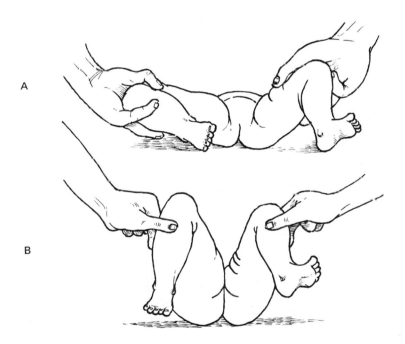

A. The left hip does not abduct fully because the femoral head is caught up in the rim of the acetabulum.

B. Asymmetry of knee level and skin folds indicate dislocation of the left hip.

Figure 6.29 Congenital hip dislocation.

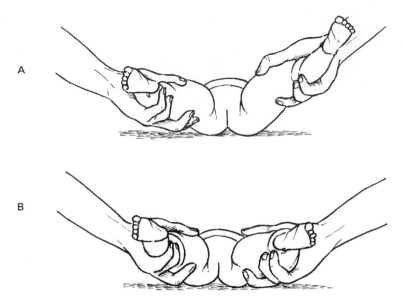

A. Ortolani's test: The examiner feels resistance to abduction on the side of the dislocated hip (left). If pressure is applied by the fingers over the greater trochanta a clunk is felt as it reduces and the hip abducts fully.

B. Barlow's test: To detect an unstable (dislocatable) hip in which the femoral head is normally in the reduced position the examiner attempts to lever the femoral head in and out of the acetabulum.

Figure 6.30 Diagnostic manoeuvres for congenital dislocated hips.

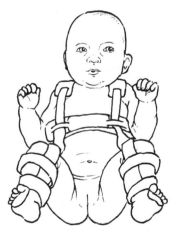

Figure 6.31 The Pavlick harness. The knees are well flexed and the hips are maintained in abduction up to 60^0.

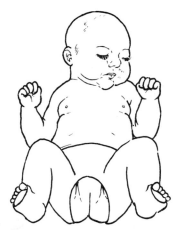

Figure 6.32 Abduction cast for congenital hip dysplasia: Reduction is maintained in a plaster of paris cast when more rigid splintage is required.

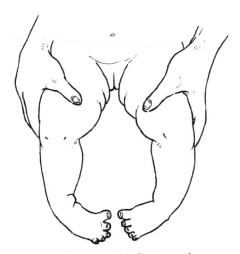

Figure 6.33 Congenital club foot: bilateral talipes equino-varus.

and family teaching in order to achieve optimal results. The Ilizarov apparatus consists of tensioned Kirschner wires that are attached to a series of full or half rings that encircle the affected limb. Once the wires are attached to the rings the rings are connected to one another by threaded or telescoping rods. A corticotomy is performed at the time of application of the device through a small incision. Corticotomy is confirmed by image intensifier and the patient is returned to the ward.[4] Distraction is begun 2 to 4 days post-operatively. This delay allows callus to form. The rate of subsequent distraction of the callus varies but 0.25 mm 4 times a day is typical[5] (**Figure 6.35**). Weight bearing is not only encouraged, it is considered essential to the healing process. The patient is discharged when the patient and family are able to manage the complete treatment process safely. This involves care of the pin sites, regular increases in distraction by correct

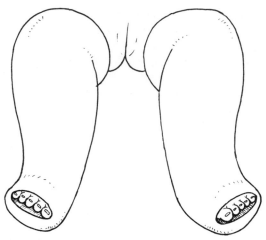

Figure 6.34 Congenital club foot. Plaster of paris splints hold up the feet in the corrected position.

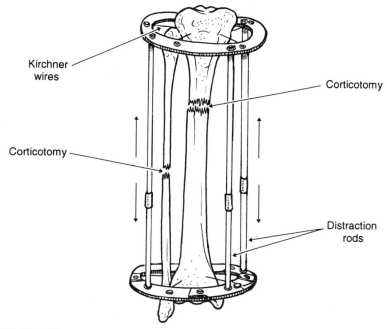

Kirchner
wires

Corticotomy

Corticotomy

Distraction
rods

Figure 6.35 The Ilizarov apparatus showing the encircling rings, tensioned wires and telescoping rods in place. The tibia and fibula have been divided (corticotomy) and distraction of the callus has begun.

adjustments to the apparatus and adherence to a prescribed regimen of weight-bearing exercise. When the desired limb length is achieved the distraction is ceased, but the apparatus is left intact until consolidation takes place. Healing is considered complete when there is no pain, limp or oedema and x-rays show evidence of sufficient bone density to bear weight. The apparatus is then removed. This procedure can be performed on a day only or short stay admission basis under general anaesthesia.

The Ilizarov process is intensive, and almost totally patient centered. The patient and family need to be involved in daily adjustments to the apparatus to achieve the correct rate of distraction and pin site care to prevent infection. The patient is required to undertake physical therapy for as much as 3 to 6 hours a day for 3 to 5 days a week. Treatment time on average is 6 months to a year. The postoperative hospital stay is from 7 to 10 days. After discharge, patients need to be seen by the surgeon weekly during the distraction phase and every 2 to 3 weeks during the period of consolidation.[6] There will need to be a major commitment on the part of the patient and family who undergo this treatment program. The physical and mental demands of the program approach those of coping with a chronic illness due to the extent to which the household routines are disrupted, assistive devices are used, clothing adapted and activities of daily living are altered. For these reasons the nurse is challenged to provide an effective education program to meet the patient and family needs in this regard. This can be achieved by the nurse organising and implementing a special program that provides a structured, multidisciplinary approach to managing the Ilizarov treatment program.

A major role of the nurse is one of coordination and collaboration with all members of the health care team as well as professionals in other fields such as employers and schoolteachers. This role demands good organisational and communication skills in order to avoid the problems and difficulties that might interfere with a successful outcome. The actual teaching of the patient and family requires the provision of written and video material as well as demonstration and explanation. Jauernig suggests introducing the patient to a person who has already undergone the treatment for additional support and encouragement.[7] This is an excellent strategy and one which could be incorporated into a group teaching session with prospective patients and members of the health care team.

ACKNOWLEDGMENTS

The assistance of Ms Anne Fallon RN BEd(Nurs) DNS Ortho Cert, Senior Educator, St Vincent's Private Hospital in preparation of this section, and of Ms Sally Pannifex with the illustrations, is gratefully acknowledged.

REFERENCES

1. Scoles PV. *Pediatric orthopedics in clinical practice.* 2nd ed. Chicago: Year Book Medical, 1988.
2. Joy C. *Pediatric trauma nursing.* Rockville: Aspen Publications, 1989: 119–120.
3. Taylor I. *Ward manual of orthopaedic traction.* Melbourne: Churchill Livingstone, 1987.
4. Greene S. Ilizarov orthopaedic methods. *AORN* 1989; 49: 215–230.
5. Newschwander GE, Dunst RM. Limb lengthening with the Ilizarov external fixator. *Orthopedic Nursing,* 1989; 8: 15–21.
6. Paley D. Problems, obstacles and complications of limb lengthening by the Ilizarov technique. *Clin Orthopedics Related Res* 1990; 250: 81–104.

7. Jauernig PR. Organizing and implementing an Ilizarov program. *Orthopedic Nursing* 1990; 9 (5): 47–55.

Disturbances in Gastrointestinal Function

Trish Comerford and Margaret Yates

Cleft Lip and Palate

The major nursing considerations when caring for an infant or child with **cleft lip** include the child's ability to feed and nutritional status, the degree of the defect and the cosmetic appearance. Assessment of the family's acceptance of the infant's deformity and the effect on their relationships is central to planning appropriate interventions.

The predominant difficulty for the infant with cleft lip and/or palate is the ability to attach and suck. Normal sucking requires the infant to push its tongue and the nipple or teat against the palate to create sufficient pressure for breast milk or formula to be delivered. These infants are more susceptible to swallowing air and therefore need to be burped for a longer period in order to minimise abdominal discomfort.

If the infant has adapted to an effective, alternative feeding method in the postnatal period, the maintenance of a sound nutritional status after surgery will be more readily achieved. The method of feeding should be individualised. Generally, breast feeding can be established successfully in the postnatal period with support and guidance from nursing staff and lactation consultants. The use of plastic droppers or artificial nipples for delivering formula also affords the infant appropriate nourishment to optimise growth and development.

A child with a **cleft palate** may undergo more than one surgical correction to repair the defect successfully. This may be done in stages at different ages, usually at 9, 12 and 18 months. Children with cleft palate will require speech therapy and orthodontic consultation on an ongoing basis for some years.

Cleft lip is a congenital defect as a result of the primary palate failing to fuse during the 7th to 8th week of gestation. Unilateral cleft lip is invariably left-sided. Bilateral cleft lip is usually associated with cleft palate.[1]

The palatine process is a horizontal extension of the maxilla which forms three-fourths of the anterior hard palate, (i.e., the anterior section of the roof of the mouth). If the palatine processes of the maxillary bones do not unite, cleft palate results. The separation can extend to the roof of the nose. The severity of the separation deformity will determine the infant's ability to feed.[2] Surgical correction is performed after the infant has an established feeding pattern of either breast feeding or use of a soft nipple, and demonstrates a satisfactory weight gain. A Z-plasty closure is performed and a Logan bow, a wire frame, is attached and kept in place with adhesive tape. The bow reduces tension on the repaired upper lip, reduces scarring and promotes healing.

PREOPERATIVE NURSING CARE

Nursing diagnosis

Nutritional compromise related to poor feeding technique.

Intervention

- Weigh the infant or child to determine if weight is within normal limits.
- If the weight is low, inform the surgeon and arrange a consultation with a dietitian.
- Ascertain whether the infant's feeding method is breast, pipette or bottle, and assess competence.
- Apply arm restraints to the infant or child the day before surgery so that the child experiences the restriction before the postoperative period. Remove them every 4 hours for 30 minutes.
- Explain to the family the necessity for splints in the postoperative phase.
- Prepare the family for postoperative care, including a description of the infant's lip and mouth. The use of photographs will increase their level of understanding.

POSTOPERATIVE NURSING CARE

Nursing diagnoses and intervention

Maintenance of patient safety related to oral surgery

- Nurse the infant or child in a high dependency unit if nasopharyngeal tube(s) are *in situ*. Suction the tubes frequently to secure patency.
- Nurse the infant or child on his/her side to promote drainage of secretions.
- Administer intravenous fluids to maintain hydration.
- Maintain nil by mouth as determined by the anaesthetist.
- Refrain from placing objects in the infant's mouth, for example a suction catheter, tongue depressor, straws or any other sharp objects.
- Remove sharp or hard objects from the infant or child's cot or bed.
- Observe closely for haemorrhage and notify the surgeon in the event of a change in vital signs or an actual bleed.
- Keep arm splints in place to prevent the infant or child from touching the wound site.
- Observe closely the circulation in fingers for digit colour and warmth.
- Release the splints every 4 hours to inspect, move and massage the arms.
- Observe for signs of pain and administer analgesia as needed.
- Provide diversional therapy such as mobiles or music.

Susceptibility to infection following surgery

- Explain to parents the importance of washing their hands before handling the child.
- If a Logan bow is *in situ*, maintain and repair anchoring tape as necessary.
- Rinse the infant or child's mouth with sterile water after each feed until the palate is free of food particles. Depending on the infant or child's age use a pipette or feeding cup.
- Clean the suture line with normal saline when necessary as well as after feeding. If there is crusting of the suture line, clean with hydrogen peroxide applied with a cotton bud.
- Inspect the palate frequently to observe for signs of healing.

Less than adequate nutrition related to pain and difficulty with feeding

- Administer analgesia approximately 30 minutes before feeding.
- Commence oral feeding using the method the infant is familiar with, i.e., breast feeding, pipette or bottle. For a child, commence with clear fluids and graduate to a very soft diet using soft plastic utensils and a cup.
- Encourage and support the parent feeding the infant or child.

Alteration to family relationships related to an infant or child with a visible physical imperfection

- Actively promote the parents' involvement in the infant or child's care and the re-introduction of diet.
- Invite the parents to voice their thoughts and feelings about the infant's appearance and progress.
- Establish an atmosphere of acceptance of the infant.
- Promote age-appropriate play to occupy and therapeutically stimulate the infant or child.
- Provide information about lip and/or palate care and diet and refer the parents to the local cleft lip/palate support group.
- Incorporate the speech therapist in the infant or child's care.

Gastro-oesophageal Reflux

Regurgitation and vomiting are common features of early infancy. Mild degrees of gastro-oesophageal reflux and associated regurgitation are sufficiently common in infants for them to be considered physiologic.[3] In only a small percentage of infants will vomiting, regurgitation or reflux indicate or be the cause of significant health problems.[4]

Gastro-oesophageal reflux refers to a group of symptoms which interrupt normal gastrointestinal motility where there is no known aetiology.[5]

NURSING ASSESSMENT

The nurse can determine and evaluate the presence of reflux by obtaining a comprehensive history of effortless vomiting or regurgitation after feeding. Where a large volume of the feed is frequently vomited, weight loss will occur, caloric intake is insufficient and normal growth will be compromised.

Other infants may present with a history of apnoeic episodes, recurrent respiratory tract infections, oesophagitis or failure to thrive with little or no history of vomiting or regurgitation. Severe gastro-oesophageal reflux may result in oesophagitis with a slowly evolving anaemia caused by constant exposure of the oesophageal tissues to gastric acid and subsequent erosion of the mucosa. The physical signs of gastro-oesophageal reflux are indicative of the complications rather than the reflux itself.[6]

The distal end of the oesophagus has an area of contracted circular smooth muscle known as the lower oesophageal or cardiac sphincter. Normally the relaxed smooth muscle facilitates peristaltic propulsion of food into the stomach.[5] Gastro-oesophageal reflux is a result of lower oesophageal sphincter incompetence, which permits the return of gastric contents to the oesophagus.

Medical investigations aim to rule out anatomic anomalies such as tracheo-oesophageal fistula, pyloric stenosis, hiatus hernia or oesophageal stricture. For the infant with typical effortless vomiting after feeding who is otherwise healthy, diagnosis will be readily achieved. Careful physical examination, attention to the history related by the parents and a barium swallow to rule out intestinal obstruction such as pyloric stenosis, will confirm the diagnosis. In the infant with respiratory signs of apnoea or recurrent respiratory tract infections which may be indicative of gastro-oesophageal reflux, pH monitoring will be required and is the preferred definitive diagnostic tool.[7] PH probe studies can be implemented over long periods of time, thus allowing the infant to function normally while being investigated. The probe is inserted via the naso-pharynx so that the tip of the probe sits above the lower oesophageal sphincter. Probe studies are able to determine the frequency and duration of acid reflux episodes and the number of prolonged episodes. Data are collected in a miniaturised portable pH meter attached to the probe. In conjunction with the meter, a data log is kept which identifies feedings, periods of vomiting, respiratory distress, crying, coughing and the infant's position. With both sets of data the relationship between reflux, clinical signs and symptoms and the infant's behaviour can be determined.

The aims of treatment are to protect the mucosal lining of the oesophagus from ulceration, prevent aspiration and the complication of pneumonia and maintain the infant's normal growth and development.[1] Interventions are determined by the severity of the reflux.

MEDICATION

Metoclopramide increases gastric motility and has been shown to increase the pressure of the lower oesophageal sphincter. The common side effects include drowsiness and restlessness. The more serious reactions are extrapyramidal disturbances manifest as neck pain and stiffness, trismus (tonic spasms of the jaw muscles) and oliguric crisis. These adverse reactions are more prevalent in infants and children than adults. **Cisapride** has a more specific action on the gastrointestinal tract with fewer side effects. Clinical studies indicate enhancement of gastric emptying and increased pressure of the lower oesophageal sphincter. In paediatric studies cisapride has been shown to be more effective in comparison to other pharmacological agents.[8]

In common with other medical interventions, the aim of using medication is to decrease the number of episodes of reflux.

The indications for surgical intervention are:

1. No improvement in growth after 6 weeks of aggressive medical management.
2. Persistence in symptoms for more than one year.
3. Recurrent respiratory problems such as pneumonia or diagnosed reflux-related apnoea.

If oesophagitis is suspected, endoscopy and biopsy is performed to confirm the diagnosis.

SURGICAL TECHNIQUE

A Nissen fundoplication involves wrapping the muscle from the fundus of the stomach around the distal oesophagus to tighten the lower oesophageal sphincter. This technique is the most commonly used successful surgical intervention.[5]

NURSING DIAGNOSIS AND INTERVENTION

Compromised nutrition and growth related to vomiting

- If the infant is breast fed, negotiate with the mother to express her milk, which is then thickened with an appropriate substance such as cornflour. Formula should be thickened in the hospital's formula room where facilities are available or in the unit using a clean technique.
- The infant is fed slowly in an upright position, and 'winded' frequently. Do not place the infant in a prone position immediately after the feed.
- The infant's growth is monitored through ongoing measurement and documentation in accordance with unit policy.
- An accurate record of the infant's oral intake and output is maintained.
- The nature of posseting or regurgitation, when it occurs, and the volume of feed lost is documented.
- The infant is positioned in accordance with observation of the individual infant's comfort.
- Episodes of apnoea and alterations in respiratory status in relation to feeding are documented.
- The infant's behaviour is observed for evidence of irritability, restlessness or discomfort indicative of pain associated with oesophagitis. In particular, the infant's facial expressions, such as grimacing, are observed.

Thickened feeds are advocated on the premise that semi-solid food is more difficult to regurgitate than liquid. Recent studies suggest that thickened formula decreases reflux in one-third of infants, has no effect in one-third and causes reflux to significantly increase in another third.[1] Thickening with additives such as rice cereal alters the caloric density of the formula. This poses a potential risk for not delivering adequate calories for normal growth. The thickening of feeds is still the preferred treatment. For breast-fed infants, a thickening agent is mixed with water or expressed breast milk and administered to the infant before feeding.

The infant should be placed on the right side at a 30° angle after feeding. Sitting at a 60° angle will increase abdominal pressure and exacerbate the reflux.[1]

Parental anxiety related to an infant with gastrointestinal disturbance

Explain and discuss with the parents all aspects of anti-reflux management and care.

- Explain the importance of positioning the infant so that gravity assists the retention of feeds.
- Explain the action of medications such as metroclopromide and cisapride and demonstrate to the parents how to administer the drugs orally with a teaspoon.
- Explain how to thicken the infant's feeds and what agent to use.
- Teach the parents to observe for posseting, which usually ceases after the first 8 weeks of life. In infants where posseting continues beyond 8 weeks, most will improve by 6 months of age and 90% of infants will have improved by 18 months of age.
- In the event the infant experiences apnoea, instruct the parents to seek medical attention urgently.
- Explain investigations such as pH monitoring and why this is undertaken.
- Assure the parents that their infant's condition is not a reflection of their parenting. Listen for any clues that may indicate that the parents are blaming themselves or feel they have failed in their care and responsibilities.

- Assist the parents to adjust to having an infant who vomits or regurgitates by encouraging them to express their thoughts and feelings.
- If the infant is to be discharged on the above management regimen, make sure the parents understand all the above aspects of care. Confirm with them that if at any time they are in doubt about managing their infant at home they should make contact with unit nursing staff, the community nurse or their local doctor for assistance.

NURSING CARE OF THE INFANT UNDERGOING PH STUDIES

- After insertion, maintain the security of the pH probe with a compatible adhesive tape.
- Record pH data sheet by describing: the time of commencement and completion of feeding; the position of the infant during the feed; evidence of crying, vomiting or coughing; additional comments on behaviour or any events perceived to be relevant to the study.

NURSING CARE OF THE INFANT UNDERGOING FUNDOPLICATION

See nursing care summary of infant/child undergoing abdominal surgery at the end of this chapter.

Special needs

- During the postoperative phase when feeding is reinstituted, offer small frequent amounts to avoid bloating.
- Consider and explain to the parents that the infant is unable to vomit as a result of the surgical correction which enhances the function of the lower oesophageal sphincter.
- In some instances where gastro-oesophageal reflux has been severe and/or chronic, the infant may have a temporary gastrostomy tube inserted. The gastrostomy tube will serve 3 purposes: to rest the upper gastrointestinal tract, permit feeding and decompress the stomach.

Pyloric Stenosis

Pyloric stenosis is a narrowing of the pyloric canal.

On admission to hospital, the nurse will establish from the parents a history of the infant. The infant with pyloric stenosis usually has a history of being well in the first few weeks of life. The parents will describe episodes of regurgitation and occasional vomiting with the vomiting becoming progressively projectile in nature. Characteristic of this projectile vomiting is the forceful ejection of gastric contents which may land anywhere up to a metre away from the infant and which occurs during or shortly after feeding. Significantly, in these infants, the vomitus contains no bile, only gastric contents. If the infant has been symptomatic for longer than one week, vomitus may be blood stained, indicating a degree of gastritis.

On physical assessment, the nurse will most often observe a scrawny, thin infant who has lost or failed to gain weight. The mother may describe the infant's stools as being much smaller or less frequent than usual. The infant is usually a greedy feeder who demonstrates discomfort and irritability arising from hunger rather than pain.

Dehydration will occur rapidly as fluid is unable to reach beyond the pyloric sphincter. The nurse will be able to determine the extent of dehydration by checking for a sunken anterior fontanelle and eyes, dry mucous membranes, reduced skin turgor and decreased urine output.

INVESTIGATION

A test feed will be given in order to scrutinise the clinical signs of visible peristaltic waves across the abdominal wall. A palpable pyloric tumour and distended epigastrium may be observed. The diagnosis is invariably confirmed by these clinical signs. If the pyloric mass can not be palpated, radiographic investigations may be required to confirm the diagnosis. In some instances, barium meal and x-ray may be performed. Surgical intervention by pyloromyotomy is performed to release the stricture in the circular muscle band.

PATHOPHYSIOLOGY

Pyloric stenosis occurs when the circular band of muscle around the pylorus hypertrophies. This causes significant narrowing of the lumen of the pyloric canal between the stomach and the duodenum. This leads to obstruction with gastric distension and dilatation.[1] In time, gastric inflammation and oedema will contribute to total obstruction of the lumen.[4]

PREOPERATIVE NURSING CARE

See care of the child undergoing abdominal surgery at the end of this chapter.

Fluid deficit related to prolonged vomiting

- Administer intravenous fluids, including electrolyte additives. Excessive vomiting will lead to serious depletion of chloride, sodium and potassium and electrolytes contained in gastric secretions. Loss of hydrogen ions is subsequent to electrolyte depletion and will result in metabolic alkalosis.
- Monitor a strict fluid balance chart.
- A nasogastric tube may be introduced in order to decompress the distended stomach. The patency is maintained by flushing the tube with 1 mL of sterile water and the drainage is recorded hourly.
- Keep the infant nil by mouth. There is a temptation with these infants who are characteristically unsettled because of hunger to put glycerine on a dummy to help them settle. Glycerine with its high osmolality will draw fluid from the gut and exacerbate the infant's vomiting. The use of glycerine is controversial and its use should be minimal.
- Observe and document the frequency of vomiting and the volume. Include a description of content, such as the presence of blood, which may have a coffee ground appearance.
- Record the number and description of the stools.

Parental anxiety related to infant's illness

- Comprehensively describe to the family the mechanical malfunction in feeding due to the presence of the pyloric tumour. Assure the parents, the mother in particular, that the infant's illness is not a reflection on parenting ability.
- Encourage the family to continue to render love and care to the infant. In so doing the parents will retain control and involvement with their new infant without interruption to the process of bonding. By encouraging 'hands on' care, the parents' confidence in handling their sick infant will be enhanced.
- Confirm the family's understanding of, and consent for surgery.
- Ensure the family is fully informed about diagnostic investigation results.
- Inform the family of the time the infant is scheduled for surgery. Include an estimation of the duration of the operation, where the family can wait and seek refreshment and the recovery room routine.

POSTOPERATIVE NURSING CARE

See care of the child undergoing abdominal surgery at the end of this chapter.

Vomiting related to anaesthesia and residual gastric irritation

- Reinstitute breast feeding or formula in accordance with the surgeon's recommendation.
- Ensure the parents are alerted to the possibility of further vomiting for the first 24 to 48 hours. Explain to the parents that if this occurs it is not related to feeding, or a recurrence of the preoperative condition.
- Observe closely for frequency of vomiting; how the infant vomits, i.e., projectile or simply regurgitation; whether the vomitus contains old blood.
- Encourage the parents to touch and hold the infant. Assist the parents in re-establishing the infant's routine, including play, which can include the use of activity sets and musical mobiles.

Short Bowel Syndrome

Short bowel syndrome involves a loss of up to 50% of small bowel as a result of surgical resection. The consequence is a diminished capacity for normal digestion and an acquired malabsorption. The major reasons for substantial small bowel resection are:

1. Gastrointestinal disorders or malformations of early infancy, e.g., necrotising enterocolitis, intestinal atresias, gastroschisis.
2. Intussusception with gangrenous small bowel or Crohn's disease, which occur in age groups beyond the neonatal period.

If more than 75% of the small bowel is removed, malabsorption will occur. The remaining intestine will hypertrophy, increasing in length and diameter, and adapt to a compensatory function of absorption.[4]

NURSING MANAGEMENT

In addition to routine postoperative care, the nursing management for short bowel syndrome can be classified according to short and long-term considerations. The immediate priority of care is to establish and maintain the child's nutritional status. The ultimate aim is to eventually achieve a normal diet. This may take years, depending on the degree of bowel resected.

For both the infant and older child, a healthy diet and adequate nutrition will be related to the degree of malabsorption. As intestinal adaptation can take up to 12 months after initial bowel resection, long-term hyperalimentation and lipid infusion will supplement the gradual re-introduction of diet. The infant will begin oral feeds of dilute formula, the strength of which will be increased in accordance with the infant's ability to tolerate feeding. This is also the case with the older child's ability to tolerate the re-introduction of food. The infant's or child's progress is gauged by the amount, consistency and frequency of diarrhoea as evidence of malabsorption and daily measurement of weight, height and head circumference as indicators of growth and development.

Where diarrhoea is a persistent problem, close monitoring of electrolytes and fluid balance is essential.

Nursing care in the acute phase involves immediate post abdominal surgery care and ongoing care of the child:

- with central venous access
- who is nutritionally compromised as a result of malabsorption
- with a potential for dehydration and electrolyte imbalance as a result of chronic diarrhoea
- who is at risk of infection as a result of prolonged hospitalisation, presence of a central venous access, and abdominal suture line.

Long-term care includes ongoing nutritional supplementation. To achieve this, the cooperation and daily involvement of the parents and family is essential. A nutritional regimen will need to be planned in conference between dietitian, social worker, medical officer, nursing staff in both the hospital and community, and the family.

The infant or child with short bowel syndrome will need long-term ongoing care requiring continuous contact and consultation with the above mentioned health care professionals. The impact on the lifestyle of the infant or child and the family will be considerable. These families need particular support and assistance once the infant or child is discharged from hospital and care begins at home. Discharge planning should commence when the diagnosis of intestinal disorder is first made.

The parents will need comprehensive education about:

- Nutrition, including what total parenteral nutrition (TPN) consists of and why it is the method of choice.
- Central line care and how to recognise and avoid potential infection, connect and administer TPN and troubleshoot when difficulties such as a blocked line arise. Parents and the child are advised about daily living activities such as bathing and the need to keep the line dry.
- The nature of diarrhoea including the colour, consistency and frequency.
- The signs of impending dehydration such as dry skin and mucous membranes, dark circles around sunken eyes and reduced urinary output.
- The importance of contacting nursing staff if they have any worries or queries is reinforced to the parents.

Intussusception

Intussusception is the invagination of one portion of the bowel into another. The most common site is at the ileocaecal valve where the ileum telescopes into the caecum and then into the colon. This is termed ileocolic intussusception. Other classifications include: colocolic, where the colon invaginates into colon; and ileoileum, where the ileum invaginates into ileum though this is uncommon.

The invagination compresses the bowel and restricts the blood supply. The bowel involved becomes oedematous and friable. Incarceration causes necrosis and haemorrhage, resulting in the passing of stool which contains blood and mucus, classically described as 'red current jelly' stool. If left untreated, the bowel may perforate, resulting in peritonitis and death. Intussusception is the most common cause of intestinal obstruction in infants and small children. The incidence is more frequent in boys.[1]

NURSING ASSESSMENT

The classical presentation is one of paroxysmal abdominal pain in an otherwise healthy child. The infant or child may scream, drawing the knees up during the spasm. Between spasms the child will appear to be normal and comfortable. During this episode the child may vomit and pass a normal stool. The longer the obstruction is present, the more the vomiting will increase, the child will pass red current jelly stools and become pale, lethargic and weak. The abdomen becomes tender and distended, and a sausage-shaped mass may be palpated in the right upper quadrant.[1]

MEDICAL INTERVENTION

If the obstruction is diagnosed within 24 hours and there is no evidence of perforation and peritonitis, reduction by air under pressure is undertaken. Reduction by air is the preferred method of treatment. A catheter is inserted into the rectum. The child's buttocks are taped firmly together to prevent leakage. Air is delivered into the bowel by a small positive pressure pump to insufflate the bowel. The process observed via an image intensifier to identify reflux of air into the small bowel. Alternatively, barium may be used and is administered via the same method. The force of the flow of air or barium is sufficient to force the telescoped portion of bowel back to its original place. At the same time serial radiographs monitor the procedure. Charcoal may be administered orally. Once the charcoal has been passed as a bowel motion, this indicates that the reduction of the intussusecption has taken place. This is usually referred to as a 'charcoal marker'.

In fewer than 10% of cases who have undergone air or barium enema, reduction will the condition recur. Parents should be informed that surgical intervention may prove necessary.[1]

NURSING INTERVENTION

Nursing care of the child who has had reduction of intussusception is consistent with care of the child undergoing abdominal surgery. In addition, the nurse should monitor the child closely for signs of further intestinal obstruction. These may include vomiting, abdominal distension, abdominal pain and increased restlessness. In the event of a recurrence of the obstruction, bowel resection and anastomosis will be necessary. A stool chart should be maintained, recording the description of the stool, colour and consistency. If the infant has had a charcoal marker, once the charcoal is seen in the bowel motion the result is documented and the medical officer notified. A normal stool with or without charcoal may indicate a spontaneous resolution.[1]

Inguinal Hernia

PATHOPHYSIOLOGY

Inguinal hernia occurs when there is a complete or incomplete failure of the processus vaginalis to obliterate. There is a potential for bowel to enter the inguinal canal and be manifested as a palpable bulge or mass in the groin. Inguinal hernia is more common in males, and especially in pre-term infants. Like hydroceles, inguinal hernias are painless and the infant or child remains asymptomatic. The palpable mass is prominent during periods of activity and disappears after a period of rest.

Unlike hydrocele, inguinal hernia is repairable. Occasionally, the portion of bowel which has entered the inguinal canal becomes obstructed and strangulates. The infant or child will demonstrate signs and symptoms of bowel obstruction such as colicky abdominal pain, abdominal distension, vomiting and dehydration. Immediate surgical intervention is necessary to release the strangulated bowel and prevent gangrene.[4]

The anatomical location of a mass and a detailed history supplied by the parents will confirm the medical diagnosis. In the infant, the mass will suddenly appear during activity, particularly crying. In the older child, the mass appears during exercise. The size of the mass fluctuates as bowel enters and leaves the sac. There are also periods when the mass intermittently returns to the abdomen completely.

The infant or child will not become symptomatic unless the bowel strangulates.[6] On confirmation of a diagnosis of strangulation, surgical intervention must be prompt to prevent complications. At operation the surgeon may choose to explore both inguinal canals as bilateral occurrence is common.[4] See care of the infant or child undergoing abdominal surgery at the end of this chapter.

Hydrocele

PATHOPHYSIOLOGY

Hydrocele is a common cause of painless swelling of the scrotum.[6] It occurs when there is a fault in the closure of the lumen of the processus vaginalis.[1]

There are 2 types of hydrocele in children:

1. Non-communicating, common in infants, occurring when the tunica vaginalis contains peritoneal fluid and the processus vaginalis has been obliterated.[4]

Non-communicating hydroceles usually resolve spontaneously.

2. Communicating, where the processus vaginalis remains intact, peritoneal fluid may gravitate or be forced by intra-abdominal pressure down the processus to collect around the testes. Scrotal swelling appears greater after episodes of crying or general activity. The swelling subsides after a period of rest as the fluid is reabsorbed into adjacent tissues.[6]

NURSING ASSESSMENT AND INTERVENTION

Inadequate parental understanding of hydrocele

The nurse rendering care to the infant or child with a hydrocele should assess the parents' understanding of the malady and provide information regarding the temporary nature of a hydrocele and that there is invariably spontaneous resolution.

Hydroceles are not surgically reducible. If they do not spontaneously resolve after 12 months, surgical intervention is indicated to prevent further accumulation of fluid in the scrotum and to reduce the risk of herniation.[4] Surgical repair involves closure of the connecting defect to prevent any further collection of fluid in the scrotum.[1] In the event the infant or child requires surgical correction, it is commonly performed as a day-stay procedure.

Abdominal Surgery

PREOPERATIVE NURSING CARE

Maintenance of patient safety related to undergoing abdominal surgery

The aim of preoperative care is to fully prepare the infant or child and their family in order to optimise a safe postoperative outcome and a positive experience during hospitalisation.

- Record vital signs, including temperature, pulse, respirations and blood pressure as well as weight as baseline parameters for comparison in the postoperative phase.
- Confirm by checking in the patient's notes that written consent for surgery has been given by the parent or guardian. If no consent has been signed, request the child's personal physician and/or a resident medical officer to explain the procedure in order to have informed consent.
- Carry out any procedural preparation such as bowel washouts, skin preparation, blood tests, preoperative medication, which are necessary and document the outcome.
- Bath or shower the infant or child, check for loose teeth, clothe in accordance with the policy of the hospital. Where possible, keep the child in their own pyjamas if this is preferred.
- Arrange for any additional information necessary for surgery, such as x-rays and ultrasound, pathology results to be readily available before transferring the child to the operating suite.

- Check that the child is identified correctly with identification bracelets and, where necessary, has an allergy alert. If the child has a favourite toy, make sure this too is identified and labelled and ready to go to operating suite with the child.
- Spend as much time as possible with the child and family in order to develop a relationship centred on mutual trust.

Apprehension and fear related to hospitalisation and surgery

Honest, accurate information will better equip the child and family to contend with the unknown of a therapeutic treatment regimen.

- Encourage the child and family to ask questions and give them explanations about hospitalisation. During the discussion, explain the likely outcomes of the surgical procedure. For example, children admitted with appendicitis should be informed that they may have some soreness postoperatively.
- Include in the interview questions which will help to establish the child and family's understanding of the underlying disease process and the necessity for surgery.
- Provide additional information which will enhance the child and family's sense of involvement and control over the events they will experience. Make it very clear that the parents will take an active role in helping the infant or child recover.
- Discuss the postoperative phase and how the child's recovery will be experienced. Describe what they can expect when waking up in the recovery room such as feeling drowsy and being attached to monitoring devices, infusion pumps and other equipment. Confirm with the family that parents are allowed to be with the infant or child once in the recovery room.
- Describe the presence of drainage tubes, nasogastric tube, stoma, intravenous therapy and medication which are anticipated in accordance with the child's condition.

Pain/discomfort related to preoperative preparation and surgical procedure

Both child and parent need to have a realistic view of pain and pain control. By facilitating their understanding the family will be confident and reassured about comfort and a pain-free recovery.

- Discuss the physical discomfort which will be experienced as the result of drainage tubes and other devices *in situ*. Mention the effect this will have on mobility and movement. Reinforce the fact that it will be temporary.
- Explain that there will be pain postoperatively. Describe the efficiency of methods of analgesic relief such as a patient-controlled analgesia systems, epidural narcotic infusion or peripheral narcotic infusion. Where possible, establish which method will be used and explain it more fully. Make it quite clear that all efforts will be made to keep the child pain-free.

POSTOPERATIVE NURSING CARE

Maintenance of patient safety in the immediate recovery phase

Being fully cognisant of the infant or child's condition after surgery will enhance the efficiency of total patient care. This is best achieved by close observation of the child. Involving the parents in the care will reinforce that they have an important and equal role in the care of their child.

*Patient-controlled
analgesia.*

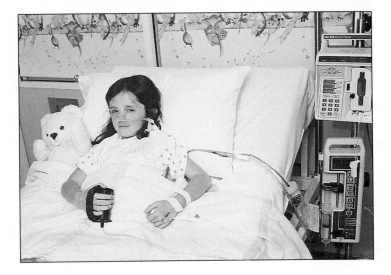

- On return from the recovery room, assess and document hourly temperature, pulse, respirations and blood pressure. Using a stethoscope, listen for presence of bowel sounds.
- Take a comprehensive verbal handover report from the recovery nurse. Check the documentation from the operating suite relating to the surgeon's summary of the operation and the presence of drainage tubes, intravenous fluids and condition of the wound.
- Inspect the suture line and wound. Observe the number of sutures, colour and consistency of wound discharge, presence of oedema, and any signs of infection.
- Determine the presence of drainage tubes, drainage or suction systems.
- Inspect the stoma, if applicable, for position and colour (a healthy stoma is pink). The colour and consistency of discharge are noted.
- Check that the nasogastric tube is secured to the child comfortably and without tension. If attached to suction, check the connections and suction pressure. Maintain suction intermittently or continuously. Observe the volume of drainage and record hourly on the fluid balance chart.
- Attend nasal toilets to both nostrils each shift or as necessary to keep the nares free of mucus.
- Re-introduce oral intake in accordance with the protocol of the surgeon. Begin with ice chips, follow with clear fluids and graduate to a normal diet.
- Maintain peripheral or central venous therapy for fluids and the administration of drugs.
- Ascertain the method of pain management and monitor its initial and ongoing effectiveness.
- Provide a quiet and comfortable environment for the infant or child.
- Involve the parents by encouraging them to be present with the infant or child. Give them the opportunity to view the suture line or wound during a dressing. Reiterate the specific technical aspects which are necessary and advantageous to recovery.
- Using age-appropriate language or terminology with which the child is familiar, ascertain initially if flatus has been passed and later when a bowel motion has been passed. Explain to the parents the importance of these observations as confirmation that

normal bowel activity has returned. For the infant, ask the parents to notify nursing staff when these events have taken place.

Pain related to abdominal surgery

- Maintain analgesia with prescribed method, for example, patient-controlled analgesia, epidural infusion, peripheral narcotic infusion.
- Record observations of pulse, respirations and blood pressure to monitor the effectiveness of analgesia.
- Use a pain rating scale to have the child indicate the presence or absence of pain and document accordingly.
- Encourage the child to move and breathe deeply. Teach the child how to use an incentive spirometer and praise the child for effort and cooperation.
- Facilitate the parents holding the baby or young child to give comfort and to maintain their bond and relationship.
- Assist children to change their position in the bed frequently. Turn the baby from side to side.

Possible fluid volume loss related to surgery

- Monitor closely and record fluid balance.
- Maintain intravenous therapy. Ensure the volume of fluid administered hourly is correct for the child's weight.
- Record urine output. Urine output should equal 2 mL/kg/hour.
- Measure and record volume of wound and nasogastric drainage.
- Measure and record vomitus. Observe and document the colour and content.
- Observe for signs of haemorrhage.
- Monitor for dehydration.
- Keep the child or baby nil by mouth until intestinal function is re-established. Gradually re-introduce oral intake. Begin with ice chips and clear fluids as tolerated. Record fluids on the fluid balance chart.
- Re-introduce a light diet, graduating to a normal diet, once bowel activity is established. This is carried out in accordance with the postoperative plan and the individual needs of the infant or child.

REFERENCES

1. Mott SR, James SR, Sperhac AM. *Nursing care of children and families.* 2nd ed. Menlo Park: Addison-Wesley, 1990.
2. Tortora GJ, Anagnostakos NP. *Principles of anatomy.* 7th ed. New York: Harper and Rowe, 1993.
3. Dodge J. Vomiting and regurgitation disease. *In:* Walker WA, Durie PR, Hamilton JR, Walker-Smith JA, Watkin JB. *Paediatric gastrointestinal disorders: pathophysiology, diagnosis, management.* Vol. 1. Toronto: Becker, 1991.
4. Wong D. *Whaley and Wong's nursing care of infants and children.* 5th ed. St Louis: Mosby, 1995.
5. Hillemeier C. Paediatric gastrointestinal disease. *In:* Walker et. al. *Pathophysiology, diagnosis, management.* Vol. 1. Toronto: Becker, 1991.
6. Hutson J, Beasley S. *The surgical examination of children.* Oxford: Heinemann Medical Books, 1988.

7. Sonheimer J. Paediatric gastrointestinal disease. *In:* Walker et. al. *Pathophysiology, diagnosis, management.* Vol. 1. Toronto: Becker, 1991.
8. Spino M. Paediatric gastrointestinal disease. *In:* Walker et. al. *Pathophysiology, diagnosis, management.* Vol. 1. Toronto: Becker, 1991.

Disturbances in Genitourinary Function

Jill Farquhar

Renal Biopsy

Percutaneous renal biopsy is a relatively simple investigative procedure performed to diagnose renal disease, monitor the disease progress and plan the most appropriate therapy.[1]

A small cylindrical piece of kidney tissue is obtained by passing a fine needle through the skin and into the kidney. Although simple, the procedure is potentially hazardous and therefore is not a routine investigation for children presenting with renal disease.

In most centres, transplanted kidneys are biopsied routinely during the immediate post-transplantation period and whenever graft rejection is suspected.

RENAL BIOPSY PROCEDURE

Once the child is sedated he or she is positioned face down on the bed or examination table with a sandbag underneath the abdomen. The purpose of the sandbag is to immobilise the child's kidney against his or her back.[2]

Children undergoing a biopsy of a transplant kidney lie on their backs for the procedure, because the graft is placed in the iliac region.

The child's skin is prepared with antiseptic lotion before administering local anaesthetic. After administration of local anaesthetic, a small skin incision is made with a scalpel blade. An exploring needle is inserted to assess the depth of the kidney below the skin. The needle will display a characteristic swing when it is in the kidney.[2]

The biopsy needle is inserted through the incision and pushed into the kidney tissue when the child inspires. The biopsy needle either has cutting blades which grasp tissue from the kidney, or cuts the tissue with the aid of suction.[3] The needle is usually inserted twice, so that 2 cores of tissue may be obtained.[4]

The needle is removed and the biopsy tissue is placed into saline and then preservative. Renal tissue may be examined by light microscopy, fluorescence microscopy and electron microscopy.[5]

NURSING RESPONSIBILITIES BEFORE RENAL BIOPSY

Blood pressure recordings

- On admission.
- Every four hours before the biopsy.
- Abnormally high blood pressure must be reported to medical staff.

Rationale: High pressure within the blood vessels may make it difficult to control blood loss from the vessels that are cut by the biopsy needle.[3]

The biopsy would most likely be postponed until the blood pressure is controlled.

Urinalysis

Test urine with a dipstick for the presence of blood.

Rationale: Haematuria is a reasonably common complication following a renal biopsy. Testing the urine before the biopsy enables the nurse to assess whether haematuria occurs as a result of the child's disease process, or as a complication of the procedure.

Skin preparation

The child should be bathed before the biopsy, and be dressed in pyjamas or a gown which is easily removable to prepare the skin for the procedure.

Rationale: Prevent bacteria entering the kidney from the skin via the biopsy needle.

Sedation

Children undergoing renal biopsy are usually sedated before the procedure. The nurse responsible for assisting with the biopsy should remain with the child at all times after the sedation has been administered. Oxygen and resuscitation equipment must be readily accessible.

Rationale: Sedation prevents the child from becoming distressed and ensures that the child does not struggle or move during the procedure. The child requires constant observation following the administration of sedation because the sedative may decrease the child's respiratory rate.

Informed consent (medical intervention)

Informed consent must be obtained from both child and parents prior to the procedure.

Rationale: To ensure that the child and family have a clear understanding of this invasive procedure and it's potential complications.

NURSING CARE AFTER RENAL BIOPSY

Pressure dressing

A pressure dressing is applied to the renal biopsy site. The dressing should remain in place for 48 hours. In the case of renal transplant biopsy, a small sandbag is applied over the biopsy site for 4 hours after the biopsy.

Rationale: The pressure dressing promotes healing of kidney tissue and prevents bleeding by occluding small blood vessels which may have been cut by the biopsy needle.

Bed rest

The child must rest in bed for 24 hours. If macroscopic haematuria is present, then bed rest should continue.

Rationale: Haemorrhage is prevented by reduced activity because cardiac output is lowered at rest. Damaged tissue and vessels heal more readily when less energy is spent on physical activity.

Observation of vital signs

Blood pressure, pulse and respiratory rate should be checked every 5 minutes for the first 15 minutes following the renal biopsy, and then every 15 minutes for one hour. If vital signs are within normal limits after the first hour, observations of pulse and respirations should continue every hour for 24 hours. Blood pressure and temperature should be recorded every 4 hours.

Rationale: If bleeding occurs due to perforation of blood vessels by the biopsy needle, signs of haemorrhage will occur in the immediate post biopsy period. Signs of haemorrhage are a weak and rapid pulse rate and low blood pressure. These symptoms must be referred to medical staff immediately.

Test all urine for blood

All urine voided during the 24-hour-period following the biopsy must be tested with a dip stick to check for the presence of blood. If macroscopic haematuria occurs, then 25 mL of the blood-stained urine should be poured into a container which is labelled with the date and time the urine was voided.

Rationale: Haematuria indicates that trauma has occurred to the kidney during the biopsy. Macroscopic haematuria indicates more severe trauma or serious haemorrhage and must be referred to medical staff for emergency intervention.

Urine should be saved for inspection so that the severity of bleeding may be estimated.[4] Dark blood indicates old blood and that bleeding has ceased. Bright red blood in the urine indicates that the child is still losing blood from the kidney.

Record urine volume

All urine voided after the biopsy should be measured and recorded on a chart.

Rationale: A sudden drop in urine output, or no urine output following the biopsy may indicate a clot in the ureter or urethra causing obstruction to the flow of urine.

Report pain

If the child complains of loin pain or colic the complaint must be referred to medical staff.

Rationale: Pain or colic following a renal biopsy indicates clots in the ureter.[6]

Increase fluid intake

Oral fluid intake should be encouraged during the 24 hours following the biopsy.

Rationale: Increased fluid intake prevents clot formation by encouraging an increased production of dilute urine.[4]

INVESTIGATIONS

Ultrasound

Ultrasound is performed prior to a renal biopsy to ensure that the child has two kidneys of normal size. A repeat ultrasound is performed just before the biopsy to check the position of the kidneys and mark the lower pole of the kidney so that the biopsy tissue can be obtained from an area away from the major blood vessels.[7]

Clotting studies

Clotting studies and a skin bleeding time must be performed before the biopsy. The child must have normal clotting and skin bleeding times. If bleeding time is prolonged, the biopsy is postponed. Vitamin K may be administered to promote clotting. The medical officer admitting the child to the ward should ensure that the child has not taken aspirin, nor any other anticoagulant during the week before the biopsy. If so, the biopsy is postponed and anticoagulant medication withheld until clotting study results are normal.

POTENTIAL COMPLICATIONS OF RENAL BIOPSY

Haemorrhage

There is a risk that minor bleeding will occur following renal biopsy because the kidneys contain numerous small blood vessels which may be punctured by the biopsy needle. Bleeding presents as microscopic or in some cases macroscopic haematuria and usually does not persist beyond 24 to 48 hours after the biopsy. A pressure dressing is always applied over the biopsy site and this is usually effective in controlling minor bleeding.

Rarely, a larger blood vessel may inadvertently be punctured during the biopsy and more serious haemorrhage may occur. Blood transfusion or surgical intervention may be required to control blood loss in these cases. On extremely rare occasions a kidney may be severely damaged during a renal biopsy and may have to be removed if bleeding cannot be controlled.

Clot formation

Haematuria following a renal biopsy may occasionally cause clot formation. If blood clots occur they are usually small and passed in the child's urine, larger clots may obstruct the ureter. The child's fluid intake should be increased in an effort to prevent clots forming.

Arteriovenous fistula formation

Although rare, the insertion of the biopsy needle may cause a fistula to form between a renal arteriole and venule. This complication is suspected when hypertension develops after the biopsy in a child who has previously had normal blood pressure. An audible bruit may be heard over the kidney. The fistula may close spontaneously or require surgical closure.

Infection

Infection may be introduced into the kidney and then spread into the systemic circulation. This complication is prevented by careful preparation of the child's skin and by the use of aseptic technique by the nephrologist performing the biopsy.

Pain

Children often complain of mild discomfort over the biopsy site. However, in some cases the pain is more severe and may indicate bleeding or clot formation.[8] Loin pain may indicate that a clot is obstructing a ureter.

INDICATIONS FOR PERFORMING RENAL BIOPSY IN CHILDREN

- Steroid-resistant nephrotic syndrome.
- Haematuria or proteinuria of unexplained origin.
- Glomerulonephritis (except post-streptococcal glomerulonephritis).
- Hypertension.
- Renal transplant rejection.

CONTRAINDICATIONS TO PERFORMING RENAL BIOPSY IN CHILDREN

- Polycystic kidneys (the cysts may bleed).
- Children with advanced renal failure (biopsy has no therapeutic value).
- Single kidney.[7]
- Children with bleeding disorders.[9]
- Hydronephrosis.
- Severe, uncontrolled hypertension.[9]
- Children that have taken aspirin, or anticoagulant medication.

REFERENCES

1. Brown CB. *Manual of renal disease*. Melbourne: Churchill Livingstone, 1985.
2. Hamilton HK. *Nurses clinical library. Renal and urology disorders*. Pennsylvania: Springhouse Corporation, 1984.
3. Uldall R. *Renal nursing*. 3rd ed. Oxford: Blackwell Scientific, 1988.
4. Montgomery Possey B, Guzzella CE, Vaderstaay Kernery C. *Critical care nursing*. 3rd ed. Philadelphia: Lippincott, 1990.
5. Davison AM. *Nephrology*. London: Heinemann Medical Books, 1988.
6. Brunner LS, Suddarth DS. *Textbook of medical — surgical nursing*. 7th ed. Philadelphia: Lippincott, 1992.
7. Newsam JE, Petrie JJB. *Urology and renal medicine*. 3rd ed. Edinburgh. Churchill Livingstone, 1981.
8. Davison AM. *A synopsis of renal diseases*. Bristol: John Wright, 1981.
9. Evans DB, Henderson RG. *Lecture notes on nephrology*. Oxford: Blackwell Scientific, 1988.

Renal Replacement Therapy

When a child's kidneys are destroyed by disease over a period of time (chronic renal failure), or fail temporarily because of acute, reversible renal failure, medical and nursing staff are presented with the challenge of replacing kidney function by artificial means in an effort to restore homeostasis and maintain life.

A variety of renal replacement therapies is available and the therapy of choice will depend on the child's clinical status, physician or client preference, equipment available and the medical and nursing expertise available at the treatment centre.

The following renal replacement therapies will be discussed: peritoneal dialysis; haemodialysis; haemofiltration; and renal transplantation.

Dialysis is a term used to describe a process of filtering accumulated waste products of metabolism, and controlling fluid and electrolyte balance in the blood by artificial means. Three physical principles are used in dialysis — diffusion, osmosis and hydrostatic pressure.[1] These processes filter accumulated solutes and water in the child's blood from one side of a semipermeable membrane into an artificial solution which has been introduced to the opposite side of the semipermeable membrane. The use of a semipermeable membrane ensures that substances which are required by the body such as red blood cells and proteins are not removed from the blood because the membrane is impermeable to them.

Dialysis replaces some of the functions performed by the kidneys, but it cannot replace renal function completely. Dialysis can not reverse renal failure, activate Vitamin D or correct renal anaemia. The goals of dialysis are to:

1. Remove accumulated waste products from the blood. Examples of waste products which are removed by dialysis are urea, creatinine, potassium and phosphate.
2. Correct acidosis by the addition of buffers such as sodium bicarbonate, lactate and acetate to the dialysate.
3. Remove excess fluid from the blood.
4. Remove drugs that are normally excreted by the kidneys in acute poisoning.

Indications that children require dialysis are:

1. Chronic renal failure where kidney function has fallen to between 10% and 25% of normal.[2]
2. Elevated serum urea and creatinine levels.
3. Hyperkalaemia which cannot be controlled by diet or medication.
4. Severe acidosis.
5. If children display complications of high blood levels of urea such as bleeding tendency, pericarditis or encephalopathy.
6. Hypertension, which is believed to be caused by intravascular fluid volume excess and cannot be controlled by medication or diet and fluid restrictions.[3]
7. Failure to thrive.
8. Reduced growth velocity.[3]
9. Head circumference not increasing.[4]
10. Lack of attainment of developmental milestones.

An understanding of the following terms provides nurses with the necessary knowledge to assess the nursing needs of children on dialysis accurately, so that safe nursing practice is performed.

Osmosis: The movement of water across a semipermeable membrane from an area of low particle concentration to an area of high particle concentration.[5] In dialysis, excess water leaves the child's blood and enters the dialysate.

Diffusion: The movement of particles from an area of high concentration to an area of lower particle concentration.[6]

Semipermeable membrane: A membrane which has tiny holes (pores) in it. When the membrane is used for dialysis, small particles (e.g., waste products and water) are able to cross the membrane, while larger molecules such as blood cells and proteins are too large to fit through the pores.

Hydrostatic pressure: The pressure exerted by the weight of a column of water in its container. This pressure may be either positive or negative.[7]

Ultrafiltration: Rapid removal of water by hydrostatic pressure.

Dialysate: A manufactured physiological solution. Dialysate and blood are on opposite sides of a semipermeable membrane during dialysis.

Peritoneum: The peritoneum is a double-layered, semipermeable serous membrane, which is rich in capillaries and lines the abdominal cavity. The space between the visceral and parietal layers of peritoneum is called the peritoneal cavity.

'Dry' (ideal) weight: This term refers to the weight the child would be if he or she had a normal urine output and did not have any fluid retention as a result of diminished renal function. Children are thought to be at their 'dry' weight when they have a normal blood pressure for age and size and have no evidence of oedema. 'Dry' weight must be reviewed regularly because it increases as children grow. If, however, a child loses his or her appetite (common in renal failure), there is a loss of body mass and therefore 'dry' weight decreases.

Dialysis disequilibrium syndrome: Changes in solute concentration occurring between the plasma and dialysate during dialysis are followed by a similar equilibration between the interstitial fluid and the plasma. As a consequence of these plasma changes, solutes in the intracellular water pass through the cell wall into the interstitial water.[8] If dialysis removes solutes from the extracellular fluid compartment too efficiently, the osmolality in this compartment drops more rapidly than the intracellular osmolality, causing the cells to swell. The cellular swelling can occur in the brain, causing raised intracranial pressure, which may be accompanied by headache, confusion, irritability, nausea, vomiting and seizures.

PERITONEAL DIALYSIS

Peritoneal dialysis is used to treat both acute and chronic renal failure. It is particularly useful for infants and small children in whom vascular access is difficult to achieve and maintain.

A catheter is inserted between the two layers of peritoneum and dialysate is aseptically administered. The dialysate remains inside the peritoneum for between 30 minutes and 4 hours, then it is drained out and fresh dialysate is administered.

Diffusion of accumulated waste products of metabolism occurs from the blood within the capillaries of the peritoneum into the dialysate. Excess fluid is removed from the child's blood by osmosis. This is achieved by raising the osmolality of the peritoneal dialysis fluid by the addition of glucose. Fluid particles move out of the blood and into the dialysate in an attempt to dilute the high particle content of the dialysate. The amount of water removed from the child's blood depends on the amount of glucose that has been

Table 6.3 Dialysate glucose concentration and indications for use

Dialysate (g/L)	Glucose (mOsm/L)	Osmolarity	Indications for use
0.5%	5 (hypotonic)	298	Children who require diffusion of solutes but no fluid removal. These children may be dehydrated and some children may absorb fluid from the dialysate into the circulation.
1.5%	15	346 (isotonic)	Children who require only a small to moderate amount of fluid removal. Children have normal blood pressure for age and size.
2.5%	25	396 (hypertonic)	Children who require a moderate to large amount of fluid removal. These children may have hypertension and moderate oedema.
4.25%	42.5	485 (hypertonic)	Children who require a large amount of fluid removal. Children may have a grossly oedematous appearance, and have hypertension. 4.25% dialysate should be used with caution as it may remove excessive amounts of fluid too rapidly.

added to the dialysate. Dialysate is presently available in 4 concentrations of glucose (**Table 6.3**).

Please note: Infants and neonates have a lower rate of fluid removal compared to adults and children over 3 years of age.[9] This is thought to be related to a more rapid absorption of glucose from the dialysate into the blood. More frequent dialysis exchanges with a higher dialysate concentration are often required in infants to prevent body fluid volume excess.

Table 6.4 lists the solute content of peritoneal dialysis fluid and aims to provide nurses with a clearer understanding of the dialysis procedure by stating the rationale for the use of each substance.

Access for peritoneal dialysis

Soft catheters for long-term dialysis

Access to the peritoneal cavity for dialysis is achieved by a surgical procedure under general anaesthesia. A soft, cuffed silastic catheter (Tenckhoff catheter), with perforations at the distal end, is inserted between the 2 layers of peritoneum (**Figure 6.36**). A variety of sizes is available with 1 or 2 dacron cuffs to secure the catheter in place and act as a barrier to infection. It should be inserted away from the nappy area to avoid infection. A guide for catheter selection is the weight of the child: 3 kg or less — neonatal catheter; 3 to 12 kg — paediatric catheter: and over 12 kg — adult catheter.

It is common practice to administer an intravenous antibiotic at the time of catheter insertion as prophylaxis against infection.

Table 6.4 Dialysis fluid content

Substance	Amount per litre	Rationale for use
Sodium	132 mmol	To maintain electrolyte balance.
Chloride	96 mmol	To maintain electrolyte balance.
Calcium	1.75 mmol	To maintain calcium balance. If the child has a low serum calcium level, calcium will move from the dialysate and into the blood.
Magnesium	0.25 mmol	Maintain normal magnesium levels in the blood.
Lactate	4 mmol	Buffers hydrogen ions.
Potassium	May be added as prescribed. (Dosage depends on the child's serum potassium level)	Added to dialysate if the child has a low serum potassium level. Potassium will move into the blood from the dialysate by diffusion across the semipermeable membrane.
Antibiotic	May be added to dialysate. (Dosage depends on the antibiotic used)	To treat infection of the peritoneum (peritonitis).
Heparin	May be added to dialysate (500 U/L is commonly prescribed).	To prevent fibrin clot formation in the catheter lumen. Heparin is usually added for 48 hours following peritoneal catheter insertion, if the child has peritonitis or whenever fibrin clots are observed in the dialysate effluent.

Note: Peritoneal dialysis fluid also contains glucose in varying amounts (*Table 6.3*).

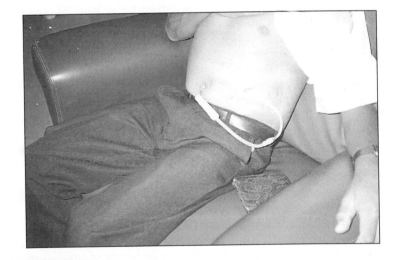

Figure 6.36 A Tenckhoff peritoneal catheter in position.

Care of peritoneal dialysis catheters

Meticulous care of the Tenckhoff catheter is important to avoid infection. A common regimen for catheter exit site care is as follows:

- Do not disturb the dressing covering the catheter for approximately 1 week after insertion unless there is leakage from the dressing or the child has a fever. A clear dressing enables daily inspection of the site.

- Curl the catheter around and tape it to avoid dragging and traction on the exit site.
- Keep the catheter site exit dry for 4 to 6 weeks. Showering or bathing is not permitted during this period. Once the dialysis nurse specialist has assessed the exit site, and has given permission for bathing, the site should be cleaned daily in the shower with antibacterial soap.
- Care should be taken to completely dry the exit site after showering.
- Apply antiseptic solution to the exit site daily.
- Apply a clean gauze dressing daily.
- Inspect the catheter exit site daily, looking for signs of redness or exudate.
- If possible, children should shower rather than bathe, but infants and small children may bathe after an initial period of healing. Swimming is at the discretion of the dialysis nurse specialist.

Acute catheters

Children not fit for general anaesthesia have a temporary catheter inserted at the bedside. This type of catheter is a semi-rigid plastic catheter with a central metal stylet which pierces the abdominal wall as it is inserted.[8] Because of the risk of infection, this type of catheter usually remains *in situ* for no longer than 48 to 72 hours.[10]

Initiating peritoneal dialysis

Peritoneal dialysis is initiated once the peritoneal dialysis catheter has been successfully inserted into the peritoneum and catheter patency has been confirmed. In children with chronic renal failure, dialysis is withheld for at least 48 hours after the insertion of the Tenckhoff catheter in order to allow healing of tissue and prevent leakage of fluid from the catheter exit site.

Peritoneal dialysis may be performed manually or by a machine specifically designed for this purpose. There are three phases to each dialysis exchange.

1. Fill (inflow) phase. The prescribed volume of dialysate is infused into the peritoneum by releasing a clamp on the dialysis tubing and allowing the fluid, which should be placed at a level above the child's abdomen, to run into the peritoneum by gravity. The duration of this phase depends on the volume of fluid to be infused, correct catheter placement and the size of the dialysis tubing. It usually takes between 5 and 10 minutes. When the prescribed amount of fluid has been delivered, the dialysis tubing should be clamped.

2. Dwell (diffusion) phase. During this phase, the dialysate remains in the peritoneum for a prescribed length of time to allow solute and water exchanges to occur from the blood into the dialysate. Dwell time varies from 30 minutes to 4 hours, depending on how rapidly solutes and fluid are to be removed.

3. Drain (outflow) phase. This is the length of time required to recover the volume of infused dialysate and any extra fluid removed from the circulation by osmosis. The roller clamp on the peritoneal dialysis drainage tubing is released and fluid is allowed to drain by gravity into a waste receptacle which must be placed at a level that is lower than the child's abdomen. The duration of this phase is dependent on the volume of fluid infused, the level of the drainage bag in comparison to the child's abdomen and correct catheter placement. The average outflow phase is 15 to 30 minutes. Usually the outflow volume is equal to or in excess of the volume infused initially.

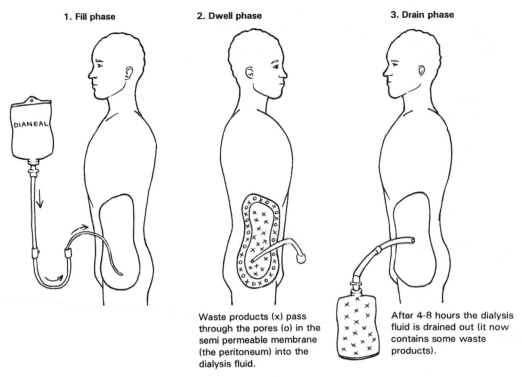

Figure 6.37 Continuous ambulatory peritoneal dialysis.

Peritoneal dialysis techniques

There are many variations of the peritoneal dialysis exchange technique. All of the systems described use a commercially available dialysis fluid (Dianeal). Dianeal is packaged in a similar fashion to solutions for intravenous administration, i.e., in sterile plastic containers. In Australia, Dianeal is available in the following volumes: 500 mL, 1 L, 1500 mL, 2 L and 3 L. Bags of 5 L are also available for use on automated peritoneal dialysis machines.

Dialysate fill volumes for children are prescribed either according to body surface area, or by body weight. In Australia it is most common to prescribe dialysate fill volumes as a dose in mL/kg of body weight.

Peritoneal dialysis techniques for children are usually the same as for adults, but there are some differences to note when performing dialysis on neonates and young infants. These differences are related to the larger ratio of peritoneal surface area to body weight, which may be twice as large in a newborn infant.[11] The larger ratio of peritoneal surface area to weight results in greater dialysis efficiency in infants, and the volume of dialysate they are able to tolerate is higher. The neonate is able to tolerate dialysate volumes of 20 to 100 mL/kg compared to 50 mL/kg in older children.

Manual exchanges using an acute peritoneal dialysis set

This system is most frequently used in the intensive care setting to treat children with acute renal failure in whom rapid removal of fluid and correction of uraemia and electrolyte

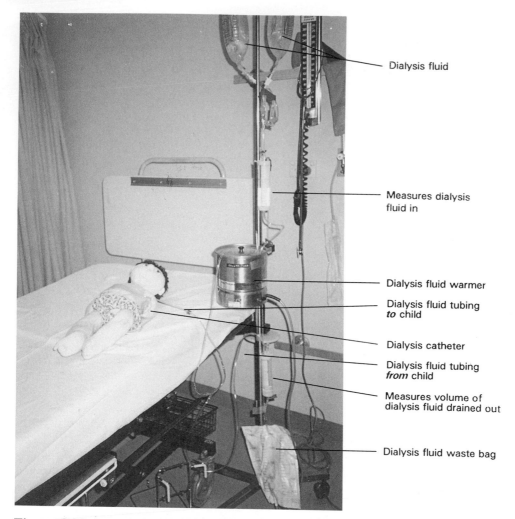

Dialysis fluid

Measures dialysis fluid in

Dialysis fluid warmer

Dialysis fluid tubing *to* child

Dialysis catheter

Dialysis fluid tubing *from* child

Measures volume of dialysis fluid drained out

Dialysis fluid waste bag

Figure 6.38 A manual peritoneal dialysis set up for acute peritoneal dialysis.

imbalance is required. 'Y' tubing with roller clamps for inflow and outflow is used, one end of the tubing is inserted into a bag of dialysis fluid using an aseptic technique (a face mask and gloves should be worn). The middle section of the tubing connects to the peritoneal dialysis catheter, and the section of tubing exiting the catheter is attached to a sterile drainage bag.

Continuous ambulatory peritoneal dialysis (CAPD)

CAPD is used for children with chronic renal failure and those children with acute renal failure who require a prolonged period of dialysis support, e.g., children with haemolytic uraemic syndrome who may require dialysis for 2 or 3 weeks. The procedure is simple and may be performed at home by the child or parents after a period of training.

- A length of sterile dialysis tubing which has a bag of fresh dialysis fluid at one end and an empty drainage bag at the other end is connected to the child's Tenckhoff catheter.
- The CAPD cycle begins by placing the drain container at a level lower than the child's abdomen. The clamp on the tubing is released and the fluid dwelling in the peritoneum drains out into the bag.
- When the drainage phase is complete, the drain tubing is clamped.
- The clamp on the fresh bag of dialysate is released to enable the fluid to run into the child's peritoneum. When the appropriate volume of fluid has run into the peritoneum, the tubing is clamped and a cap is placed on the dialysis catheter.
- The dialysate dwells for 4 hours.
- This technique is repeated 3 or 4 times during the day. For the school-aged child it is preferable to attend a bag change before school, one on return from school and then again before bed. The last exchange dwells inside the peritoneum for about 8 hours. Some children require a 4th bag change in the middle of the day to maintain optimal fluid and electrolyte balance. Unfortunately, this interrupts the school day. CAPD is performed every day of the week.

Strict attention to aseptic technique is applied when changing the dialysis bags in order to prevent bacteria entering the dialysis tubing and migrating into the peritoneum.

Continuous cycling peritoneal dialysis (CCPD)

This technique uses a specifically designed peritoneal dialysis cycling machine, which is set up to perform 4 or more complete dialysis exchanges during the night while the child is sleeping. CCPD may be performed in the home as well as in the hospital setting. The machine can be set up to deliver the correct prescription of dialysate volume, fill/dwell time and drainage time. Safety alarms are incorporated into the machine design so that if there is a problem draining the fluid in or out the machine alerts the operator by sounding an alarm. CCPD treatment is terminated each morning with a prescribed volume of fluid remaining in the child's peritoneum throughout the day.

The advantages of this system are that the child's day is uninterrupted, allowing for normal schooling and interaction with peers. Disadvantages of this system are the cost of the machine, the amount of space that the machine may take up in the child's home, and the possibility of interruption of sleep by machine alarms.

Tidal volume peritoneal dialysis

This technique uses a peritoneal dialysis cycling machine with a tidal volume option programmed into the machine.

Tidal volume peritoneal dialysis differs from other methods of peritoneal dialysis which have 3 complete cycles ending with a drain cycle of up to 30 minutes to allow the dialysate fluid to drain out of the peritoneum completely. In most cases most of the fluid drains out of the peritoneum quite rapidly within the initial half of the cycle, and the remainder drains slowly until the completion of the dwell time. It is felt that this time is wasted because solute removal is not occurring during this period. In tidal peritoneal dialysis the peritoneum is never allowed to empty.

The machine is set up to deliver an initial dialysate volume of 40 to 50 mL/kg.[12] The cycles that follow this are of a smaller volume of 20 mL/kg and are of short duration, for example the period to deliver the fresh dialysate and allow it to dwell within the

Table 6.5 Placement of an acute peritoneal dialysis catheter: nursing responsibilities

Step	Nursing responsibility	Rationale
1. Preparation.		
The child is prepared by careful physical examination by medical staff which should include palpation of bladder and abdomen to assess urinary retention or constipation.	Ensure that the child's bladder is empty by asking the child to void if possible. Insertion of a urinary catheter may be requested by the child's physician.	There is a potential for perforation of bowel, bladder or blood vessel as the catheter is inserted 1 to 10 centimetres below the umbilicus[13] An empty bladder reduces the risk of perforation.
Informed consent must be obtained from the child's parents before the procedure.	Record baseline observations (blood pressure, pulse, respirations, temperature, oxygen saturation). Bare weight.	Signs of bowel perforation, haemorrhage and shock may be recognised promptly during the procedure by alteration in vital signs. A knowledge of vital signs at the beginning of the procedure is necessary for comparison of any alterations that may occur.[14]
		It is necessary to know the child's predialysis weight and blood pressure to assess the child's fluid status so that the appropriate strength of dialysate may be ordered.
2. Administer sedation.	Monitor the child's vital signs regularly.	Children usually require sedation to allay their anxiety and to ensure that they remain still during the procedure to reduce the risk of perforation of bowel, bladder or blood vessel.
		The sedation may depress respirations, so children should be monitored closely following administration.
3. Sterile preparation of the skin before puncture.	Wash the child's skin with surgical soap before the procedure. Have antiseptic solution readily available for further skin preparation just before catheter insertion.	Preparation of the skin minimises skin bacteria and prevents bacterial invasion of the peritoneum by bacteria present on the child's skin.
4. Local anaesthesia is administered.	Reassure the child if awake (this would be unusual).	To prevent pain and distress.

Table 6.5 (*continued*)

Step	Nursing responsibility	Rationale
5. Catheter insertion. Prior to catheter insertion a large bore needle is inserted through the skin and into the peritoneum. Warmed dialysate is then infused into the peritoneum at a volume 25 to 50 mL/kg of body weight. The catheter is then inserted into the peritoneum. The catheter is secured with a purse string suture and a sterile dressing is applied to the catheter site.	Monitor child's pulse, respiratory rate and blood pressure every 5 minutes during the procedure.	The peritoneum is distended with fluid, making catheter insertion easier. Shock, haemorrhage, bladder or bowel perforation may occur during the procedure.
6. Attach dialysis tubing to catheter. The sterile peritoneal dialysis drainage — infusion set is attached to the catheter, and the drainage clamp is released to drain the dialysate out of the peritoneum.	Prior to the procedure prepare the dialysate as follows, using an aseptic technique: • add medications to the dialysate if required. • connect the dialysate to an appropriate dialysis giving set. • prepare fluid warmer and insert the coiled area of the dialysis giving set into the fluid warmer. • place the prepared dialysate by the child's bed ready for use.	Strict asepsis is required to prevent bacterial contamination of the peritoneum. Certain medications such as heparin to prevent clot formation in the catheter are administered via the peritoneal route. Fluid must be warmed to body temperature to avoid hypothermia and shock.
7. Initiate dialysis. More fluid is instilled and then immediately drained out. A 3rd volume of dialysate is instilled and allowed to dwell in the peritoneum for a prescribed time. Dialysis proceeds once catheter function is established.	Observe the drained dialysate for blood staining and volume. Observe the catheter site for leakage. Monitor vital signs.	Assess the patency of the catheter.

peritoneum could be between 20 and 40 minutes, followed by a 10-minute drain cycle. The drain cycle is time regulated rather than regulated by waiting until the peritoneum is empty. There is always a volume of dialysate dwelling in the peritoneum throughout treatment, and this enhances solute removal. At the end of the treatment the dialysate in the peritoneum is completely drained by incorporating a final drain period of a longer duration.

Acute peritoneal dialysis

Children requiring insertion of an acute peritoneal dialysis catheter are critically ill. Both the child and his or her family require a great deal of emotional support during the procedure. Clear information about the procedure may be given using diagrams, books, dolls etc.

Nursing assessment

Before performing each dialysis exchange, the nurse attending the peritoneal dialysis must carry out a careful nursing assessment of the child's current fluid status. The selection of the appropriate concentration of dialysate is dependent on this assessment.

The following observations are made at the completion of the peritoneal dialysis drain phase.

Weight: Children should be bare weighed at the completion of every drain phase. This weight should be compared to the previous weight. Weight loss between dialysis cycles indicates that fluid has been removed by dialysis. Weight gain indicates either that insufficient fluid has been removed by dialysis, which may be related to a catheter problem, or an inappropriate choice of dialysate concentration, or that the child's fluid intake is excessive. Non-compliance with fluid restriction is very common in children with renal failure.

Blood pressure: Blood pressure must be measured using a cuff with an internal bladder that completely encircles the arm and covers 75% of the child's upper arm. High or low blood pressure is reported to the medical staff. Dialysate fluid orders are reviewed carefully by the medical and nursing staff before continuing peritoneal dialysis cycles.

Respiratory effort: Attention is paid to the child's respiratory rate and effort at the completion of dialysate inflow. The presence of dialysate in the peritoneum increases abdominal pressure, creating pressure on the diaphragm and inferior vena cava which may result in hypotension, respiratory embarrassment and impaired gas exchange.[14]

Abdomen: The child's abdomen is assessed for signs of overdistension, which may be caused by the administration of too high a volume of dialysate. Abdominal distension could lead to respiratory distress. Dialysate should be drained out immediately if respiratory distress or overdistension occur. The fill volume should be reviewed to avoid these complications.

The Tenckhoff catheter exit site is examined each day. The exit site should not have any ooze or discharge from it, and there should be no inflammation around it.

Dialysate: Dialysate is examined at each dialysis exchange. The effluent should be clear, not cloudy. Cloudy fluid is indicative of infection and requires prompt initiation of treatment with an appropriate antibiotic.

The volume of fluid is measured and recorded on the dialysis fluid balance sheet. It is abnormal for the dialysate to be blood-stained. Blood staining may occur as a result of abdominal trauma, or in adolescent girls during menstruation because the fallopian tubes open into the peritoneum. Blood-stained dialysate is reported.

HAEMODIALYSIS

Unlike peritoneal dialysis, haemodialysis occurs outside the body (extracorporeal). The child's blood is pumped out of the circulation and through an artificial kidney (dialyser) by a haemodialysis machine. The processes of diffusion and ultrafiltration across a semipermeable membrane occur between the blood and dialysate compartments before pumping the blood back into the circulation. The most widely used dialyser is the hollow-fibre dialyser which consists of hundreds of hollow fibres which are placed inside a hard plastic casing. The fibres are hollow lengthways and each fibre has many tiny pores in it. The pores are permeable to the smaller molecules in the blood which have a molecular weight of up to 500 daltons.[8] Examples of molecules which diffuse across the haemodialyser are urea, electrolytes and creatinine. The dialyser is not permeable to larger molecules such as red blood cells and proteins. Blood is pumped through the inside of the hollow fibres, while dialysate flows over the outside of the fibres. The blood and dialysate do not come into contact with each other because they are on opposite sides of the semipermeable membrane. Water removal occurs by the process of ultrafiltration. An artificially created pressure gradient is applied to the dialysate. The machine applies a negative pressure to the dialysate which pulls water out of the blood and into the dialysate, the pressure can be adjusted according to the amount of fluid removal desired.

Children require haemodialysis treatments for 3 to 5 hours, 3 or 4 times weekly. Although haemodialysis techniques are similar to that of an adult, the child's smaller size and lower circulating blood volume makes haemodialysis technically more difficult. For haemodialysis to occur, blood has to pumped out of the body through sterile plastic blood lines and through the artificial kidney. A standard set of dialysis blood lines and dialyser contains 250 to 300 mL of blood, which is 2% to 5% of an adult's circulating blood volume and is reasonably well tolerated by an adult. However, this amount of blood in the extracorporeal circuit would be equivalent to 30% in a 10 kg child and would not be tolerated. Paediatric and infant blood lines and dialysers are available. The smallest lines available have a volume equivalent to 10% of the child's blood volume. Small children often experience haemodynamic instability during haemodialysis treatments because of the large proportion of their blood volume which is in the extracorporeal circuit.

Vascular access for haemodialysis

In order to perform haemodialysis, access to the child's circulating blood volume must be created to enable blood to be removed from the body and then returned. Achieving a vascular access that will provide an adequate blood flow in small children with small blood vessels is a very difficult task.

The following types of access are currently used for haemodialysis.

Arteriovenous fistula

This is the ideal access for haemodialysis. If the child's vessels are large enough, attempts will be made to create an arteriovenous fistula in children over 20 kg who require long-term haemodialysis.

Table 6.6 Complications of peritoneal dialysis

Problem	Intervention	Rationale
1. Peritonitis (infection of peritoneal membrane). Recognised by: • Cloudy dialysate effluent • Diffuse abdominal pain • Fever One or all of the above may be present in peritonitis[15] The peritoneum is at risk of infection each time the dialysis bags are changed, or the child is connected to the cycler. The most frequent route of infection is via the lumen of the catheter.	Save the first cloudy bag of dialysate and send it to pathology for culture. Add antibiotics to the dialysate before inflow. Two antibiotics to cover Gram positive and Gram negative organisms are required initially until the infective organism is identified. Administer analgesia as appropriate. Avoid infection by careful handwashing before dialysis exchanges.	The infective organism may be isolated so that appropriate antibiotic therapy is administered. Antibiotics are effectively transferred into the circulation via the peritoneal route to treat infection. Once the causative organism is identified one of the antibiotics is withdrawn and the appropriate antibiotic continues for 1 to 2 weeks. The pain of peritonitis varies from mild to severe.
2. Tenckhoff catheter leakage. Children with uraemia may have delayed wound healing. Recognised by: • Wet catheter exit site dressing. • Fluid visibly leaking from the catheter exit site.	If child is well enough avoid using the catheter for at least 48 hours after insertion in order to prevent this problem. If the dialysis must begin immediately after insertion, commence dialysis using half volume fill cycles (approx. 25 mL/kg) If leakage presents cease dialysis for approx. 2 days.	Allows time for healing and tissue growth around the cuffs of the Tenckhoff catheter which provide a seal. Reduces intra-abdominal pressure. Allows time for healing.
3. Poor dialysate inflow or outflow.	If renal replacement therapy must continue, an alternative such as haemodialysis or haemofiltration should be introduced. Change wet dressings frequently and apply antiseptic to the catheter exit site.	Reduces intra-abdominal pressure. To prevent bacterial growth around the catheter. The dialysate leakage is warm and has a high glucose content which provides a good medium for bacterial growth. Relieves obstruction. The catheter may be kinked by the child's position. Ensure that the child's abdomen is lower than the dialysis bag

Table 6.6 (*continued*)

Problem	Intervention	Rationale
	Check for kinks in the dialysis line or catheter. Reposition child.	to allow for gravity fill, and that the child's abdomen is higher than the drainage bag to allow gravity drain.
	Check roller clamp on tubing and for presence of outlet port clamp on the dialysis bag.	Tubing may still be clamped! Fibrin clots may be present in newly inserted catheters or when the child has peritonitis. Heparin prevents fibrin clot formation in the catheter. The
	Add heparin to the bags if fibrin is present. Abdominal x-ray.	catheter may have migrated out of the child's pelvis and into the upper abdomen. This can be seen on abdominal x-ray.
4. Tenckhoff catheter exit site infection: • Inflammation around the exit site. • Discharge from the exit site.	Surgical intervention. Refer to peritoneal dialysis catheter care. Swab the catheter and forward to pathology for culture.	To replace the catheter in the correct position and allow free drainage and inflow. Good exit site care is vital for prevention of infection. Identify the causative organism. Eradicate infection. Exit site infection may cause peritonitis. Addition of antibiotics to the dialysate. Chronic exit site infection can lead to infection of the subcutaneous catheter tunnel and recurrent peritonitis. Removal of catheter. Removal of the infective source is necessary to treat peritonitis.
5. Hernias are a common complication of peritoneal dialysis as a result of increased intra-abdominal pressure.[16]	Reduce dialysis fill volumes. Surgical correction.	Reduce intra-abdominal pressure. Repair hernia to prevent complications such as strangulation.
6. Constipation may be a problem for children on peritoneal dialysis and is the result of decreased peristalsis secondary to abdominal distension during the dwell phase.	Encourage the child to ambulate. Administer aperient if necessary.	Prevent constipation. Relieve constipation.
7. Pain on inflow. Dialysate is slightly acidic and may cause pain when it is infused.	Reduce the inflow rate with the roller clamp.	May help to relieve pain. Fluid that is too hot or too cold causes abdominal cramping. Ensure that the dialysate is heated to 37°C.

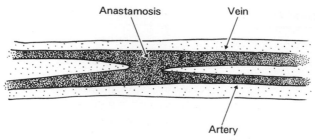

Figure 6.39 An arterio venous fistula.

A surgical procedure is performed to join an artery to a vein under the skin (**Figure 6.39**). This procedure creates a fast flow of blood through the vein. Over a period of several weeks the vein enlarges and the wall of the vein becomes thicker as a result of the arterial blood flow through it.[8] The vein must become large enough to insert 16 to 17 gauge needles into the vessel. Two cannulas are required for dialysis, one to remove blood and a second to return it.

In larger children, the radial artery and cephalic vein are joined by an end-to-side anastomosis at the wrist.[3] If this type of access fails or is not suitable, an attempt may be made to create a fistula at the elbow using the brachial artery and cephalic or basilic vein.

Saphenous vein loop

For smaller children under 20 kg, successful vascular access may be achieved by creating a fistula in the thigh. The distal end of the saphenous vein is brought round in a loop and anastomosed to the side of the femoral artery.

Synthetic grafts

If attempts at creating an arteriovenous fistula have failed, or the child does not have a suitably sized blood vessel for vascular access, a synthetic material such as poly-tetrafluoroethylene (PFTE) may be substituted. The synthetic material is grafted between an artery and a vein in the arm or leg. Synthetic grafts have the disadvantage of being more prone to infection than the child's own vessels.

Care of haemodialysis vascular access

Until the veins have dilated and thickened (1 to 6 months), trauma or a sudden reduction in blood pressure or blood flow through the fistula may cause clotting in the veins of the fistula. The following strategies must be observed when caring for a child who has internal haemodialysis access or an arteriovenous fistula:

- Avoid compression of the limb by tight clothing, jewellery and watches etc.
- Keep the fistula arm and hand warm in cold weather.
- Avoid low blood pressure and dehydration. If this occurs lay the child flat, and seek medical advice regarding fluid replacement.
- Listen to the fistula with a stethoscope twice daily in an established fistula, and every 1 to 4 hours for a new fistula. An audible flow through the fistula (bruit) should be heard, a vibration should be able to be felt over the fistula (thrill). If there is absence

of bruit or thrill report this to the child's physician immediately. It may be possible to restore fistula patency if rehydration or declotting occurs promptly.

- Do not obstruct the flow through the fistula by recording blood pressure on the fistula arm.
- Never collect blood samples, insert cannulas, or apply a tourniquet to a fistula arm.
- Report redness, swelling, discharge or pain in the fistula to medical staff. These signs may indicate infection, and if not treated promptly may lead to septicaemia.

The child's haemodialysis access is his or her lifeline. It should be treated with respect and accessed only by the haemodialysis team.

See Nursing Care of the Child with Chronic Renal Failure for additional information.

Cannulation of vascular access

Cannulation of vascular access is painful and creates tremendous stress for the child. Every effort must be made to relieve this trauma. Topical local anaesthetic cream (Emla cream) is now available and when a liberal amount is applied to the cannulation sites 1 hour before treatment, pain on cannulation is prevented. If the cream is unavailable the child will require a subcutaneous injection of local anaesthetic before inserting the cannula. Despite the use of local anaesthetic, many children find cannulation stressful. Two nurses are often required for cannulation, one to soothe and restrain the child and the other to insert the needles. It is beneficial for an occupational therapist to be involved in preparation for cannulation and to provide ways to allow children to express their anxiety through play. The therapist's presence during cannulation to provide relaxation therapy is also useful.

It may be difficult to distract the child from the procedure, but strategies such as counting, singing, reading stories, wriggling toes, television, music, and talking about positive events may be useful. Children should be told that it is acceptable to cry in order to express their feelings, but that they should try not to move their arm or leg during cannulation. Children should not be scolded for crying or screaming during the procedure.

Older children may be more cooperative and accepting of the procedure if they are allowed to participate. Strategies such as allowing the child to choose the cannula sites, making the child responsible for washing his or her own arm and applying antiseptic lotion prior to cannula insertion, applying their own local anaesthetic cream or administering the local anaesthetic injection will give them a feeling of having more control over the situation. Adolescents should be encouraged to learn self-cannulation. **Photos 6.2 and 6.3**.

Parents should be allowed to stay with their child during cannulation, but nurses must be aware that parents often experience a great deal of distress, or feelings of inadequacy or guilt about their child's illness and the painful procedures they are enduring. Nurses caring for children undergoing haemodialysis should attempt to spend time with the child's parents, to answer questions about treatment, and to allow them the opportunity to express feelings.

Central venous catheter

If it is not possible to create a subcutaneous vascular access on an infant or small child, or it is anticipated that haemodialysis will only be required for a short time, it is possible to gain access to the child's circulation through a central venous catheter specially

A 14-year-old girl performing self-cannulation.

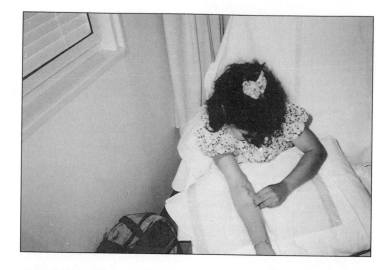

A 14-year-old girl administering heparin into a cannula which she inserted herself.

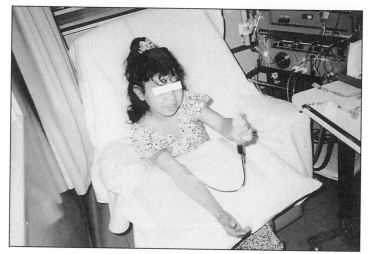

designed for haemodialysis. A surgical incision is made and the catheter is inserted into the internal or external jugular vein, the tip of the catheter is placed in the upper right atrium.[9] Catheters have been used successfully for haemodialysis for many months.

Subclavian catheter

A double-lumen catheter is inserted percutaneously into the subclavian vein. This type of access is useful for temporary access, such as for acute renal failure.

STRATEGIES FOR CARING FOR CHILDREN ON DIALYSIS

Although the number of children undergoing dialysis is small, the requirements for nursing support and interventions are great. Dialysis presents a tremendous burden and severe interruption to the lifestyle of children with renal failure and their entire family unit.

The stress that renal disease and its seemingly complex treatment modalities present to families and staff caring for these children must never be underestimated. In order to achieve a successful outcome, the care of children on dialysis requires a team approach. This team includes parents, siblings, nursing and medical staff, dietitian, social worker, occupational therapist and school teacher.

It is preferable for children to receive dialysis in the home. Parents and children undergo training programs to enable them to perform both peritoneal dialysis and haemodialysis at home. Children must be included in any training program, so that they are encouraged to take control of their lives. Even at a young age they can assist their parents in performing dialysis techniques. The nurse responsible for the training program must develop imaginative and interesting training methods, such as games, toys, videos and books.

The following nursing diagnoses are applicable to children with kidney failure requiring dialysis.

Abnormal serum electrolyte levels related to kidney failure

Hypokalaemia (low serum potassium)

Serum potassium levels may be depleted by aggressive dialysis treatments, e.g., in acute renal failure when hourly peritoneal dialysis cycles may be performed for several days.

Potassium chloride may be added to both the peritoneal dialysate solution and to the haemodialysis concentrate to prevent depletion. (See nursing care of the child with chronic renal failure for further information.)

Hyperkalaemia (elevated serum potassium)

Hyperkalaemia is more common in children undergoing haemodialysis than peritoneal dialysis, and may occur as a result of poor compliance with dietary potassium restriction. Counselling and education about the consequences of a high serum potassium level should be implemented, as well as a referral to the renal dietitian.

High serum potassium levels in the peritoneal dialysis patient may indicate that the child is omitting some of the dialysis exchanges that have been prescribed and this is a particular problem in the adolescent age group. More frequent dialysis exchanges will assist in lowering serum potassium levels. (See nursing care of the child with chronic renal failure for further information.)

Alterations to body fluid status

Potential for body fluid deficit related to rapid removal of intravascular fluid

Peritoneal dialysis: The use of dialysate fluid with a high dextrose concentration (e.g. 2.5% and 4.25% dialysate) may cause rapid intravascular fluid removal resulting in hypotension and dehydration. This may be avoided by careful nursing assessment of the child before performing each dialysis exchange. If the situation does occur, dialysis must continue to enable solute clearance to occur, but 1.5% or 0.5% dialysate should be used. The child's fluid intake should also be increased.

Haemodialysis: Attempts to remove excessive amounts of body fluid during haemodialysis can cause hypotension and cardiovascular instability.

In some instances body fluid deficit occurs because the child has gained body weight through growth and increased muscle and fat. When this occurs the dialysis regimen must be altered to avoid excessive fluid removal. The 'dry' weight should be reviewed and increased by 250 to 500 g.

Potential for body fluid excess related to inefficient dialysis

One of the kidney functions which is replaced by dialysis is the removal of excess fluid from the bloodstream. This is achieved using the principles of ultrafiltration or osmosis. If the child's fluid intake (from all sources) is greater than the amount of fluid removed by dialysis, signs of intravascular and extravascular fluid volume excess will become evident as hypertension, oedema, pulmonary oedema and cardiac failure.

The child's fluid intake must be reviewed and further fluid restriction will be imposed. Attempts to make dialysis more efficient should be implemented.

Peritoneal dialysis: Increased fluid removal with peritoneal dialysis may be achieved by increasing the number of peritoneal dialysis cycles, or increasing the strength of the dialysate concentration used.

Haemodialysis: It may be useful to prolong treatment hours, or increase the number of dialysis treatments performed each week in order to remove excess fluid from the body. If it is necessary to remove more than 60 mL/kg of the child's ideal bodyweight during a single haemodialysis treatment (e.g., more than 600 mL for a 10 kg child), a half-hour period during which pure ultrafiltration without solute removal should be performed. The pure ultrafiltration process exerts a negative suction pressure on the dialysate lines and artificial kidney, but dialysate flow through the dialyser is ceased. As a result of this technique there is only fluid removal, and no solute removal. Pure ultrafiltration allows quite large volumes of excess fluid to be removed from the child without lowering the plasma oncotic pressure. This means that as fast as fluid moves out of the blood compartment into the dialysate more water will enter the blood from the interstitial space, hence hypotensive episodes are avoided.[8]

Poor nutritional status

Dietary interventions are individualised for children. Unlike adult renal patients, children should not automatically be placed on a 'renal diet'. They require constant review by the dietitian involved in the renal team. Adequate energy and protein intake to achieve growth is extremely difficult to achieve in children who are anorexic as a consequence of uraemia. In many cases dialysis must be adapted to the child's diet rather than restricting the diet to fit in with dialysis.

Dietary restrictions are only ever implemented as a last resort, when other measures have failed. When a child with renal failure is on a restricted diet, it is a nursing responsibility to ensure that the diet is followed rigidly while the child is in their care. (See nursing care of the child with chronic renal failure for further information about diet.)

Peritoneal dialysis: Peritoneal dialysis provides constant fluid and solute removal, 7 days per week, enabling a more liberal daily fluid allowance than is possible when haemodialysis is used. If a child has some residual renal function which provides some urine output, and he or she is on peritoneal dialysis free access to fluids in some instances may be permitted. If the child has little or no urine output then fluid intake will be restricted to between 500 mL and 1 L daily. Apart from the avoidance of excessively salty foods, diet is not usually restricted. It is important to provide a diet which will provide a protein intake of 2 to 3 g/kg daily,[11] because protein diffuses into peritoneal dialysate. During episodes of peritonitis, protein requirements are even greater because protein losses increase.

Children on peritoneal dialysis may experience a reduction in their appetite because of an elevated intra-abdominal pressure and feelings of fullness related to the presence of dialysate in their peritoneum. Strategies to avoid this are to reduce the volume of dialysate instilled to prevent abdominal distension, and increase the number of dialysis cycles performed each day to maintain dialysis efficiency.

Haemodialysis: Because haemodialysis is intermittent and children do not have constant fluid removal, most children on haemodialysis require a fluid restriction. The fluid restriction imposed is more severe than for peritoneal dialysis, and is more difficult to adhere to. Fluid intake is restricted to slightly more than the child's insensible losses each day. A typical fluid restriction is 300 to 500 mL/m^2 of body surface area. This restriction makes it difficult to provide enteral feeding supplements should they be required. Children on haemodialysis must avoid foods which are rich in potassium and sodium.

Potential for dialysis disequilibrium syndrome due to rapid removal of solute from the blood

Nurses caring for children with both acute and chronic renal failure who are undergoing their first dialysis must be aware of this complication and plan interventions which will prevent it.

Methods of preventing disequilibrium are a slow blood flow rate and lower dialysate flow to prevent rapid solute removal; intravenous Mannitol infusion during dialysis, which raises the serum osmolality and prevents disequilibrium; and anticonvulsant therapy as prophylaxis.

Family stress and fatigue

Having a child on dialysis creates tension in a family unit. Well siblings may feel their parents' attention and time is devoted to the child on dialysis and they are being forgotten.

Table 6.7 Technical considerations for the child on haemodialysis

Dialysis order	Rationale	Child	Adult
1. Blood Flow Rate through the inside of the dialyser fibres (calculated in mL/min.)	Blood is pumped out of the circulation by the machine and pushed through the dialyser so that dialysis can occur. The blood flow rate through the dialyser must be fast enough to prevent clotting in the dialyser, and to allow the entire blood volume to pass through the dialyser several times to enable removal of waste products from the blood.	Blood flow rate is calculated by aiming to remove 1 to 3 mL/kg of urea each minute. The faster the blood flow the more urea is cleared. If urea is cleared too quickly, disequilibrium syndrome may occur.	200 to 300 mL/min.

Table 6.7 (*continued*)

Dialysis order	Rationale	Child	Adult
2. Allowable extra-corporeal blood volume.	Blood is pumped from the circulation outside of the body so that dialysis may occur in the artificial kidney. Careful consideration must be given to the amount of blood required to fill the dialysis blood lines and artificial kidney. If too much blood is taken from the circulation, shock and hypotension will occur.	No more than 8% to 10% of the child's circulating blood volume. The child's circulating blood volume is calculated as 60 to 80 mL/kg of body weight. A 10 kg child has a circulating blood volume of 800 mL. Therefore the dialysis lines and dialyser must have a priming volume of not more than 60 to 80 mL.	250 to 300 mL (2% to 5% of the average adult's circulating blood volume)
3. Dialysate flow rate (expressed as mL/min.)	Fresh dialysate must continually flush through the dialyser to allow for adequate diffusion to occur. The more rapid the dialysate flow rate, the more efficient the dialysis.	500 mL/min. If dialysis efficiency needs to be reduced to prevent disequilibrium syndrome, this flow may be lowered.	500 mL/min.
4. Heparin loading dose and heparin hourly infusion rate.	When the child's blood comes into contact with the artificial membrane, the body's clotting mechanism is stimulated. Heparin is given to prevent clotting in the dialysis circuit and thus large volume of blood loss.	Heparin doses are individualised according to the child's needs. Considerations in heparin doses are the length of time venipuncture sites take to clot when cannulas are removed after dialysis and if there is any visible clotting in the dialyser at the completion of dialysis.	As for children. A guide for both children and adults is: Loading dose: 25 to 50 U/kg. Hourly infusion: 25 to 50 U/kg.

This is often true! Having a child on dialysis creates marital tension because the responsibility of the treatment often falls on one parent who feels resentful that their spouse is not sharing the burden. Even family outings and holidays are disrupted because of dialysis schedules. Recognising family stress is an important part of paediatric renal nursing. Because it is usually the nurse who has had the most contact with both the child and parents during the dialysis training period and at follow-up visits, it is usually the nurse with whom the parents feel most comfortable, and are able to express their feelings. Nurses can help families in a number of ways. These include:

- Offering suggestions of ways to readjust dialysis schedules to fit in with family activities.
- Training other family members, such as grandparents, to attend dialysis to enable the parent to have some respite.
- Having the child attend hospital-run holiday camps which provide the family with a respite from dialysis for at least 1 week of the year.

Poor self-esteem

Chronic renal failure and dialysis severely affect psychosocial development of children and adolescents. Their lives are dependent on machines and hospital staff. They are subjected to complicated and often painful medical regimens such as dialysis, repeated venipunctures, unpleasant medications (which often have unpleasant side effects), restrictions on eating and drinking freely, while many are reliant on gastrostomy or nasogastric feeding. Their body image is impaired by short stature, bony deformities as a result of renal osteodystrophy, numerous surgical scars, urinary diversion devices, peritoneal catheters, fistula or haemodialysis catheters, which make it impossible for the child not to feel different from siblings and peers. Children of all ages regularly display acting out behaviour and non-compliance, particularly in the adolescent age group.[17] It is important that nurses caring for children on dialysis allow them to express their feelings and approach them in a firm but gentle and understanding manner. Strategies to help children cope with dialysis are:

- Allow children to express their frustration and fears through verbalisation and play.
- Provide education about their disease and dialysis.
- Encourage family attendance at family conferences.
- Encourage self-care in older children and adolescents. This should include listening to the child's opinions and perhaps adjusting dialysis techniques or medication schedules to allow them some control over the situation. An example is to allow second daily Tenckhoff catheter dressings in an established catheter. Second daily care is better than none at all and the child feels more in control of their body.
- Encourage attendance at support groups if they are available.[13]

HAEMOFILTRATION

Haemofiltration is a renal replacement therapy used primarily to treat critically ill children with acute renal failure or fluid overload. The technique simulates the non-specific filtration that occurs in the glomerulus by using the principle of convection rather than diffusion to remove fluid and solutes from the blood. Blood is passed through a semipermeable membrane called a haemofilter. The haemofilter is made of approximately 5000 hollow fibre capillaries.[18] The filter is permeable to solutes with a molecular weight from 0 to 30 000 daltons. As blood passes through the filter a pressure gradient is created which forces water and solutes out from the plasma and through the semipermeable membrane. Because extremely large volumes of filtrate are removed from the circulation during this process, a sterile physiological replacement fluid is administered at a rate which is slightly less than the filtration rate in order to avoid severe fluid and electrolyte depletion. The replacement fluid is designed to replace volume and solutes such as sodium, chloride, bicarbonate and glucose, but does not contain urea, creatinine, potassium and phosphorus and other waste products.

Haemofiltration mimics the normal glomerular activity in 2 ways by:

1. The production of a large volume of filtrate which is forced out of the blood by the hydrostatic pressure created in the filter.
2. Selective reabsorption which is imitated by the infusion of fluid to replace the water and solutes that the body needs to maintain homeostasis.

Nursing care

After initiating haemofiltration, nurses are responsible for hourly monitoring of the child and the extracorporeal circuit.

Selecting the haemofilter

To avoid cardiac instability, consideration must be given to the volume of blood that will be contained in the extracorporeal circuit. The haemofilter and lines must not contain more that 10% of the child's circulating blood volume.

Setting up and disconnecting the haemofiltration circuit

The nurse responsible for setting up the haemofiltration circuit, and commencing haemofiltration must adopt an aseptic technique. If bacteria enters the circuit the child may develop septicaemia.

Vital signs

The child's vital signs should be monitored every 15 minutes for the 1st hour and then every hour. Hypotension may indicate that ultrafiltration is occurring too rapidly, therefore this must be reported and the hourly ultrafiltration rate reviewed in consultation with the child's attending physician.

The haemofiltration circuit

The blood tubing should be inspected for kinks or leakage, and that the connections are secured. The vascular access should be inspected for signs of infection at the exit site.

Ultrafiltrate

The ultrafiltrate should be inspected for signs of blood leak from ruptured fibres within the haemofilter each hour. The fluid should have a clear, straw-coloured appearance. Pink or red staining indicates a blood leak. If a blood leak occurs, the haemofilter must be changed.

Fluid balance

Nurses are responsible for an accurate measurement and recording of all fluid intake and output, as well as for adjusting the ultrafiltration outflow and amount of replacement fluid each hour.

Heparin

Unless children have a coagulation disorder, they will require a continuous heparin infusion to prevent their blood clotting inside the filter. The heparin dose varies according to individual requirements, but a common rate is between 5 and 10 U/kg of body weight each hour.[19] The aim of heparinisation is to prevent clotting inside the extracorporeal blood circuit without systemic anticoagulation. Hourly clotting studies should be performed initially so that the heparin dosage may be adjusted accordingly. Signs that clotting has occurred are: the extracorporeal blood appears darker; the venous pressure reading is high, causing the blood pump alarm to sound; the ultrafiltration rate drops; clots are visible in the blood lines. If clotting occurs, the haemofiltration circuit must be changed. The child must also be observed for signs of haemorrhage such as bleeding around the vascular access.

Weight

A bare weight should be recorded before haemofiltration begins, and from then on daily. The purpose of weighing the child is to assess the degree of fluid overload that the child has so that the hourly ultrafiltration rate may be calculated.

Parental support

The parents of seriously ill children are under a great deal of stress, and when a procedure such as haemofiltration is added to the child's treatment it may be very frightening for the parents. Parents must be given a detailed, but simple explanation of the procedure, and regular reinforcements why the treatment is required. Parents must be allowed contact with the child during therapy, and should be encouraged to touch their child, and to talk to them if they wish.

Variants of haemofiltration

Continuous arteriovenous haemofiltration

Access to the child's circulation is achieved by cannulating an artery and a vein. Blood is propelled out of the artery by the child's cardiac contraction force (blood pressure). No machines are required for this procedure. Blood flow is dependent on the child's blood pressure, haematocrit, cannula position and the amount of resistance in the venous cannula creating a backflow pressure. Flows of 19 to 30 mL/min are common in children, and 70 to 120 mL/min in adolescents and adults. The blood flows via a blood line through the haemofilter and then returns to the circulation via the venous cannula. Filtration occurs through the membrane as a result of a high pressure being created as the child's blood pressure pushes the blood through the filter. The pressure increases in the filter as the blood meets a resistance in the venous return cannula (positive pressure).

The filtration rate achieved is proportional to the blood flow rate. An average of 0.7 to 1.1 mL/min is achieved in infants and children and as much as 60 mL/min in adults.

In addition, a negative pressure is created by the height difference between the haemofilter and the filtrate collection bag.[20] This pressure assists in filtration and may be adjusted by raising or lowering the bag according to the desired amount of fluid removal.

Continuous venovenous haemofiltration

This method of haemofiltration is gaining popularity for the treatment of acute renal failure. The principles of haemofiltration are the same as described above. Access to the circulation is via a double lumen venous catheter inserted into a large vein. The femoral, subclavian and internal jugular veins are commonly used.[19] As there is no arterial pressure to push the blood through the haemofilter a blood pump is used for this purpose.

Continuous venovenous haemodiafiltration (CVVHD)

In some cases, the urea clearance achieved in a standard haemofiltration system is insufficient. A technique which combines diffusion with convection has been developed to increase solute clearance. The CVVHD circuit is similar to the continuous venovenous haemofiltration circuit but dialysate fluid is added to the filter to facilitate diffusion of waste products out of the child's blood.[21]

Intermittent haemodiafiltration

Haemodiafiltration may be performed as an intermittent treatment for chronic renal failure with the use of a machine designed for this purpose. Intermittent haemodiafiltration is not a popular alternative to haemodialysis therapy at present because it is more expensive.

REFERENCES

1. Keshavich S. Equipment for haemodialysis and peritoneal dialysis. *In:* Nissenson AR, Fine RN, Gentile DE. *Clinical dialysis.* 2nd ed. Christchurch: Appleton Lange, 1990.
2. Plowman PN. *The illustrated lecture series: nephrology, electrolyte physiology and poisoning.* New York: Medical Examination Publishing, 1987.
3. Fine RN, Tejani A. Dialysis in infants and children. *In:* Daugirdas JT, Ing TS, eds. *Handbook of dialysis.* Boston: Little Brown, 1988.
4. Fine RN. Open forum: children on dialysis. *Dialysis Transplant* 1991.; 20 (6): 297–316.
5. Cree L, Rischmiller S. *Science in nursing.* Sydney: Harcourt Brace Jovanovich, 1989.
6. Tortora GJ, Anagnostakos NP. *Principles of anatomy and physiology.* 7th ed. New York: Harper and Rowe, 1993.
7. Hamilton HK. *Nurses clinical library: renal and urologic disorders.* Springhouse, PA: Springhouse Corporation, 1984.
8. Uldall R. *Renal nursing.* 3rd ed. Oxford: Blackwell Scientific, 1988.
9. Fine RN, Gruskin AB. *End stage renal disease in children.* Philadelphia: Saunders, 1984.
10. Brenner BM, Lazarus JM. *Acute renal failure.* Philadelphia: Saunders, 1983.
11. Stewart CL, Katz SP, Kaskil FJ. Unique aspects of the care of pediatric dialysis patients. *Seminars in Dialysis* 1988; 3: 160–169.
12. Doyle CL, Flanigan MJ, Mube C. Tidal peritoneal dialysis vs continuous cycling peritoneal dialysis: children's preference. *Am Nephrology Nurses Assoc* 1992; 19: 249–254.
13. Greenberg CS. *Nursing care planning guides for children* Sydney: Williams & Wilkins, 1988.
14. Blatz S, Paes B, Steele B. Peritoneal dialysis in the neonate. *Neonatal Network* 1990; 8 (6): 41–44.
15. Levy M, Williamson Bulle J. Optimal approach to the prevention and treatment of peritonitis in children undergoing CAPD and CCPD. *Seminars in Dialysis* 1994; 7: 442–449.
16. Tzamaloukas AH, Gibel LJ, Eisenberg B, Simon D, Wood B, Nevarez M, Quintana EJ, Avasthi PS, De Lavega OR, Goldman RS, Hartshorne MS, Kanig SP, Spalding CT, Zager PG. Scrotal edema in patients on CAPD: Causes, differential diagnosis and management. *Dialysis and Transplant* 1992; 21 (9): 581–605.
17. Weiss RA, Edellman CM. Children on dialysis. *N Engl J Med* 1982; 307: 1574–1575.
18. Cotton Palmer J, Koorejian K, Brown London J, Dechert RE, Bartlett RH. Nursing management of continuous arterio-venous hemofiltration for acute renal failure. *Focus on Critical Care* 1986; October: 21–30.

19. Zobel G, Trop M, Bietzke A, Ring E. Vascular access for continuous arterio venous hemofiltration in infants and young children. *Artificial Organs* 1988; 12 (1): 16–19.
20. Williams V. Continuous ultrafiltration — a new ICU procedure for the treatment of fluid overload. *Focus on Critical Care* 1984; July/August: 44–49.
21. Lievaart A, Voermann HJ. Nursing management of continuous arteriovenous hemodialysis. *Heart Lung* 1991; 20: 152–158.

Renal Transplantation

Renal transplantation is the treatment of choice for children with end-stage renal failure (ESRF). This form of treatment offers a greater opportunity for both emotional and physical growth and development. Most importantly, transplantation provides children with ESRF an opportunity to lead an almost normal life.

The transplant procedure involves the removal of a functioning kidney from a donor and placing it into the child's iliac fossa outside the peritoneal cavity.[1] The transplant kidney's renal artery is anastomosed to the iliac artery and the renal vein is anastomosed to the iliac vein. The ureter is implanted into the recipient's bladder.[2]

In small children the iliac fossa may be too small to accommodate a kidney transplant from an adult donor or their iliac vessels too small to anastomose the transplant kidney vessels. In this situation the transplanted kidney is placed intraperitoneally, with the vascular anastomoses to the aorta and inferior vena cava.[3]

DONORS

Donor kidneys may be obtained from a living relative (usually a parent) or from a non-related donor who has been declared brain dead. Less commonly, transplantation from live, unrelated donors are performed (e.g., a husband may want to donate a kidney to his wife).

Living donors must be in good health to be considered to be suitable candidates for kidney donation. Siblings are usually the best tissue match, but it is not common in paediatric units to obtain a donor kidney from a sibling because of ethical considerations. Siblings must be over the age of 18 years to be considered and it must be established that the donor has not been coerced into kidney donation by other family members.

In some Third World countries, kidneys are purchased for transplantation.[4] The ethics of this practice have been a topic for debate in recent times. Purchase of organs for transplantation is illegal in most countries, including Australia.

NURSING ASSESSMENT

Pretransplant education

The specialist renal nurse is often a primary source of information for the child and family prior to, during and after renal transplantation. It is important for the specialist nurse to have a precise knowledge of all aspects of renal transplantation to enable her or him to explain procedures and pass on relevant information.[5]

Many families perceive renal transplantation to be a cure for their child's renal failure. Unfortunately, renal transplant is not a cure for end-stage renal failure, therefore it is important that renal transplantation be presented to the child and his or her family as another form of treatment, rather than a cure. The possibility of failure of this form of treatment as a result of rejection or recurrence of the original disease in the transplanted kidney, should be addressed prior to transplantation.

Siblings

Preparation of the whole family prior to transplant surgery is important. Siblings must never be forgotten and should be included in family discussions wherever possible. Siblings may feel neglected, particularly in a live donor situation where one parent is absent from them because they are donating a kidney, and their other parent is spending most of his or her time visiting the donor and recipient. Arrangements for child care for siblings must be made before transplant surgery.

Telephone contact

The family must be informed about what to expect when they receive a telephone call from their physician informing them that a renal transplant is available for the child. The family should be aware that they should go to the transplant unit immediately they receive the call. It is important that a contact telephone number is available at all times in case a transplant becomes available. The child's school telephone number and the parents' work numbers should be recorded in their file. Should the family go away on holiday, they should always inform the hospital and a contact telephone number should be provided.

Medication compliance

Compliance with immunosuppressant therapy to prevent rejection of the transplant kidney is vital. Immunosuppressant therapy must continue for the life of the transplant. Side effects of immunosuppressant therapy should be discussed and ways to overcome them suggested as follows:

- Cyclosporine causes excessive facial and body hair growth. Information about hair removal methods such as waxing, depilatory creams and shaving may be given. Another complication of cyclosporine is gum hypertrophy and in some cases the gums cover the child's teeth to such an extent that the gums have to be trimmed by a dentist. Regular dental check-ups and good dental hygiene should begin prior to transplantation and continue for life.
- Prednisolone causes increased appetite, obesity and moon facies. A sensible eating plan should be obtained from the renal dietitian. Exercise should be encouraged.
- Azathioprine increases the risk of skin cancer. The importance of avoiding excessive exposure to the sun, applying sun screen and wearing a hat outdoors is important information to give to all Australian children. It is even more important that children on immunosuppressive therapy adhere to this advice.

Non-compliance with antirejection therapy is a reasonably common problem in the adolescent age group. Most paediatric renal units have experienced the disappointment of graft failure as a result of non-compliance in the adolescent age group.[6] Non-compliance is hypothesised to be related to the undesirable changes in body appearance that result from immunosuppressive medications.[6] Therefore the issue of non-compliance must always be addressed prior to transplantation. Children and adolescents receiving immunosuppressants may have poor body image, low self-esteem, or may be the target of teasing at school about their appearance. As a result they may find it difficult to form friendships with other children. Counselling may help overcome these problems.

If younger children are known to be non-compliant with medications prior to transplant, alternative methods of administration such as crushing tablets and offering them in a small quantity of ice cream, yoghurt, flavoured milk or fruit juice may be suggested to their parents.

Pre-transplant ward visits

Paediatric renal transplant surgery and postoperative nursing care is often performed at an adult transplant unit. This situation can present anxieties not only for the child and family, but also for the nursing staff. The child and parents may feel anxious that the child will be cared for by nurses with whom they are not familiar. Nurses with limited paediatric nursing experience may feel stressed about nursing children in the transplant ward. Good communication and rapport between the paediatric and adult renal nurses will provide a more comforting environment for everyone involved.

Pre-transplant ward visits provide an opportunity to introduce the child and his or her family to the transplant ward staff. The visit should take place just prior to the transplant and be conducted by the child's primary renal nurse.

Information about reverse barrier nursing and ward visiting policies can be given. A simple explanation about the urinary catheter, wound drains, intravenous lines, postoperative chest physiotherapy and pain relief can be provided.

In many transplant units, staff and visitors wear gowns and face masks when they are in contact with the child. The visit provides an opportunity for the child to touch or play with these articles in a non-threatening situation. Parents should be shown how to wear the gown and mask and how to dispose of them after use.

If the child is to receive a transplant from a parent, they should be informed about where their parent will be nursed after the transplant and how long it will be before the donor will be allowed to visit them.

PREOPERATIVE NURSING ASSESSMENT

The nursing assessment of a child presenting for renal transplantation is similar to nursing assessment of the child with chronic renal failure. In addition, consideration must be given to the fact that immediately prior to and following renal transplantation, immunosuppressive medications are administered to the child in an attempt to prevent the body rejecting the transplanted tissue. As these medications increase the child's susceptibility to infection, the child should be assessed closely for signs of infection before the transplant.

Peritoneal dialysis catheters

If the child is undergoing peritoneal dialysis, the catheter exit site must be carefully examined for signs of infection such as redness, pain or discharge. If infection is suspected, this must be reported to the child's physician or surgeon. The exit site should be swabbed.

Peritoneal dialysis fluid

Peritoneal dialysis fluid should be drained out of the child's peritoneum before the operation. The fluid should be inspected for clarity; if the fluid is cloudy in appearance the nurse admitting the child for transplant should notify the child's physician or surgeon. Cloudy fluid must be sent to the bacteriology department for culture and sensitivity because this symptom indicates peritonitis.

Arterio venous fistula and external haemodialysis access devices

Haemodialysis access should be inspected for signs of infection, such as redness, pain or discharge. If the child has an arteriovenous fistula the patency must be checked by listening for an audible bruit. If the nursing assessment reveals that the haemodialysis access is not patent, this must be reported, because alternative dialysis access may be created at the time of transplant in case the child requires dialysis during the postoperative period.

Nose and throat swabs

A nose and throat swab should be taken. Any recent episode of fever, throat or chest infection should be reported to the child's physician prior to surgery.

Urine specimen

A clean specimen of urine should be collected prior to surgery if possible.

MEDICAL ASSESSMENT

A medical officer should conduct a full physical examination of the child before surgery. Particular attention should be paid to the child's state of hydration. Children must be well hydrated prior to transplantation because when the vascular clamps are released intraoperatively, up to 300 mL of blood from the child's circulating blood volume may be required to perfuse an adult-sized kidney. This sudden loss of blood may result in hypovolaemia, hypotension and vascular thrombosis of the graft.[3]

INVESTIGATIONS

Psychological assessment

It is common for families to be referred to a psychiatrist for psychological assessment prior to living relative donor transplantation. Family dynamics and coping mechanisms are explored during the assessment.

There are many potential emotional stressors for both the child and their family. The following are common questions and issues to be addressed before and after transplant:

- What is the motivation of the potential donor in offering the kidney?
- Would the child feel guilty, or the parents feel angry with the child, if the kidney is rejected?
- Would the recipient feel indebted to the donor or be expected to display an unreasonable amount of gratitude to the donor?
- How does the child feel about cadaveric donor transplantation? Recipients often wonder about the donor's identity and may feel guilty about accepting a cadaveric transplant.

Some recipients wonder about the gender, age or nationality of the donor and whether or not this will have any adverse effect on them.

- Although potential organ donors are tested for human immunodeficiency virus (HIV), hepatitis B, hepatitis C and cytomegalovirus,[5] the recipient may worry about contracting HIV through transplantation.

Tissue typing

The ability of the body's immune system to recognise foreign tissue and destroy it is the major obstacle to successful organ transplantation. Successful renal transplantation involves careful matching of the recipient and donor tissue. The following investigations are performed to minimise organ rejection by the recipient's immune system.

ABO blood typing

The first criterion in the selection of a suitable donor is that the ABO blood grouping is compatible.[7]

White cell crossmatching

The recipient's serum is mixed with donor serum and then observed for cell agglutination or lysis, which indicates a positive reaction. This reaction is caused by antibodies in the recipient. Antibodies form following blood transfusions or previous transplants.[8]

If the child's serum displays a positive reaction towards donor serum the kidney would most probably be rejected. The transplant would then be cancelled. A negative crossmatch is considered necessary for successful transplantation.[9]

Human leucocyte antigen (HLA) testing

HLA antigens are carried on most cells in the body and are genetically determined. The genes which code for HLA antigens are carried on the short arm of chromosome 6.[7] Everyone has 2 sets of chromosome 6 (one set is inherited from each parent).[9]

Lymphocytes are used to detect tissue antigens because they are easy to obtain through venipuncture and they carry all HLAs. The histocompatibility antigens comprise 4 loci, A, B, C and DR.[10] About 20 HLA A, 40 HLA B, 8 HLA C and 20 HLA DR have been identified.[11]

There are 2 types of lymphocytes, B cells and T cells. T cells express high quantities of HLA A, B and C antigens and B cells have high concentrations of the HLA DR antigen.[1] The tissue typing procedure aims to detect the HLA antigens and their associated antibodies.

Tissue typing tests are performed by the Red Cross Blood Bank in each state in Australia. All patients wishing to be placed on the waiting list for a kidney transplant must have the blood tests performed. In order to perform the tissue typing, 2 separate samples of 60 mL blood, at least 1 week apart, are requested by the blood bank. It should be remembered that this is an enormous quantity of blood to take from a small child. Therefore, either the specialist paediatric renal nurse or the child's physician should negotiate with the blood bank that the tests be done on a smaller volume of blood. No more than 35 mL blood should be taken from children who weigh less than 20 kg, and no more than 50 mL from children 20 to 40 kg. Children must be well hydrated prior to collecting blood.

Monthly antibody status

Following the initial tissue typing, a 10 mL sample of blood must be forwarded to the blood bank each month in order for the child to remain on the waiting list for a kidney transplant. This blood is crossmatched against each potential donor.

Renal vasculature

It must be established that the blood vessels which will perfuse the transplant kidney are healthy and have a good blood flow. Adolescents should be discouraged from cigarette smoking if they wish to be considered as a renal transplant recipient.

Bladder function

Some children require urodynamic studies of their bladders prior to transplantation, to establish that their bladder is capable of storing urine after the transplant. If a child has a severely abnormal urinary tract, the transplanted ureter is anastomosed to a urinary diversion such as an ileal conduit. In order to prevent damage from urinary reflux to the transplanted kidney, some children require antireflux surgery prior to placement on the transplant waiting lists.

Postoperative investigations

The following investigations are performed to assess how well the transplant kidney is functioning: ultrasound; glomerular filtration rate; DTPA scan; transplant renal biopsy.

POSTOPERATIVE CARE

Immediate postoperative nursing care involves hourly monitoring of vital signs, close observation of the child's fluid status by hourly measurement of central venous pressure and hourly urine measure and observing for signs of graft rejection. The child will return to the ward with a triple lumen central venous line to measure central venous pressure and to administer intravenous fluids and medication. Wound drains will be *in situ*.

The kidney may not function immediately following renal transplantation. The child may be anuric or oliguric or experience a massive diuresis[2] and will have a urinary catheter *in situ*. Dialysis is sometimes required during the postoperative period until transplant renal function is established.

In order to assess the child's kidney function and electrolyte balance, a blood sample to measure the serum urea, creatinine and electrolyte level, is collected immediately on return to the ward.

Children require cardiac monitoring and monitoring of oxygen saturation by pulse oxymetry in the immediate postoperative period. Oxygen therapy may be ordered by the anaesthetist or paediatrician.

Monitoring of fluid status

Hourly measurement of fluid intake and output is performed for at least 48 hours. Fluid replacement therapy depends on urine output[12] and aims to encourage a forced diuresis by maintenance of central venous pressure between 5 and 8 cmH$_2$O. A sudden fall or increase in urine output must be reported to medical staff immediately.

Reverse barrier nursing

Transplant recipients receive large doses of immunosuppressant drugs prior to and following the transplant. Therefore reverse barrier nursing is implemented to prevent opportunistic infections.

Oral hygiene

The side effects of immunosuppressant drugs increase the child's vulnerability to opportunistic infections in the mouth. Therefore daily inspection of the oral cavity must be performed. Meticulous attention to oral hygiene should commence postoperatively. Strategies such as six hourly mouth washes, regular brushing with a soft tooth brush and the use of dental floss keeps the mouth clean.[13] *Candida* albicans (thrush) and herpes simplex virus are common infections for transplant recipients. Both of these conditions are uncomfortable and may lead to further complications such as candida or herpes oesophagitis.[13]

Sore gums and mouth may prevent the child from eating. A regular anesthetic mouth wash or jelly such as xylocaine viscous or Bonjella prior to meals may relieve the pain and encourage adequate nutritional intake.

Behavioural problems

When children are nursed in isolation for lengthy periods and are subjected to continual nursing and medical procedures which often cause them pain and discomfort, they become depressed and angry. The child may demonstrate anger by being uncooperative with even the simplest nursing procedures, screaming or crying, or becoming withdrawn and not talking to anyone. The following may be considered in this situation.

The child's emotional needs must never be ignored, no matter how difficult or unpleasant the child's behaviour. Attempts to prevent the anxiety occurring should be made when the child is first admitted to the transplant unit and should continue throughout the admission. Strategies such as making up a mural of family photographs, and allowing favourite toys, blankets or pillows to be brought to the ward with the child may help the child to feel more comfortable in the strange environment.

Parents should have unlimited visiting privileges, and be allowed to be involved in their child's care. Children may cooperate more if their parents are allowed to assist with bathing, toileting, administration of medications and other simple procedures. Encouraging parental involvement may also help the parent to deal with a stressful situation. Allocating the parent certain tasks not only passes time, but makes them feel useful because they are really having input into the child's recovery. However, the nurse must be astute enough to recognise when the parents are becoming tired or exasperated and should suggest that they rest while the nurse takes care of their child.

Allow siblings and peers to visit for short periods. If this is not possible then telephone contact should be available. Contact with children of their own age provides peer support and a sense of normality.

Periods for quiet time and play time should be set aside during the day. Most young children have a nap during the day and this should be allowed to continue in hospital. If possible, a recreational therapist should be involved with the child to provide play therapy. The child should not be interrupted for nursing procedures during recreation and rest periods.

Television is a good diversion, but it should not be the only recreational activity offered to the child.

Diversional techniques such as deep breathing, practising counting or the alphabet, singing or listening to favourite songs could be attempted to distract the child during procedures.

Limits of acceptable and non-acceptable behaviour should be set for the child to follow. Parents should be encouraged to discipline their child as if they were at home.

School work

School-aged children should be visited by the hospital school teacher each day (if there is one available). If this is not possible, then arrangements should be made for school work to be sent in from the child's own school. Children with chronic illness often miss a lot of their schooling and it is easy for them to fall behind in their studies. Some never catch up because they are able to manipulate parents, teachers, nurses and other health workers into believing that they are too unwell to do their school work. Nursing and medical procedures should be arranged so that the child is allowed uninterrupted schooling each day.

GRAFT REJECTION

The presence of a transplant kidney in the recipient's body may stimulate the immune system to produce an antigen — antibody reaction in an attempt to destroy the foreign tissue (the transplant kidney).[2] This reaction may lead to rejection of the transplant. The T lymphocytes are the main cells responsible for recognition of the foreign antigen and generation of cytotoxic cells directed against donor tissue.[12]

There are 3 kinds of rejection that may occur.

Hyperacute rejection occurs immediately or within a few hours of the transplant kidney being revascularised. This type of rejection is irreversible and necessitates removal of the transplant.

Acute rejection occurs within the first few months after transplant. This type of rejection is common within the first few days after transplant. The usual treatment is large doses of intravenous methylprednisolone. More severe episodes of acute rejection are treated with OKT3 or antilymphocyte globulin (ALG).

Chronic rejection may occur at any time after the first 6 months after renal transplant. Chronic rejection results in a gradual deterioration of the transplant kidney function and may follow a course of several months or years.

Children must be monitored closely for signs of rejection as follows:

- Daily measurement of serum creatinine level. An elevation in creatinine level indicates transplant rejection.
- Close monitoring of urine output. A sudden drop in urine output indicates rejection.
- Bare weigh children daily. A sudden increase in weight indicates fluid retention as a result of a decreased urine output.
- Observe for pain over the area of the kidney transplant. Rejection causes swelling and inflammation of the transplant kidney.
- Daily urinalysis. The presence of blood or protein in the urine may indicate rejection.
- Record temperature at least every 4 hours; fever is a sign of graft rejection.

IMMUNOSUPPRESSION

Immunosuppressant medication is given following transplant in an attempt to prevent the body from recognising the transplant kidney as foreign tissue, and allow the kidney to be accepted. Immunosuppressive therapy must continue daily for the life of the transplant. The drugs most commonly used are prednisolone, azathioprine and cyclosporin A. Nurses responsible for administration of these potentially toxic medications should be aware of their mode of action, as well as the more common adverse effects of the drugs.

Prednisolone

Prednisolone is administered once daily by mouth for routine therapy and should be given with food to prevent gastric irritation. It is administered in larger, once-only doses by mouth or intravenous infusion as treatment for acute rejection.

Prednisolone suppresses the body's inflammatory response to foreign tissue by preventing leucocyte infiltration into tissues, decreasing antibody production and inhibiting antibody — antigen complex formation.[8]

Side effects of prednisolone include increased susceptibility to viral, fungal and bacterial infections, delayed wound healing, Cushingoid appearance, gastric irritation and ulceration, hypertension, increased appetite, obesity and stunted linear growth.[14]

Cyclosporin A

Cyclosporin A is administered by intravenous infusion for the first few days after transplant. Cyclosporin should not be administered in a standard PVC giving set since the drug may adhere to the plastic and an incorrect dose may be delivered. The most frequently used giving sets are manufactured from polypropylene or ethylene vinyl acetate.

Once gastric absorption has been established, oral administration twice daily is the maintenance dose. As absorption of oral cyclosporin is often slow it is suggested that it be administered on an empty stomach.[14] It is available in capsule or liquid form. If liquid is given, the medication is mixed with milk or fruit juice to disguise the unpleasant taste. Administer cyclosporin in a glass container as the medication adheres to plastic.

Cyclosporin A suppresses the body's immune response by acting predominantly on T lymphocytes.[15] It is commonly administered as routine daily therapy. Children metabolise Cyclosporin A more quickly than adults, and therefore require twice daily administration.[16]

Cyclosporin A may be nephrotoxic, so serum levels of this drug must be monitored closely to avoid toxicity. Other side effects include hirsutism, tremor, gum hypertrophy and, less commonly, lymphoma.[17]

Azathioprine

Azathioprine is administered once daily by mouth. Azathioprine should be administered in the afternoon, so that the dosage can be adjusted according to the day's blood test results. The dosage may be reduced or withheld if the child has a white blood cell count below 4×10^9/L.[12] Azathioprine diminishes the body's immune response by interfering with cellular purine synthesis, and therefore decreasing antibody production.[8]

Side effects include bone marrow depression, increased risk of infection, increased risk of skin cancer (children must be advised against excessive exposure to the sun) and viral warts. Liver toxicity is also a side effect. Parents should be advised to report any dark urine or pale stools or signs of yellowing of the skin or eyes.[17] Parents must also be warned that the child should avoid contact with people who may have chickenpox, measles etc. If the child accidentally comes into contact with one of these contagious viruses, parents should be told to advise their physician so that immunoglobulin may be administered.

Antilymphocyte globulin

Antilymphocyte globulin (ALG) is administered by intravenous infusion over a period of at least 4 hours and is restricted to a course of 10 days' therapy.

Antilymphocyte globulin is an immunoglobulin produced by injecting human lymphocytes into a horse or rabbit. The animal then produces antibodies to the human cells. When the animal serum is refined and administered to humans by intravenous infusion, their T and B lymphocytes and monocytes become coated with the medication and are then susceptible to destruction by the immune system.[8] It is effective in treating transplant rejection.

Side effects include anaphylaxis (rare) (premedication with hydrocortisone, phenergan and paracetamol is usually administered to prevent anaphylaxis); serum sickness (rare); fever, thrombocytopenia; and predisposition to viral infections, including herpes and cytomegalovirus.

Orthoclone OKT3

OKT3 is administered by intravenous injection for a period of 10 days. Cyclosporin therapy is usually withheld during the period in which OKT3 is being administered.[18] OKT3 is an immunoglobulin G antibody that reacts in T lymphocyte membranes with a molecule referred to as CD3. CD3 is necessary for antigen recognition. OKT3 therefore blocks the T cell functions involved in rejection.[19] OKT3 is efficient in reversing rejection episodes and prevents the onset of rejection.[20]

If OKT3 is administered to children who are fluid overloaded it may result in severe pulmonary oedema. Therefore dialysis or diuretic medication may be required before therapy. Side effects such as fever, chills, dyspnoea and chest pain may be prevented by premedication with intravenous hydrocortisone. Increased susceptibility to infection, particularly cytomegalovirus and herpes are other side effects.

COMPLICATIONS OF RENAL TRANSPLANT

The reader should refer to a renal nursing text book for a full explanation of the following potential complications of renal transplant.

- Initial non-function of renal transplant (may be due to acute tubular necrosis, rejection, renal vein thrombosis, or obstruction of urine flow).
- Haemorrhage.
- Urine leak.
- Recurrence of original disease in the transplant kidney.
- Viral infections such as cytomegalovirus or herpes.
- Yeast and fungal infection (especially of the mouth).
- Protozoal infection.
- Hypertension.
- Increased risk of malignancy and lymphoma.

REFERENCES

1. Uldall R. *Renal nursing.* 3rd ed. Oxford: Blackwell Scientific, 1988.
2. Greenberg CS. *Nursing care planning guides for children.* Sydney: Williams & Wilkins, 1988.
3. Fine RN, Gruskin AB. End-stage renal disease in children. *End stage renal disease in children.* Philadelphia: Saunders, 1984.
4. Dosselor JB. Ethics in transplantation *In:* Morris PJ, ed. *Kidney transplantation. The principles and practice.* 4th ed. London: Harcourt Brace Jovanovich, 1994.
5. Shiel AG, McCaughan GW, Thompson JF, Dorney SFA, Stephen MJ, Bookallil MJ. The first five years clinical experience of the Australian National Liver Transplant Unit. *Med J Aust* 1992; 156: 9–16
6. Shaben TR. Psychosocial issues in kidney transplanted children and adolescents: Literature review. *American Nephrology Nurses Association Journal* 1993; 20: 663–668.
7. Ting A. Welsh, K. HLA matching and crossmatching in renal transplantation *In:* Morris PJ. *Kidney transplantation the principles and practice.* 3rd ed. London: Harcourt Brace Jovanovich, 1994.
8. Hamilton HK. *Nurses clinical library. Renal and urological disorders.* Springhouse, USA: Springhouse Corporation, 1984.
9. Noreen J. Tissue typing for renal transplantation. *The Lamp* 1980; 37: 57–60
10. Gower PE. *Nephrology.* London: Grant, McIntyre, 1983.
11. Terasati PI, Park MS, Danovitch GM. Histocompatibility, testing, crossmatching and allocation of cadaveric kidney transplants *In:* Danovitch GM, ed. *Handbook of kidney transplantation.* Boston: Little Brown, 1992.
12. Davison AM. *Nephrology.* London: Heinemann Medical Books, 1988.
13. Campton CM. Oral care for the renal transplant patient. *American Nephrology Nurses Association Journal.* 1991; 18: 39–41.
14. Shaefer MS, Collier DS. Immunosuppression for solid organ transplantation. *Dialysis and Transplantation.* 1993; 22: 542–553.
15. Keown PA. Cyclosporin in organ transplantation and autoimmunity. *Current Therapeutics* 1990; November: 75–83.
16. Cutler RE. Cyclosporine revisited, part 1: structure and function, pharmacokinetics, and mechanism of immunosuppression. *Dialysis Transplant* 1990; 19: 440–443.
17. Duffy MM, Uber L. Immunosuppressive medicine. *Dialysis and Transplantation* 1994; 23: 571–574.
18. Palmer J, Slook P. Successful use of Orthoclone OKT3 for steroid resistant acute rejection in pediatric renal allograft recipients. *American Nephrology Nurses Association Journal* 1992; 19: 375–377.
19. Thistlethwaite JR, Cosini AB, Delmonica FL, Rubin RH, Tulkoss-Rubin N, Nelson PW, Fang L, Russell PS. Evolving use of OKT3 monocolonal antibody for treatment of renal allograft rejection. *Transplantation* 1984; 38: 695–701.
20. Shield CF. *Orthoclone OKT3 in transplant rejection.* Amsterdam: Excerpts Medica, 1990.

Disturbances in Sensory Function

Alteration to Structure of the Eye

Julie Bleasdale and Jill Molan

The principles of paediatric ophthalmic nursing have been stated in Chapter 5, to which the reader is referred. Visual assessment of a baby or child is an important component of paediatric assessment. The child's visual assessment includes the family history and identification of prenatal, perinatal and developmental influences, as any alteration to the eye structures may lead to an alteration in function. It is therefore important to test visual function. This is possible for an infant or child of any age. Each eye must be tested separately, as a defect in a one eye may be masked by use of the 'good eye'. Visual testing can be carried out by nurses, orthoptists and medical officers.

Simple examinations that may be used to assess visual function in an infant are: eye contact, size and clarity of corneas, corneal light reflexes, pupillary responses to light, eye movements (following objects), preferential looking, and red reflex. In addition to these methods, children aged 2 to 3 years and older may be tested formally by the use of picture cards requiring verbal responses.

ANOMALIES

Congenital anomalies may occur in any part of the eye structure including the sclera, cornea, anterior chamber, iris, lens, lens zonules, vitreous, retina and optic nerve. Anomalies can also involve the whole eye, and these include anophthalmia, which is the congenital absence of the whole of the eye/s.

Coloboma

A coloboma is a gap or notch in any ocular structure, reflecting the incomplete closure of the embryonic ocular fissure. The most common form occurs in the eyelid. Surgery is usually required to prevent corneal exposure. Iris and retinal colobomas can also occur and may lead to visual impairment.

LACRIMAL DUCT OBSTRUCTION

Lacrimal duct obstruction is a very common problem in early infancy. It is usually caused by an imperforate nasolacrimal duct which is present at birth. The obstruction causes tears and mucus to pool in the sac above the obstruction and results in a watery eye. The stagnation of this material leads to chronic discharge and sometimes acute infection. The majority of these obstructions will resolve spontaneously by 6 to 9 months of age, when the duct becomes patent.

Nursing action

Parent education consists of teaching about eye toilets, massage of the lacrimal sac and instillation of antibiotic drops following massage.

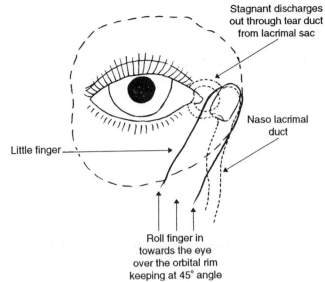

Figure 6.40 Massaging the lacrimal sac.

Massaging the lacrimal sac:

- Wash hands.
- Place the little finger at 45° angle below the inner canthus, so that the finger can feel the orbital rim.
- Roll the finger over the orbital rim towards the eye. This expresses stagnant material in the sac out through the tear duct.
- Repeat until no discharge is expressed.
- Clean the eye with normal saline and instil eye drops if prescribed.

Obstruction of the lacrimal duct which does not resolve will require probing of the nasolacrimal duct under general anaesthesia. The infant is admitted as a day stay patient. Blood-stained ooze from the tear duct and nose can be expected after probing, and the tear duct area may be red for several days.

CATARACT

A cataract is an opacity of the lens which can be either unilateral or bilateral. The causes of cataract in children are multiple and may be congenital (e.g., intrauterine rubella) or acquired (e.g., following trauma). Surgery is the only effective treatment and may be undertaken as early as 1 week of age.

Specific preoperative care

- Prophylactic antibiotic drops may be ordered preoperatively.
- The pupil must be dilated to allow the surgeon access to the lens. More that one type of mydriatic (dilating drop) may be ordered. Wait 10 minutes between each drop for maximum effect.

Specific postoperative care

- Some haemoserous ooze may be present. Discourage rubbing of eyes. Arm splints may be needed.
- Dressings are removed the next morning, the eye cleaned and treatment commenced in the form of eye drops, usually an antibiotic and an anti-inflammatory.
- Parents are instructed on eye assessment and instillation of eye drops.

Two major problems occur following surgery. Aphakia is the absence of the lens which makes it impossible for the child to focus an image on the retina. Aphakia is usually corrected by either glasses or contact lenses which can be prescribed for babies as young as 1 week old.

Postoperative amblyopia is a potential problem which is more likely to develop in children with unilateral cataract. The image projected onto the retina, in the eye without the lens, is larger than the image in the eye which still retains the lens. It is impossible for the brain to fuse the 2 images when they are so different in size, so the image from one eye is suppressed, resulting in an impairment in the visual development in that eye. Visual development in these children is therefore closely monitored by the ophthalmologist. Management of amblyopia is outlined in the section on strabismus.

GLAUCOMA

Glaucoma is a condition of raised intraocular pressure (IOP) leading to pressure on the optic nerve head (optic disc) which can result in loss of vision. Normal IOP is 10 to 22 mmHg.

Nursing assessment

- Eye/s appear large (buphthalmos), stretched.
- The child will show signs of photophobia by watery eyes, avoidance and sensitivity to light.
- The corneas may have a hazy appearance.
- The child may be irritable because of the increased intraocular pressure which may cause eye discomfort.

Normally, intraocular pressure is maintained by the volume of aqueous humour in the eye. The aqueous humour is filtered constantly from the blood in the epithelium of the ciliary body. It flows out of the eye at a similar rate, through the drainage angle back into the bloodstream. The drainage angle is located where the iris and cornea meet and consists of the trabecular meshwork and canal of Schlemm. In children, sometimes a membrane covers the trabecular meshwork and obstructs the aqueous outflow, resulting in a decreased outflow and consequently an increased IOP.

Glaucoma may be a unilateral or bilateral condition and may be present at birth or develop within a few months after birth. It can occur in isolation or in association with other congenital ocular abnormalities or systemic disorders. An examination under anaesthesia (EUA) is necessary to carry out the following diagnostic tests:

- Measurement of intraocular pressure (IOP).
- Measurement of corneal diameters. Sometimes the high pressure causes stretching of the cornea.
- Gonioscopy (looking into the drainage angle).

- Optic disc assessment.
- Surgery is usually required. Goniotomy is a procedure where the membrane is removed by incision and an opening is created in the trabecular meshwork to increase the outflow of aqueous humor.
- Other surgical procedures such as trabeculectomy may be required if goniotomy is unsuccessful.

Follow-up at regular intervals by the ophthalmologist to monitor IOP and adjust treatment is essential, as an eye which appears to be normal on inspection may still have raised IOP. These check-ups require an EUA and may be as often as every 3 months. Sometimes eye drops are needed to help control IOP. Parents should be instructed to watch for raised pressure between medical check-ups. The main signs are photophobia, clouding of the cornea/s and red, irritable eyes.

PTOSIS

Ptosis is a condition in which the eyelid droops and the child is unable to elevate it. It is usually caused by an underaction of one of the muscles in the eyelid, usually the levator palpebrae. Ptosis can be unilateral or bilateral and is most commonly hereditary. The severity of the condition varies from hardly noticeable to so severe that the lid occludes the pupil (and the line of vision). The child may tilt the head in order to see from beneath the drooping lid. Amblyopia may develop. Surgical correction is necessary. This may involve resection of the levator muscle or brow suspension where a muscle sling using donor fascia lata or synthetic mersilene is constructed.

After surgery the lids will be swollen and may not close initially. The upper lid suture is usually removed the morning after surgery. Brow sutures will fall out in about 3 weeks. Lubricant ointment should be instilled at night to protect the cornea.

STRABISMUS (SQUINT)

Strabismus is also referred to as a turned eye or a lazy eye. It is a misalignment of the eyes so that only 1 eye can look at a chosen object at a given time. The misalignment can be caused by an underaction or overaction of any 1 of the 6 extra ocular muscles. The eye/s may be deviated in an inward, outward, upward or downward direction. Some squints are present all the time, others are latent and will manifest themselves only when the child is tired. Strabismus is a very common eye disorder in children and can be unilateral or bilateral. The major complication of strabismus is the risk of amblyopia. The aims of treatment are to:

- Restore optimum visual acuity in the affected eye while maintaining good vision in the unaffected eye.
- Encourage binocular vision to develop where images from both eyes are able to provide depth perception.
- Improve the child's appearance. Treatment is very complex and must be individualised to each child.

Orthoptists work in conjunction with ophthalmologists to diagnose which muscles are involved and monitor visual development. Organic causes of the visual loss, for example retinoblastoma, are eliminated. The most appropriate treatment is then chosen from occlusion therapy (patching), glasses or exercises. These treatments may be used singly or in combination.

Occlusion therapy is very difficult and frustrating for both the child and family. It remains, nevertheless, the most effective way to improve the visual acuity in amblyopia. An occlusion patch is applied to the good eye for a prescribed amount of time per day. This forces the child to use the affected eye which, in turn, improves the visual acuity in that eye.

Surgical correction of the deviation is often necessary. Surgery on its own, however, will not improve the vision. There are 2 main surgical methods. Muscle recession is a weakening procedure, whereby the muscle insertion is moved posteriorly towards its origin. Muscle resection is a strengthening procedure, whereby the muscle is shortened, enhancing its pull. Strabismus surgery is often a day-stay procedure or the child may be required to stay overnight.

After surgery, the white of the affected eye/s will be red. This redness may take up to 4 weeks to resolve. There will be some blood-stained ooze/tears from the affected eye during the first night. The child may have some double vision, but this should resolve.

Specific postoperative care

- Eye toilets for hygiene and comfort.
- An antibiotic ointment will be prescribed and parents/caregivers need to be instructed in the instillation of eye ointment.
- The eye will not be padded postoperatively.
- Refer to the ophthalmologist regarding the need to resume preoperative treatment, for example patching.

AMBLYOPIA

Amblyopia can be defined as 'unilateral defective vision, incorrectable by glasses, in an otherwise normal eye' which 'develops in young children in whom visual information received by the brain from one eye is inadequate or conflicts with information from the other eye'.[1] Blindness caused by amblyopia is preventable. With early detection and treatment it is possible for normal vision to be restored, but treatment must be given during childhood. Treatment for amblyopia consists of an occlusion program, usually prescribed by the orthoptist. The good eye is covered, usually by a stick-on patch, to encourage use of the amblyopic (weaker) eye, thereby improving visual acuity. Close monitoring by the orthoptist and ophthalmologist ensures visual development is regularly assessed and treatment is then tailored to the particular child.

RETINAL PROBLEMS

Retinal problems can be hereditary, vascular or related to detachment.

Hereditary

The most familiar hereditary retinal problem is retinitis pigmentosa, a progressive deterioration of the rods and cones in the retina. It first reduces the ability to adapt to the dark, and eventually affects the visual acuity, usually in adolescence.

Vascular — retinopathy of prematurity

The retinopathy observed in premature infants, previously known as retrolental fibroplasia, is now called retinopathy of prematurity (ROP). ROP is characterised by retinal ischaemia, a consequence of the immature vasculature of the retina. It may resolve spontaneously, or may progress rapidly leading to retinal detachment and subsequent visual loss. All infants born prematurely with a low birthweight should have an ophthalmic assessment within 4 to 6 weeks of delivery to assess the retinal state.

Retinal detachment

The choroid underlies the retina and its blood vessels supply nutrients to the rods and cones of the retina, but are not firmly attached to it. Hence the choroid can become separated from the retina, leading to ischaemia and eventual necrosis of the rods and cones. Trauma, such as a blow to the eye, is the most common cause of retinal detachment in children, although the child may not present with symptoms for months or years after the initial trauma. The child may complain of seeing flashing lights, or a curtain or fog ('spider webs') over his or her vision. There is no pain. Children with retinal detachment usually require surgery.

PERSISTENT HYPERPLASTIC PRIMARY VITREOUS

The primary vitreous develops in the first few weeks of pregnancy. Persistent hyperplastic primary vitreous (PHPV) is a developmental abnormality of the vitreous which is usually unilateral and associated with a small eye (microphthalmos). Parents may notice a white pupil (leukocoria) and that the affected eye appears small. Differentiation from a retinoblastoma is essential and is usually undertaken by ultrasound, CT scan or an examination under anaesthesia.

PHPV is caused by a failure of regression of the primary vitreous. The primary vitreous forms a retrolental mass which occupies the anterior vitreous cavity. With time the vitreous contracts, causing dehiscence of the lens leading to a cataract. Swelling of the lens may also lead to glaucoma. Early surgical intervention is necessary for removal of the mass and the lens, and is undertaken in an operation called a lensectomy and anterior vitrectomy. Limited vision can be restored in mildly affected eyes.

OCULAR TRAUMA

The history of the injury is important as it provides clues as to the nature of the injury. For example: 'playing cricket and hit in the eye with the ball' would describe blunt trauma; 'watching dad hammering a nail and something flew into the eye' would cause a high-velocity intraocular foreign body to be suspected; and 'walking in the wind' would result in dust in the eye.

Ideally, visual acuity should be assessed before treatment, except where a chemical has been splashed in the eye. The eye is assessed as described in Chapter 5. X-ray, ultrasound or computed tomography scans may be necessary to locate intraocular foreign bodies. Any ocular injury should be assessed by a medical officer.

Types of injuries

Lid lacerations

Lid lacerations in children are mostly the result of a dog bite or cat scratch. If lid margins or tear ducts are involved, surgical repair by an ophthalmologist is necessary to realign the lid margins and tear ducts.

Chemical burns

Alkali is more damaging to the eye than acid as it penetrates the cornea more readily and damages intraocular structures. Prompt and effective first aid may determine visual prognosis. It is essential that copious continuous irrigation be carried out at the scene, en route and after arrival at the hospital. The lids are everted to remove any material trapped under them.

The child may be admitted to hospital in order to monitor for complications and to observe the healing process in the eye.

Corneal foreign body or abrasion

If a foreign body under the upper lid is suspected, the lid must be everted. It is common for a subtarsal foreign body to cause corneal abrasions. After removal of a foreign body, antibiotic ointment is instilled and a firm pad is applied. The eye is reviewed daily. An embedded foreign body may require the child to be hospitalised for general anaesthesia in order to facilitate removal. Pain is relieved by keeping the eye closed, usually with the support of an eye pad, and the administration of appropriate pain relief. Under no circumstances should local anaesthetic drops be administered regularly as these delay healing and aggravate inflammation, thus compounding the problem.

Superglue in the eye

Rapidly bonding glue is not usually irritating to the eye and its presence usually will not cause permanent damage. As old skin cells are shed the glue will be removed with them. Lashes may need to be cut to increase comfort and will regrow in a matter of weeks.

Blunt injuries with hyphaema

A hyphaema is blood in the anterior segment of the eye, that is, in front of the lens and behind the cornea. It is usually caused by a blunt blow to the eye with, for example, a ball, which tears the blood vessels of the iris. A hyphaema is a serious eye injury, and may be associated with concomitant injuries caused by the blow, for example, retinal damage, orbital fractures. A simple hyphaema, however, does not cause permanent visual disturbance. Loss of vision is the result of associated injuries, or secondary complications.

In an uncomplicated hyphaema, the blood is absorbed within 3 to 7 days, depending on the size. To assess any damage to the retina or optic nerve, the pupil is dilated and the internal structures inspected, usually immediately before discharge or at a follow-up appointment.

The treatment for hyphaema aims to promote resorption of the haemorrhage and monitor for signs of complications, for example, raised IOP or a secondary bleed. Medical treatment is usually conservative, varies with individual preference and includes:

- Bed rest in hospital for 3 to 7 days. The child may be positioned with the head elevated at 45° so that blood in the anterior chamber forms a level or lying flat which allows the blood to drain more readily.
- Eye pad which may be unilateral or bilateral.
- Prophylactic antibiotic eye drops. In some circumstances, steroid eye drops, mydriatics (dilating drops) and surgery to drain the blood is carried out.

The complications of hyphaema include:

- A secondary haemorrhage, which occurs 2 to 5 days after injury. The secondary haemorrhage is often larger than the initial bleed and may fill the anterior chamber, requiring surgery to drain it. The patient may complain of sharp pain if a secondary bleed has occurred.
- Secondary glaucoma, which occurs when damage to the drainage apparatus impedes aqueous outflow, leading to increased IOP. This may develop months or years after the initial injury.
- Corneal staining where iron from the red blood cells stains the endothelial cells of the cornea and which may take months to clear.

Prognosis is directly related to the size of the hyphaema. The larger the hyphaema, the greater the risk of complications. Penetrating eye injuries are not discussed and the reader is referred to the bibliography at the end of this section.

REFERENCE

1. Martin F. Current paediatric ophthalmic problems. *In:* Procopis PG & Kewley G. eds. *Current paediatric practice.* Sydney: Harcourt Brace Jovanovich, 1991: 267–273.

BIBLIOGRAPHY

Kanski JJ. *Clinical ophthalmology: a systematic approach.* London: Heinemann, 1994.
Nelson LB, Calhoun JH, Harley RD. *Paediatric ophthalmology.* Philadelphia: Saunders, 1991.
Spalton O. *Atlas of clinical ophthalmology* 2nd ed. London: Wolfe Publishing, 1994.

Ingestion of a Foreign Body

Lynne Brodie

The ingestion of a foreign body is a common occurrence in children, particularly in the toddler age group. Coins and other disc-shaped objects are the most frequently swallowed. Other than food, the next most frequently swallowed objects include nuts, pins and small batteries.[1] The parent may witness the event or the child may confess. In either case, oesophagoscopy is indicated unless the object is known to be radiopaque and can be shown on x-ray. The child may present with no clinical features unless the object is large or sharp. Operation is usually delayed until a safe fasting time has elapsed and the child can be safely anaesthetised.

POSTOPERATIVE NURSING CARE

In most cases, the child will experience little or no discomfort following removal of the foreign body and may be allowed home the same day. A sip test is given one hour after surgery and if the child is able to swallow easily, fluids and food are gradually offered. If the child is febrile, or has persistent dysphagia, a longer stay may be required. Paracetomol is generally sufficient to relieve discomfort. Some children are reluctant to swallow and in a small number of cases this may continue for several weeks after surgery.

REFERENCE

1. Royal Alexandra Hospital for Children data. *Foreign body ingestion excluding poisoning.* Childsafe New South Wales, 1992.

Aspiration of a Foreign Body

Lynne Brodie

Although not as common as ingestion, aspiration also presents a problem in the paediatric population, particularly in the toddler age group.[1] Symptoms may vary according to the size and position of the aspirated body, but persistent cough and wheeze are frequent presenting symptoms. Physical examination may reveal unequal air entry, which may be localised to one lung or lobe. In a small percentage of children, there may be no symptoms despite a clear history of aspiration. In cases where the history is unclear, endoscopy may be required for definitive diagnosis. X-ray may be helpful if the foreign body is radio-opaque, but approximately 20% of x-rays are normal and the remainder are often misinterpreted as unresolved upper respiratory tract infections.[2] Before endoscopy, the child may be in some degree of respiratory distress and the nurse should observe the child closely and report worsening symptoms immediately. Pulse and respirations should be monitored every half hour if the child is distressed. Following endoscopy, there may be persistent symptoms which require short-term hospital admission for antibiotic treatment and physiotherapy. However, in most cases, removal of the foreign body will result in immediate relief of symptoms and the child will be discharged following routine postoperative recovery.

REFERENCES

1. Royal Alexandra Hospital for Children data. *Inhaled foreign bodies.* Childsafe New South Wales, 1992.
2. Evans JNG. Foreign bodies in the Larynx and trachea. *In: Scott-Browne's otolaryngology.* London: Butterworth, 1987: 438–447.

Cochlear Implant

Lynne Brodie

The bionic ear, developed by Professor Clark at Melbourne University, was initially used on adults. Paediatric implants were first performed in Sydney in 1986 under a trial program involving the Children's Cochlear Implant Centre (NSW), The University of Sydney and The Royal Alexandra Hospital for Children, Camperdown. The Australian 22 Channel Cochlear Implant, manufactured by Cochlear Pty Ltd in Sydney, was approved in June 1990 as a safe and effective device for children aged 2 to 17 years.

At selected centres throughout Australia, the device is implanted by specialists who work in conjunction with a highly skilled team of health professionals. They include audiologists, habilitationists, speech pathologists, counsellors, administrative staff and research personnel.

Following initial assessment by the specialist, a series of medical tests is performed. Tests include specialised CT scans, promontory stimulation tests (for older children), electrocochleography and assessment by a paediatrician and neurologist if indicated. Further assessments include extensive testing of audiology, speech, language and general physical and psychosocial development.

All children undergo a 10-week trial period of using a hearing aid/vibrotactile aid. Only children who show no benefit from such aids are eligible for implant. Family commitment and support are essential and parents are required to attend preoperative counselling and assessment sessions.

Parents are fully informed of the benefits, limitations and possible complications of surgery. Once all assessments have been completed and the child is accepted for the program, parents sign a contract. A comprehensive protocol has been developed by the Children's Cochlear Implant Centre (NSW) and other centres involved in such programs.[1]

Medical tests

Before the actual implant surgery, the child will be admitted to hospital on a day-stay basis for CT scans and electrocochleography. The scans are taken to diagnose osteogenesis (new bone growth) which may obliterate the lumen of the cochlear, preventing insertion of the cochlear device.

Electrocochleography, also performed under light anaesthesia, determines whether the child has high frequency hearing, and provides an indication of the intactness of the haircells of the cochlea. The eardrum and middle ear are also examined at the same time to detect any abnormalities.

Implant surgery

The child enters hospital the day before surgery. Admission procedure and assessment is routine and the parents and child are seen again by the specialists to discuss any questions and obtain written consent. The parents are told of potential risks to the facial nerve, the dangers of infection and that a small section of hair will be shaved on the affected side of the head.[2]

Nursing care following cochlear implant surgery

Postoperative observations will be determined by hospital protocol. At The Royal Alexandra Hospital for Children in Sydney, temperature, pulse and respiration are recorded on return from the recovery ward and hourly pulse and respirations are monitored for the first 4 hours. Any sign of facial weakness should be reported immediately. Thereafter, vital signs are monitored every 4 hours if satisfactory.[3]

The child has a head bandage and the nurse notes and reports any bleeding or swelling. The dressing is left intact and in the early postoperative period is only removed on the surgeon's instructions if there is concern over excessive exudate or pain. Narcotic analgesia is provided as necessary for the first 24 hours and thereafter paracetamol is usually sufficient to relieve discomfort. Intravenous therapy is maintained until the child is tolerating oral fluids. In some cases, antiemetics may be required for excessive vomiting, but this is generally only a short-term problem. Prophylactic antibiotic cover is required. This is initially given intravenously and then changed to oral once the child is tolerating oral fluids. The cannula can then be removed.

Experience has shown that children recover very quickly and are anxious to resume their normal activities by the 1st or 2nd postoperative day when they may generally be discharged. The dressing is removed by the surgeon before discharge. If the suture line is clean and dry it may be sprayed with plastic skin and a clean bandage reapplied to protect the wound. It is recommended that the wound be protected by a bandage or beanie. This measure also alerts others to the need for care when playing with the child.

Parents are advised to restrict their child's activity for 1 week and to avoid exposing the child to others with upper respiratory tract infections. They are instructed to ensure the child completes the course of antibiotics. School-age children can return to school after the follow-up appointment 7–10 days after discharge. Contact sports such as football are not recommended.

Approximately 4 to 5 weeks after implant, the child is readmitted as a day-stay patient and the functioning of the implant is tested while the child is lightly anaesthetised. If the implant evoked brainstem auditory potentials (IMEBAP) are satisfactory, the child attends the Children's Cochlear Implant Centre in Naremburn NSW for 'switch on'. This process marks the beginning of an intensive 5-year program which is detailed in the protocol. Although the program is still in its infancy, the results to date are extremely promising and the future for deaf children and their families has been considerably enhanced by the dedication of those involved in the development of this new technology.

REFERENCES

1. Department of Otolaryngology, University of Sydney, The Children's Hospital, Camperdown & The Children's Cochlear Implant Centre, NSW. *The protocol for children eligible for cochlear implantation*, Sydney, 1991.
2. Cochlear Pty Ltd. *Issues and answers: a guide to cochlear implants.* 1990.
3. Royal Alexandra Hospital for Children. *Nursing policy and procedure manual.* Sydney: RAHC, 1991: 06. 06.

in 5 children who have asthma are sensitive to orally administered aspirin.[2] Parents should be advised to avoid aspirin, as paracetomol offers a suitable and readily available alternative for pain relief and temperature reduction in children.

Other factors

Although a complete list of potential triggers to the asthma sufferer is impossible to compile, there are several that are worthwhile mentioning, even though they are not always avoidable.

Weather change has been noted by many parents to be responsible for exacerbations of asthma. These observations are well supported by an increase in hospital attendance and admission rates for asthma which correlate with changes in weather.[2] Phelan proposes that 'sudden weather change may be responsible for the sudden release into the atmosphere of large amounts of aero-allergen, which may be a factor in the association of weather and exacerbations of asthma'.

Air pollution is also considered by a substantial portion of the general public to cause respiratory illness. The evidence, however, is inconclusive and it is suggested that the influence of atmospheric pollution on childhood asthma is small.[2] While air pollution is not considered a cause of asthma, high levels of photochemical smog and airborne particulates may well be a trigger factor in susceptible individuals.[25]

TYPES OF ASTHMA

Asthma covers a broad spectrum and is usually described according to its pattern and severity. The severity is generally described as mild, moderate or severe,[14,15] while the pattern is classified according to type and frequency. The most common classifications being infrequent episodic, frequent episodic and chronic or persistent.[2] Optimal management is dependent upon recognising the severity and the pathological processes,[26] and needs to be specific to the type of asthma and severity.[19,21]

During the acute phase, the nurse's primary roles include assessment, administration of prescribed treatments and providing support for the child and family.

NURSING ASSESSMENT IN AN ACUTE PRESENTATION

In order to determine the presence and severity of airways obstruction, the assessment should combine collecting a relevant history, conducting a physical assessment and gathering clinical data.[27,28]

The assessment will be enhanced by using age-appropriate strategies when dealing with the child and family. Reducing parental anxiety will assist in reducing the anxiety of the child. Consideration of age-related signs of respiratory distress will facilitate accurate assessment.

History

The nursing history should be conducted briskly but thoroughly, focusing on aspects related to asthma and the current episode including: length of current attack; severity; recent medications; exposure to potential triggers; night cough; previous history related to asthma and other relevant information. In addition, a more general history may elicit further information to assist in care of the child.

Clinical assessment

The clinical assessment is aimed at gathering data to determine the severity of the asthma and to monitor response to interventions. The assessment should focus on parameters such as: behaviour, conscious state, colour, respiratory rate, respiratory effort and heart rate.

Additional information that will further enhance the assessment includes: peak expiratory flow rates (PEFR); oxygen saturations; respiratory sounds; measurement of pulsus paradoxus; and response to bronchodilators. The use of an asthma severity score based on the above may further improve the assessment.

Changes that may signify an early change in the child's clinical status should be noted. These could include cough, restlessness, anxiety, inability to speak, irritability, colour changes, respiratory changes, exhaustion or loss of consciousness. Airflow may still be compromised even in the absence of these signs.[27,28]

Assessment of colour

The child's colour may vary depending on the severity of the airway obstruction. The subtle colour changes that occur provide vital clues to alteration in clinical status.

Accurate oxygen saturations measured with a pulse oximeter provide useful data that may reflect the severity of the asthma as well as providing information relating to the child's response to interventions.[29,30] Accurate readings will only be achieved if factors that may interfere with the oximeter, such as movement of the child, cool extremities, nail polish and poor signal are minimised.

Oxygen saturation readings can fluctuate widely during an episode of asthma and have a tendency to fall during a coughing bout.[31] Inspection of the mucous membranes and fingernail beds will assist in distinguishing central from peripheral cyanosis. Cyanosis in the child with asthma occurs at a late stage and is a serious finding (see physiological changes in asthma).

Respiration

Assessment of respiration involves observing the respiratory rate, the chest movement, the depth of respiration, and use of accessory muscles.

The respiratory rate will vary, but generally reflects the severity of the airway obstruction, increasing breathlessness with tachypnoea indicates increasing severity and reducing airflow. The more effort required to maintain adequate ventilation by the child the greater the possibility of exhaustion.

During the normal respiratory cycle, expiration time is twice that of inspiration. Increasing airway obstruction causes inspiration to become shorter and expiration prolonged,[32] causing respiratory effort to increase. Wheezes, if present, tend to occur initially during expiration, and as the condition worsens, become generalised.

The increase in depth of respiration is related to the increased effort required to exhale expired air. The accessory muscles may become active to support respiration, involving additional use of the intercostal muscles, supraclavicular with sternal retraction, as well as use of the abdominal muscles. This may indicate a degree of respiratory distress. The extent of accessory muscle use further reflects the severity of the airway obstruction.[33,34]

Children less than 7 years of age tend to be diaphragmatic breathers so their abdomen naturally rises on inspiration.[35]

The chest should be observed to determine if chest movement is symmetrical. Loss of symmetry may indicate diminished air entry, possibly due to lobar collapse, air entrapment, mucus plugging and, less commonly, pneumothorax.[2]

Auscultation

As part of a respiratory assessment, the child's chest should be auscultated to distinguish normal from abnormal breath sounds and to ensure that air entry is satisfactory. The abnormal sound in asthma is usually a wheeze, although this is not always the case. Other possible causes of wheeze include aspiration of a foreign body, bronchiolitis and pneumonia.

The chest should be auscultated before and after inhaled medications in order to monitor the child's response.

An extreme situation may develop when the air entry diminishes so significantly that the amount and velocity of the air passing through the lungs is generating insufficient energy to produce a sound, this is termed a 'silent chest'.

The findings associated with acute airflow limitation include tachycardia, tachypnoea, wheeze, cough, poor air entry, use of accessory muscles, sweating and pulsus paradoxus. Changes may occur in some or all of these parameters at any time. Concern will be evident if the child exhibits a silent chest, cyanosis, bradycardia, exhaustion, confusion or unconsciousness.[36]

Behaviour

The parents are a valuable resource in distinguishing normal from abnormal behaviour. The child's general appearance, behaviour, and ability to cope with activities provides significant data which assist in determining the severity of the airway obstruction. Restricted airflow may reduce the child's ability to perform normal functions such as playing, talking and concentrating on simple tasks.

Assessment of behaviour will generally reflect the clinical status; the irritable, uncooperative or drowsy child may be associated with a degree of cerebral hypoxia. The conscious state may deteriorate with worsening asthma. Frequent assessment is therefore important.

Peak flow

During an acute attack, peak flow measurements which are easy to teach and relatively simple to perform may assist in determining severity of airways obstruction.

The procedure for performing the peak flow usually involves the child having 3 attempts and the best result is recorded (**Figure 7.1**).

The age of the child needs to be considered, but most children 6 years and older should be able to learn and perform a satisfactory technique and provide a reliable reading. Predicted values are based on height, sex and weight. If possible, the peak flow recording should be compared with the child's previous recordings when well.

If the child has no previous experience with PEFR, the interpretation of the recording can be difficult. A low reading may be related to poor technique, rather than airway obstruction; on the other hand, a good reading tends to provide additional worthwhile data.[28] In the child who is inexperienced, multiple attempts should be avoided to prevent distress.

DEVICES

Peak flow meter (Figure 7.1)

Ensure the meter gauge is returned to zero. Hold meter up to mouth, keep horizontal. Breath out completely.

Take one large breath in to fill lungs and place lips around the mouthpiece, ensuring a firm seal, then breath out hard and fast. Note reading. Repeat twice more and record the best of the 3.

Advantages

Gives an objective measure of lung function and thus enables the child, parent and/or staff to better assess severity of asthma. The peak flow meter is a useful tool that can aid in decision-making related to increasing medication, seeing the doctor or going directly to hospital.

Turbuhaler (Figure 7.2)

Suitable for children 4 years and onwards.[75]

Technique

Remove cap and hold turbuhaler vertically; prepare dose by twisting dial at base until a click is heard; hold up to the mouth and seal lips around mouthpiece; breath in deeply. Remove from the mouth, reload and repeat for further doses. Note: Turbuhaler must be kept dry at all times.

Advantages

No coordination required, very portable.

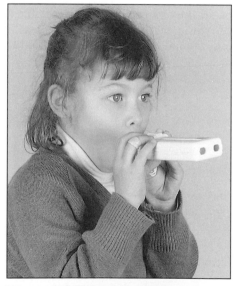

Figure 7.1 Peak flow meter.

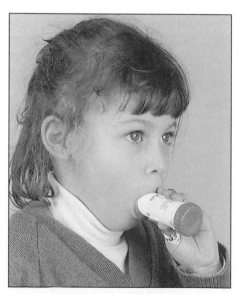

Figure 7.2 Turbuhaler.

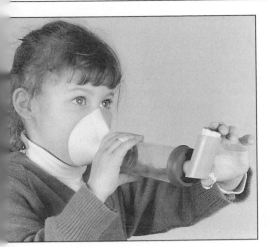

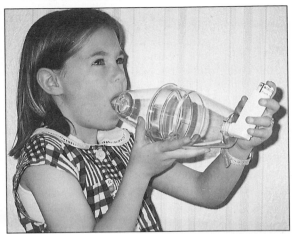

Figure 7.3a Small-volume spacer.

Figure 7.3b Large-volume spacer and metred-dose inhaler.

Small-volume spacer with mask and metered-dose inhaler (Figure 7.3a)

Suitable for very young children, including infants.

Technique

Shake the canister and insert into spacer. Place mask over the child's nose and mouth and press canister. Hold mask in place for 4 to 6 tidal breaths. Repeat if more than 1 puff is required.

Advantages

As for the large-volume spacer and MDI. Much less expensive and cumbersome than a nebuliser pump, which does not require a power source for operation.

Large-volume spacer and metered-dose inhaler (Figure 7.3b)

Suitable for a child 4 to 5 years onwards.

Technique

Shake the canister and insert in spacer. Get the child to: breathe out and press canister; take 1 long, slow breath in and hold for about 5 seconds (or, alternatively, take several slow breaths in and out).

Advantages

Minimal coordination required, reduced mouth deposition of drug and greater deposition deep within the lung due to smaller particle size and low aerosol velocity when compared with metered-dose inhaler alone (MDI).[74]

It is suggested that reduction in PEFR by 20% to 30% equates to mild asthma symptoms, by 30% to 50% moderate symptoms, and greater than 50% severe symptoms.[12] Multiple peak flow recordings should not be performed too frequently in children with moderate/severe asthma, particularly if distressed.

If possible, more specific pulmonary function tests should be performed, particularly once the acute phase has passed and the child is deemed to be well.[12]

Pulsus paradoxus

Pulsus paradoxus is another parameter used to determine severity of airway obstruction. Pulsus paradoxus is a marked variation of pulse pressure with respiration. During the respiratory cycle there are changes in arterial pressure, the pressure falls during inspiration and rises during expiration. As respiratory effort increases the changes become more marked,[37] and when the changes result in a drop in systolic blood pressure of more than 10 mmHg during inspiration, pulsus paradoxus is present.[38]

HOSPITAL ADMISSION

The criteria for children to be admitted to hospital generally include symptoms of moderately severe asthma unresponsive to emergency therapy, a recurrence of symptoms within 4 hours or peak flow less than 60% of predicted.[28,39] In addition other factors need to be considered such as: age of the child, previous history, time of day, psychosocial factors, distance from the hospital as well as the perceived families coping abilities.[28,40]

Oxygen saturations measured with a pulse oximeter are of value in predicting the need for hospital admission as the level reflects the severity of the airway obstruction and the likelihood of relapse if the child is sent home.[8,41,42] Specific levels are hard to determine, but it is suggested that an accurate oximetry reading of 91% or less in air on presentation usually requires hospital admission,[28,41,42] even if there is initial improvement. In contrast, a child presenting with oxygen saturations greater than 95% rarely requires admission and relapse is unlikely.[41]

Severe asthma or acute, life-threatening asthma (status asthmaticus) may warrant admission to an intensive care unit.[2] The frequency of assessment will vary according to the child's condition and actual findings on examination. In general, the more severe the asthma, the more frequently observations will be necessary.

Nursing staff must be able to assess accurately and interpret all designated parameters, as well as accurately document findings.[43]

MANAGEMENT

The management of asthma is aimed at improving respiration by reducing the narrowing of the airways. Treatment should address both the inflammatory process and the bronchospasm that contribute to the narrowing of the airway (see physiological changes in asthma).

Medications

There is a wide variety of medications available for the management of asthma. The actual medications and dosages will be dependent upon the type, pattern and severity of asthma. Treatment with medications is aimed at using the least drugs and smallest doses to prevent or relieve symptoms with the minimum of side effects.[12,21]

Various medications can be administered by different routes — inhaled, oral or intravenous. The most widely prescribed route currently is inhaled, and there are many delivery systems available for administering medications to the child via this route. These include metered dose inhaler, turbuhaler (**Figure 7.2**), dry powder and wet nebulisation. Additionally, large and small volume spacers (**Figures 7.3a and 7.3b**) are available (Volumatic, Nebuhaler, Fisonair, Brethotec, Areochamber) to facilitate the administration of metered-dose inhalers. The appropriate medication and delivery system will be chosen according to the type and pattern of asthma, the individual's and the family's needs, the age of the child, physical capabilities and the medication of choice.

Bronchodilators

The mainstay of asthma management are the beta-2 agonist bronchodilators, salbutamol (Ventolin, Respolin), terbutaline (Bricanyl), and fenotrol (Berotec), administered via the inhaled route.

Beta-2 agonist medications are believed to produce bronchodilation by raising the cyclic AMP level through stimulation of the beta-2 receptors and stabilising the mast cells causing chemical mediators to be released.[2]

Side effects from beta-2 agonists may include tachycardia, rise in blood pressure, muscle tremors, hyperactivity, hypokalaemia and hyperglycaemia.[28]

Salbutamol and terbutaline, the most commonly used medications in this group, are usually prescribed on an as-needed basis for infrequent episodic asthma when the child is symptomatic[44] and before exercise to prevent exercise-induced asthma.

Recent developments include longer acting beta-2 agents such as salmeterol (Serevent) and formeterol. These may be used in children, although more research is needed to determine the benefits and disadvantages of this group of drugs in children.[2]

Ipratropium bromide (Atrovent) is another inhaled bronchodilator that may be administered for moderate to severe asthma. It is used in the acute phase. Ipratropium bromide acts very specifically by reducing bronchoconstriction caused by cholinergic input. It appears that the best response from ipratropium bromide is achieved when it is administered mixed with beta-2 agonist bronchodilator.[45]

Corticosteroids

The recognition of the inflammatory response that occurs in the airways in asthma has led to an increase in the use of steroids, although the action is poorly understood. It is proposed that steroids provide an anti-inflammatory component as well as improving the response to beta-2 agonist.[46]

Steroids are seen to contribute to a shorter period of treatment and early discharge,[48,49] but have the potential for numerous side effects, including growth and adrenal suppression[44] when administered for long periods or very frequently over a period of time.

Inhaled steroids may be used prophylactically for frequent episodic asthma. Inhaled steroids include beclamethasone (Becotide, Becloforte, Aldecin) and budesonide (Pulmicort). If metered-dose inhalers are used then it is advisable to use a spacer with them to improve the quantity of drug absorbed. After administration of inhaled steroid, the child should rinse his or her mouth out to reduce the risk of oral and throat side effects such

as candidiasis. If budesonide is administered using a nebuliser, the eyes must be protected and the face must be washed after each treatment.

Oral corticosteroids tend to be prescribed for acute exacerbations when the response
to nebulised beta–2 agonists alone is poor.[44]

Methylxanthines

Methylxanthines are bronchodilators whose specific mechanism is unknown, although a
number of theories are postulated.[50]

Theophylline may be used in persistent asthma, particularly if night symptoms are a
problem,[2] or may be prescribed for acute severe asthma.

Sodium cromoglycate

Sodium cromoglycate (Intal) is used as a prophylactic agent in the management of children with frequent episodic asthma,[2] but does not have a role in the treatment of an acute
episode.

It appears that cromoglycate sodium stabilises the mast cell[47] and inhibits the release
of mediators responsible for bronchoconstriction.[50]

ACUTE MANAGEMENT

The pathophysiology of asthma is complex and includes an inflammatory process as well
as bronchospasm. The initial treatment, though, is aimed at relieving the bronchospasm
and ensuring adequate oxygenation.

If the child has previously had asthma then initial management should begin at home
in accordance with a previously organised individualised action plan. This may include
metered-dose inhalers with spacers or nebulisation of a bronchodilator.[51] In the older
child, it appears that metered-dose inhalers used with spacers are as effective as nebulised
beta-2 agonists.[52] Metered-dose inhalers are mainly used in mild to moderate asthma,
as in more severe cases the severity of the airway obstruction may prevent effective
technique.[51]

Treatment regimes for inhaled bronchodilators vary; 2 commonly used regimens are:
a fixed dose of salbutamol, irrespective of age or weight, diluted with normal saline to
4 mL[2] and nebulised though 8 to 10 L oxygen over 10 minutes,[28,51] based on the rationale
that the dose absorbed will be guided by the child's minute volume, which is related to
the child's size and weight.[2,8,28] Alternatively, a prescribed dose according to the child's
weight[2,28,53] up to a maximum of 1 mL and then diluted may be given.

The frequency of the dose will be dependent upon the severity of the asthma and the
response to interventions. If presenting symptoms on assessment indicate moderate or
severe acute asthma, a recommended regimen could be 3 nebulisers in 1 hour, prescribed
and administered in a pattern of 10 minutes of treatment and 10 minutes without treatment.[2,28,54,55] In some situations continuous nebulisation may be necessary.[28]

The response to inhaled bronchodilators in children under 2 years of age is variable,
and the reasons for this are not clear. It is recommended that a trial of these medications
be prescribed at each presentation or exacerbation.[2]

Oral bronchodilators are not recommended in an acute attack as they are of minimal
value and the inhaled route using spacer devices enables children of all ages to use this
preferred route[19,56]

Steroids

Oral (prednisolone) or intravenous (methylprednisolone, hydrocortisone) steroid administration is likely in children with moderate/severe asthma when response to beta-2 agonists is not achieved or there is deterioration after initial improvement. The oral route is the preferred route, where possible, as response time is similar in both methods.[40,57,58] A situation in which an intravenous doses may be necessary could be the vomiting child.

Various regimens of steroids have been used.[29] Currently, a course of steroids is usually administered for 3 to 5 days.[2]

The inhaled route for steroids is not considered to be effective in the management of acute asthma at this time.[59,60]

Other bronchodilators

Ipratropium bromide may be added to the treatment regimen in moderate/severe asthma.[28,28a]

Methylxanthines (Aminophylline), a mainstay of medication for many years, has declined in routine use in recent times. Studies have indicated that there is no additional benefit using Aminophylline when maximal nebulised bronchodilator is used[61,62] and that the risk of adverse side effects are increased while not shortening hospitalisation time for the child with moderately severe asthma.[63]

Aminophylline may, however, still be prescribed in the treatment of severely ill children who are not responding adequately to nebulised beta-2 agonists and corticosteroids.[28,61,64] If theophylline is used, serum concentrations should be monitored as toxic levels can easily be reached.[15] Aminophylline may cause unpleasant side effects, the most common being nausea, vomiting, headache and abdominal pain.[64]

When prescribed, it is administered slowly by intravenous infusion either as a bolus every 6 hours over 20 to 30 minutes, or in a continuous infusion.[65]

Oral theophylline is not recommended for an acute attack.[28]

ADDITIONAL NURSING CONSIDERATIONS

Aspects of nursing management necessary to support medical management and provide support care for the child and family include observation and documentation (as previously discussed) oxygen therapy, positioning of the child, nutrition, play and education.

Oxygen therapy

The benefits of oxygen in the management of acute severe asthma are well recognised.[51] Hypoxaemia is a common finding and administration of oxygen improves gaseous exchange.[14,32,51]

Oxygen will generally be administered via a face mask. Different types of masks produce different concentrations of oxygen according to the flow rate. The flow rate needs to be greater than 4 L/min to prevent rebreathing of carbon dioxide. A disadvantage of the oxygen mask is the feeling of suffocation experienced by the child. An alternative method of administration available is nasal prongs.

Oxygen will be prescribed on an individual basis to maintain oxygen saturations. Specific oxygen saturations for children having oxygen administered are hard to determine, so parameters within a specified range are usually prescribed. In general, an oxygen saturation maintained above 93% is usually acceptable, although it needs to be recognised that normal oxygen saturations can occur even when the child has respiratory failure.[28]

An increase in oxygen demand may be demonstrated by the necessity to increase flow rates to maintain previously attained oxygen saturation levels. The child's oxygen saturation levels should be monitored using pulse oximetry.

Positioning

Children tend to place themselves into positions of comfort, which may support optimal lung expansion. This will be facilitated if the child can be encouraged to sit up and is well supported by pillows. To reduce exposure to potential allergens, pillows should be made of non-allergenic material or have plastic covers.

Diet and fluids

Mouth breathing is often a consequence of dyspnoea or breathlessness, causing the child's mouth to become very dry. This is further exacerbated by oxygen administration. Mouth care will promote the child's comfort. Diet and fluids are important, but should not be forced on the child, particularly if it causes the child to become distressed. Small, frequent drinks are preferable to occasional large volumes.

A mild degree of dehydration is common in children with moderate/severe acute asthma,[66] and is further exacerbated in the vomiting child. The increased metabolic rate of the child during acute asthma may cause problems with hydration. An intravenous infusion may be needed if measures taken to maintain adequate hydration are unsuccessful. If an intravenous infusion is inserted, overhydration must be avoided to prevent pulmonary oedema.[39] Diet may be offered as desired. An accurate record of input and output needs to be maintained.

Play

Quiet play, appropriate for age, should be organised for the child and is necessary in order to restrict activity and reduce oxygen consumption and demand. A reduced activity level may be indicative of worsening airflow obstruction.

Education

Education within the hospital setting is aimed at preparing the child and family to manage asthma at home. For children admitted with asthma for the first time, education for child and family should involve information related to a basic understanding of asthma, medications, correct use of devices, and when to seek medical help. For others it is a time for reviewing current status of asthma management at home and a time to check the child's technique with devices and promote the importance of compliance. Education and discharge information should be supported with written information. All families should have an individualised action plan for the ongoing management of their child's asthma.

INVESTIGATIONS

Chest x-ray

In the acute phase, a chest x-ray is not a routine investigation, but it may be necessary in children responding poorly or if the child has other abnormal respiratory signs, and to exclude non-asthmatic causes.[2,28,67,68] It has been suggested that chest x-rays are performed too often,[8] and they do not appear to alter the management of the child in the emergency area.[69]

Pulmonary function tests

Pulmonary function tests are used to provide objective data, and can be performed effectively by most children of 6 years of age and older. Pulmonary function tests are used to measure the forced expiratory volume in one second (FEV1). This is the child's ability to breathe out forcefully and rapidly and can be measured using simple equipment such as a peak flow meter, or more elaborate equipment such as a spirometer.

Pulmonary function tests can be used in conjunction with inhaled asthma medication to assist in confirming the diagnosis and are useful in ascertaining the pattern of asthma. They may be repeated at regular intervals to monitor the child's asthma. Underdiagnosis of airflow obstruction in asthma may occur if spirometry is not performed.[70]

Pulmonary function tests may be useful, particularly in older children/adolescents, in assisting them to develop a better perception of the severity of their asthma.[2] Peak flow monitoring may provide data that reflects changes in respiratory status as well as providing information to assist in diagnosis.[39] At home, twice daily peak flow monitoring combined with accurate record keeping may assist the child and family in recognising changes in airflow as well as identifying the pattern and severity of asthma.

A better guide for detecting airflow obstruction than peak flow monitoring is spirometry,[21] which is useful in differentiating between obstructive and restrictive airway problems as well as the presence of small airways disease.[71]

Allergy testing

Allergy testing is not performed routinely in children with asthma,[11] but may be useful in children whose symptoms are caused by specific allergies. Skin testing may produce positive results in the radioallergosorbent test (RAST) to various stimuli which are not associated with the asthma.[2]

Immunological tests

Immunological testing is not routinely performed,[11] except in circumstances where clear unavoidable allergic triggers are suspected. If these triggers are identified, immunotherapy may be instigated under specialist supervision.[15,15a]

Provocation tests

Provocation tests such as histamine and metacholine challenge are not necessary in children with established airways obstruction which is bronchodilator responsive. The test, if used, usually determines whether there is bronchial hyperreactivity in the child.[2]

EDUCATION AND MANAGEMENT AT HOME

The main aims in managing children with asthma at home include the following:

- Maintain optimal lung function.
- Promote a normal lifestyle with minimal interruption from symptoms or side effects from drug therapy.

- Prevent exacerbations through adequate education of the child and family regarding the disease and its management.
- Develop a precise plan for intervention in the event of an exacerbation.

Many families have difficulties coping with and adapting to the problems associated with asthma. This is probably due to worry and anxiety surrounding the uncertainty of asthma and the threat of exacerbation rather than any serious underlying disturbance. The principal concerns are related to 'the nature and outcome of the disorder; the effect asthma may have on the child's schooling, health and social activities; the parents problems in management of attacks and knowing when to seek medical help; the prevention of attacks; and permanent effects of long-term medication'.[2] These concerns establish the obvious necessity for improved education of both parents and children. Few parents have a clear understanding of the aetiology of asthma and a lack of certainty and knowledge invariably leads to anxiety. Evidence suggests that poor parental knowledge is a contributing factor to childhood morbidity.[60]

Education of the parents and the child is vital if the asthma is to be managed successfully. Information should be provided in a language the parents understand and cover the nature of the disease, methods of assessing the severity, the aims or goals of treatment and explanation about the drugs used and their side effects. This takes considerable time and the more anxious the parents, the more time it will take. Repeated explanation and reassurance may be necessary before parents feel confident in their ability to manage attacks. There is a range of written literature available for educational purposes from such organisations as the Asthma Foundation and Thoracic Society. Audiovisual material is also available for teaching inhaler techniques.

Parents commonly become confused by the various prescribed drugs. It is therefore important that they are given information about each drug and the side effects which might occur. Failure to do this often results in poor control as parents may think it correct to increase the use of prophylactic agents when symptoms occur, and subsequently fail to see improvement. Lack of information may also lead to non-compliance as confidence in maintaining control of attacks wanes. The consequences, usually, are more recurrent acute episodes which often require hospital admission. Furthermore, anxiety may be heightened both in the child and the family. It is important that the regimen of drugs prescribed be as simple as possible and readily understood as this enables parents to control their child's asthma, greatly helps the parent's and child's morale and relieves anxiety.[2]

Crisis management should be discussed, and a written plan of instructions given so that parents know exactly what to do if there is an exacerbation and when to seek medical assistance. This is called the Action Plan.

Once the child is old enough to understand simple explanations, then it is important to discuss the asthma and his treatment with him, and to teach him how and when to administer his medication. Children become aware of their own breathing and can differentiate between inspiration and expiration by about the age of 3 years.[72] Until this time, inhalation devices, such as a nebuliser or a spacer with a face mask attached which can be applied during tidal breathing, are the only alternatives. Correct use of inhalers is essential to ensure optimal effect from inhaled medications. Once the appropriate inhaler has been chosen for a child, the technique should be checked regularly.

Children should be give the opportunity to discuss their fears and worries about their asthma, how they feel about it, how it affects them and so on. This will promote independence in the child and minimise the occurrence of non-compliance where the child is difficult or unwilling to cooperate with the treatment regimen.

Community nurses, in conjunction with the treating doctor, are in an ideal position to provide the necessary education to the families of children with asthma. It is recognised that retained knowledge and understanding following the acute episode when the diagnosis of asthma was been made, will at best be sketchy. The anxiety accompanying diagnosis of an illness will usually inhibit learning. However, given time, the need for information and the ability to absorb and understand information will increase. The opportunity to learn more about asthma can be offered by community nurses in a number of different settings. One-to-one education may be the most appropriate form of teaching. This was found in a study of low income and migrant communities in Melbourne, who showed a noticeable reluctance to discuss personal issues in a group situation.[73] Others, however, benefit from exposure to people in similar situations. Feelings of isolation and helplessness are ameliorated through sharing a common problem and discussing issues of concern in small groups. Such small groups also allow the opportunity for skills training through explanation, demonstration and skills practice in a supervised setting. Information giving or knowledge education sessions can be delivered in both the above settings, as well as in lecture form to larger groups. The knowledge gained in this latter forum is limited, but it may be sufficient to stimulate and encourage individuals to seek further advice specific to their own needs.

In summary, the main objectives of asthma education are twofold — to teach management skills to improve asthma control, and to increase confidence in the ability to use these skills.

CONCLUSION

It has been highlighted that successful management of children with asthma is not simply a matter of prescribing drugs. It is a disease that is extremely variable, for which there is no cure, and control of symptoms while promoting as normal a lifestyle as is possible, will require health care professionals to consider each child and family individually, to plan a regimen that suits their needs.

Families should be encouraged to discuss asthma with relatives, friends and school teachers. Pamphlets should be made available to assist not only the family, but also those outside the family in understanding how to manage the problem, if and when the child is in their care.

Encouraging the child and family to take control through reassurance and education while providing appropriate back-up in times of need and regular review for reassessment and re-education is the key to success. This requires a team approach on the part of the health care givers.

REFERENCES

1. Robertson CF, Rubinfeld AR, Bowes G. Deaths from asthma in Victoria. *Med J Aust* 1990; 152: 511–517.
2. Phelan PD, Olinsky A, Robertson CF. *Respiratory illness in children.* 4th ed. Melbourne: Blackwell Scientific, 1994.
3. Mecoy RJ. The patient with life threatening asthma. *Aust Family Physician* 1989; 18: 791–799.

4.   Kelly W, Mitchell C. Why are people dying of asthma? Perspective 2. *Modern Medicine* 1991; May (suppl): 7–9.

5.   Robertson CF, Heycock E, Bishop J, Olinsky A, Phelan PD. Prevalence of asthma in Melbourne schoolchildren over 26 years. *BMJ* 1991; 302: 1116–1118.

6.   Bauman A, Mitchell CA, Henry RL, Robertson CF, Abramson MJ, Comino EJ, Hensley MJ, Leeder S. Asthma morbidity in Australia: an epidemiological study. *Med J Aust* 1992; 156: 827–831.

7.   Landau LI. Evolution of asthma. *J Paediatr Child Health* 1993. 29: 4–5.

8.   Barnett PJ, Oberklaid F. Acute asthma in children: evaluation of management in a hospital emergency department. *Med J Aust* 1991; 154: 729–733.

9.   National Asthma Campaign. *The asthma management plan.* Melbourne: National Asthma Campaign, 1990.

10. Henry RL, Fitzclarence CAB, Henry DA, Cruikshank D. What do health care professionals know about childhood asthma? *J Pediatr Child Health* 1993; 29: 32–35.

11. Henry RL, Landau L, Mellis C, Van Asperen PV, Morton J, Cooper P, et al. Childhood asthma: application of the international view of management in Australia and New Zealand. *J Paediatr Child Health* 1990; 26: 72–74.

12. Henry RL, Sly P, Godfrey S, et al. Assessment and treatment of childhood asthma. *J Paediatr Child Health* 1991; 27: 218–220.

13. Bauman A, Young L, Peat JK, Hunt J, Larkin P. Asthma under recognition and under-treatment in an Australian community. *Aust NZ J Med* 1992; 22: 36–40.

14. Warner JO. Asthma: a follow-up statement from an international pediatric asthma consensus group. *Arch Dis Childh* 1992; 67: 240–248.

15. Rachelefsky GS, Warner JO. International consensus on the management of pediatric asthma: a summary statement. *Pediatr Pulmonol* 1993; 15: 125–127.

15a. Frank MO. Skin testing and immunotherapy in children. [Letter] *J Allergy.* Clinical Immunology 1995: 96 (1): 138.

16. Tinkelman D, Falliers C, Naspitz C. *Childhood asthma; pathophysiology and treatment.* New York: Marcel Dekkar, 1987.

17. Traver G, Martinez M. Asthma update. Part I. Mechanisms, pathophysiology and diagnosis. *J Pediatr Health Care* 1988; 2: 221–226.

18. Clark T, Godfrey S. *Asthma.* 2nd ed. London: Chapman & Hall, 1983.

19. Sly P, Robertson CF. Managing childhood asthma. *Current Therapeutics* 1989; Dec: 47–56.

20. Barnes D. Asthma education: current concepts. *Current Therapeutics* 1990; Oct: 33–37.

21. Isles A. Management of childhood asthma. *Modern Medicine* 1991 May (Suppl): 25–29.

22. Allen D. Causes and triggers of asthma. Paper presented at The Inaugural National Asthma Conference: Asthma into the 21st Century. Brisbane, Oct 2–4, 1991.

23. Sly P. Patterns of asthma in children. *Modern Medicine* 1991; May (Suppl): 17–20.

24. Walls R. Controversies regarding trigger factors in asthma. *Patient Management* 1991; June: 59–65.

25. Abramson M. Air pollution and asthma. *Modern Medicine.* 1992; July: 84–90.

26. Smith L. Childhood asthma diagnosis and treatment. *Cur Problems Paediatr* 1993; 23: 271–305.

27. Kerem E, Canny G, Tibshirani R, et al. Clinical—physiologic correlations in acute asthma of childhood. *Pediatrics* 1991; 87: 481–486.

28. Henry RL, Robertson CF, Asher I, Cooper DM, Cooper P, Dawson KP, et al. Consensus view management of acute asthma. *J Paediatric Child Health* 1993; 29: 101–103.

28a. Schuh S, Johnson DW, Callahan S, Canny G, Levison H. Efficacy of frequent nebulised ipratropium bromide added to frequent high-dose albuterol therapy in severe childhood asthma. *J Pediatr* 1995; 126 (4): 639–645.

29. Ho L, Landau LI, Le Souef PN. Lack of efficacy of single-dose prednisolone in moderately severe asthma. *Med J Aust* 1994; 160: 701–704.

30. Bishop J, Nolan T. Pulse oximetry in acute asthma. *Arch Dis Childh* 1991; 66: 724–725.

31. Hoskyns EW, Heaton DM, Beardsmore CS, Simpson H. Asthma severity at night during recovery from an acute asthmatic episode. *Arch Dis Childh* 1991; 66: 1204–1208.

32. Nelson DR, Sachs MI, O'Connell EJ. Approaches to acute asthma and status asthmaticus in children. *Mayo Clinic Proc* 1989; 64: 1392–1402.

33. Commey JOO, Levison H. Physical signs in childhood asthma. *Pediatrics* 1976; 58: 537–541.

34. Fitzgerald JM, Hargreave EH. The assessment and management of acute life-threatening asthma. *Chest* 1989; 95: 888–894.

35. Engel J. *Pocket guide to paediatric assessment*. 2nd ed. St Louis: Mosby Year Book, 1992.

36. Hetzel M, Modell M. *Asthma*. Occasional paper 58 — Royal College of General Practitioners, 1992: 14–20.

37. McGregor M. Current concepts pulsus paradoxus. *N Engl J Med* 1979; 301: 480–482.

38. Sulzbach LM. Measurement of pulsus paradoxus. *Focus Critical Care* 1989; 16: 142–145.

39. Warner JO, Gotz M, Landau LI, Levison H, Milner AD, Pederson S, Silverman M. Management of asthma: a consensus statement. *Arch Dis Childh* 1989; 64: 1065–1079.

40. Mitchell EA, Bland JM, Thompson JMD. Risk factors for readmission to hospital for asthma in childhood. *Thorax* 1994; 49: 33–36.

41. Geelhoed GC, Landau LI, Le Soeuf PN. Predictive value of oxygen saturation in emergency room evaluation of asthmatic children. *BMJ* 1988; 297: 395–396.

42. Geelhoed GC, Landau LI, Le Soeuf PN. Evaluation of SaO2 as a predictor of outcome in 280 children presenting with acute asthma. *Ann Emergency Med* 1994; 23: 1236–1241.

43. Dawson KP, Penna AC. Observations on the management of childhood acute asthma in a large hospital. *Med J Aust* 1992; 156: 845–846.

44. Isles AF, Robertson CF. Treatment of asthma in children and adolescents: the need for a different approach. *Med J Aust* 1993; 158: 761–763.

45. O'Driscoll BR, Taylor RJ, Horsley MG, et al. Nebulised salbutamol with and without ipratropium bromide in acute airflow obstruction. *Lancet* 1989; 1: 1418–1420.

46. Phelan PD, Landau LI, Olinsky A. Respiratory illness in children. 4th ed. Melbourne: Blackwell Scientific, 1994.

47. Wynn SR. Alternative approaches to asthma. *J Pediatr* 1989; 115: 846–849.

48. Gleeson JGA, Loftus BG, Price JF. Placebo controlled trial of systemic corticosteroids in acute childhood asthma. *Acta Paediatrica Scand* 1990; 79: 1052–1059.

49. Connett GJ, Warde C, Wooler E, Lenney W. Prednisilone and salbutamol in the hospital treatment of acute asthma. *Arch Dis Childh* 1994; 70: 170–173.

50. Noche ML. Prophylaxis in childhood asthma. *Acta Paeditrica Japan* 1990; 32: 176–182.

51. Murphy S, Kelly HW. Management of Acute Asthma. *Pediatrician* 1991; 18: 287–300.

52. Freelander M, Van Asperen PP. Nebuhaler versus nebulisers in children with acute asthma. *BMJ* 1984; 288: 1873–1874.

53. Landau LI. Asthma in childhood. *In:* Robinson MJ. *Practical paediatrics*. 3rd ed. Melbourne: Churchill Livingstone, 1994.

54. Mellis CM. Important changes in the emergency management of acute asthma in children. *Med J Aust* 1988; 148 (5): 215–217.

55. Robertson CF, Smith F, Beck R, Levison H. Response to frequent low doses of nebulised salbutamol in acute asthma. *J Paediatr* 1985; 106: 672–674.

56. Phin S, Oates RK. Variations in the treatment of childhood asthma, *Med J Aust* 1993; 159: 662–666.

57. Harrison BD, Stokes TC, Hart GJ, Vaughan DA, Ali NJ, Robinson AA. Need for intravenous hydrocortisone in addition to oral prednisolone in patients admitted with severe asthma without ventilatory failure. *Lancet* 1986; 1: 181–184.

58. Kelly HW, Murphy S. Corticosteroids for acute severe asthma. *Pulmonary and Allergy* 1991; 25 Jan: 72–79.

59. Phelan PD. Childhood asthma — the role of corticosteroids. *Current Therapeutics* 1992; Aug: 11, 13, 14.

60. Van Asperen PP, Mellis CM, Sly PD. The role of corticosteroids in the management of childhood asthma. The Thoracic Society of Australia and New Zealand. *Med J Aust* 1992; 156: 48–52.

61. Carter E, Cruz MC. Efficacy of intravenously administered theophylline in children hospitalised with severe asthma. *J Pediatr* 1993; 122: 470–476.

62. Fanta CH, Rossing TH, McFadden ER. Treatment of acute asthma. Is combination therapy with sympathomimetics and methylxanthines indicated? *Am J Med* 1986; 80: 5–10.

63. Strauss RE, Wertheim DL, Bonagura VR, Valacer DJ. Aminophylline therapy does not improve outcome and increases adverse effects in children hospitalised with acute asthmatic exacerbations. *Pediatrics* 1994; 93: 205–210.

64. McKenzie SA. Aminophylline in the hospital treatment of children with acute asthma. *BMJ* 1994; 308: 1384–1385.

65. Lilley B, McDowell J, Munari G, Parsons B, eds. *Paediatric pharmacopoeia*. 11th ed. Melbourne: Pharmacy Department, Royal Children's Hospital, 1994.

66. Potter PC, Klein M, Weinberg EG. Hydration in severe acute asthma. *Arch Dis Childh* 1991; 66: 216–219.

67. Dawson P, Capalda N. The chest x-ray and childhood acute asthma. *Aust Clin Rev* 1993; 13: 153–156.

68. Gershel JC, Goldman HS, Stein RE. The usefulness of chest radiographs in first asthma attacks. *N Engl J Med* 1983; 309: 336–339.

69. Rushton AR. The role of the chest radiograph in the management of childhood asthma. *Clin Pediatr* 1982; 21: 325–328.

70. Bye MR, Kerstein D, Barsh E. The importance of spirometry in the assessment of childhood asthma. *Am J Dis Child* 1992; 146: 977–978.

71. Olinsky A. The child with a persistent cough. *In:* Robinson MJ. *Practical paediatrics*. 3rd ed. Melbourne: Churchill Livingstone, 1994.

72. Rees J, Price J. *ABC of asthma*. Cambridge: Cambridge University Press, 1989.

73. Crockett S, Pepper S. *Asthma and heath education: A research project*. Melbourne: Collingwood Health Centre, 1990.

74. Bowler SD. Spacers vs Nebulisers. *Asthma News*. Asthma Foundation of Queensland, December 1989.

75. Goren A, Noviski N, Avital A, Maayan C, Stahl E, Godfrey S, Springer C. Assessment of the ability of young children to use a powder inhaler device (Turbuhaler). *Pediatr Pulmonol* 1994; 18: 77–80.

Cystic Fibrosis

Sandra Wales

Cystic fibrosis is the most common genetic disease found in a Caucasian population. It was first described in the 1930s.[1] Cystic fibrosis is a disease that affects the exocrine glands in that they secrete thick, sticky mucus. The respiratory, digestive, reproductive systems and sweat glands are affected.

There is no cure for cystic fibrosis. The survival rate, however, is improving with new methods of treatment and management and many people with cystic fibrosis are living well into adult life. The disease is manifested in many ways, hence diagnosis is not always made at birth. It is a chronic disease which requires continual assessment and management at a specialised cystic fibrosis clinic. The incidence of cystic fibrosis is approximately 1 in 2000 to 2500 births in Australia. The autosomal recessive gene is carried by 1 in 20 people. When both parents carry the gene, there is a 1 in 4 chance with each pregnancy that a child will be born with cystic fibrosis.

The gene was discovered in 1989 on the long arm of chromosome 7. The common mutation is identified as delta F508, that is the 508th position on the protein chain. As the discovery of the gene is recent, more mutations are gradually being identified. The significance of the disease severity and gene mutation is unknown at present.

Studies are continuing to investigate the function of the gene with the view of improving management and eventually finding a cure. The cystic fibrosis gene produces a protein called cystic fibrosis transmembrane conductance regulator (CFTR). Evidence suggests that this protein in healthy people probably acts as a channel for chloride to pass in and out of the epithelial cell. When this is defective, as in cystic fibrosis, it causes the mucus to become thick and sticky.[2] Scientists are working on therapies to stimulate the defective channel, and on gene therapy.

The discovery of the gene has made it possible for prenatal testing to be offered to high-risk couples, by performing chorionic villi testing at 10 to 12 weeks' gestation or amniocentesis at 16 to 19 weeks' gestation. Carrier status is also available for these families. Genetic counselling is offered to all families with an affected member.

MEDICAL DIAGNOSIS

In most states of Australia, the newborn screening program is available. The test, carried out on day 4 of life, screens for the presence of immunoreactive trypsin (IRT) in the blood. In NSW (at the Oliver Latham Laboratory), if this is found to be elevated, DNA testing for the common mutation delta F508 will be performed. In cystic fibrosis the levels of IRT are raised because of the pancreatic involvement. DNA testing will provide the following information:

- Homozygous delta F508/delta F508 means the child has cystic fibrosis and is referred to a cystic fibrosis clinic, where a sweat test is performed.
- Heterozygous delta F508/N means the child could be a carrier or have cystic fibrosis, hence the child is referred for a sweat test (N being a normal gene or an undetectable mutation).
- A raised IRT but delta F508 is not detected. The family is told that cystic fibrosis is not detected. About 2 to 3 children per year are missed on screening as they have two uncommon mutations of the cystic fibrosis gene.
- A negative IRT. This indicates normal pancreatic function. The child may have two uncommon genes which will not be detected.

The sweat test will confirm the diagnosis of cystic fibrosis in the case of the heterozygous presentations. A certain percentage of these babies will have the disease as N will be an undetectable mutation. The remaining babies will be a carrier for the disease as N will represent a normal gene.

The most common procedure for the sweat test is the pilocarpine iontophoresis test, which should be performed at a recognised laboratory. An electrical current is passed into the forearm to produce sweat, which is collected on a filter impregnated with pilocarpine. The amount of sodium is measured in the sample.[3] The test is painless and gives an accurate result in an hour.

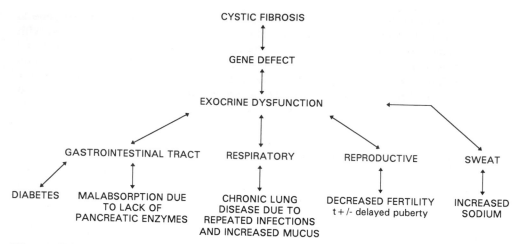

Figure 7.4 The pathology of cystic fibrosis.

PATHOPHYSIOLOGY

Cystic fibrosis is characterised by a dysfunction of the exocrine glands, the glands that secrete into ducts or onto the body surface. The disease affects the respiratory, gastrointestinal and reproductive systems and the sweat glands (**Figure 7.4**).

The lungs are normal at birth, but over time, the secretion of thick, sticky mucus clogs the airways, predisposing the child to infection, inflammation and chronic lung damage, which can eventually cause death.

In the upper airway, the effects can cause sinusitis and nasal polyps. In the lower airway, obstruction from the mucus can cause wheezing and coughing, which increases as the child grows older. The amount of sputum produced increases as well. Chronic infectious conditions such as bronchitis, bronchiolitis and bronchiectasis are frequently seen in the child with cystic fibrosis.[4] As the disease progresses the airways become more narrowed and the alveoli overinflated due to the mucous plugs trapping air. This causes the chest to become barrel-shaped. Clubbing of the fingers may occur.

Overinflation of the airways in time can lead to emphysema. In the later stage of the disease, pneumothorax and haemoptysis related to repeated chest infections may occur. The infections in the airways are caused by both viral and bacterial organisms. The viral infection usually starts in the upper respiratory tract and is followed by a secondary bacterial infection in the lower airways. The most common organisms are *Staphylococcus aureus*, *Haemophilus influenzae*, non-mucoid and mucoid *Pseudomonas aeruginosa*, *Pseudomonas cepacia*, and fungal infections caused by *Aspergillus fumigatus* and *Candida albicans.*[5]

In cystic fibrosis, the disease affects the gastrointestinal system through the malfunction of digestion and the absorption of food. The symptoms of the gastrointestinal malfunction usually appear before the symptoms of respiratory involvement.

The major organ involved is the pancreas. The deterioration of this organ begins in utero. The pancreatic cells are replaced with an excessive formation of fibrous scar tissue. Thick mucous secretions block the ducts and impede the passage of the pancreatic enzymes lipase, trypsin and amylase[1] causing an abnormal amount of fat and protein in the stool. Also, the fat-soluble vitamins A,D,E and K are not absorbed. The result is foul-smelling, bulky stools (steatorrhoea) which are frequently passed. The destruction of the pancreas may further be demonstrated in the presentation of diabetes mellitus. The fibrosis of the organ tissue impairs the blood supply to the Islet of Langerhans. Diabetes mellitus usually presents in adolescence.

Complications of the bowel include meconium ileus, which occurs in 10% to 20% of newborns with cystic fibrosis.[5] The meconium is thick and bulky and blocks the small intestine. This often requires intervention, either radiological or in some cases surgical. Rectal prolapse occurs occasionally in children because of the secretion of frequent, fatty stools. This resolves once pancreatin supplement is corrected. Surgical intervention is rarely needed. 'Meconiun ileus equivalent' or distal intestinal obstruction syndrome can occur and is characterised by a complete or partial blockage of the bowel. This is usually managed with an enema or oral preparations that will soften and act as a laxative to move the stool. Intussusception is rare but may occur.

The liver may develop cirrhosis because of the blockage of the bile ducts in approximately 5% to 10% of children with cystic fibrosis.[6] Cirrhosis may in turn cause oesophageal varices. A common bile duct stricture may occur and sometimes surgery is performed.

The sweat contains an increased amount of sodium, but is not more viscous than normal. The sweat glands are normal.

The reproductive system is affected in both males and females. Puberty is occasionally delayed. In males there is an abnormality of the vas deferens and epididymis in that they are obliterated and atretic.[4] These abnormalities result in sterility in most males. The semen therefore does not contain sperm. Sexual function is normal. In females, reduced fertility may occur. The cervical mucus may be thicker, making it difficult for sperm to reach the ovum. Depending on general health, the menstrual cycle may be irregular, however sexual desire and performance are normal. Many women with cystic fibrosis have given birth, but close monitoring by both medical and gynaecological teams is needed.

Hypertrophic pulmonary osteoarthropathy occurs in some children with cystic fibrosis but the cause is unknown. The joints become swollen and there is a potential for fever. These effects abate over time, usually as a result of treatment.

NURSING DIAGNOSIS

The first contact a nurse has with a child and family can be in any of the 3 following settings.

Firstly, in a neonatal ward where an infant may present with a meconium ileus, which occurs in approximately 10% to 20% of children with the disease. Secondly, the child may be admitted to hospital for confirmation of a diagnosis following a positive sweat test, or for investigation leading to diagnosis if there is a history of infections, failure to thrive and loose stools or rectal prolapse. Thirdly, a nurse in the community setting may see a child who displays the above symptoms and is undiagnosed, or provide support and education to a family with an affected child or children.

The nursing diagnoses of a child with cystic fibrosis would include the following.

Potential for ineffective airway clearance related to increased mucous secretions leading to chest infections

The most distinctive sign of the disease is the presence of a cough. The child may have a history of recurrent colds associated with an increase in cough, wheeze and sputum production. The younger child, however, may have a non-productive cough. The older child may present with a barrel chest and clubbing of the fingers. There may be a decrease in exercise tolerance.

Potential for impaired gas exchange related to infection and inflammation of the lungs

The child may display symptoms of dyspnoea, tachypnoea and possibly cyanosis. The adolescent may complain of morning headaches and restless sleep. There may be a need for oxygen therapy.

Potential for chest infections related to increased bacteria, tenacious mucus and decreased body defences

The child may present with a history of persistent cough, weight loss, decreased exercise tolerance and minimal response to oral or inhaled antibiotics. These symptoms, sometimes with a fever and being generally unwell, are the most common presentation to hospital.

Potential for poor digestion of food related to malabsorption leading to weight loss and poor growth and development

On admission, the child may appear thin and malnourished. The mother of a newly diagnosed child will often report how well the child feeds, but always appears unsettled. The child may pass frequent bulky stools. It is best for the nurse to examine the stool for consistency, fat streaks, or oil and colour. Often the stool is bright yellow/green. Many first-time mothers do not know what a 'normal' stool is. In a toilet-trained child the stool may float or have an oily film. These signs suggest malabsorption. A 3-day faecal fat collection may be ordered. A diet history is obtained to determine the amount of fat ingested.

The older child may complain of abdominal pain and experience excessive flatus and on examination have a distended abdomen (pot belly). Bulky and fatty stools may cause a rectal prolapse; the nurse should check for this. Occasionally, the child may have severe constipation leading to a bowel obstruction. The child in this instance may present with nausea and vomiting and abdominal pain. In the adolescent, a history of weight loss and polyuria with excessive drinking should alert the nurse to the possibility of diabetes mellitus. The child may also have a loss of appetite and weight due to a chest infection. Excessive coughing can cause vomiting.

Potential for excessive salt loss through sweat

The mother of a newborn child may state her child tastes salty when kissed. On assessment the older child may be lethargic, weak or have muscle cramping, abdominal pain, headaches, vomiting and nausea. The child may appear dehydrated where there is inadequate salt replacement. The excess salt in the sweat is the reason for the diagnostic sweat test.

Potential for family anxiety and stress related to the diagnosis of a chronic, life-threatening illness

As the whole family is involved when the child is diagnosed with cystic fibrosis,[5] many long-term social and emotional problems can be created. Parents will often mourn the loss of their healthy child and display emotions of bereavement.[5] Each time the child experiences a deterioration in health, the family's anxieties are increased.

In the adolescent, the following diagnoses may be considered

Potential for non-compliance related to having a chronic illness leading to exacerbation of symptoms.

Potential for delayed puberty related to disease process.

Potential for low self-esteem relate to poor body image and effects of a chronic illness.

Potential for fear of dying related to a deterioration in health.

Potential for isolation from peers related to increased hospital admissions.

MANAGEMENT AND TREATMENT

It is well known that life expectancy is improved when treatment for cystic fibrosis is delivered at a specialised centre.[5] Management and treatment is best delivered by a multidisciplinary team, which consists of a respiratory physician, gastroenterologist, geneticist, specialist nurse, physiotherapist, social worker and dietitian. The nursing management is multifactorial. The following can be considered.

Respiratory aspects

The goal of treatment is to promote effective airway clearance and prevent infection. Chest physiotherapy is commenced at diagnosis. The parents are taught to perform chest physiotherapy in the required positions. Daily physiotherapy is recommended, and should be increased to twice daily if an infection is present. The child, when old enough, is taught breathing exercises. Various techniques are the active cycle of breathing and the forced expiratory technique (FET) or huffing. This assists with the clearance of mucus from the lungs and can promote independence. A positive expired pressure (PEP) mask may be used. The child is also encouraged to partake in a regular exercise program such as swimming, running or team sport. This enables children to increase their fitness level and exercise can induce coughing. Many children, and especially adolescents, find physiotherapy a chore so a combination of techniques and exercise can work well.

Bronchodilators, when prescribed, are usually given before physiotherapy or if the child has an increased wheeze. The nurse may need to instruct the parents and older child on the use of nebulised medication and the care of the equipment. Nebulised antibiotics are commonly prescribed and are administered after physiotherapy. The use of nebulised antibiotics enables the treatment to continue at home and reduces the need for frequent hospitalisation and intravenous antibiotics. However, if after a reasonable course of inhaled antibiotics the child's condition does not improve, hospitalisation is indicated. If diagnosed with CF under 1 year of age, the child receives an anti-staphylococcus antibiotic which is prescribed for the first year of life. This is given as a prophylactic measure.

While in hospital the patient will receive intravenous antibiotic therapy, usually for a period of 2 to 3 weeks. The care of a long line or implantable device (a port implanted subcutaneously attached to a central venous catheter) should be instigated. Sputum may need to be collected so that pathogens can be isolated and sensitivities determined for the appropriate drug therapy. If collecting a sputum specimen from a child, oropharyngeal aspiration is preferred. Pulmonary function tests and chest x-rays are routinely ordered. It should be noted that cough suppressants are not recommended. Coughing is a natural mechanism for clearing mucus from the lungs. If the ability to cough is reduced and mucus is retained, lung function can ultimately be impaired.[6] The intravenous antibiotics most commonly used are B lactam drugs, such as penicillins (e.g., ticarcillin, timentin) and aminoglycosides (e.g., tobramycin) . These antibiotics are usually given together. Oral antibiotics are broad spectrum and quinoline derivatives. Oral and perianal thrush and diarrhoea are side effects of oral antibiotics. Anti-fungal preparations should be administered orally and applied to the perianal region when thrush occurs.

If the child is unwell on presentation to hospital, oxygen saturations should be recorded and oxygen therapy given as required. The child may also need supplemental oxygen during physiotherapy or exercise treatment during an exacerbation of a chest infection.

The frequency of hospital admissions depends on the severity of the disease and philosophy of the attending team. Some centres admit their patients on a regular basis whereas others await an exacerbation of symptoms. Home intravenous antibiotic therapy is also an option. This can reduce the disruption to the family and child and improve the lifestyle. The program needs to be well structured and support services must be in place to enable the same care and outcome as hospitalisation.

Immunisation is encouraged for all children with cystic fibrosis.

Heart–lung and double-lung transplantation is being offered to those who have severe lung disease. This is not a cure for cystic fibrosis. There is a problem with the supply and demand of donor organs in Australia. As the donor population is relatively small, many potential recipients do not receive a transplant.

Gastrointestinal aspects

The goal is to maintain normal growth and development. The principal management of the digestive system is with pancreatin supplements which are supplied in enteric-coated capsules, which are administered orally with each food intake. They are activated in the alkaline environment of the small bowel. Half the number of required capsules should be taken at the beginning of the meal and remainder halfway through the meal. For infants who are unable to swallow a capsule, the capsule can be opened and the beads mixed with an acidic medium such as pureed apple or gel. This medium is used because its acidic pH prevents the breakdown of the enteric-coated beads by the saliva.

On and during admission, weight should be recorded and compared with previous measurements. Children with cystic fibrosis have an increased calorie requirement. This increased amount can be achieved by using foods high in fat, protein and carbohydrate content. The dietitian can educate the patient and family on nutritional needs and the necessary vitamin and salt supplements.

The stool consistency and frequency should be noted. Constipation can occur. For children who, despite eating a high caloric diet, do not gain weight because of their high energy need, enteral feeding is an option. Usually this is given as an overnight feeding via a gastrostomy tube. Educating the family about the procedure is important so the feeding can continue at home. Pancreatin supplement is given at the beginning of the feed. The management of the adolescent with diabetes mellitus requires a sugar-free and carbohydrate managed diet and generally insulin. Blood sugar levels are monitored before meals.

Psychosocial aspects

In the initial nursing assessment the need for support and advice will be determined. Many families, on diagnosis, only manage to absorb information about the necessary treatment. Long-term and crisis management is dealt with at a later stage.

The nurse may enable the family to express their feelings and anxieties and refer them, if needed, to appropriate sources. Each time a child becomes unwell, and especially if hospitalisation is required, stress is placed on the family and their coping mechanisms. Siblings always need to be considered when caring for these families. The day-to-day management of the disease creates demands on the family in areas such as time, financial resources, emotional aspects and relationships. Children with cystic fibrosis are able to attend pre-schools and mainstream schools. School teachers should be educated on the condition and the particular needs of that child.

The child and adolescent may wish to discuss concerns and anxieties about death. The nurse should listen, answer questions honestly, and refer to another professional if need be. This referral should be in consultation with the child or adolescent who will often state with whom they have a good rapport.

As treatments have improved over the years, longevity has increased for people with this disease and many adult hospitals are now providing services. The transition from a paediatric to an adult hospital or service is not always easy for the patient, family or health team. The change needs to be handled slowly to allow all concerned to adjust. Clear guidelines of how and when the transition will take place need to be instituted. Joint clinics can work well. Adolescents with cystic fibrosis are encouraged to further their education and seek suitable employment. Government assistance is available for all families with a child with cystic fibrosis. Reassessment is then made once the adolescent has left school.

When repeated treatments do not arrest the disease process, death will result and is usually caused by chronic obstructive respiratory disease and right-sided heart failure.[1] Treatment is usually reassessed after consultation by the health team with the family and the patient. The team can provide palliative care in hospital or at home. Ongoing support for the family is usually provided after a child's death by the specialist nurse and social worker.

REFERENCES

1. Goodchild M, Dodge JA. *Cystic fibrosis: manual of diagnosis and management.* 2nd ed. London: Balliere Tindall, 1985.
2. Davies K. Cystic fibrosis: the quest for a cure. *New Scientist* 1991; 7 Dec: 22.
3. Jackson ADM. The natural history of cystic fibrosis. *In:* Goodfellow P. *Cystic fibrosis.* Oxford: Oxford University Press, 1989: 7.
4   Mott SR, James SR, Sperhac AM. *Nursing care of children and families.* 2nd ed. Menlo Park: Addison-Wesley, 1990. 1034.
5. Dodge JA. Management of cystic fibrosis. *In:* Goodfellow P. *Cystic fibrosis.* Oxford: Oxford University Press, 1989.
6. Harris A, Super M. *Cystic fibrosis. The facts.* Oxford: Oxford University Press, 1987.

Disturbances in Blood Volume, Pressure and Flow

Carmel McQuellin

Common degenerative processes affecting the myocardium in infancy and childhood are the cardiomyopathies. The problems of hypertropic cardiomyopathy, dilated cardiomyopathy, of which endocardial fibroelastosis is a form, and glycogen storage disease are briefly discussed.

Cardiomyopathy

Although the aetiology of cardiomyopathy is unknown, three groups are recognised — hypertropic, dilated and restrictive cardiomyopathy. Assessment and care of children with hypertrophic and dilated cardiomyopathy, which include endocardial fibroelastosis, form the discussion that follows. Children who develop myocardial degenerative problems ultimately present in cardiac failure. The goal of treatment is control of the failure through supportive and pharmacological approaches. Cardiac transplantation is, however, recognised as an acceptable approach for treatment of cardiomyopathy of congenital or acquired aetiology.[1,2]

HYPERTROPHIC CARDIOMYOPATHY

Hypertrophic cardiomyopathy (HCM) is a genetically inherited disease affecting twice the number of males as females. The prominent characteristic of HCM is the development of left ventricular hypertrophy, which may affect the volume of blood pumped by the left ventricle.[3]

Nursing assessment

The outcome and degree of debilitation from HCM in infants and children is highly variable. Once the clinical signs of cardiac failure become established, the long-term outcome is poor. Reports indicate that when cardiac failure develops in the first months of life, the infants die before the age of 2 years.[4] Sudden collapse is a characteristic feature noted in older children with HCM following strenuous activity. It is postulated that the alteration in the myocardial cellular structure may account for the abnormal conduction of impulses that result in life-threatening dysrhythmias.[4]

Pathophysiology

The cardiac muscle cells are notably abnormal in shape and alignment, deviating from the characteristic parallel arrangement.[4] In HCM, the hypertrophy causes narrowing of the left ventricular outflow tract which results in further hypertrophy of the left ventricle.

Treatment modalities

In infants with HCM in whom left ventricular functioning is satisfactory but where an elevation in pulmonary venous pressure increases the workload of the heart, the use of digoxin is generally contraindicated and therapeutic support is provided through the use of beta blockade or calcium channel blocking agents.[4] When heart failure attributed to HCM develops in infancy, poor left ventricular function and cardiac dilatation develops and therapeutic manipulation is dependent upon the effectiveness of the ventricular myocardium to maintain the cardiac output. This group of infants may require the support of digoxin and diuretics to alleviate the symptoms.[3]

Results of surgical resection for the relief of obstruction to left ventricular outflow are excellent, with recent studies indicating a 90% to 98% reduction in the children's symptoms.[4–6] The postoperative risks of resection are associated with persistent symptoms in up to 10% of children, with late deaths in 5% attributed to cardiac failure and arrhythmia.[4]

DILATED CARDIOMYOPATHY (IDIOPATHIC)

Idiopathic cardiomyopathy is a disease which affects the myocardium, characterised by dilation of the ventricles and resulting in poor myocardial contractility. When undertaking a nursing assessment in a child with this form of cardiomyopathy, the nurse will detect the clinical signs of heart failure, which include the signs of pulmonary congestion and liver enlargement.

Clinical assessment of the child with dilated cardiomyopathy is at times indistinguishable from those with myocarditis and endocardial fibroelastosis. The children's prognosis is poor, especially when associated with heart failure. Current data suggests a 1-year survival in two-thirds of children, with only one-third surviving to 5 years.[4]

Treatment for the children is aimed at relieving their heart failure and includes the use of digoxin and diuretics, with or without the addition of vasodilator medication.[4]

Endocardial Fibroelastosis

A form of dilated cardiomyopathy, endocardial fibroelastosis (EFE) is a rare, degenerative process affecting the heart which results in myocardial failure.

Nursing assessment

The highest incidence of EFE in childhood occurs in infants between 3 and 6 months of age and often causes severe and rapid decompensation in the clinical state. Clinical assessment of these infants reveals the characteristic features of myocardial failure, in addition to skin rash, fever, leucocytosis and anaemia.[4]

Pathophysiology

The process responsible for the development of cardiac failure in these children is the diffuse, endocardial thickening from excessive amounts of collagen and elastin fibres, which particularly affects the left ventricle and, to a lesser degree, the left atrium and right ventricle. Although the exact mechanism for development of EFE in infants and children remains undetermined, evidence suggests a link with myocarditis of viral aetiology.[4,7]

Treatment modalities

These infants require early recognition and prompt support of their failing circulation with digoxin and diuretics. Fatal embolisation of the cerebral, cardiac or pulmonary vasculature can occur, the result of thrombus formation within the dilated cardiac chambers.[4]

Glycogen Storage Disease

Glycogen storage disease (GSD) is an inherited, degenerative, metabolic disorder, the result of deficient enzyme activity causing glycogen of abnormal chemical structure to be deposited into body tissues, notably cardiac and muscle tissue.[8] There are 22 classifications of GSD, although severe myocardial compromise is associated with only 3 of the groups.

The heart in infants with GSD becomes globular in nature and may increase in weight 3 to 10 fold. There is a 100% incidence of mortality by 2 years of age for infants presenting with Type II GSD, known as Pompe's disease, despite interventional support to control the infant's cardiac failure.[8]

From a nursing perspective, an ability clinically to assess and analyse findings in infants with cardiovascular dysfunction due to an alteration in cellular function is essential from an early stage and facilitates prompt management of the heart failure. A detailed review of the nursing assessment and principles of management of cardiac failure are included in the subsection 'Failure of Control Mechanisms' included in Chapter 11, to which the reader is referred.

REFERENCES

1. Johnston J. Cardiac transplantation in early infancy. *Crit Care Nursing Clin North Am* 1992; 4: 521–525.
2. O'Brien P, Hanley FL. New directions in pediatric heart transplantation. *Crit Care Nursing Clin North Am* 1992; 4: 193–203.
3. Hazinski MF. Cardiovascular disorders. *In:* Hazinski MF, ed. *Nursing care of the critically ill child.* 2nd ed. St Louis: Mosby, 1992: 117–394.
4. Maron B. Cardiomyopathies. *In:* Adam FH, Emmanoulides GC, Riemenschneider TA, eds. *Moss' heart disease in infants, children and adolescents.* 4th ed. Baltimore: Williams and Wilkins, 1989: 940–964.
5. Kirklin JW, Barratt-Boyes BG. Hypertrophic obstructive cardiomyopathy. *In:* Kirklin JW, Barratt-Boyes BG. *Cardiac surgery: morphology, diagnostic criteria, natural history, techniques, results and indications.* 2nd ed. New York: Churchill Livingstone, 1993: 1239–1262.
6. Mohr R, Schaff HV, Puga FJ, Danielson GK. Results of operation for HOCM in children and adults less than 40 years of age. *Circulation* 1989; 80 (Suppl 1): 191–196.
7. Pereira Baretto AC, Lemos da Luz P, De Olivera SA, Stolf NAG, Mady C, Bellotti G, Jatene AD, Pileggi F. Determinants of survival in endomyocardial fibrosis. *Circulation* 1989; 80 (Suppl 1): 177–182.
8. Caddell JL. Metabolic and nutritional diseases. *In:* Adams FH, Emmanoulides GC, Riemenschneider TA, eds. *Moss' heart disease in infants, children and adolescents.* 4th ed. Baltimore: Williams and Wilkins, 1989: 750–778.

Disturbances in Neuroendocrine Function

The Epilepsies

Laurence Dubourg

An epileptic seizure is a symptom which occurs as a consequence of an uncontrolled electrical discharge of neurons from a sudden disturbance of the central nervous system. The cause may remain of unknown origin, but lesions such as cerebral tumours, scarring of the cerebral cortex, metabolic or electrolytic disturbances are commonly identified to be the origin of the seizures. In most instances, the correction of the disturbance will prevent the symptom from recurring and the child will not require further anti-epileptic therapy. Only children with recurrent seizures will be investigated to identify the epileptic syndrome. This is done by correlating the medical history of the child and the family, the seizure types (**Table 7.1**), their frequency, any electroencephalographic abnormalities, the child's age and overall psychomotor development. The diagnosis of one epilepsy syndrome (**Table 7.2**) allows appropriate treatment and counselling to be undertaken.

In general, the public perception of epilepsy is limited to the generalised seizure, where the patient falls to the floor, loses consciousness and has extreme clonic movements. Awareness of subtle epileptic manifestations experienced by many patients is poor. This chapter discusses the epilepsies and emphasises the differences between the various seizure types and nursing approaches.

NURSING ASSESSMENT

History taking

Parents and children will form an initial impression on the quality of care during the admission and it is essential they rapidly develop a feeling of trust. Ideally, the setting for obtaining the history requires privacy. The skilled nurse, who is a good listener, will

Table 7.1 Classification of the seizure types from the International League Against Epilepsy (ILAE), in 1981

Partial seizures (focal)

Simple partial seizures
Complex partial seizures
Secondarily generalised partial seizures

Generalised seizures

Absence seizures
Myoclonic seizures
Clonic seizures
Tonic seizures
Tonic–clonic seizures
Atonic seizures

Adapted from *Epilepsy in children.*[1]

Table 7.2 Some epileptic syndromes

Syndromes	Seizure types	Onset	Outcome
Neonates			
Benign neonatal familial convulsions	Repeated convulsions	2nd or 3rd day	In a low percentage of cases, seizures can occur in childhood or later in life
Early myoclonic encephalopathy	Massive myoclonic seizures, tonic spasms or partial seizures	Before 3rd month	Severe course: complete lack of psychomotor development, frequently death before 1 year
Infancy and childhood			
Febrile convulsions predisposition (Genetic response to sudden temperature rise)	Brief, generalised, can be partial	6 months to 5 years	Overall excellent but less hopeful before 1 year. Less than 4% develop epilepsy later A seizure of > 15 to 30 minutes' duration can damage the brain
Infantile spasms (West syndrome)	Spasms	Before 1 year, peak 3 to 7 months	Mental retardation
Infantile myoclonic epilepsies with variable outcomes	Variable: from several head nods through to several generalised myoclonic fits a day to generalised unilateral clonic, tonic/clonic seizures or status epilepticus	7 months to 6 years. Peak to 5 years	Variable: • controlled by treatment, normal development • inefficacy of treatment, normal 1st stage of psychomotor development which slows down after 2 years • unfavourable outcome with development of dementia
Lennox Gestaut	Axial tonic seizures Atypical absences Atonic seizures also frequently myoclonic, general tonic–clonic and partial seizures	1 to 8 years, rarely after 8 years	Unfavourable with slowing in mental development and personality disorder
Childhood			
Childhood absence epilepsy	Absence seizures	6 to 7 years	Remission. Tonic-clonic seizures in 40% of cases
Benign partial epilepsy with centrotemporal spikes	Brief hemi-facial motor, somatosensory symptoms, nocturnal, sometimes become generalised	3 to 13 years	Recovery before 15 to 16 years
Benign partial epilepsy of childhood with occipital paroxysms	Visual symptoms followed by hemiclonic seizures or automatisms Migraine follows		Benign

Table 7.2 *(continued)*

Syndromes	Seizure types	Onset	Outcome
Landau Kleffner syndrome	Language disorder: regression of previously acquired language skills		No intellectual deterioration Language improvement in majority ceases prior adolescence
Epilepsy with continuous spike waves during sleep	Atypical absences Rare nocturnal partial or generalised motor seizures, never tonic seizures		Benign but various neuropsychosocial disturbances
Childhood and adolescence			
Juvenile absence epilepsy	Absences, tonic-clonic mostly on awakening		Low seizure frequency
Juvenile myoclonic epilepsy	Irregular bilateral myoclonic jerks predominantly in the arms. Conscious, may fall. Often tonic-clonic shortly after awakening. Increases with sleep deprivation		
Epilepsy with tonic–clonic seizures on awakening	Tonic–clonic, for 90% on awakening Absences Myoclonic		65% complete seizure control but relapse rate high on cessation of medications
Benign partial seizures of adolescents	Partial motor/sensory seizures, secondary generalised	10 to 20 years Peak 13 to 14 years	Normal neurological and mental status

Adapted from *Epileptic syndromes in infancy, childhood and adolescence.*[2]

question in a caring and non threatening manner and encourage questioning from the family.

As a fundamental component of the nursing assessment, the comprehensive nursing history provides invaluable information that facilitates developing a plan of care to meet the needs of child and family. It is important to include the family because the efficacy of the treatment regimen is based on their cooperation. Issues raised by the caregiver and the child will therefore be given special consideration.

The nurse must acquire astute clinical assessment skills and attain in-depth knowledge of the various seizures as each of them will present with specific signs and symptoms.

Partial seizures (focal)

A partial seizure has a focal origin within the cerebral cortex. This localised area leads to specific related clinical manifestations. The excessive electrical activity during a seizure may spread to nearby brain structures, increasing the clinical manifestations.

Table 7.3 Examples of questions which help identify the effect epileptic seizures may have on the life of the child and the family

---

1. The child's experience of the epileptic syndrome.

   Perception of the epileptic syndrome

   What is the child's anxiety related to?
   What will the outcome of the epileptic syndrome be?
   Does the child tell others about the epileptic syndrome?

   Child's quality of life

   What are the dos and don'ts imposed?
   What do the family members say/think?
   What do school teachers say/think?
   How do the peers react if they are told?
   How does the epilepsy affect school performance?

   Child's compliance with treatment

   What medications are taken?
   Are the medications good?
   What do they do to the child?
   Which ones does the child prefer and why?

   Child's habits in relation to the epilepsies

   What do you do that might bring on a seizure?
   When do the seizures occur (a.m. seizures contraindicate an a.m. bath)?

2. The family's experience of the epileptic syndrome

   Has life changed since your child has epilepsy?
   What has changed?
   How do you feel about it?
   What do you do about it?
   The siblings must be allowed to discuss issues from their own perspective.

Simple partial seizures

During a simple partial seizure, the child is conscious and the clinical signs exhibited are related to the site of the epileptic focus within the brain, as represented in **Figure 7.6**. A child with an epileptic focus localised in the motor cortex will present with motor signs such as hand movement or leg movement. A speech disorder may occur if the dominant cerebral hemisphere, most commonly on the left, is involved. When an epileptic focus is localised in the sensory cortex, a child will experience sensory disturbances such as tingling or numbness of a part of the body. Additional sensory experiences related to a focus localised in other parts of the cortex may take the form of hallucinations, a feeling of 'déjà vu', vertigo, gustatory, olfactory or auditory experiences. Autonomic symptoms and signs such as sweating, flushing of the face, increased salivation, abdominal sensation or nausea may also occur. A child may present with several types of simple partial seizures in a cluster.

Complex partial seizures

The child loses awareness during a complex partial seizure. The seizure may have a warning sign and, for example, commence as a simple partial seizure. The clinical signs

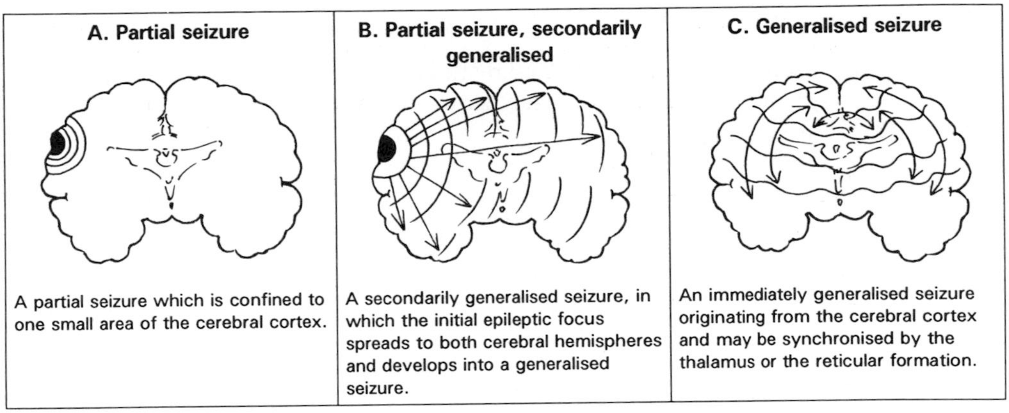

A. Partial seizure	B. Partial seizure, secondarily generalised	C. Generalised seizure
A partial seizure which is confined to one small area of the cerebral cortex.	A secondarily generalised seizure, in which the initial epileptic focus spreads to both cerebral hemispheres and develops into a generalised seizure.	An immediately generalised seizure originating from the cerebral cortex and may be synchronised by the thalamus or the reticular formation.

Figure 7.5 Diagrammatic representation of seizures.

are also related to the site of the epileptic focus within the cerebral cortex. Automatisms, which are repetitive actions such as trying to stand up, mouthing or wiping the nose, are quite common.

Partial seizures becoming secondarily generalised

Simple or complex partial seizures may both evolve into a generalised seizure. A simple partial seizure, which spreads to surrounding brain structures may evolve into a complex partial seizure and then become generalised. The progression of the seizure is related to the spreading of the epileptic activity throughout both sides of the brain.

Generalised seizures

Generalised seizures occur following general electrical abnormalities from the whole cerebral cortex, throughout the brain. No specific localised focus can be found.

Absence seizures

In an absence seizure (previously called 'petit mal'), a brief (usually 5 to 15 seconds) impairment of consciousness occurs with subtle signs. The seizure may take the form of a staring attack or a brisk cessation of speech. Automatisms such as mouthing, chewing, minor jerking of eyelids or head movement may occur. Occasionally, there is a loss of bladder control. There will be little, if any, confusion after the event, and falling does not occur.

Myoclonic seizures

Myoclonic seizures are brief, shock-like muscle contractions that may be isolated or occur repeatedly and irregularly, for a few seconds' duration. These jerks may be bilateral and symmetrical or may be irregular, moving from limb to limb. They usually involve the arms, but when they involve the legs they will cause the child to fall. Consciousness may not be affected.

Clonic seizures

During a generalised clonic seizure, bilateral rhythmic jerks occur in a symmetrical manner. When the rate of the seizure progressively slows down, the jerks become increasingly more violent.

Tonic seizures

Tonic seizures are brief attacks of rigidity lasting 1 to 10 seconds and are typically activated by sleep. The axial part of the body is involved and autonomic signs such as tachycardia, apnoea, flushing of the face, cyanosis, salivation and lacrymation are commonly associated.

Tonic–clonic seizures

These were previously called 'grand mal' seizures. During the tonic phase, the child lies rigidly in an extensor posture. The diaphragm and the intercostal muscles are involved and as a consequence the child's respiration is inhibited. The clonic phase of rhythmic jerking then follows.

Atonic seizures

The briefest attacks may only be a head nodding or sagging of the knee. Others can be drop attacks when the children fall and then immediately pick themselves up to resume activities. There is no alteration of consciousness or period of postictal confusion. A child suffering from Lennox–Gastaut epilepsy (**Table 7.2**) has this type of seizure and repeatedly injures the face and head.

NURSING INTERVENTIONS

General safety aspects

A child with **an acute illness** such as meningitis, encephalitis or brain trauma (surgical or accidental) and experiencing a seizure which can further compromise his/her brain must be aggressively treated. A child with **chronic epilepsy** who experiences a seizure of different clinical manifestation (longer or of greater intensity) must also be treated aggressively.

If in doubt about the child's condition, the safest interventions apply:

- the airway must be protected by positioning child on the side;
- the airway must be cleared with suction; and
- oxygen must be administered.

The nurse will always maintain the equipment ready.

In other instances, children with simple partial seizures will require different safety measures to children with multiple seizure types. It is therefore essential to identify the individual child's safety needs relating to specific seizure and intervene with preventive measures (**Table 7.4**) that afford appropriate protection.

The balance between providing safety measures and restricting the child's life is difficult to gauge. For example, the use of oxygen, although reassuring, may increase the parents' sense of helplessness. Oxygen is rarely available at home, at school or in the

Oxygen and suction are checked daily.

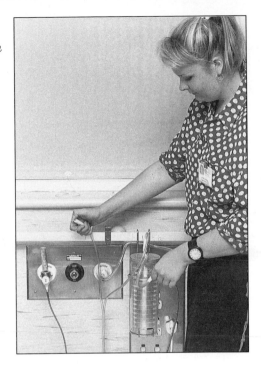

Table 7.4 Safety measures for various seizure types

Seizures types	Cot sides	Supervision		Oxygen	Suction*	Helmet
		Bath	Shower			
Partial seizures						
Simple partial		Sometimes	Sometimes			
Complex partial	Sometimes	Always	Sometimes			
Secondarily generalised	Always	Always	Preferably	Yes[†]	Yes	
Generalised seizures						
Absences		Sometimes	Sometimes			
Myoclonic	Sometimes	Sometimes	Sometimes			Sometimes
Clonic	Always	Always	Preferably	Yes[†]	Yes	
Tonic	Always	Always	Preferably	Yes[‡]		
Tonic–clonic	Always	Always	Preferably	Yes[†‡]	Yes	
Atonic	Always	Always	Preferably			Always

* Suction must be used if there is a risk of aspiration pneumonia.

† Oxygen is required if cyanosis is present.

‡ Oxygen may assist after the tonic–clonic seizure, but during the tonic attack, the intercostal muscles are also involved and oxygen may not be inhaled.

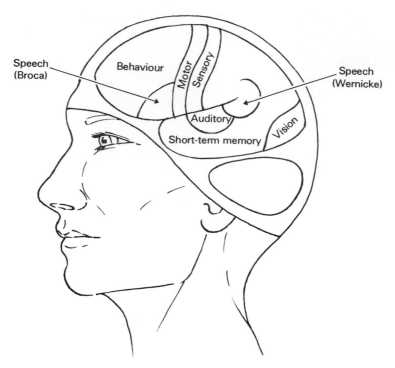

Figure 7.6 Areas of the brain and their related function. The left side of the brain, dominant in most of the population, contains Wernicke's area and Broca's area grouped as 'speech' areas.

community and by creating a need for it, the child's independence may be dramatically restricted.

Similarly, suction equipment is not generally available in the community and renders the child's care quite technical in the eyes of the family. Its use must be limited to the need to clear upper airway obstruction and prevent aspiration pneumonia. Commonly, after a seizure, the child can go to the bathroom to brush the teeth or rinse the mouth.

Of equal importance as a safety aspect in children with numerous atonic or myoclonic seizures is the child's need for a helmet. The design must be appropriate if the helmet is to provide effective protection. Therefore assessing the way the child falls (on the face or on the back of the head) and questioning about past injuries may assist in identifying the proper design. To date, no perfect helmet design is available and children having drop attacks still suffer numerous, repeated nose injuries, facial and head lacerations, and abrasions. It is rare, however, for serious head injuries to occur as a sequel of a seizure fall.

Additional measures regarding bathing and showering include supervision in the bath to prevent drowning and temperature control of hot water to prevent scald burns.

Description of the seizures

The nurse, in addition to intervening and providing support during the seizure will, with the family, collect visual data. This accurate record will be an invaluable contribution to the making of a medical diagnosis and the prescribing of appropriate treatments. Specific information should include the description of the preictal phase (moment immediately preceding the seizure), the ictal phase (the seizure itself) and the postictal phase (the time between the end of the seizure and full recovery). The frequency and the length of the seizures will also be recorded.

Preictal phase

The description should include:

- Precipitating factors if applicable.
- Activity when the seizure started.
- Feeling, sensation before the seizure.
- Reaction when aware of the oncoming seizure.

Ictal phase

1. The description should include:

- Initial clinical signs of the seizure (twitching of eye lid or corner of the mouth, jerking of one limb, head turning to one side, eye movement, vocal noise or sudden fall).
- Progression of the seizure (parts of the body which become gradually involved).
- Autonomic system involvement (sweating, salivating, flushing of the face, vomiting).
- Time and length of the seizure.

2. Neurological observations performed in a simple manner will consider:

- Consciousness — the child will be asked to obey simple commands during the seizure, such as touching the nose.
- Memory — the child will be asked to remember a word or an object.
- Pupils — can be pin-point, large or medium size.

3. Additional observations are recorded if they occur:

- Respiration — can be fast, deep, shallow or irregular.
- Pulse — can be rapid or unchanged.
- Incontinence — urine and faeces.
- Emotional status — fear, aggressive behaviour or post-event withdrawal.
- Cyanosis — length and extent.

Postictal phase

The following should be recorded:

- Residual weakness, confusion and or drowsiness.
- Length of time before full recovery occurs.
- Child's memory of the event or of part of it.
- Child's feelings about the seizure.
- Feelings of the family.

A seizure type which is observed for the first time is described thoroughly. When the same seizure type is repeated, it is acceptable to number it (type 1, 2 or 3) and record it as such. Differences in clinical manifestation must always be recorded. The description can be discussed with other witnesses to ensure accuracy.

A fitting chart, as in **Figure 7.7**, is used prior to the child's discharge and continued at home. It has the advantages of being easy to fill in and it provides the medical staff

NAME				SEIZURES CODE AND DESCRIPTION									
				....	....								
				....	....								
				....	....								

DATE	YEAR											
	Jan	Feb	Mar	Apr	May	Jun	Jul	Aug	Sep	Oct	Nov	Dec
1												
2												
3												
4												
5												
6												
7												
8												
9												
10												
11												
12												
13												
14												
15												
16												
17												
18												
19												
20												
21												
22												
23												
24												
25												
26												
27												
28												
29												
30												
31												

Figure 7.7 Fitting chart. Each seizure is given a code, which can be selected by the child or the caregiver. The code is entered in the calendar when a seizure occurs.

with a graph to correlate frequency of seizures with medication changes or life experiences such as holiday, menstruation or sleep deprivation.

Nursing actions during seizures

The registered nurse will attend the child confidently but will never dramatise the event. Nursing actions depend on the type of seizure, whether the child suffers from chronic epilepsy or is acutely ill and the environment where the seizure occurs.

Brief generalised seizure

The nurse will avoid dramatisation, keep calm and act as in a home environment.

Protect the child, but do not restrain since this often induces an aggressive response. Initially the environment is assessed and protective measures are taken. If the child has a seizure in a bath, the plug must be pulled immediately and the airway maintained out of the water. A child having a seizure in a swimming pool, should have the head maintained out of the water and should be taken out of the water. A child having a seizure on a chair, can be positioned safely on the floor if necessary. The environment should be manipulated to allow for the seizure to occur without causing injuries. Sharp objects must be removed or padded. Finally, the head should be protected from repetitive minor injuries with a pillow, a folded jacket or a soft toy placed underneath.

Objects are not inserted into the mouth to maintain the airway patency as it is sufficient to position the head on the side The tongue, which cannot be swallowed, may be bitten but will heal rapidly. The attempt to separate the teeth and insert an object in the mouth may lead to additional damage of the teeth, the gum and the tongue and is therefore unnecessary. The child requires supervision till the end of the seizure, which includes the phase of postictal confusion. In the eventuality of postictal drowsiness, the nurse will check that its duration is normal for the child and is not related to a head injury.

Parental teaching. The family will gain confidence by gradually becoming involved during seizures. Parents facing a seizure for the first time may initially be involved by describing the seizure. This useful exercise will teach them to observe their child well, detailing eye twitching, mouth, head or limb movements as well as other events such as salivating, sweating or facial flushing. When parents demonstrate their familiarity in observing the seizure, they will be involved in positioning their child appropriately on the side. Issues in regard to protecting the child from injuries will be discussed to help parents learn appropriate and simple actions. The child's needs for reassurance with cuddling or talking will be emphasised. Parents will clean their child's mouth, if required, after the seizure. Gradually parents will learn to handle the event more confidently. Potential caregivers such as grandparents and friends of the family, who are likely to offer some parental relief, should be taught how to care for the child. It is also important to remember that children interact together while playing and siblings therefore must be taught what to do during a fit. Consistent family independence in caring for the child will permit a safe discharge home. Following the seizure, while acknowledging the child's tiredness, caregivers encourage the return to previous activities to avoid taking a sick role.

Prolonged generalised seizure or status epilepticus

As stated earlier, children experiencing an acute sickness such as meningitis, encephalitis or acute medical illness leading to seizures must be immediately treated to prevent additional intracerebral damage to a brain already compromised by the acute illness.

First aid: The child is initially positioned on the side. The head on the side permits the tongue to fall forward, prevents the aspiration of vomitus and allows good air entry to occur. The airway is cleared of obstructive material by suctioning oropharyngeal material. Suction, when performed on babies, must be gentle to prevent ulceration of the fragile mucosa.

The colour of the child will direct the administration of oxygen, which is required should the infant be pale or cyanosed. A sustained cyanosis requires the child to be assisted with oxygen via a bag and mask.

The infant is safely positioned and closely monitored during a seizure.

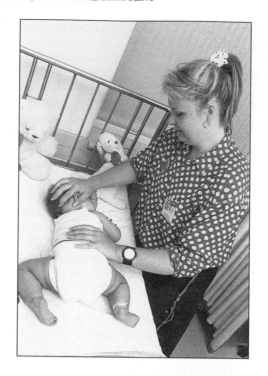

Parents are involved in the nursing care, shown here positioning the infant during a seizure.

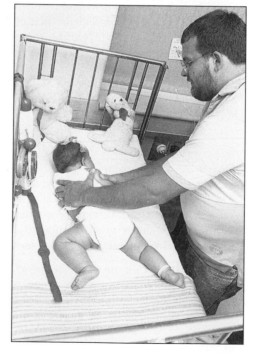

The infant can be nursed prone in the parent's arms.

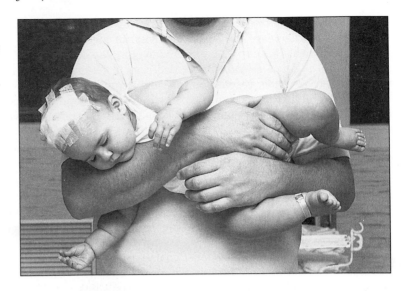

Oxygen can be administered by holding the oxygen tubing in front of the infant's mouth or nose.

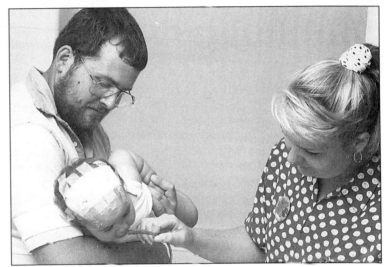

Seizure control: Generalised seizures may induce marked cardiovascular changes, transient respiratory changes, autonomic nervous system responses, endocrine events and metabolic changes. In animals, it is suggested that intraneural metabolism is not able to meet the energy demands of seizure activity and ischaemic neuronal changes follow. Anti-epileptic medications are administered. Diazepam, given rectally, is used when a venous access is not available. Intravenous clonazepam or diazepam will have a rapid action. Jerking movements make the administration of the intravenous anti-epileptic medication difficult. An intravenous cannula may be sited to permit further intravenous administration.[7]

The effect of the anti-epileptic agent will be recorded and correlated with the dosage given and the time of administration.

Respiratory status monitoring: Anti-epileptic agents may depress the respiratory centres and while they decrease the seizure activity, in high doses they can gradually lead to respiratory arrest. *The nurse is prepared to clear the child's airway, administer oxygen and provide manual ventilation.* A decrease in jerking movements is observed along with oxymetry reading, respiration rate and depth.

Some children can receive high doses of anti-epileptic agents without the seizure ceasing. The continual epileptic activity can be demonstrated by twitching of the eyelids, the mouth or some muscles. In these extreme cases of status epilepticus, following intubation and ventilation, barbiturates are given, sometimes in large quantities, to control the seizure. The absence, decrease or continuity of the seizure must be reported. Electroencephalographic monitoring may be used to guide a gradual lightening of the barbiturate therapy. In most cases, nursing monitoring of seizures guides the decrease of doses. Should seizures recur, further barbiturate therapy will be required.

Family teaching: Children with chronic epilepsy having experienced status epilepticus without apparent reason may be at risk for further similar seizures following recovery and discharge home. Caregivers must be prepared for the recurrence of status epilepticus and taught the appropriate actions before the child is discharged.

A rectal diazepam kit will be given to the parents if the child is frequently experiencing status epilepticus or if the parents live in an area distant from medical support. Parents should store the drug appropriately and maintain its constant availability. Importantly, they should know when the drug is required and how to prepare the prescribed dose. They must understand that overdosing, without medical support, is in fact more dangerous than the seizure as it can stop the child's breathing. Caregivers must demonstrate competency in drug administration before discharge. Should readmission occur following a long seizure, the timing of administration and the problems faced will be assessed. Encouragement is given on the aspects well handled while acknowledging the difficulties and the parental anxiety in facing such a crisis alone.

Parents should be taught confidently to perform first aid actions such as positioning the child on the side to prevent aspiration, mouth to mouth resuscitation and protecting the child from additional injuries.

It is important for the caregivers to identify when to seek medical assistance. The local medical facilities must be investigated before discharge to clarify accessibility to local medical services. In some instances, a general practitioner nearby will be the preferred alternative, while a rapid means of transport to a hospital or the ambulance services can be the optimum choice in other circumstances.

Medication compliance

The registered nurse is required to develop a good knowledge of anti-epileptic medications, as well as skills in assisting and promoting compliance.

General nursing considerations

Anti-epileptic drugs decrease epileptic activity by affecting (slowing or stopping) the conduction of the impulse or raising the threshold of neurons so that they require greater electrical stimulation to fire. Drugs control symptoms only if they are consistently taken.

A child does not usually require this therapy after a single seizure; only recurrent seizures are treated. The appropriate drug will be selected following identification of the epilepsy syndrome and through a degree of trial and error. Dosages may be altered according to clinical efficacy, side effects or blood levels. Events such as diarrhoea and vomiting may decrease absorption, while alcohol or additional drugs may interact with the therapy and destabilise the control. An abrupt cessation of medication can lead to status epilepticus. Compliance with medications is encouraged at the earliest stage of the therapy. The preparation will be made available to the child in the most appropriate or preferred form such as syrup, chewable tablet, ordinary tablet or capsule. Nursing strategies such as dribbling the medication into an infant's mouth, while talking and playing, rather than force feeding it, are adopted. Observations reported by the parents in regard to behavioural changes are reported to the medical staff as these unpleasant effects may lead to a lack of compliance. The whole family may suffer from a child becoming hyperactive. A pill bag can be given to adolescents, set around the neck and hidden under the shirt if discretion is important for them. A pill dispenser (e.g., dosette) obtained from a pharmacy can help with remembering when tablets are to be taken. A child who wants to stop medications, disbelieving the need for them, may require hospitalisation and the video technique may be used here, to show the seizures and convince the child of the need for anti-epileptic therapy.

Special queries about medications can be discussed with the pharmacist.

Details of the commonly used anti-epileptic drugs and the nursing considerations in their administration are given in **Table 7.5**.

Discharge planning

Misconceptions about epilepsy are identified by questioning the child and the family. Their perceptions of living with epilepsy are clarified. A personalised discharge plan is developed to provide the family with the required knowledge. Because ongoing support will be required, each admission provides an ideal opportunity for the family to obtain information and seek appropriate help.

The subsequent strategies of care aim to establish a realistic quality of life, with emphasis on the child's social integration. Nursing actions target education of the entire family. Role playing with siblings and peers can be used and an 'epilepsy certificate' can be given.

Referral to social work services may be required to provide family support or therapy. Nurses must discuss problems brought to their attention by parents with the medical staff, as the neurologist will continue to treat and review the child in outpatient services.

Epilepsy support groups are recommended to parents. These groups encourage parents to address safety issues in the home to protect the child. Issues related to school and community integration, child support, social activities, career development, sexuality and planning for the future can be discussed as well as the legal requirements for obtaining a driving licence. Strengthened by the organisation, the families' self-esteem may grow to the degree that they participate to support other families.

Details of support service and educational sessions must be recorded to ensure continuity of care. The ongoing objectives will aim for quality of life and acceptance of the seizures if they cannot be controlled by drugs or surgery. The child will learn to live with the epilepsy syndrome and the family will learn to avoid dramatising it.

INVESTIGATIONS

Investigations aim at identifying the presence of epileptic activity, and to localise the site of origin within the brain. A defined epileptic focus, with or without a structural lesion, may be removed surgically with a subsequent cure of the epilepsy.

Table 7.5 Main aspects of the administration of antiepileptic medications

Medications	Nursing considerations	Dosage
CARBAMAZEPINE		
Dosage forms available: Mixture Tablets	The drug must be introduced at a low dosage as carbamazepine is likely to cause neurotoxic adverse effects. Carbamazepine also induces enzymes within the liver, and increases its own metabolism and that of some other drugs. The dose of the other drugs should be maintained or reduced gradually. ***Common Adverse Effects:*** nausea, drowsiness, dizziness, ataxia, diplopia, nystagmus, blurred vision, skin rashes. ***Occasionally:*** pulmonary problems, blood disorders.	**No loading dose.** *Oral:* Commence 5 mg/kg/24 hours (maximum 200 mg) in 1 or 2 doses, increase to 10–15 mg/kg/24 hours in 2 or 3 doses, over two weeks. (Increase dosage slowly to allow for enzyme induction upon initiation of therapy.)
CLONAZEPAM		
Dosage forms available: Injection Tablets Mixture	*Rate of intravenous administration:* minimum time 2 minutes. ***Common Adverse Effects:*** Drowsiness, sedation, ataxia, behavioural disturbances, (aggression, hyper-activity, irritability), skin rashes, gastro-intestinal disorders, increased salivation, enuresis. **Repeated intravenous doses may cause respiratory depression, therefore the respiratory status must be monitored and equipment for ventilatory support must be prepared.**	***Neonates:*** *Intravenous during seizures:* up to 0.25 mg. Less for premature babies and infants not on ventilators (0.1–0.2 mg). ***Infants and children:*** *Intravenous:* up to .5 mg *Oral:* Initially give 0.01–0.03 mg/kg/24 hours in 2–3 doses. Doses should be increased by no more than 0.25 mg or 0.5 mg every third day until control is achieved (maximum: 2 mg/kg/24 hours). ***Adults:*** *Intravenous:* 1mg per dose which may be repeated up to 13 mg. *Oral:* Initially no more than 1.5 mg/24 hours. Increase gradually to a maximum of 20 mg/24 hours.

Table 7.5 (*continued*)

Medications	Nursing considerations	Dosage
DIAZEPAM		
Dosage forms available: Tablets Injection Rectal preparation	**Administration:** During administration observe for hypotension and respiratory depression. **Caution:** *Intravenous:* give as a slow bolus usually over 2–5 minutes. Not greater than 5 mg/minute. Injection into small veins may extravasate into subcutaneous tissue and inflict pain, phlebitis or necrosis. Do not store Diazepam in plastic syringes as this will decrease the availability of the infused drug. *Rectal:* delayed respiratory depression may occur after rectal administration. *Intramuscular:* Erratic absorption ineffective for status epilepticus. **Common Adverse Effects:** Drowsiness, respiratory depression, confusion, depression, lethargy, hangover effect, ataxia, dizziness, slurred speech, tremors, muscle cramps, euphoria, blurred vision, weakness, dysarthria, impaired memory, headache, sleep disorders, vertigo, incontinence, nystagmus, cardiac arrest, skin rash, urticaria, constipation, nausea, vomiting, abdominal discomfort.	*Intravenous:* 0.1–0.3 mg/kg dose (maximum 10mg). Repeat every 1–4 hours as needed (maximum 30 mg in 8 hours). *Oral:* 0.1–0.3 mg/kg/dose, 8 to 12 hourly, starting at lower dose and gradually increasing. *Rectal:* 0.3 mg to 0.5 mg/kg/dose. **Adults:** *Oral:* 5 to 40 mg/day in divided doses.
PARALDEHYDE		
Dosage forms available: Injection Rectal preparation Oral preparation	**Administration:** Paraldehyde must be diluted before administration. *Intravenous:* Give over 15 minutes or by continuous infusion. Dilute with normal saline. *Oral:* Dilute in milk or fruit juice to disguise taste and minimise gastrointestinal irritation.	*Intravenous:* 0.2 millilitre/kg over 15 minutes then 0.02 millilitre/kg/hour. *Intramuscular:* 0.2 millilitre/kg stat. (maximum 10 millilitres), then 0.1 millilitre/kg/dose, 4–6 hourly. *Rectal:* 0.3 millilitre/kg/dose (maximum 5 millilitres) every 4–8 hours.

Table 7.5 (*continued*)

Medications	Nursing considerations	Dosage
PARALDEHYDE (*Cont.*)	*Rectal:* Dilute 1:10 with isotonic sodium chloride immediately before use or in 1:3 with olive oil. *Intramuscular:* Painful and can cause muscle necrosis. **CAUTION:** Discard preparations that have a brownish colour of acetic acid. Decomposed paraldehyde has produced a few cases of severe corrosion of the stomach and/or rectum. Metabolic acidosis and fatalities have occurred. **Do not use any plastic equipment for administration. The drug dissolves plastic.** ***Common Adverse Effects:*** drowsiness, gastric irritation, rectal irritation, erythematous rash, toxic hepatitis, necrosis.	
PHENOBARBITONE *Dosage forms available:* Injection Mixture Tablets	***Administration:*** Intravenous: Dilute and infuse slowly by intravenous push at a rate not exceeding 1 mg/kg/minute. ***Adverse Effects:*** *Premature infants:* Depressant effects because of immature hepatic metabolism. Overdose occurs easily in premature and small babies which can result in respiratory depression requiring ventilation. ***Common Adverse Effects:*** drowsiness, lethargy, headache, agitation, hyper excitability in children, nightmares, respiratory depression, nystagmus, ataxia.	*Febrile convulsion prophylaxis:* 3–4 mg/kg/dose at night. ***Neonates:*** *Intravenous during seizure:* loading dose 20 mg/kg given as two doses of 10 mg/kg 3–4 hours apart. *Intravenous/oral (maintenance):* 3–4 mg/kg/24 hours in 1 or 2 doses. ***Infants and children:*** *Intravenous/intramuscular: Emergency:* loading dose 20–30 mg/kg/dose. *Maintenance with intravenous, intramuscular or oral:* 3 to 5 mg/kg/day, in 1 or 2 doses.

Table 7.5 (*continued*)

Medications	Nursing considerations	Dosage
PHENYTOIN		
Dosage forms available: Injection Capsule Chewable tablet Mixture	*Rate of administration:* Under 50 kg: up to 1 mg/kg/minute. Over 50 kg: up to 50 mg per minute Loading dose: over 60 minutes. *Administration:* *Intravenous:* Inject slowly to minimise incidence of hypotension and circulatory collapse. ***Incompatible with Dextrose.*** Preferably dilute with 0.9% sodium chloride to 5 millilitre or to a maximum dilution of 1 mg per millilitre. Do not use if cloudy or if crystals are visible. *Intramuscular:* Irregularly and incompletely absorbed. *Subcutaneous:* Possibility of local tissue damage. *Enteral:* A very marked reduction in absorption occurs when given with enteral feeds. This is successfully managed by stopping the feeds 2 hours before and after the Phenytoin administration. ***Common adverse effects:*** Skin rashes (drug should be stopped), excess hair growth, accentuation of acne, gingival hyperplasia, lethargy, nystagmus, ataxia, increase seizures, vertigo, confusion, slurred speech, hallucination.	***Neonatal:*** Pre-term: 2 mg/kg/dose, 12 hourly First week of life: 4 mg/kg/dose, 12 hourly Second week of life to 12 months of age: 4 mg/kg/dose, 6 hourly ***Infants and children:*** 4–8 mg/kg/24 hours in two or three doses, adjusted to achieve therapeutic effects or levels. ***Adults:*** 7 mg/kg/24 hours in 2 or 3 doses, adjusted to achieve therapeutic levels or effects. *Loading dose:* 15 to 20 mg per kg
SODIUM VALPROATE		
Dosage forms available: Tablets Mixture	Drug should be discontinued if signs of hypersensitivity, hepatic dysfunction, or coagulation abnormalities (bruising or haemorrhage) occur.	*Oral:* Commence 5–7.5 mg/kg/dose 8–12 hourly, increasing to a maximum of 50 mg/kg/24 hours (in 2–3 doses).

Table 7.5 (*continued*)

Medications	Nursing considerations	Dosage
SODIUM VALPROATE (*Cont.*)	***Common Adverse effects:*** Jaundice, severe hepato-toxicity have been reported; abnormal bruising, sedation, lethargy, tremors, ataxia, nausea, vomiting, diarrhoea, increased appetite and/ or thirst, and weight gain, anorexia, inhibited platelet aggregation, thrombocytopenia, increased bleeding time, alopecia insomnia.	***Adults:*** 1–2 g/24 hours in divided doses.
VIGABATRIN		
Dosage forms available: Tablets	Oral administration only. Efficacy is not related to serum levels. ***Common Adverse Effects:*** Psychosis with high dosages or withdrawal. Excitation, insomnia, fatigue, dizziness, depression, confusion, drowsiness, weight gain, nausea, vomiting.	*Infantile Spasms:* *Oral:* May require up to 150 mg/kg/ 24 hours. *Oral:* Initially, 40 mg/kg/24 hours in 1 or 2 doses, increased to maximum 80 mg/kg/24 hours. ***Adults:*** *Oral:* Initially, 2 g/24 hours in 1 or 2 doses, gradually increased to 3 g/24 hours if required.

Electroencephalography

An electroencephalogram (EEG) is the interictal recording, usually by means of scalp electrodes, of the electrical potentials generated by neurons in the brain. The EEG may reveal slow wave activity or focal or general presence of electrical discharges. EEG is not so much used in diagnosis of epilepsy but to attempt to gain additional information to type the seizures and define the epilepsy syndrome.

The nurse's aim of care is to inform the child about the test in an age-appropriate manner to gain cooperation. A diagram showing the mapping of the electrodes may be useful (**Figure 7.9**). The child, if able to understand, requires the explanation that no pain will occur during the procedure, that no electrical sensation will be generated, that the technologist does not read thoughts and that movements induce artefacts. The child's cooperation may be encouraged by offering rewards such as stickers or certificates.

Sedation may be used, sometimes to enable the test to be performed in a distressed child, at other times when a sleep recording is required in order to observe certain aspects of brain wave activity which only occur during sleep. It is relatively uncommon to record an actual attack during a routine EEG.

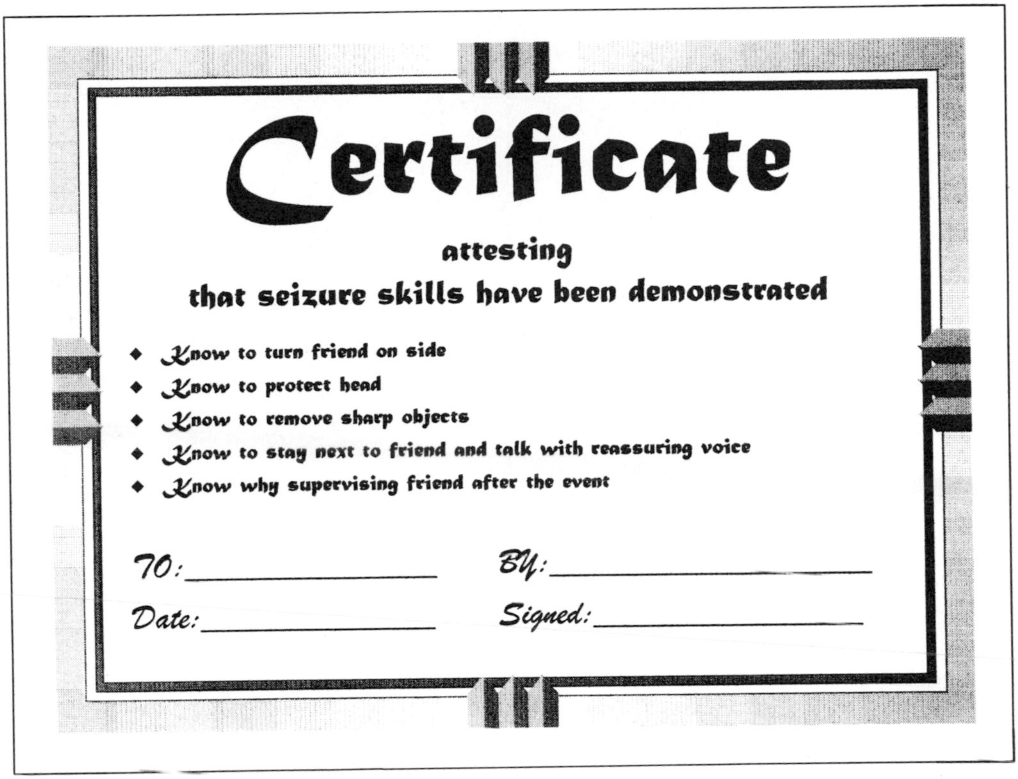

Certificate

attesting

that seizure skills have been demonstrated

- ♦ *Know to turn friend on side*
- ♦ *Know to protect head*
- ♦ *Know to remove sharp objects*
- ♦ *Know to stay next to friend and talk with reassuring voice*
- ♦ *Know why supervising friend after the event*

TO: _____   *BY:* _____

Date: _____   *Signed:* _____

Figure 7.8 This epilepsy certificate is given to children who learn through role playing how to look after their sibling or friend who is having a seizure. The sibling or friend is asked to role play a seizure while a second child demonstrates the following skills: The child having the seizure is turned on the side to avoid food or saliva 'going the wrong way'. The child's head is protected and she is reassured. After the seizure, the sibling or friend explains what happened to the child who had the seizure and watches to see that he is all right. Children then reverse the role.

Video-EEG monitoring

Video-electroencephalographic monitoring (VEM) is a continuous EEG recording using glued scalp electrodes and video camera filming of the child. The EEG data and video pictures are recorded on a video tape via a data encoder. The tape can be played back for analysis and to correlate clinical information with the EEG.

Parental and child anxiety

Children undergoing VEM are in the frightening situation of awaiting a seizure. To achieve this, they may be taken off their anti-epileptic medications. This conflicts with lifetime education which emphasises the danger of abrupt anti-epileptic medication withdrawal and the risk of having a prolonged seizure. Preparation for rapid intervention should a seizure occur is made. Anti-epileptic medications for emergency use should be readily

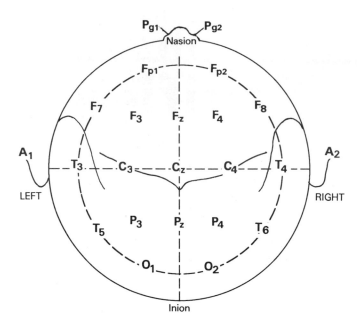

TOP OF HEAD

Figure 7.9 Position of skin electrodes.

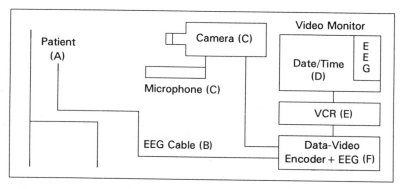

(A) is seated in an armchair or resting in bed. The EEG technologist positions the scalp electrodes with a strong glue which permits conductions of brain potential activity. The cable (B) transfers the EEG to a data encoder (F) which correlates the video with the EEG. The video cassette recorder (E) tapes the EEG and video allowing them to be played back together. The data encoder can also be connected to an EEG printer to review the seizure activity more precisely. The TV monitor (D) displays the date, time, child's activity and EEG if required. The camera and microphone (C) record the child 24 hours a day.

Figure 7.10 Video EEG setup.

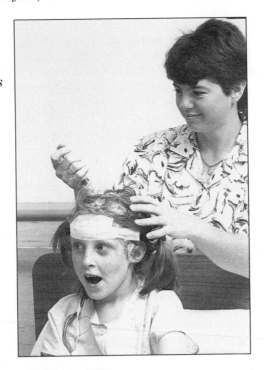

The EEG technologist checks the scalp electrodes daily and adds glue as required.

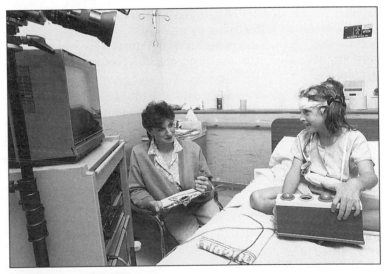

The child under VEM is given activities. A parent is observing and documenting the time of the seizures. With the use of a switch the video tape is marked and the event found easily.

accessible. The child must stay in the camera field all the time and this immobilisation is an added source of stress. Maintaining privacy when attending physical needs such as washing and toileting must be considered.

The parent attending the child for the prolonged hospital stay may experience additional domestic concerns such as work, other children and home. These issues considered, volunteers or social workers may become involved as required.

The anxiety of the parents and the child can only be alleviated by shortening the length of investigation. It is therefore beneficial to identify triggering factors inducing epilepsy. If it is boredom, leave the child without activities; if it is school work, call the hospital teacher in or ask the parents to bring school activities; if it is physical exercise, ask the physiotherapist to provide an exercise bike. Seizures occurring with sleep deprivation will be induced by keeping the child awake as long as possible.

The waiting time for a seizure is unpredictable. The child must be provided with age-appropriate activities to tolerate this long (sometimes weeks) investigation time.

Information for parents and child

Parents and child must be aware of the possible length of the investigation. The ideal time for these investigations is therefore school holidays and weekends.

In preparation for VEM, the child will wear a top garment which buttons up at the front and can be easily changed. This simple initiative will permit a continued recording when the child's clothes are changed and thus prevent missing the recording of a seizure. Toilet privileges are discussed with the medical staff and the family. They are discouraged when seizures are rare.

The permanent caregiver (usually a parent) is the best witness to identify a seizure, having seen many of them in the past. The switch which labels the event on the tape is shown, practiced and readily accessible. This electronic marker is important as it permits the automatic rewinding of the tape to the actual event when reviewing the seizures. As previously stated, the length of the recording may vary, therefore parents must have some time out. The nurse can plan at the beginning of each shift for these breaks. Another family member or a volunteer can be taught and relieve the parent.

The recorded seizure may be used to show the child what happens when the event occurs. Criteria to decide whether or not the seizure can be shown to the child vary and must be discussed with the team and the parents. Factors in favour of showing the seizure are:

- The seizure is not extravagantly generalised and frightening.
- The child is confabulating and dramatising the seizures.
- The child has been told fearful descriptions of the seizure.
- The child denies having seizures and is not compliant with the treatment.

Factors against showing the seizure are:

- The child has been using the seizures to manipulate the family and will simulate seizures more realistically.
- The seizure is frightening.
- The child copes well with the seizures and is not curious about them.

Provide quality recording

The nurse will know the type of seizure to capture on VEM and will monitor the set-up. The part of the body to be filmed is in the video field and the picture is clear as the light and the focus are appropriate. For example, should the neurologist need to investigate a seizure where the early clinical manifestation is eye twitching, the camera will be set on the face and the lighting will come from eye level instead of the ceiling, so eyebrows do not make a shadow over the eyes and mask the seizure. Similarly, the entire body may need to be in the video field if the seizure involves the limbs. The nurse will ensure that

MRI showing a lesion in the temporal lobe. This lesion is localised in an area of the temporal lobe which is prone to epilepsy.

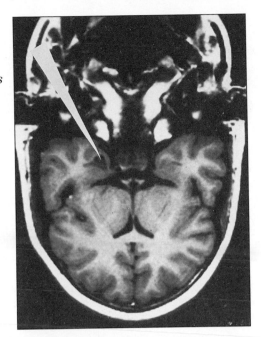

CT showing a lesion in the temporal lobe.

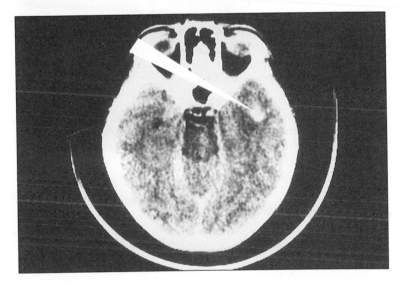

the camera is not obstructed by any object and will control well-intentioned helpers who may inadvertently obstruct the camera during the seizure. The EEG electrodes are checked and if disconnected, the EEG technologist is notified. Essential care during the seizure must be given and the appropriate safety measures taken. EEG technologist and nurse monitor the overall quality of VEM because missed seizures or bad quality recording increase the length of stay, prolonging a stressful investigation for the child and the family.

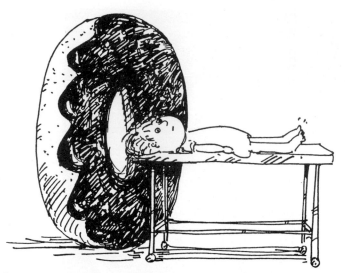

Figure 7.11 Cartoon to help prepare a child who will have a head CT. The child can be shown that the character having a CT wriggles the toes but not the head.
(With the kind permission of Jocelyn Bell — Educational Resources Centre, Royal Children's Hospital, Melbourne)

Computed tomography and magnetic resonance imaging

Computed tomography (CT) and magnetic resonance imaging (MRI) are used to identify anatomical abnormalities such as:

- brain tumour
- cerebrospinal fluid obstruction
- calcified lesion (tuberous sclerosis, necrosis, tuberculosis, vascular lesions)
- scarring (often of one temporal lobe)
- oedema (as with herpes encephalitis)
- demyelination
- other tissue abnormalities.

Except for bone and calcified lesions which are better demonstrated on CT, MRI provides data enabling study of the internal brain structures and types of tissue. Pathologies such as demyelination are well demonstrated on MRI with greater differentiation between white and grey matter than is possible with CT.

Nursing care objectives and strategies

The need to prepare children in an age-appropriate manner before the radiological test cannot be over-emphasised. Preparation aims to effectively reduce the trauma of the experience, as well as the need for sedation and general anaesthesia. Well prepared children will accept radiological tests better, the time required for a test will decrease and the throughput of children will increase, reducing the overall cost of these investigations. The child is more likely to cooperate during the radiological test if the test is understood.

A cartoon can be shown to describe a CT (**Figure 7.11**). Similarly, the MRI can be described as being like a sausage in a hot dog to the youngsters. To reduce the fear of the unknown, the room where the CT or MRI is performed can be visited or shown on photograph. Before sending the child for a procedure requiring contrast, a local skin anaesthetic to numb the skin and alleviate the trauma of the injection can be used, or a cannula can be sited to permit rapid injection without disturbing the child during the test. The parents are valuable judges of their child's tolerance and will help in identifying:

- The need for sedation of their baby or toddler.
- The need for general anaesthesia if the child is likely to refuse to cooperate because of a previous bad experience, a hyperactive response to sedation, irritability or inability to tolerate the lengthy procedure.
- The strategies required to decrease the trauma of the procedure.

Before consenting, parents must understand the test, the reason for it and, if applicable, know the potential complications related to general anaesthesia.

The pre-procedure preparation requires that the child is fasted should general anaesthesia be required. After confirming this with the anaesthetist, it is often possible to fast for 3 hours with breast milk, for 2 hours with clear fluids, for 4 hours with other drinks and for 6 hours with semi-solid or solid food.

Appropriate nursing documentation must accompany the child to assist the radiology nursing staff in providing continuity of care. The child's experience of the test is monitored and recorded by the radiology nursing staff, to facilitate the management of further tests. Allergy to contrast, if known, must be accurately recorded.

The child is encouraged to describe the experience of the test and issues of concern are discussed.

Continuity of care is achieved when the ward nurse understands the test to be performed, and understands the organisation of the radiology department, and when the radiology nurse appreciates the preparation undertaken and uses the suggested strategies to satisfy the child's special needs.

Single photon emission computed tomography and positron emission tomography

Single photon emission computed tomography (SPECT) and positron emission tomography (PET) are used to identify physiological abnormalities such as abnormal blood flow and abnormal metabolism.

SPECT permits the study of the cerebral blood flow during seizures (ictally) or between seizures (interictally). There is an increase of cerebral blood flow in the region of the epileptogenic focus ictally. Interictally, the blood flow to the epileptic focus is lessened. When used to identify an epileptic focus, this technique requires the injection of a radio-isotope during a seizure. This is achieved with the video EEG monitoring (VEM) set up to identify the seizure at its onset while administering an ictal injection. Interictal studies appear less reliable in determining the epileptic focus than ictal studies, but ictal studies are technically more difficult to perform as the injection must occur during the seizure.

Safety considerations relate to the isotope storage. As it must be injected as soon as the seizure starts, it needs to be stored in close proximity of the child, in a lead box, out of children's reach. The storage cupboard will display a nuclear medicine warning sign. The nursing responsibilities relate to the IV cannula flushing at least every 4 hours to ensure continued patency and maintain the accessibility to the injection port, (the success of this investigation relies on the extreme rapidity of the isotope injection). Some seizures last seconds and the nurse responsible for the isotope administration is notified via an emergency calling system. While handling the isotope, the nurse makes maximal

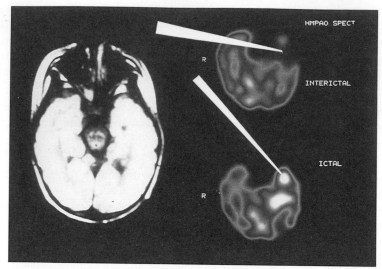

CT showing the temporal lobe on the left and the SPECT study on the right. The upper SPECT, taken between seizures, shows a decrease of cerebral blood flow to the anterior pole of the right temporal lobe. The lower SPECT, taken during a seizure, shows an increase of cerebral blood flow to the area previously less irrigated. The upper interictal SPECT is a base line study which when compared to the lower ictal SPECT, can reveal the epileptic focus.

use of the syringe's protective lead shielding, uses appropriate gloves and reduces the exposure time to the minimum. After the injection, gloves are worn when handling the child's body fluids for the 6 hours of the isotope's half-life.

The child must go to nuclear medicine for the SPECT scan within hours because the radioisotope has a short half-life and delayed SPECT may reduce the quality of the picture obtained.

Positron emission tomography (PET) provides regional interictal quantitative information on brain perfusion and metabolism.

CONCLUSION

A number of nursing interventions are necessary to assist the child and the family to live with epilepsy. Most children will grow out of their epilepsy or will have it controlled with their medication, rarely requiring hospitalisation. Others will not respond well to their anti-epileptic medications and following extensive investigations may be selected for surgery if they fulfil the criteria. They will be identified to have one unilateral epileptic focus and preoperative investigation will demonstrate that no morbidity will be created by the surgery. The neurosurgeon will surgically remove the identified focus of the brain, commonly in one temporal lobe. Seventy-five per cent of the patients selected for surgery can expect to be seizure-free and may later be taken off their anti-epileptic medication. The minority of children whose condition is not controlled by medications and cannot benefit from surgery, will require constant medical interventions and nursing support.

The neuroscience nurse must take on the role of patient's advocate and from that perspective assist epilepsy sufferers in gaining optimum independence and self-confidence.

The successful outcome will be demonstrated by the acceptance of the epilepsy where children and their families acquire greater understanding of epilepsy, achieve a greater degree of independence or are linked to specific services to receive on-going support. The reading of *Ragged Owlet* by Sue Goss,[8] which gives the point of view of a person with epilepsy, may assist nurses in understanding family needs and is recommended.

REFERENCES

1. Aicardi J. *Epilepsy in children*. New York: Raven Press, 1986.
2. Roger J, Davet C, Bureau M, Dreifuss FE, Wolf P. *Epileptic syndromes in infancy, childhood and adolescence*. Paris: John Libbey Eurotext, 1985.
3. Lindsay KW, Bone I, Callander R. *Neurology and neurosurgery illustrated*. Edinburgh: Churchill Livingstone, 1986.
4. Pagliaro LA, Pagliaro AM. *Problems in paediatric drug therapy*. Hamilton: Hamilton Press Drug Intellignce, 2nd ed 1987.
5. Hickey JV. *The clinical practice of neurology and neurosurgical nursing*. Philadelphia: Lippincott, 1992.
6. Lilley B, McDowell J, Munari G, Parsons B. *Pharmacy Department Royal Children's Hospital: Paediatric Pharmacopoeia*. 11th ed. Melbourne: Sands and McDougall, 1994.
7. Laidlaw J, Richens A, Oxley J. *A textbook of epilepsy*. 3rd ed. Edinburgh: Churchill Livingstone, 1988.
8. Goss S. *Ragged Owlet*. Australia: Houghton Mifflin, 1989.

Raised Intracranial Pressure

Angela M Jones

Intracranial pressure (ICP) may increase in the presence of tumour, haemorrhage, infection, oedema or congenital anomalies of the brain. Neurological deficits develop as intracranial volume increases and compensatory mechanisms fail to maintain ICP within normal limits. Neurological assessment skills and the implementation of an appropriate care plan are critical in the management of a child with raised ICP and fundamental to neuroscience nursing practice.

ANATOMY AND PHYSIOLOGY

Protection of the brain

The brain is afforded protection from injury by the skull, the *meninges* and the *cerebrospinal fluid* (CSF). The three meninges, the *dura mater*, the *arachnoid* and the *pia mater*, provide a continuous sheath of protection around the brain and spinal cord. (**Figure 7.12**) Within the cranium, the dura mater is anchored to the skull, thereby limiting movement of the brain.[1] The brain floats in CSF, a clear liquid found within the meninges. The CSF supports and cushions, creating a buoyant effect which reduces momentum and acceleration of the brain during sudden displacement of the cranium.[2]

The dura mater, the outermost meninge, is a dense and tough membrane. Two potential spaces, one on each side of the dura, may develop in the presence of haematoma or

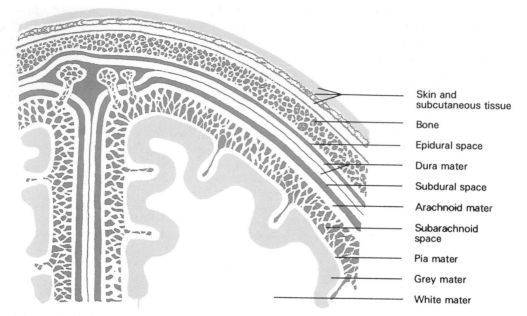

Skin and subcutaneous tissue

Bone

Epidural space

Dura mater

Subdural space

Arachnoid mater

Subarachnoid space

Pia mater

Grey mater

White mater

Figure 7.12 Protective coverings of the brain.[29] (Reproduced with permission)

infection. They are the *extradural* space between the dura and the skull and the *subdural* space between the dura and the arachnoid. The arachnoid, a delicate and non-vascular membrane, lies next to the dura. The pia mater, the innermost meninge, adheres closely to the external surface of the brain. The *subarachnoid* space is between the arachnoid and the pia mater and contains the cerebrospinal fluid.

At 4 points within the cranium, sheet-like extensions of the dura called dural septa extend inward and divide the cranial cavity into freely communicating compartments.[3] The dural septa also prevent injury to the brain by limiting its movement within the cranial vault. The main septa include the tentorium cerebelli and the falx cerebri. The tentorium cerebelli is a tent-like structure which is higher in the centre than on the sides of the skull. It separates the occipital lobes of the cerebral hemispheres from most of the brainstem and creates 2 compartments within the cranium: the *supratentorial* compartment which contains the cerebral hemispheres and the *infratentorial* compartment which contains most of the brainstem and the cerebellum. The falx cerebri lies in the longitudinal fissure between the left and right cerebral hemisphere.

The cerebrospinal fluid

The CSF is secreted by choroid plexus located in fluid-filled cavities within the brain, called ventricles. The rate of CSF production by the choroid plexus is highly variable. The total volume of CSF ranges from 5 mL in neonates to 150 mL in adults. CSF flows from the lateral and 3rd ventricles via the cerebral aqueduct into the 4th ventricle. It then circulates through the subarachnoid space around the brain and spinal cord. Absorption of CSF occurs via *arachnoid granulations* which project from the subarachnoid space through the dura and into venous sinuses. These granulations enable one-way flow of

CSF into the venous system. Blockage of these granulations, obstruction of the CSF pathways or overproduction of CSF may lead to *hydrocephalus*, a cause of raised ICP.

The blood supply to the brain

The brain requires a constant supply of oxygenated blood. Ischaemia and permanent neurological deficit are the outcomes of cerebral hypoperfusion and hypoxia. The child's clinical presentation varies according to the functional area of the brain affected during the hypoxic episode.

The *cerebral perfusion pressure* (CPP) is defined clinically as the difference between the mean arterial pressure (MAP) and the intracranial pressure. It is a measure of the adequacy of the cerebral circulation and the blood pressure gradient across the brain.[5] The CPP is responsible for maintaining the blood flow to the brain, referred to as the cerebral blood flow.[6] Systemic hypotension and raised ICP compromise both cerebral perfusion and cerebral blood flow. Under normal conditions CPP is in the range of 70 to 100 mmHg. While data specific to children are lacking, 50 mmHg is considered to be the minimal adequate CPP in adults.[7]

Fluctuations in cerebral perfusion occur with changes in body posture, intercranial pressure and blood pressure. The process of autoregulation preserves cerebral blood flow over a wide range of cerebral perfusion pressures. Autoregulation is achieved through physiological changes to the cerebral vasculature. Cerebral vasodilation maintains cerebral blood flow and increases the cerebral blood volume (CBV), thereby restoring the CPP. Trauma or ischaemia to the brain can cause localised destruction of the autoregulatory mechanism.

The cerebral vasculature is exquisitely sensitive to changes in pCO_2, and less so to fluctuations in pH and pO_2.[6] A high level of CO_2 or hydrogen ions, either in the blood or localised areas of the brain, causes vasodilation and increased cerebral blood flow. In the presence of an elevated CO_2, cellular metabolism may produce substances such as lactic acid which also cause vasodilation.

The cerebral venous system

The venous system within the cranial vault has a number of unique features. Firstly, it is the only system for drainage of excess intracranial fluid. Unlike many other areas of the body there is no lymphatic system within the intracranial vault. Secondly, cerebral veins do not contain valves which prevent backflow of venous blood. Any increase in thoracic pressure during coughing or straining impedes venous drainage from the brain, thereby increasing cerebral venous pressure and ICP.

THE PATHOPHYSIOLOGY OF RAISED INTRACRANIAL PRESSURE

ICP rises when one of blood, CSF or brain tissue increases in volume.

Normally, brain tissue accounts for 80% of the volume of the cranial vault while CSF and blood each comprise 10%.[5] Beyond infancy, the bony and rigid skull functions as a semi-closed box and the volume of the cranial vault is fixed. A state of dynamic equilibrium exists when the volume of each of these non-compressible components remains constant.[8] The modified Monro Kellie doctrine states that any increase in the volume of one component must be accompanied by a decrease in the volume of the other components to maintain ICP within normal range.

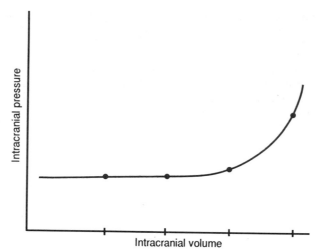

Figure 7.13 The volume-pressure curve.[25]

Figure 7.13 illustrates the relationship between volume and pressure within the cranial vault. In the flat part of the curve, ICP remains fairly constant as intracranial volume increases. During this period ICP is maintained within normal range by the following compensatory mechanisms[9,10]:

- Displacement of CSF from the ventricles and cerebral subarachnoid space into the spinal subarachnoid space.
- Increased reabsorption of CSF.
- Displacement of blood into the venous sinuses, decreasing cerebral blood volume.

In the steep part of the curve, compensatory mechanisms fail and small increases in intracranial volume produce large increases in ICP.

Compensation for raised ICP in infants

Unlike children and adults, infants are able to compensate for increases in intracranial volume. The volume of the cranial vault is not fixed and the skull can expand to accommodate increases in intracranial volume. During infancy, the fontanelles remain open and the skull is soft and unfused. In the absence of raised ICP, the fontanelles feel soft and the brain falls slightly below the level of the skull when the infant is upright. It is normal for the anterior fontanelles to feel slightly fuller when the infant is sleeping and in the supine position. Bulging fontanelles are a normal sign in a crying infant. When the ICP is raised, the infant's anterior fontanelle remains full, tense or bulging, both at rest and in the upright position. The head circumference increases and the cranial sutures may split.

Normal ICP values

The pressure within the intracranial vault is not constant, it increases in response to activities such as coughing and straining, which initiate Valsalva's manoeuvre and decrease venous drainage. In the absence of intracranial pathology, these elevations are brief and ICP returns to normal in a short period. In an adult normal ICP ranges between

Table 7.6 Cerebral herniation syndromes and their clinical manifestations

Cerebral herniation syndromes	Clinical manifestations
Tentorial herniation (lateral)	
An expanding pathology in one cerebral hemisphere causes the medial edge of the temporal lobe to push through the tentorial notch. If ICP continues to rise, central herniation may occur.	Entrapment of the oculomotor nerve causes pupillary dilation. Level of consciousness (LOC) deteriorates due to pressure on the reticular formation within the midbrain. Contralateral hemiparesis or hemiplegia. If ICP remains untreated alterations in vital signs and respiratory arrest may occur.
Tentorial herniation (central)	
Diffuse swelling of both cerebral hemispheres or a midline lesion causes displacement of the cerebral hemispheres, midbrain and diencephalon through the tentorial notch. Surrounding blood vessels may become stretched, compromising blood supply.	LOC deteriorates due to mechanical distortion of the midbrain and diencephalon. Eye movement is impaired, the pupils are initially small but dilate and fail to respond to light. A contralateral hemiplegia may develop.
Tonsillar herniation	
A consequence of untreated central herniation or an expanding infratentorial lesion. The cerebellar tonsils protrude through the foramen of magnum in response to rising ICP. Upward herniation of the cerebellar tonsils through the tentorial notch may also occur.	Compression of the brainstem by the cerebellum causes a decrease in LOC and respiratory dysfunction due to pressure on the centre for respiration in the medulla. Respiratory arrest will occur without prompt reduction of ICP. Neck stiffness due to meningeal irritation and head tilt may be present.

Data based on Lindsay KW, Bone I, Callander R. *Neurology and neurosurgery illustrated*. Edinburgh: Churchill Livingstone, 1986: 76–78. Hickey JV. *The clinical practice of neurological and neurosurgical nursing*. 3rd ed. Philadelphia: Lippincott, 1992: 262–267.

0 and 10 mmHg and a mean KP > 15 mmHg is considered abnormal. In infants and children these values are considerably lower. Mean values of 2 to 4 mmHg are found in the newborn, rising to 6 to 13 mmHg in the older child.

CEREBRAL HERNIATION SYNDROMES

Cerebral herniation is life threatening and occurs when all compensatory mechanisms have been depleted and ICP continues to increase. During herniation, pressure within a compartment of the cranium causes a part of the brain to protrude through a break in the dura, such as the tentorium cerebelli (the tentorial notch) or a boney opening like the foramen of magnum. The clinical presentation varies according to the location of the pathology and the rate at which intracranial volume and pressure increase.

A wide range of clinical manifestations is possible with each of the herniation syndromes. The clinical presentation herniation syndromes associated with infratentorial lesions is extremely variable and no clear-cut syndromes are present.[8] This herniation syndrome may occur more frequently in children due to the higher incidence of posterior fossa pathology.

CAUSES OF RAISED INTRACRANIAL PRESSURE

The ICP rises when the volume of one of the intracranial components increases. Some of the major causes of raised ICP include the following.

Brain tumour

Brain tumour is the most common solid tumour and the second most common neoplasm found in children. Brain tumours account for approximately 20% of all childhood cancers.[12] The anatomical distribution of paediatric brain tumours differs from the adult population. In children, almost 70% of brain tumours are located infratentorially within the posterior fossa, while a smaller proportion arise from the cerebral hemispheres.

Table 7.7 Common posterior fossa tumours of childhood

Tumour	Location	Clinical Presentation	Diagnosis and Medical Management
Medulloblastoma			
Fast growing and highly malignant, accounts for 20% of all brain neoplasms. The five year survival rate is approximately 50%.[1]	Originates in the cerebellum, extends to the fourth ventricle. Readily seeds into the spinal cord via the CSF pathways. May metastasise to the bone, bone marrow and lymph.	Vomiting, lethargy headache and papilloedema. The ataxia may become so severe that the child is unable to stand or walk without support.	Diagnosis: CT or MRI scanning. Treatment: The child's age, the residual amount of tumour following surgery and the risk of seeding of tumour cells guide decisions about radiotherapy and chemotherapy treatment options.
Cerebellar astrocytoma			
Generally benign and cystic. Carries the best prognosis of any childhood intracranial neoplasm.	Originates in the cerebellum. Tumour growth may cause occlusion of the fourth ventricle.	Headache and vomiting due to the raised ICP. Ataxia, papilloedema and dysmetria are other clinical features.	Primary treatment: complete surgical removal offers a very high cure rate if tumour is well differentiated. Diffuse tumours have a poorer survival rate.
Ependymoma			
The five year survival rate for children with ependymoma is approximately 60%.[1]	Arises within any part of the ventricular system. Occurs twice as frequently in the posterior fossa as in supratentorial areas.[2] Infratentorially, originates within the roof or floor of the fourth ventricle.	Vomiting, headache and unsteadiness of gait. Hydrocephalus due to obstruction of CSF flow. Neck pain and stiffness due to encroachment of the tumour on the upper cervical nerve roots.	Initial treatment: surgical debulking which is rarely curative, followed by craniospinal radiation due to seeding of the tumour in the spinal cord. Chemotherapy can also be offered.

Table 7.7 (*continued*)

Tumour	Location	Clinical Presentation	Diagnosis and Medical Management
Brainstem glioma			
The most common of all brainstem tumours. The clinical course is short and rapid, the overall 5 year survival rate being 20% to 30%.[3]	Classified as diffuse because they rapidly extend throughout the entire brainstem.	Cranial nerve deficits including extraocular muscle paralysis, facial nerve weakness, diplopia, dysphagia and a diminished gag reflex.[3] Ataxia and spastic hemiparesis due to involvement of the corticospinal tracts.	Surgical removal carries a high risk of morbidity due to the many vital functions of the brainstem. A stereotactic biopsy is less dangerous and assists in the selection of treatment options. Radiotherapy is the primary treatment modality.

[1] Anti-Cancer Council of Victoria. *Childhood cancer in Victoria*. Melbourne: Anti-Cancer Council, 1993: 24–31.
[2] Cohen ME, Duffner PK. Neoplastic Diseases. *In:* David RB, ed. *Pediatric neurology for the clinician*, Norwalk, CT: Appleton and Lange, 1992: 358.
[3] Shiminski-Maher T, Abbott R, Wisoff JH, Epstein FJ. Current trends in the management of brainstem tumours in childhood. *J Neurosci Nursing* 1991; 23: 356.

Signs of raised ICP occur early in children with posterior fossa tumours.[13] The posterior fossa itself is a small area and there is little room for an expanding mass. Tumours in this area can increase ICP through compression of neighbouring structures. Hydrocephalus may develop due to obstruction of the 4th ventricle.

This discussion is limited to the most common posterior fossa tumours of childhood — medulloblastoma, cerebellar astrocytoma, ependymoma and brainstem glioma.

Intracranial haematoma

The causes of intracranial haematoma include trauma to the head and haematological diseases such as sickle cell disease, haemophilia and idiopathic thrombocytopenic purpura. The haematoma may have a mass effect which causes brain compression, raised ICP and brain herniation.

An *extradural or epidural haematoma* is a collection of blood in the extradural space. It frequently arises from a blow to the temperoparietal region of the head, which fractures the skull and tears an underlying artery, often the middle meningeal artery. Extradural haematoma may develop following trauma to a venous sinus or vein. Small collections, in the absence of underlying brain compression, may not require surgical evacuation.[14] However, surgical evacuation is essential with larger haematomas to prevent herniation and significant injury to underlying brain tissue.

Subdural haematoma results from tearing of the cerebral veins which occupy the subdural space. The shearing forces which cause formation of the haematoma often disrupt underlying cortical fibres leading to the development of cerebral oedema.[15] Medical management consists of evacuation of the haematoma via a subdural tap or an open craniotomy. These children require close neurological observation and repeat CT scanning due to the tendency for recollection of subdural haematomas.

Intracerebral haematoma is often associated with focal contusion or laceration of the brain and accompanied by diffuse brain oedema. Bleeding occurs within the cerebral hemispheres due to shearing of small perforating blood vessels. In some cases bleeding may be delayed by a period ranging from hours to days. Craniotomy and evacuation of the haematoma is only beneficial in a small number of children.

Head injury

Significant injury to the brain may occur with trauma to the head, but without evidence of gross intracranial haematoma. This type of injury is often called a 'closed head injury'. Direct contusion of the brain frequently occurs at the point of impact and is accompanied by *contre-coup* injury to the opposite side of the brain.

During sudden displacement of the head the brain is contused on the undersurface of the temporal and frontal lobes. This results from contact with the boney prominences at the base of the skull. Head trauma due to shearing forces often causes extensive injury to the white matter of the brain.[15] Secondary brain damage from oedema and hypoxia may be significant.

Cerebral oedema

Cerebral oedema or 'brain swelling' accompanies many neurological conditions, including head injury, brain tumour and CNS infection. Oedema may be focal or diffuse and lead to brain displacement, herniation syndromes and an acute increase in ICP. In some cases, the effects of oedema are more harmful to the child than the primary injury itself. There are 3 major types of cerebral oedema: vasogenic, cytotoxic and interstitial oedema.

Vasogenic oedema may be caused by brain tumour, abscess, haemorrhage, contusion or radiation in a localised area of the brain.[16] There is disruption of the blood — brain barrier which performs a protective function by controlling the movement of substances from the general extracellular fluid of the body into the extracellular fluid of the brain.[1] Vascular permeability is altered and plasma filtrate and water accumulate in the extracellular space around the area of injury. Vasogenic oedema may be treated with osmotic agents such as mannitol.

Cytotoxic oedema may develop following a cerebral hypoxic episode. Failure of the intracellular sodium pump produces accumulation of water and sodium within the cell and shrinking of the extracellular space. There is no pharmacological agent effective in the treatment of this type of oedema.

Interstitial oedema is caused by leakage of CSF into the extracellular space of brain tissue. It occurs in the presence of hydrocephalus.

Hydrocephalus

Hydrocephalus is an increase in cerebrospinal fluid volume associated with ventricular dilatation and elevation of the intraventricular pressure. Hydrocephalus occurs when there is an imbalance between the formation and absorption of CSF. Impaired absorption is almost always due to an obstruction of the CSF pathways.[17] Overproduction of CSF is rare, but does occur in the presence of a tumour of the choroid plexus, the CSF secreting cells of the ventricles.

Communicating hydrocephalus	Non communicating hydrocephalus
1 Arachnoid granulations, where CSF is absorbed into the blood stream are blocked by protein, blood or bacteria. *A shunt system will be required if multiple lumbar taps do not stabilise the condition.*	**4** Cerebral aqueduct obstruction often results from a congenital anomaly but may complicate infection, haemorrhage or tumour. *The treatment consists of a shunt system or endoscopic fenestration of the third ventricle.*

2 Post meningitic, inflammation leads to adhesions which impair CSF circulation in the subarachnoid space. *A shunt system will be required unless the condition becomes stable.*

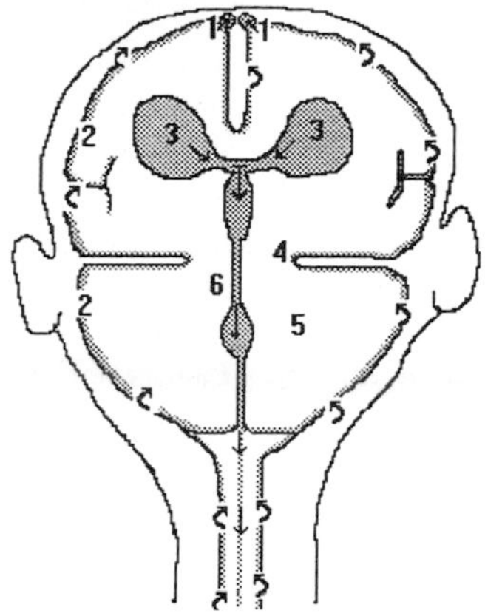

Arrows show CSF flow
Numbers show site of pathologies described in surrounding table | **5** Dandy Walker syndrome is a congenital condition where, usually, the foramina of Magendie and Lushka are absent and the fourth ventricle becomes a large cyst and blocks the overall CSF flow. *A shunt will be required either from the cyst, the lateral ventricle or both.* |

Communicating hydrocephalus	Non communicating hydrocephalus
3 A choroid plexus papilloma increases CSF production which exceeds absorption. *The total surgical removal of the tumour is likely to correct the hydrocephalus.*	**6** A midline tumour, particularly of the posterior fossa region may obstruct CSF flow and cause hydrocephalus above the site of obstruction. *Surgical removal of the tumour restrores the CSF pathways in most instances*

Figure 7.14 Diagram showing the types of hydrocephalus and the treatment options.

Treatment of hydrocephalus

Insertion of a ventriculoperitoneal shunt is the most common treatment for hydrocephalus. The shunt consists of a silastic catheter with a valve. One end of the shunt is positioned in a lateral ventricle via a Burr hole incision. The other end of the shunt is tunnelled under the skin and placed in the peritoneal cavity within the abdomen where CSF absorption occurs.[17]

The neurosurgeon will select a shunt according to the age of the child and the type of hydrocephalus. The most commonly used shunts are:

- Low-pressure valve: the valve offers little resistance to CSF flow.
- Medium-pressure valve: the valve offers medium resistance to CSF flow.
- High-pressure valve: the valve offers a greater resistance to CSF flow.
- Flow valve: a regulated flow (20 mL/hour) circulates through the shunt regardless of the child's position.
- Variable-pressure valve: a magnet or computer can change the gradient of the pressure to suit the child's needs after the shunt has been inserted.

Table 7.8 Postoperative nursing care of the child with a ventriculoperitoneal shunt

Nursing problem and actions	Rationale
Potential for alteration in neurological observations:	
Monitor the child's level of consciousness, vital signs, head circumference, anterior fontanelle. Observe for fever, neck stiffness and photophobia.	Shunt blockage, cerebral haemorrhage, infection, CSF leak, and overdrainage or underdrainage of CSF may occur.
Check the wound dressing and skin integrity over the valve site.	The very thin skin of neonates may breakdown if pressure is applied over the valve site.
Potential for inadequate nutritional intake:	
Oral intake resumes when bowel sounds have returned.	A paralytic ileus may occur.
Potential alteration in comfort:	
Assess the child's behaviour, vital signs and pain score hourly, consult with parents, administer relevant analgesia.	Pain is not ethically acceptable. The child in pain may be irritable.
Level of mobility:	
The level of mobilisation is determined by the neurosurgeon, but must be gradual. The child must be monitored for headache, dizziness, colour and tone and the anterior fontanelle should be palpated.	The brain tolerates gradual changes. However, rapid ventricular over-drainage can lead to brain collapse. This sudden collapse causes enlargement of the subdural space. Subdural haematoma may develop due to stretching of cerebral vessels within the subdural space.
A pale, floppy baby with a markedly depressed anterior fontanelle needs to return to the supine position. A child complaining of a low pressure headache or dizziness must sit up slowly.	
Inadequate functioning of shunt:	
Continue neurological observations.	
Infant — observe for full fontanelles, poor feeding, irritability, vomiting, and a continual increase in the head circumference.	The shunt may be blocked. Underdrainage of the ventricles may occur. Overdrainage may have caused formation of a subdural haematoma.
Child — observe for irritability, headache, drowsiness, loss of upward gaze, nausea or vomiting. The child feels better sitting up.	

Pressure-regulated shunts drain more CSF when the child is in the upright position because gravity induces a syphon effect. A high-pressure valve would not be inserted into an infant as the soft skull offers less resistance than the shunt itself. In this instance, rather than CSF flowing through the shunt the head would continue to expand to accommodate the increasing CSF volume. Shunt selection affects the postoperative management of the infant or child with hydrocephalus, therefore the nurse must know which type of device has been used. Signs of overdrainage, underdrainage or shunt blockage must be reported to the medical staff.

The most common complication following insertion of a ventriculoperitoneal shunt is blockage or infection of the shunt. The signs and symptoms of hydrocephalus and shunt blockage are as follows.

- *Infant*: Impaired conscious level; vomiting and/or poor feeding; impaired upward gaze, 'sun setting' eyes; tense anterior fontanelle; widening cranial sutures; increase in head circumference — the child's curve is growing out of the birth head circumference percentile; irritability; lid retraction; thin scalp and dilated veins; 'cracked pot' sound on head percussion; and high pitch cry.
- *Child*: headache; vomiting; papilloedema; change in level of consciousness; visual changes; behavioral changes — irritability, poor concentration, tiredness; and squeaky voice.

The valve or reservoir of a normally functioning shunt is easily depressed and refills rapidly. CSF flows to the peritoneal cavity when the valve is depressed and CSF is aspirated from the ventricles when the valve is released. A valve which is hard to depress is suggestive of a blockage at the peritoneal end of the shunt. A valve which fails to refill after it has been depressed indicates an obstruction at the ventricular end of the catheter. Shunts may be blocked by the choroid plexus or accumulated debris within the ventricles. It has also been suggested that constipation may intermittently impair drainage of CSF from the shunt.[18]

Discharge education for the child with a shunt

The quality of the discharge education is paramount to the safety of the child with a shunt. The signs and symptoms of failure of the shunt system must be thoroughly explained to the parents, child, maternal health nurse, paediatrician and general practitioner. When parents and children present to the emergency department, they must be listened to carefully because their subjective observations may have clinical relevance. Children have been known to state: 'My shunt feels blocked'. A parent's observation that their child 'is not himself' should not be ignored. However, it is also common for parents to underestimate the signs of a blocked shunt or to have mistaken gastroenteritis or viral illness for a shunt problem.

Hydrocephalus is a condition which can be successfully treated and by itself does not lead to mental retardation. However, the outcome is less satisfactory if structural brain anomalies are associated with the hydrocephalus and complications such as shunt obstruction and infection are inadequately treated.

Central nervous system infection

Bacterial or viral infection of the brain or meninges increases ICP by causing cerebral oedema, obstructing the flow and reabsorption of CSF and impairing venous outflow.[19] For a full discussion of the management of the child with central nervous system infection, see Chapter 5.

Vascular malformations

An *arteriovenous malformation* (AVM) consists of a tightly tangled collection of dilated blood vessels which shunt arterial blood directly into venous channels without the usual connecting capillary network.[8] AVMs occur within the cerebral hemispheres, brainstem or spinal cord. The child with an AVM may present with acute intracranial haemorrhage, either subarachnoid or intracerebral, although seizures are the more common presenting sign.[20] Neurological signs vary with the size and location of the AVM. Angiography provides a definitive diagnosis of an AVM while CT scanning is used in the event of intracranial haemorrhage.

A cerebral *aneurysm is* a balloon-like structure which arises from a weakness in the wall of an artery. Aneurysms commonly occur at the bifurcation of major arteries at the base of the brain. Rupture and subsequent subarachnoid haemorrhage is rare before 10 years of age.[19] Haemorrhage is confirmed by lumbar puncture and angiography reveals the size and location of the aneurysm. Treatment consists of surgical clipping, excision or embolisation.

Near drowning

Near-drowning is a major cause of mortality and morbidity in children. The neurological complications that accompany near-drowning are related to the duration of the submersion, the temperature of the water and the time that elapses before cardiopulmonary resuscitation is commenced. Irreversible neurological damage due to cerebral hypoxia and ischaemia[21] may occur if the period of submersion extends beyond a couple of minutes. For a full discussion of the management of the child following near-drowning, see **Chapter 12**.

Reye's syndrome

Reye's syndrome is characterised by toxic encephalopathy with hepatic dysfunction. Clinically, the child presents with protracted vomiting, fever, impaired liver function, lethargy, and agitation proceeding to coma with raised ICP.[22] ICP increases due to the presence of cerebral oedema. While the exact aetiology of the condition is unknown, it often develops following viral infection of the influenza or varicella virus. In recent years, an association between aspirin administration and Reye's syndrome has been established.[23] For a full discussion of the management of the child with Reye's syndrome, see **Chapter 5**.

Shaking injuries

In the infant, intracranial haemorrhage and raised ICP may arise following non-accidental injury such as violent shaking. While there may be an absence of external trauma, the shaking causes significant acceleration–deceleration injury to the infant's brain. The term acceleration-deceleration injury refers to injury due to rapid increases and decreases in the velocity of the brain within the cranial vault. Cerebral oedema and haemorrhage in the subarachnoid space, cerebral cortex and retinal and preretinal areas may be present on CT scan, along with evidence of previous contusion. Child abuse must always be suspected when the history does not concur with the clinical findings.

NEURODIAGNOSTIC PROCEDURES

Cranial ultrasound, computed tomography and magnetic resonance imaging allow direct visualisation of the brain. They are indicated in the child with raised ICP, enlarging head circumference, progressive focal neurologic signs, coma of uncertain aetiology, vascular malformation, intracranial haemorrhage or a mass lesion.[24]

General preparation

Adequate preparation of the child and family is central to the success of all neurodiagnostic procedures. While many of these procedures are non-invasive, the equipment itself may be frightening and accurate visualisation of the brain is only achieved when the child remains still. Planning, answering questions and visual aids may promote cooperation and remove the need for sedation in school-aged children and adolescents. These children should be aware of some of the devices (e.g., chin or cheek pads) which may be used to immobilise the head during the procedure. Sedation or general anaesthesia is required in infants or developmentally impaired children. Parents should be encouraged to remain with their child.

Cranial ultrasound

Cranial ultrasound is an imaging technique performed through the open anterior fontanelle of an infant using a hand-held transducer head. The technique is only useful up until about 12 months of age, when the anterior fontanelle closes. Ultrasound is frequently used to screen premature infants for ventricular dilatation and intraventricular haemorrhage. It is also sensitive to congenital anomalies of the central nervous system.[24]

Cranial ultrasound has a number of advantages. The equipment is small and portable, allowing the procedure to be carried out at the bedside of a critically ill infant. Cranial ultrasound does not use ionising radiation, therefore serial scans may be safely performed to follow the course of the intracranial pathology. Because the transducer head is handheld it is easily manipulated according to the infant's position. Sedation is rarely needed and repositioning of the infant may not be necessary.

Computed tomography (CT)

CT scanning is based on the premise that tissues of different densities absorb varying degrees of radiation. The child lies motionless on a table while images are taken at 1° intervals via a circular frame which surrounds the head. CT scanning is often the first choice for imaging of the brain in trauma and emergency settings.

A contrast medium may be used to improve the clarity of the images obtained. This is administered by intravenous injection and carries the risk of allergic reaction. The child may be required to fast for 4 to 8 hours. Both the nurse and the parents should know that some patients experience a feeling of warmth, transient headache, a salty taste in the mouth or nausea or vomiting during injection of the contrast medium. If appropriate, the parents may inform their child of these side effects. After the procedure, adequate hydration is essential to promote excretion of the contrast medium.

Magnetic resonance imaging (MRI)

MRI detects both structural and biochemical abnormalities of the brain and spinal cord. Images may be obtained from multiple angles, providing clearer visualisation of the brainstem and posterior foss structures than has been possible with other imaging techniques. MRI is a useful diagnostic tool in the evaluation of degenerative disorders of the central nervous system.

During the procedure, the child lies on a bed within a long cylindrical magnet that looks like a tunnel. High-frequency radio waves are delivered in precise bursts to the child and absorbed by atomic nuclei which in turn generate their own weaker radio frequency signal. These signals from the body's nuclei are processed and a video image is produced on a monitor.

It is difficult to reach the child or monitor cardiorespiratory function during the procedure. A thumping noise may be created as the radio waves cross the magnetic field. The child should be informed of this as it may be distressing and delay the procedure. Ear plugs may be used to reduce this noise. The child must be capable or remaining still for an extended period of time. Images are obtained in repetitive sequences, therefore movement affects the entire sequence. Unlike CT scanning, individual slices cannot be repeated. For this reason general anaesthesia is necessary in the infant, developmentally impaired or claustrophobic child. Fear may be decreased by having the child imagining that the MRI system is a spaceship.

The strong magnetic field created during an MRI scan may cause movement of implanted metallic objects. For this reason, MRI is contraindicated in patients with pacemakers, valve prostheses, internal surgical clips, bullet fragments or orthopaedic pins. All jewellery and metal objects must be removed prior to the procedure.

Cerebral angiography

Cerebral angiography allows visualisation of the intracranial and extracranial blood vessels. A catheter is inserted into the femoral artery and guided to the point of origin of the carotid and vertebral systems under x-ray control. A contrast medium is injected via the catheter and films are taken of the cerebral circulation. Angiography may be used to define the blood supply to a cerebral tumour, to make a differential diagnosis between an aneurysm or tumour or if haemorrhage into a tumour bed is suspected.

SIGNS OF RAISED INTRACRANIAL PRESSURE

Level of consciousness

A decreased response to procedures that are normally frightening or painful to a child is abnormal and may be indicative of an alteration in level of consciousness.[25] The child with raised ICP may be drowsy when woken and sleep constantly, even while venepuncture is performed. On the other hand, some children are extremely placid and never complain. This underscores the need for constant evaluation of behaviour in relation to the child's normal response pattern. Lethargy, lack of interest and poor feeding habits can also be related to a change in level of consciousness.

Anterior fontanelle

Bulging fontanelles are a normal sign in a crying, distressed infant but they may also be an early sign of cerebral pathology and raised ICP. The normal fontanelle is clearly demarcated from the bone edges, falls below the surface, and pulsates under the examining finger.[19] The fontanelle that bulges above the level of the bone edges and is tense such that it is difficult to determine where bone ends and fontanelle begins is abnormal and indicates raised ICP.[19] In the infant with raised ICP, the scalp veins are distended and the eyes deviate downward giving the 'sunset eye' appearance. In the presence of a slow-growing pathology, the cranial sutures may separate to accommodate the increasing volume and maintain ICP within normal limits. In this instance, these sutures may be palpable.

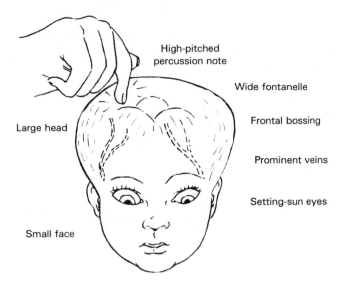

High-pitched percussion note

Wide fontanelle

Large head

Frontal bossing

Prominent veins

Setting-sun eyes

Small face

Figure 7.15 Child with enlarged head.

Head circumference

An increase in head circumference may be a clinical sign of raised ICP in the child under 3 years of age. Regular measurements of head circumference are performed and evaluated in the context of other clinical signs and the child's growth percentile.

Vomiting

Vomiting due to raised ICP is typically worse in the morning and unrelated to meals. Vomiting on awakening is explained by the mild hypercapnia which develops during sleep and increases cerebral blood flow and ICP. This is part of a normal physiological event secondary to hypoventilation during sleep. In addition, cerebral blood flow and ICP increase during periods of REM sleep. These events may be poorly tolerated in the child with cerebral pathology and elevated ICP.

Papilloedema

Papilloedema is oedema of the optic nerve or disc. It is caused by impaired venous drainage from the cranial vault and identified by examining the child's optic disc using an ophthalmoscope. This examination may be difficult to complete because children must remain still while a bright light is flashed in their eyes. If the child is given a general anaesthetic for a neurodiagnostic procedure, the examination may be more easily performed at that time.

Ophthalmoplegia

Ophthalmoplegia is impairment of eye movement. It results from damage to the muscle itself or to the cranial nerve nuclei (III, IV or VI) in the brainstem which control eye movement. Paralysis of these cranial nerves often develops in the presence of raised ICP.

Loss of upward gaze occurs with lesions of the upper part of the brainstem. Paralysis of the 6th cranial nerve, the abducens nerve, may cause diplopia and strabismus. Compression of the 3rd cranial nerve, the oculomotor nerve, produces pupil dilation, a decreased response to light stimulus and a *ptosis*, drooping of the eyelid. *Proptosis* or exopthalmos consists of abnormal protrusion of the eyeball and may occur when ICP is raised.

Behaviour

In both the infant and child, subtle changes in behaviour may be an indicator of neurological dysfunction. All behaviour is evaluated in the context of the child's normal behaviour pattern and routine. Involvement of the parent is essential in this process. *Irritability* is a common finding in a child that is tired, hungry or overstimulated. However, excessive irritability which does not subside with parental comforting is a common and non-specific sign of cardiopulmonary or neurologic dysfunction.[25]

Vital signs

The *Cushing reflex* consists of a triad of physiological responses which attempt to preserve the blood supply to the brain during an acute rise in ICP. The systolic blood pressure rises to maintain cerebral perfusion pressure and causes a widening of the pulse pressure, the difference between the systolic and diastolic blood pressure. Bradycardia and a decrease in respiratory rate are secondary to ischaemia of the vasomotor centre within the brainstem. This ischaemia results from downward displacement of the brain against the brainstem. The Cushing reflex is a late sign of raised ICP and may be absent in certain pathologies. This response may occur more frequently in children due to the increased incidence of posterior fossa pathology.

Cry

Crying is normal for an infant or child, but the nurse and parent should observe for changes in the quality of the cry which accompany raised ICP. The child with raised ICP and cranial nerve dysfunction due to infratentorial pathology often presents with a very weak cry. It may be that it is the parent that detects a different crying sound from their child. A high-pitched cry is often present in infants with raised ICP.

Pain

Headache that wakes a child from sleep or occurs on rising in the morning is suggestive of intracranial pathology. Supratentorial lesions produce pain in the frontotemporal region while posterior fossa lesions cause pain in the occiput and neck. Coughing, sneezing and straining initiate Valsalva's manoeuvre and may exacerbate the pain. Valsalva's manoeuvre occurs when the child exhales through a closed epiglottis. Children often lack knowledge of pain and therefore are unable to recognise or talk about it.

FACTORS THAT INCREASE ICP

A thorough knowledge of factors that are known to influence ICP is essential in caring for the child with a neurological disorder.

Carbon dioxide is a powerful dilator of cerebral blood vessels. During periods of *hypercapnia*, vasodilation occurs, raising ICP by increasing cerebral blood flow and blood volume. In the child with a neurological condition, the causes of CO_2 retention include hypoventilation, sputum retention, aspiration and pneumonia. The child with a weak cough, gag or swallow reflex and an impaired conscious state has a high risk of developing these complications. Pallor and sweatiness are clinical signs of hypercapnia and may appear despite normal oxymetry readings.

Suctioning increases ICP by increasing CO_2, decreasing O_2 and stimulating the cough reflex. Coughing increases intra-abdominal and intrathoracic pressure and impedes venous drainage from the brain. These factors combine to increase ICP. The child with raised ICP may be suctioned regularly but for short periods. This ensures that ICP rapidly returns to normal and avoids sustained periods of elevated ICP. While suctioning has an adverse effect on ICP, aggressive airway clearance is necessary to promote effective gas exchange and prevent respiratory complications.

Valsalva's manoeuvre occurs when the child exhales against a closed epiglottis. The child may perform this manoeuvre unknowingly while straining at stool, using a bedpan and sneezing. This may be avoided by having the child breath out during these activities.

Positive end expiratory pressure (PEEP) may be delivered at the end of the respiratory cycle to prevent atelectasis in the ventilated child. This is used cautiously in the child with raised ICP because PEEP causes an increase in intrathoracic pressure, central venous pressure and ICP. An Ambu bag may be used to increase pO_2 before suctioning in the unventilated child. Improper use of this device produces a physiological response similar to that described with PEEP. This occurs when delivery of oxygen from the Ambu bag is not synchronised with the child's respiratory cycle.

There are a number of *body positions* which adversely affect ICP. Because venous drainage from the cranial vault is facilitated by gravity, flexion of the neck may impede venous return from the brain and increase cerebral blood volume and ICP. Similarly, Trendelenburg's position is rarely used without medical orders because of the dependent position of the head and the risk of increasing cerebral oedema.

ASSESSMENT OF THE CHILD WITH RAISED ICP

Assessment skills are crucial in the management of a child with raised ICP. Failure to identify and report an early change in neurological observations may delay intervention essential in preventing cerebral ischaemia and permanent neurological deficit.

The neurological assessment of preverbal children and infants presents a special challenge. In this group, the parameters of normal behaviour vary with age and responses must be evaluated with a knowledge of normal growth and development. Playing is a very effective way of assessing the child.

History

The history given by the parent or primary caregiver provides baseline information regarding the child's normal pattern of behaviour. The child's level of motor and language development; sleeping, eating and elimination patterns; reactions to separation; likes, dislikes and daily routine should be documented. Documentation is vital for the purposes of comparison should the child's neurological signs change.

It is important that the mechanism of injury is established and evaluated in the context of the child's level of physical and motor development. Brain injury may have an accidental or non-accidental cause. The parent of an unconscious child should be asked about any recent falls or injuries. The nurse should also check for contact with or ingestion of neurotoxic substances or chemicals. If this information is not available from the child

Table 7.9 The Modified Glasgow Coma Scale

Eyes open	4		Spontaneous
	3		To speech
	2		To pain
	1		None
Best verbal response	5		Orientated
	4	*Words*	Confused
	3	*Vocal sounds*	Inappropriate
under 4 years	2	*Cries*	Vocal sounds
	1	*None*	None
Best motor response	6		Obey commands
	5		Localises to pain
	4		Withdrawal
	3		Abnormal flexion
	2		Extension
	1		None
Total score			

or parent, the nurse initiates contact with the child's school. The child's peers may be a valuable source of information, recent sickness among other children may aid clinical diagnosis. The child is also examined for insect or animal bites. These aspects of the history are particularly important because they may provide information which explains the child's neurological status.

Level of consciousness

Consciousness relates to the child's level of wakefulness and awareness and the degree to which he or she can interact with and interpret the environment in an age-appropriate manner.[26] Consciousness cannot be measured directly, but is estimated by evaluating behavioral responses to the environment and other types of stimuli. The tool most widely used in the assessment of level of consciousness is the Glasgow Coma Scale.

The Glasgow Coma Scale

The Glasgow Coma Scale (GCS) was first developed for the assessment of level of consciousness in adult patients following head injury.[27] The scale has been modified by the Adelaide Children's Hospital and the chart reproduced below is now used in many Australian paediatric centres.

The GCS uses 3 parameters to assess level of consciousness: eye opening, motor response and verbal response. Many hospitals use a standardised chart to plot responses graphically. This chart provides a visual record of any deterioration, improvement or stabilisation in the child's neurological observations. Numerical values may be assigned to each response.

Eye opening

The child is observed for *spontaneous* eye opening. If the child's eyes are not open at the start of the examination, *speech* may be used to wake the child, or gentle touch in the infant. *Pain* is only applied if the infant or child does not open its eyes in response to verbal and tactile stimulation.

The painful stimulus may consist of a gentle pinch on the infant's calf or the application of pressure to the child's nail bed or supraorbital ridge. If pressure to one side of the body does not illicit a response the opposite side should be checked. Painful stimuli must be used consistently among staff to ensure that assessment results are accurate.

Verbal response

Assessment of verbal response can be difficult in all children, irrespective of age. Parental involvement is often helpful in gaining the child's cooperation. Verbal response must be assessed with a knowledge of normal speech and language development.

The child 4 years or older: An orientated child that has a developmental age of 4 years or more should be able to answer questions such as: 'Where are you? How old are you? Are you at home? Are you at school? Is it night or is it before breakfast? Is she a doctor or is it Mum? What is the name of your teddy?' The questions should assess orientation to time, place and person. Questions which can be answered with a yes or no response may be more appropriate if the child is shy or does not answer in a full sentence. However, caution must be used with this approach to ensure that the child is giving an accurate response.

A confused child may not know where she is or give an inaccurate response. The verbal response is inappropriate if the child gives an answer which is unrelated to the question. Vocal sounds may consist of moans and groans or attempts at vocalisation which cannot be understood. The 'none' box is charted if the child gives no verbal response.

Verbal response is evaluated with a knowledge of the child's normal activities, including favourite toys, family pets, friends, and even an invisible friend. A nurse may feel that a child is confused when the child is talking about an invisible friend or the family pet.

The child under 4 years: produces recognisable words but does not give correct answers to questions. This is a normal response between 1 and 4 years of age. The presence of vocal sounds, such as 'DaDa' and 'MaMa' is normal for an infant between 6 and 12 months of age. In the first 6 months, the infant cries but does not produce recognisable words. The 'nil' box is charted if the infant neither cries nor makes sounds.

Motor response

This part of the assessment tool focuses on the child's ability to perform a simple motor task. The best response is recorded. Actual limb strength is addressed at a later stage in the assessment.

The child 4 years or older may be asked to perform a simple, purposeful movement such as: 'lift up your arms,' 'clap your hands' or 'pop your tongue out'. The child is charted as *obeying commands* if the motor response is appropriate. The infant should be observed for the ability to reach out for toys or objects. The ability to perform reflexive activities such as squeezing a hand is an inappropriate gauge of motor response and level of consciousness. Such a response is integrated at spinal cord level.

Pain is only applied when there is no motor response to verbal stimulus. A *localising* response occurs when the child moves its limb toward the source of the painful stimulus. If supraorbital pressure was applied, the child's arm would come up towards its forehead. A *withdrawal* response consists of the child moving the limb laterally, away from the source of the pain. *Abnormal flexion* is flexion of the arms towards the chest. *Extension*

Table 7.10 Normal coma scale scores

Age	Eyes open	Verbal response	Motor Response	Total
0–6 months	4	2–3	4	10–11
6–12 months	4	3	5	12
1–2 years	4	4	5	13
2–4 years	4	4–5	6	14–15
>4 years	4	5	6	15

manifests as extension of the arms and rotation of the wrists. A painful stimulus should never be used in the conscious child with motor dysfunction secondary to a spinal cord lesion.

The most accurate response is often obtained by playing with the infant or child. There are a number of factors which may affect the child's response during the assessment process. They include fear, a new environment, unfamiliar voices and anxiety around strangers. The child's cooperation may be gained by having the primary caregiver present during the assessment. Neurological assessment also includes evaluation of motor function and pupillary response.

Motor function

Impaired motor function in the infant or child presents as a decrease in spontaneous limb movement, failure to achieve milestones or regression from previously established behaviours. The term *hemiparesis* is applied to a motor weakness that is confined to one side of the body. *Hemiplegia* implies total loss of motor function in one side of the body. A lesion within a motor area of the left hemisphere of the brain produces motor dysfunction in the right side of the body. This is explained by the crossing over or decussation of all descending motor fibres in the medulla of the brainstem.

The tools used to assess motor function in many paediatric centres remain subjective, however, a number of points are worthy of discussion. It is important that left and right sided motor function are compared. This allows the examiner to differentiate between a generalised motor weakness and a hemiparesis. The findings should always be compared with those of the previous health worker responsible for the child's care, particularly at the end of each shift. If differences are found both staff should reassess the child. An established deterioration in motor function should be promptly reported to the child's physician.

A cooperative child may be asked to lift the leg and hold it for the count of 10. The child counts to create consistency in the technique. An infant can be observed while crawling. Ataxia, incoordination of voluntary movement, is a common feature in children with posterior fossa pathology. The ability to walk is impaired and safety is often an issue because these children do not understand that their level of activity should be restricted.

The child with impaired motor function may develop abnormal posturing. *Decorticate* rigidity and posturing presents as flexion of the fingers, wrists and elbows with extension of the legs and ankles and plantar flexion of the feet. It is an outcome of extensive ischaemia of the cerebral hemispheres. The child with *decerebrate* rigidity and posturing extends the elbows, legs and ankles. This is due to diffuse metabolic injury to the cerebral hemispheres or ischaemia to the diencephalon, midbrain and pons.

The child may show these postures in response to painful stimulus. Decorticate rigidity, of the 2 postures, represents a higher level of reflexive functioning. A change from decorticate to decerebrate posturing in the acute phase of injury should be reported. It may indicate that the child's neurological status has deteriorated. In both of these postures the child's body will be very rigid and difficult to move.

Babinski's reflex may be used as a tool in the assessment of motor function in the infant or child. A positive reflex consists of flexion of the great toe and fanning of the other toes when the sole of the foot is stroked. This response is normal in an infant before walking is established. In other children it is abnormal and may be symptomatic of damage to the motor pathways of the brain and spinal cord.

Eye observations

Normally, the pupils are round, equal in size and constrict briskly in the presence of light. This constriction occurs when the 3rd cranial nerve, the oculomotor nerve, is intact. The appearance of a difference in pupil size and a sluggish response to light indicates entrapment of the 3rd cranial nerve and rising ICP. This finding should be reported to the physician immediately.

The eyes should be assessed from a direct, midline position. Both eyes are assessed in equivalent conditions with windows and lights midline rather than towards one side. The child is observed for impairment of eye movement, which may signal a cranial nerve palsy.

MEDICAL MANAGEMENT OF RAISED ICP

The medical management of the child with raised ICP aims at supporting and preserving brain function by: identifying and removing underlying causes; supporting all body systems; preventing secondary complications; and maintaining ICP within normal limits. A number of treatment modalities will be reviewed in this section. The medical management is individualised according to the child's condition and the physiological data that are available.

Airway management and control of respiration

Adequate oxygenation is essential in the child with raised ICP. Intubation may be indicated to maintain a patent airway in the following circumstances: impaired airway clearance due to compromised protective reflexes (e.g., cough and gag); hypoventilation or breathing irregularities; shock, pulmonary failure and raised ICP itself.[7,25] Oral, rather than nasal, intubation is performed in the child who has sustained head trauma, until a fractured base of skull has been excluded. A nasally inserted endotracheal (or nasogastric) tube may travel into the cranial cavity via a break in the dura resulting from this specific fracture.

Mechanical ventilation facilitates adequate oxygenation and prevention of hypercarbia. Hyperventilation is the most rapid and effective method of reducing ICP.[28] In the ventilated child, this is achieved by increasing the rate of respiration and maintaining a constant tidal volume. Excessive volumes are avoided because they increase intrathoracic pressure and adversely affect ICP. The pO_2 is maintained above 90 mmHg and the pCO_2 between 25 and 30 mmHg.[7] This reduction in carbon dioxide decreases ICP through vasoconstriction of the cerebral arteries and a decrease in cerebral blood flow and intracranial volume. Arterial blood gases are monitored frequently to assess oxygen saturation and the adequacy of ventilation.

In the unventilated child, hyperventilation may be carried out using an Ambu bag. The bag is connected to a tracheostomy or endotracheal tube or a face mask placed over the child's face.

Maintenance of circulation

Hypovolaemia and hypotension must be corrected due to their potentially adverse effect on cerebral perfusion. The blood pressure must be kept sufficiently high so that cerebral perfusion is maintained and ischaemia is avoided. However, severe hypertension may aggravate cerebral oedema in injured cerebral tissue where the blood — brain barrier has been destroyed.[28]

Drug therapy for raised ICP

Osmotic diuretics and corticosteroids are 2 groups of drugs which may be included in the treatment plan for a child with raised ICP.

Osmotic diuretics

Mannitol is the osmotic diuretic used most widely in Australian settings in the management of raised ICP. Mannitol does not cross the blood — brain barrier. After intravenous administration, the plasma becomes hypertonic in relation to the extracellular fluid. This creates an osmotic gradient that draws water away from the cerebral extracellular space into the plasma. Mannitol may rapidly reduce ICP in emergency situations when herniation is occurring or pending.

Mannitol is administered using a filter due to possible crystallisation of the drug in the giving set. Dosage is titrated according to the child's ICP, cerebral perfusion pressure and serum osmolality. The onset of action is within 20 to 60 minutes and the peak effect is observed 1 to 3 hours following administration. The side effects of mannitol therapy include dehydration and hypokalaemia. For these reasons, a urinary catheter is inserted and a strict fluid balance chart maintained. Mannitol is contraindicated in hypovolaemic shock, congestive cardiac failure, dehydration and kidney disease.

Corticosteroids

Corticosteroids have an established role in the management of oedema associated with cerebral tumours, but their use in other instances of raised ICP remains controversial. Dexamethasone is the mainstay of corticosteroid therapy. It must be withdrawn slowly due to the risk of adrenal insufficiency. Side effects include gastric irritation and a rise in the serum glucose level.

Fluid management

Cerebral oedema is a common consequence of central nervous system pathology. Fluid intake may be restricted to half or three-quarters of the child's daily requirements so that a state of controlled dehydration exists. This promotes a decrease in extracellular fluid and ICP. It is imperative that the child's serum electrolyte levels, osmolality and blood pressure are closely monitored.

Sedation and paralysis

Neuromuscular paralysis facilitates control of ventilation and prevents increases in ICP due to coughing, straining, and 'bucking' the ventilator, which increase intrathoracic and venous pressure and ICP.[28] 'Bucking' occurs when the child is unable to breathe synchronously with the ventilator. Evaluation of neuromuscular function is not possible in the paralysed child, therefore pupil observations, EEG and ICP recordings, and diagnostic tools such as CT scans are used to monitor the child's neurological status. The drug of choice in most clinical settings is pancuronium.

Sedation and analgesia are used to decrease fear, anxiety and pain and promote an optimal level of comfort for the child during invasive and painful procedures. The ideal sedative has minimal side effects and a short duration of action or is easily reversed to permit accurate evaluation of the child's neurological status.[28] Barbiturates, benzodiazepines and narcotics are the drugs in current use. It should be noted that only narcotics have an analgesic effect.

Temperature control

Because the cerebral metabolic rate increases with temperature, hyperthermia should be controlled in the child with raised ICP. This may be achieved through the appropriate use of antipyretic agents. Shivering must be avoided due to its adverse effect on ICP.

Seizure control

The cerebral metabolic rate also increases during seizures, thereby raising the brain's oxygen demands. During this time cerebral blood flow and ICP are also increased. Phenytoin is the drug of choice for the initial management or prophylaxis of seizures. A loading dose may be administered intravenously, followed by a regular regimen.

Drainage of cerebrospinal fluid

Drainage of CSF may reduce increased ICP secondary to obstruction of the CSF pathways. This is achieved by inserting a catheter through a hole in the skull into the lateral ventricle or, in some instances, through an open anterior fontanelle in emergency and life-threatening situations. It is a temporary measure that carries a significant risk of infection.

Surgery

Surgery may be indicated in the presence of a mass lesion such as a cerebral tumour, abscess or haematoma.

Barbiturate coma

Barbiturate coma remains a controversial treatment modality in the management of the child with raised ICP. Cerebral metabolism decreases during barbiturate administration. This parallels a decrease in cerebral blood flow and blood volume and ICP.

MONITORING OF ICP

Intracranial pressure monitoring techniques allow for measurement and control of ICP before clinical deterioration and irreversible brain damage occur. The effects of nursing care and therapy on ICP are quantified so that activities are planned and sustained increases in ICP are avoided. In some cases, a child may be monitored to establish or confirm a diagnosis of raised intracranial pressure.

General nursing considerations

Each of the invasive methods described below carries a significant risk of infection, therefore stringent nursing measures are required. Extreme care must be exercised when repositioning a child with an ICP monitoring device in place. The child may be sedated to reduce the risk of pulling on the monitoring device. Restraints should be avoided as ICP is increased in an agitated and fighting child. Tension of the tubing may cause movement of the monitoring device and trauma to the underlying brain tissue or dislodgement. Pulling or stretching the cable from the transducer may cause inaccurate readings of ICP.

The following invasive monitoring techniques are currently in use.

Ventricular catheterisation

Ventricular catheterisation involves the insertion of an intraventricular catheter into one of the lateral ventricles. A direct measurement of ICP is obtained by connecting the catheter to pressure tubing and a transducer, which provides a reading of ICP. Sampling and drainage of CSF are possible and a major advantage of this technique. The risks associated with ventricular catheterisation include infection, clogging of the catheter or tubing, haemorrhage as the tube penetrates the cerebral cortex, and ventricular collapse if CSF drains too rapidly. The child should be monitored for infection and leakage of CSF around the insertion site.

Subarachnoid bolt or screw

The subarachnoid bolt or screw is placed near the subarachnoid space via a burr hole in the skull. The dura is penetrated but the arachnoid is left intact and the subarachnoid space is not entered. This technique does not allow for sampling or drainage of CSF to reduce ICP and also carries the risk of infection.

Extradural sensor

The extradural sensor consists of a fibreoptic sensor which is placed between the skull and the dura. Sampling or drainage of CSF is not possible, but the risk of infection is reduced. An advantage of this technique is that the agitated child may be disconnected from the monitoring equipment and allowed to play for a period. The leads are rolled and secured safely with a head bandage. The monitor may be reconnected for sleep recording.

NURSING MANAGEMENT OF THE CHILD WITH RAISED ICP

The child's neurological condition dictates the frequency of neurological observations. Observations may be performed every 15 minutes in the child who is unstable or in the immediate postoperative period. Observation of the child with a neurological condition occurs not only when the scheduled observations are due, but whenever the nurse interacts with the child. Subtle changes in the child's motor function may be observed during bathing or play periods or reported by the parents. Changes in neurological status may occur over a period of time; therefore astute observation skills are central to the management of the child with raised ICP. All observations are carefully documented so that trends may be identified.

The child with a compromised gag and swallow reflex requires careful positioning and chest physiotherapy to prevent aspiration and respiratory complications. The child is placed laterally with the head in a neutral position. This position prevents the tongue from obstructing the airway and aspiration should vomiting occur. It also facilitates drainage of saliva. The head of the bed is elevated and the child is positioned in an upright position for meals. Close nursing supervision is essential during this time to prevent aspiration. Thickened fluids and a pureed diet are easier for the child with a swallowing difficulty.

The unconscious child is repositioned at regular intervals to prevent pressure sores. The skin is examined for redness and broken areas during bathing and each time the child is moved. The head of the bed is maintained at 30° to facilitate venous drainage. The child with a neurological condition may have poor control of their head position. The head must be fully supported at all times and caution must be used, especially during transfers.

Activities which initiate Valsalva's manoeuvre and are known to affect ICP are avoided. This includes constipation and straining, which adversely affect ICP by increasing intra-abdominal and cerebral venous pressure. The unconscious and immobile child is especially at risk of constipation. Bowel function is monitored and documented each day. Codeine is avoided due to its effect on bowel motility. Stool softeners may be administered, but high-volume enemas are avoided because they increase intra-abdominal pressure.

Nursing activities are spaced to permit regular rest periods and the child is approached in a calm manner. Clustering of nursing activities may cause sharp increases in ICP. Sedatives are used cautiously in the child with raised ICP due to their depressant effect on level of consciousness and respiratory function.

Oxygen administration is guided by regular determination of pulse oxymetry and arterial blood gas analysis. Oxygenation is performed both before and after suctioning. Blowing bubbles may reduce a high CO_2 level in the child with raised ICP.

Table 7.11 Nursing care plan for the child with raised intracranial pressure

Nursing problem and actions	Rationale
Hypoventilation and airway obstruction	
Causes: depressed level of consciousness; weak or absent cough, gag or swallow reflex; sputum retention.	
Assess respiratory pattern, rate and depth; breath sounds and oxymetry.	Indicates airway is patent, lung expansion is present and oxygen saturation.
Place the child laterally in a neutral position. The head of the bed or the entire bed may be elevated.	Prevents aspiration and the tongue obstructing the airway, allows drainage of respiratory secretions.
Administer oxygen therapy with humidification as ordered	Prevents hypoxaemia and drying of respiratory secretions.
Suction pharynx and nasopharynx as required, for no longer than 10 seconds. Suctioning must be gentle to avoid damaging the very soft tissue of infants and children.	Maintains a patent airway, prevents chest infection and promotes gas exchange.

Table 7.11 (*continued*)

Nursing problem and actions	Rationale
Monitor saturation during suctioning, if not maintained, use bagging before and after with short periods of suctioning.	Oxygenate to prevent hypoxaemia and increases in ICP.
Reposition child regularly, encourage deep breathing and coughing.	Prevents pooling and mobilises secretions.
Monitor arterial blood gases and pulse oximetry.	Indicates effectiveness of ventilation.

Potential for alteration in neurological status

Assess an document baseline neurological observations: level of consciousness, pupillary size and response, eye observations, motor function. Perform serial observations and compare with previous findings.	Neurological observations are an indicator of improvement or deterioration in neurological status.
Assess vital signs and compare with previous findings.	A change in vital signs may occur with a deterioration in neurological status.
Assess temperature with vital signs.	A high temperature increases the cerebral metabolic rate and oxygen consumption. Shivering should be prevented.

Potential for increase in intracranial pressure

Elevate head of bed 30°.	Increases venous drainage, reduces cerebral oedema and ICP.
Avoid head and neck flexion and extreme hip flexion.	Impedes venous drainage, increases intrathoracic and intra-abdominal pressure and ICP.
Encourage the child to exhale during movements which may initiate Valsalva's manoeuvre.	This manoeuvre increases ICP.
Maintain fluid restriction which includes intravenous fluids and fluid balance chart. Monitor electrolytes, urine output and blood pressure.	Restricting fluids decreases extracellular fluid and ICP. The child is monitored for signs of dehydration, hypovolaemia and diabetes insipidus.
Monitor bowel elimination.	Constipation and straining increases intra-abdominal pressure and ICP.
Plan rest periods and avoid clustering of nursing activities.	Clustering of activities may have a cumulative effect, causing sharp increases in ICP.

REFERENCES

1. Nolte J. *The human brain. An introduction to its functional anatomy.* 2nd ed. St Louis: Mosby, 1988: 34.
2. Carpenter MB. *Core text of neuroanatomy* 4th ed. Baltimore: Williams & Wilkins, 1991: 1–22.
3. Snell RS. *Clinical neuroanatomy for medical students.* 2nd ed. Boston: Little Brown, 1987: 491.
4. Swaiman K. *Pediatric neurology: principles & practice.* 2nd ed. St Louis: Mosby, 1994: 123.

5. Ropper AH, Rockoff MA. Physiology and clinical aspects of raised intracranial pressure. *In:* Ropper AH, ed. *Neurological and neurosurgical intensive care.* 3rd ed. New York: Raven Press, 1993: 11–27.
6. Cole GF. Acute encephalopathy of childhood. *In:* Brett EM, ed. *Paediatric neurology.* 2nd ed. London: Churchill Livingstone, 1991: 667–699.
7. Yatsiv I. Central nervous system support techniques. *In:* Holbrook PR, ed. *Textbook of pediatric critical care.* Philadelphia: Saunders, 1993: 170–175.
8. Hickey JV. *The clinical practice of neurological and neurosurgical nursing.* 3rd ed. Philadelphia: Lippincott, 1992: 249–287.
9. Martins AN, Wiley JK, Myers PW. Dynamics of the cerebrospinal fluid and the spinal dura mater. *J Neurol Neurosurg Psychiatry* 1972; 35: 468–473.
10. Langfitt TW. Increased intracranial pressure. *Clin Neurosurg* 1969; 1: 436–471.
11. Minns RA. Intercranial pressure monitoring. *Arch Dis Child* 1984; 59: 486–488.
12. Anti-Cancer Council of Victoria. *Childhood cancer in Victoria.* Melbourne: Anti-Cancer Council of Victoria, 1993: 24.
13. Cohen ME, Duffner PK. Neoplastic diseases. *In:* David RB, ed. *Pediatric neurology for the clinician.* Norwalk, CT: Appleton and Lange, 1992: 385–406.
14. James HE. Head trauma. *In:* Holbrook PR, ed. *Textbook of pediatric critical care.* Philadelphia: Saunders 1993: 205.
15. Hutchison HT. Traumatic encephalopathies. *In:* David RB, ed. *Pediatric neurology for the clinician.* Norwalk, CT: Appleton and Lange, 1992: 169–184.
16. Speers I. Cerebral edema. *J Neurosurg Nursing* 1981; 13: 102–113.
17. Klug G. The child with a large head. *In:* Robinson MJ, Roberton DM. eds. *Practical paediatrics.* Melbourne: Churchill Livingstone, 1994: 475.
18. Bragg C, Edwards-Beckett J, Eckle N, Principle K, Terry D. Shunt dysfunction and constipation: could there be a link?. *J Neurosci Nursing* 1994: 26: 91–94.
19. Fenichel GM. *Clinical pediatric neurology. A signs and symptoms approach.* Philadelphia: Saunders, 1993: 89–114.
20. Golden GS. Cerebrovascular disease. *In:* Swaiman K, ed. *Pediatric neurology. Principles and practice.* St Louis: Mosby, 1989: 787–803.
21. Fields AI, Holbrook PR. Near-drowning in the pediatric population. *In:* Shoemaker W, Ayres S, Grenvik A, Holbrook PR, Thompson WL, eds. *Textbook of critical care.* Philadelphia: Saunders, 1989; 67–69.
22. Breningstall GN. Diseases of ammonia metabolism. *In:* Swaiman K, ed. *Pediatric neurology. Principles and practice.* 4th ed. St Louis: Mosby, 1994: 1233–1242.
23. Barrett MJ, Hurwitz ES, Schonberger LB, Rogers MF. Changing epidemiology of Reye syndrome in the United States. *Pediatrics* 1986; 79. 598 602.
24. Filipek PA, Blickman JG. Neuroimaging techniques. *In:* David RB, ed. *Pediatric neurology for the clinician.* Norwalk, CT: Appleton and Lange, 1992: 134–150.
25. Hazinski MF. *Nursing care of the critically ill child.* 2nd ed. St Louis: Mosby Year Book, 1992: 521–628.
26. Lower J. Rapid neuro assessment. *Am J Nursing* 1992; 92 (6): 38–45.
27. Teasdale G, Jennett B. Assessment of coma and impaired consciousness. Lancet 1974; 2: 81.
28. Ropper AH. Treatment of intracranial hypertension. *In:* Ropper AH, ed. *Neurological and neurosurgical intensive care.* New York: Raven Press, 1993: 29–52.
29. Wong DL. *Whaley and Wong's nursing care of infants and children.* 5th ed. St Louis: Mosby Year Book, 1995.

BIBLIOGRAPHY

Goodman LR, Putman CE. *Critical care imaging.* Philadelphia: Saunders, 1992.
Pallett PJ, O'Brien MT. *Textbook of neurological nursing.* Boston: Little Brown, 1985.

Raimond J, Taylor JW. *Neurological emergencies — effective nursing care.* Rockville: Aspen, 1986.

Shiminski-Maher T. Brain tumors in childhood: implications for nursing practice. *J Pediatr Health Care* 1990; 4: 122–130.

Wagner MB. Neurologic emergencies in the young. Part 1. Evaluation and stabilisation. *Emergency Med* 1992; 24: 204–224.

Diabetes Mellitus

Katrina Brereton, K. Meei Chen, Helen Dickinson, Paul Longridge, Jane Lush, and Mary Perisanidis-Douros

The word diabetes comes from the Greek and means siphon or excessive flow of urine. Mellitus is derived from Latin and means honey. Diabetes mellitus is a condition where there is an excessive amount of sugar (glucose) in the bloodstream and urine.

Diabetes has been attributed to various factors. In children it is most commonly due to a lack of the hormone insulin. This type of diabetes is known as insulin-dependent diabetes mellitus (IDDM) or type I diabetes.

Diabetes may also result when there is either insufficient quantity of insulin present in the body or when it is unable to be utilised by the body. In this situation the binding process of insulin to the receptor is impaired.

Mature-onset diabetes of youth (MODY) is hyperglycaemia diagnosed before the age of 25, which remains treatable for at least 5 years without insulin in patients who do not show immune or human leucocyte antigen (HLA) markers of IDDM. MODY is usually inherited as an autosomal dominant gene.

CAUSES OF DIABETES MELLITUS

In a person with diabetes mellitus (Type I) the pancreas fails to secrete insulin because the beta cells in the islet of Langerhans have been destroyed by the autoimmune system. The exact aetiology of this destruction is still unclear, but it is known that individuals can be genetically predisposed to diabetes mellitus type I and that environmental factors such as viruses seem to trigger the onset. The destructive autoimmune response can actually be triggered months before diabetic symptoms present themselves (Warne G. RCH, Melbourne. Personal communication, 1990).

Statistics

Approximately 1 out of every 1000 children has diabetes. At the Royal Children's Hospital in Melbourne, newly diagnosed children with diabetes are admitted at a rate of 2 per week and the current clinic population exceeds 800. Only one of these 800 is not insulin dependent. The vast majority of children with diabetes has classic type I, or insulin dependent diabetes, caused by destruction of the beta cells of the islets of Langerhans. The 2 peak ages of onset are 5 and 12 years and 50% of all type I diabetes is diagnosed before the age of 20 (Warne G. RCH, Melbourne. Personal communication, 1992).

Table 7.12 Types of diabetes

Type	Also known as	Usual treatment
Diabetes mellitus Type I	Insulin dependent diabetes mellitus or juvenile diabetes	Subcutaneous synthetic insulin injection given daily or twice daily in conjunction with exchange diet.
Diabetes mellitus Type II	Non-insulin dependent diabetes mellitus or mature onset diabetes	Normally controlled by oral hypoglycaemic preparations in conjunction with sugar-free diet. If condition becomes unstable, regular insulin injections may be commenced.
MODY	Mature onset diabetes of youth	Initially controlled with oral hypoglycaemic agents, progressing to regular insulin injections as blood sugar levels become more difficult to control.

DIAGNOSIS

The diagnosis of diabetes mellitus (type I) is confirmed by:

- The clinical manifestations.
- A random blood glucose estimation (capillary or venous) which shows abnormal elevation.
- Preprandial and postprandial blood glucose levels, which are compared with a fasting blood glucose which displays abnormal elevation when taken 2 hours after a large carbohydrate meal.

The HbA1C test is an additional test which can be performed when the diagnosis needs to be substantiated, or a known diabetic child's glucose level control is uncertain. In the bloodstream, glucose circulates and attaches to haemoglobin and other proteins. Over several weeks the glucose accumulates, becoming fixed to the haemoglobin. The HbA1C test measures the percentage of glucose which has attached to the haemoglobin. The more elevated the blood glucose level has been, the more glucose will have attached to the haemoglobin. A diabetic child with poor control will therefore have an elevated HbA1C. The aim of the test is to indicate how long the child has had an elevated blood glucose level, and to estimate the control of diabetes over the previous 1 to 3 months.

CLINICAL ASSESSMENT

The classic signs of diabetes are: hyperglycaemia; glycosuria; ketonuria; polydipsia; polyuria; polyphagia, which may be followed by anorexia; weight loss; and lethargy.

Some children will be well on admission to hospital and others will present in diabetic ketoacidosis of varying severity. Many children who are diagnosed with diabetes may have already presented to their local general practitioner with the common classic signs of diabetes.

A child with diabetes mellitus admitted to hospital for management has the potential to developing ketoacidosis or may already be in ketoacidosis, thus it is imperative the child is assessed appropriately by the admitting nurse.

The nurse will be aware that if ketoacidosis is present and not accurately assessed and promptly treated, diabetic coma can result. It is important for the nurse to understand the pathophysiology of both diabetes mellitus and ketoacidosis, thus gaining a clear understanding of why specific clinical manifestations result. The nurse will maintain consultation with medical staff, frequently recording and reporting the child's progress.

The nurse instigates a comprehensive nursing assessment. A complete clinical assessment of the child is made and an accurate and informative nursing history is ascertained from the patient, if old enough and well enough, or from the parents or guardian.

A comprehensive nursing assessment enables the nurse to establish priorities of care and implement the nursing care accordingly. Vital signs and neurological observations are necessary, especially when a child is in diabetic ketoacidosis, to establish a baseline for ongoing assessment. A detailed nursing history will identify the areas of care required during the initial management, when stabilisation of the blood glucose level will be the focus, and ongoing care, with needs such as diabetic education. As the nurse is the health care team member who will spend the most time with the child, he or she has a very important role. Specific responsibilities of other members of the health care team are shown in **Table 7.13**.

CLINICAL MANIFESTATIONS OF KETOACIDOSIS

It must be noted that not every child will exhibit all the clinical manifestations of diabetes mellitus. If a child is diagnosed early and appropriate management is implemented, ketoacidosis should be prevented. In this case, the child will only display the classic signs of diabetes. If ketoacidosis develops, the following clinical manifestations will result.

Head

Metabolic acidosis and the accompanying hyperglycaemia results in dehydration, which alters electrolyte balance and mental status, resulting in drowsiness, lethargy, disorientation and coma. These changes in physiology also cause the child to feel listless and suffer headaches.

In infants, the nurse may find through palpating the head that the fontanelles are depressed. This change is the result of dehydration. It must be remembered that infants and children can become dehydrated rapidly, so their hydration status needs to be assessed immediately, reported and acted on quickly. It is important to note that dehydration has many causes, which include the inability to tolerate fluid orally because of nausea, vomiting; extracellular and intracellular changes relating to electrolyte imbalance; polyuria; and water lost through laboured breathing.

Eyes

Metabolic acidosis results in electrolyte disequilibrium, which causes blurred vision and a glassy-eyed appearance. The nurse may note that the pupils are equally dilated, but with depressed reflexes. This is a result of acidosis and poor hydration and may lead to the eyeballs becoming sunken and soft.

Mouth

On examination of the child's mouth, the nurse will often observe dry, cracked lips, dry mucous membranes and a white-coated tongue which is furry in appearance. These signs relate to the child being unable to tolerate oral fluids.

Table 7.13 Specific responsibilities for each member of the medical and allied health team in the management of a child or adolescent with diabetes mellitus

Consultant	A consultancy position where the RMO and registrar can seek advice in regard to individual diabetic care and control in patients. Responsible for ensuring families have a clear understanding of hypoglycaemia.
Medical registrar and resident doctor	Provide continued medical supervision during patient stay in hospital, authorise appropriate medical treatment.
Community health nurse or community specialist	Offer school visits for all diabetic schoolchildren in order to provide some community awareness and acceptance of diabetes in the child's normal environment. Demonstrate blood glucose monitoring and the importance of doing so. Provide example of various types of blood glucose machines so that patients and their families can choose one which best suits their needs. Act as a liaison between hospital, outpatient clinic and home for families who have a child with diabetes mellitus.
Dietitian	Explain fully the exchange diet (15 grams carbohydrate = 1 exchange). Educate family on the various food groups and help work out dietary programs suitable for each patient and family. Provide sample menus.
Social worker	Act as a intermediary for patients and their parents to express their fears and worries. Arrange financial assistance where necessary. Help to organise accommodation for out-of-town families while their child remains an inpatient.
Play therapist	Will help to understand diabetes and deal with their frustrations through play. Many diabetic children have been able to deal with their emotions about diabetes through medical play, ie giving dolls insulin injections and finger pricks.
Outpatient clinic	Provide ongoing care through the diabetes clinic. Ensure regular review of insulin doses, exchange diet and blood glucose levels. Opportunity for HbA1C tests to be carried out. Also opportunity for patients and families to see dietitian or ancillary staff.

Chest

The human body has an in-built buffering system which attempts to eliminate excessive carbon dioxide in the bloodstream related to acidosis.

The child's respiration rate and depth will be altered as the body attempts to blow off through respiratory effort the excess carbon dioxide and ketone bodies in order to regain equilibrium. This type of respiration pattern is known as Kussmaul breathing. Kussmaul breathing can be identified by characteristics such as deep but rapid breathing with sighing sounds.

Ketotic (acetone) breath is another result of acidosis. Excess ketone bodies are excreted from the lungs, thus the child's breath is tainted with the smell of ketones.

Abdomen

Initially, the body cells and tissues are unable to obtain the necessary energy for daily activities, so the child feels tired, hungry and lethargic. In an effort to gain some energy the child frequently consumes large amounts of food. The body still remains depleted of energy as there is no insulin to make the cell membranes permeable to glucose. The body tries to compensate and breaks down fat and protein, which causes weight loss but again, because of the body's lack of insulin, these cannot be used as energy sources.

As more glucose and ketones accumulate in the bloodstream, the child feels very unwell and becomes anorexic. Anorexia also results from the nausea and vomiting the child may experience.

The child often has abdominal pain which is generalised in nature. The abdomen is tender on palpation. The exact cause of these symptoms is unknown, but is thought to be related to hyperglycaemia, acidosis, dehydration and anorexia.

Nausea and vomiting accompany the above signs and symptoms. Again the cause is not established, but thought to be related to electrolyte imbalances as a result of acidosis. A later sign which may appear from dehydration and anorexia is constipation.

Skin

If dehydrated, the child will have dry skin and poor skin turgor. A subnormal body temperature may also be noted. This is related to hypotension and shock. When this sign is present, the child is very sick and requires immediate expert assessment and appropriate medical treatment.

The child may have muscular aches. Such a symptom arises from dehydration, which in turn results in haemoconcentration. A decrease in blood circulating volume occurs which leads to tissue anoxia. The body then produces excess lactic acid, which accumulates in the tissues causing aching and fatigued muscles.

Endocrine

Hyperglycaemia results from an accumulation of excess glucose in the bloodstream. This leads to dehydration as high levels of glucose exert an osmotic effect which pulls cellular water into the bloodstream.

Renal

One of the first clinical manifestations to be noted occurs when a urine sample from the child is tested. The urine is positive for both glucose and ketones, definitive signs of ketoacidosis.

Glycosuria occurs when the serum level of glucose exceeds the renal threshold and glucose spills over into the urine. Glycosuria contributes to extracellular dehydration because glucose has a strong osmotic effect which prevents the kidney tubules from re-absorbing water.

Ketones are by-products of fat oxidation and metabolism and accumulate in the bloodstream. When oxidation of fat occurs at an abnormal rate, the body attempts to regain equilibrium by trying to rid itself of these ketone bodies and excretes them in the urine.

The body attempts to excrete both glucose and ketones by diuresis (polyuria), which in turn causes excessive thirst (polydipsia) and if not compensated will result in dehydration. It is often noted when testing a child's urine sample that the specific gravity is high. This is because the urine contains glucose and ketones.

Genitourinary

Vaginitis and penile irritation are related to hyperglycaemia, which changes the body's pH level. An overgrowth of *Candida albicans* can follow.

Circulatory

Metabolic acidosis is related to a lowered blood pH level, which is a result of the cumulative effects of ketones and subsequent electrolyte disequilibrium. Hypotension results from dehydration. The severity of this clinical sign is related to the degree of dehydration.

If a child is vomiting, unable to tolerate oral fluids and has polydipsia, the electrolyte balance is compromised. The body's compensatory mechanism is to increase the pulse rate as the circulatory blood volume decreases. Such circulatory problems can lead to peripheral shutdown.

Cerebral oedema is a controversial issue. Many factors are cited as the cause. It must be noted that cerebral oedema is life threatening as it may lead rapidly to brain herniation.

In conclusion, it is extremely important to assess the patient thoroughly, as the baseline assessment will enable medical and nursing staff to give appropriate ongoing care. A child with diabetes mellitus or in ketoacidosis cannot regain equilibrium unless assessed and reassessed frequently to identify actual and potential nursing and medical problems as they arise.

NURSING MANAGEMENT

Nursing diagnosis

Actual or potential fluid volume deficit, related to acidotic state and osmotic diuresis.

Nursing intervention

Monitor vital signs half-hourly, and observe for decreasing skin turgor and a deterioration in hydration status. Perform neurological observations half-hourly and report any abnormalities immediately. Maintain a strict fluid balance chart.

Test all urine for ketones until urine is free of ketones. Continue to test for glucose when blood sugar readings are above 15 mmol/L. Monitor blood glucose every 2 hours in order to evaluate the effect of insulin therapy.

If the child is vomiting then nil orally is instigated. If tolerating fluids, small frequent amounts of carbohydrate-free fluids are given. Assist, if necessary, with blood sample collection for acid base, urea and electrolyte levels. Ensure that appropriate changes to fluids are made according to blood test results.

Nursing diagnosis

Potential alteration in conscious state related to dehydration and electrolyte imbalance.

Nursing intervention

Monitor vital signs and neurological signs half-hourly. Report immediately an alteration in orientation, conscious state, motor response, pupillary reaction or headache. Ensure oral airway, suction and oxygen equipment is available.

Nursing diagnosis

Potential for hypoglycaemia related to insulin infusion.

Nursing intervention

Test blood glucose levels every 2 hours. Report any increase or decrease. Observe child for symptoms of hypoglycaemia such as pallor, restlessness, shakiness, lethargy and headache. If the blood glucose level drops below 5 mmol/L, treat symptoms and report to medical staff. If intravenous therapy is *in situ*, a reduction in the amount of infused insulin and an alteration in the intravenous rate is needed.

Nursing diagnosis

Altered dietary requirements for the toddler with diabetes.

Nursing intervention

Consult with the dietitian and arrange for the provision of an adequate exchange diet (1 exchange equals 15 g carbohydrate). Allow flexibility with exchanges. Allow flexibility in the timing of meals. Plan a daily routine that follows the one at home and encourage family to participate during meal times.

Nursing diagnosis

Anxiety of the child, parents and family related to admission to hospital and diagnosis of diabetes mellitus. Knowledge deficit related to management of the diabetic child.

Nursing intervention

Arrange suitable times for nursing staff to talk with family about various aspects of diabetic care. Provide suitable learning material such as pamphlets, videos and encourage the family to familiarise themselves with the information. Ensure patient and family have the opportunity to discuss any issues relating to diabetes of which they are unsure. Reinforce good techniques in diabetic management by demonstrating and encouraging participation during the patient's stay in hospital.

PATHOPHYSIOLOGY

In a healthy child the hormone insulin is released from the pancreas to aid the digestion of carbohydrates and, in addition, it plays a role in protein and fat metabolism. The pancreas is a salmon-coloured, soft, lobular, leaf-shaped organ, which will eventually weigh 60 to 120 g and have a length approximately 24 cm and a width of 15 cm. It is situated just below the stomach.

The pancreas produces 2 main hormones, insulin and glucagon. Insulin is secreted from the beta cells in the islets of Langerhans, which is located in the body and tail of the pancreas and makes up nearly 2% of the pancreatic tissue. Insulin travels through the bloodstream and binds to the receptors located in the membrane wall of individual cells in order to facilitate the transfer of glucose into the intracellular space. Glucagon is secreted by the alpha cells in the islets of Langerhans and is released in response to low blood glucose levels or stimulation by growth hormone. Its function is to increase the blood glucose level by stimulating glycogenesis in the liver.[1]

When food is eaten and digested by the stomach it moves through the duodenum into the small intestine (jejunum and ileum) where the carbohydrate is broken down into glucose, which is absorbed into the bloodstream. The higher levels of glucose in the bloodstream stimulate the pancreas to secrete insulin, which enables the glucose to be transferred to muscle cells and other tissue cells in order to provide energy. Insulin also accelerates the conversion of glucose to glycogen to be stored in the liver. In a healthy infant or child, the insulin maintains a blood glucose level between 1.0 mmol/L and 8 mmol/L.

In a person with type I diabetes, carbohydrates are broken down in the normal manner and absorbed as glucose into the bloodstream, but the pancreas fails to secrete insulin in response to high bloodstream glucose levels. When this abnormality occurs, the body responds in 2 main ways: the blood glucose level continues to rise; the body looks for other sources of energy for its cells. In order to maintain its state of equilibrium, the body tries to flush the excess glucose out through the kidneys in the urine and therefore glycosuria develops. An osmotic diuresis occurs as a result of the glycosuria and therefore results in polyuria. The polyuria stimulates thirst, leading to polydipsia. These effects are characteristic clinical findings.[2]

In response to the cells' demand for energy, protein is rapidly metabolised into amino acids which are then liberated into the bloodstream. On reaching the liver the amino acids are converted into urea and glucose. As a consequence of protein metabolism, blood glucose levels rise even higher. At the same time fats are broken down into glycerol and fatty acids to be used as energy by cells. Glycerol converts to glucose and follows the glucose path. When fatty acids are catabolised, ketone bodies are released as a byproduct. Ketone bodies are mainly acids and must be buffered by the body to maintain a stable pH level. If too many ketones accumulate in the blood, the buffers are unable to cope and blood pH falls, leading to metabolic acidosis.[2]

Ketoacidosis

Diabetic ketoacidosis is an acute complication of hyperglycaemia, which may initially occur in the patient with undiagnosed type I diabetes or may occur as a complication. Precipitating factors such as illness, infection, stress or non-compliance with insulin doses, diet and general care, may also lead to ketoacidosis.

Hypoglycaemia

To counteract the lack of insulin in a child with diabetes mellitus type I, synthetic insulin is injected subcutaneously to meet the body's needs. (Note: insulin preparations cannot be taken orally as they are destroyed by gastric juices in the stomach.)

Synthetic insulin cannot mimic the response of natural insulin perfectly. It is essential, therefore, to distribute the carbohydrate intake evenly throughout the day to offset the action of the synthetic insulin. If an imbalance in carbohydrate and insulin levels occurs, hyperglycaemia or hypoglycaemia will result. In hypoglycaemia the insulin level is in excess relative to the carbohydrate level. Low blood sugar levels will result. Hypoglycaemia is the result of too much insulin, too little food or too much exercise without extra carbohydrate intake.

In response to lowered blood sugar levels the body's cells break down fatty and amino acids into adenosine triphosphate (ATP) for energy. (Note: the brain cells cannot use ATP for energy, therefore mild cerebral disfunction occurs which can show itself as symptoms including headaches, dizziness and restlessness. Early glucose deprivation of brain cells also stimulates the autonomic nervous system and produces symptoms such as hunger, tachycardia, pallor, sweatiness and tremors.)

Unless carbohydrate is given, the body's compensatory mechanisms will fail, resulting in cerebral hypoxia, cerebral oedema, coma and death.

Each child will experience individual signs and symptoms when blood sugar levels are lowered and learn to identify them quickly.

Somogyi phenomenon

The Somogyi phenomenon is characterised by swings of blood glucose levels which result from the administration of more insulin than is needed. Severe hypoglycaemia occurs followed by a rebound hyperglycaemia. Treatment is the reduction of insulin dose.

EDUCATIONAL NEEDS OF CHILDREN, PARENTS AND FAMILIES

The initial aim of a diabetic teaching program is to inform each child and family of the different aspects of diabetes mellitus within a period of 5 to 7 days, thus allowing them to return to the community with confidence and a thorough understanding of diabetes mellitus.

Each family is treated individually, in that they have their own special needs and these needs are accommodated in a flexible teaching program. Generally, teaching begins the 2nd day after admission to hospital. This provides the family with some time to accept the diagnosis and prepare for the future. If the teaching program were to commence immediately after admission, the family may have difficulties concentrating on new information, a state not conducive to learning.

A teaching program has no restrictions as to who is educated on the aspects of diabetes. Grandparents, babysitters and neighbours are encouraged to attend teaching sessions, in order that care by these extended family members and friends can continue.

An education program which consists of daily teaching with an introduction about diabetes mellitus using a simple format and incorporating a short slide presentation has been found to be successful. A short overview of the areas of diabetic care to be covered during the teaching sessions is also included. The introduction is designed so that the family is gradually introduced to the latest information about a disease of which they may have little knowledge.

Preparation and administration of insulin

The goal of teaching is for the family and child (if old enough) to understand the need for insulin treatment, the action of insulin and be able to prepare and inject insulin.[3]

During teaching, nursing staff provide explanations and answers to questions such as:

- What is insulin?
- What happens to the body when insulin does not work?
- How is insulin replaced?
- Where does insulin come from?
- Why is an oral insulin preparation not possible?
- What are the types of insulin available?
- Which types of insulin are being used for the child's management?

Parents and family members are then taught how to administer insulin by way of a step-by-step demonstration. They are taught about mixing insulins, air pressure within the vials, correct insulin temperature and the removal of air bubbles from the syringe before injecting.

Additional diagrams are provided to indicate where the insulin is injected and its effect over a 24-hour period.

What is insulin?

Insulin is a hormone produced in the pancreas and ensures that carbohydrates that have been digested by the stomach can be turned into energy in the body's cells.

What happens to the body when insulin does not work?

If the insulin does not work, carbohydrate (or glucose) that has been digested by the stomach builds up in the bloodstream, raising the blood sugar level. The body will attempt to get rid of the extra glucose by flushing it out via the kidneys, which results in glycosuria (sugar in the urine). At the same time the body's cells become starved of the glucose needed to make energy and function efficiently. Tiredness, weight loss and increased appetite become apparent.

How is insulin replaced and where does it come from?

The insulin is replaced by regular measured dose injections once or twice a day. Until fairly recently the insulin was obtained from animals — mainly cows and pigs — but now synthetic insulin can be produced which more closely resembles human insulin.

Why is an oral preparation not possible?

At present an oral insulin preparation is not possible because it is destroyed by the gastric juices in the stomach before it can be absorbed into the bloodstream to be used by the body.

What types of insulin are available?

There are many different trade names for insulin but basically there are three types of insulin: short-acting insulin; intermediate acting insulin; and long-acting insulin. There are also single bottles which have a premixed combinations of short and long-acting insulin.

Honeymoon phase

It is common for some newly diagnosed diabetic children to go through a period of time where the pancreas attempts to produce insulin again. This is known as the honeymoon phase. When this occurs, the need for exogenous (synthetic) insulin is reduced. Usually, this period is only temporary and children will require an increasing dose of insulin as they become older.

Blood glucose monitoring

The goal of this teaching is for the family to become familiar with the many types of blood glucose monitors in order to select one appropriate to their child's needs and to learn how to use and care for the machine chosen.

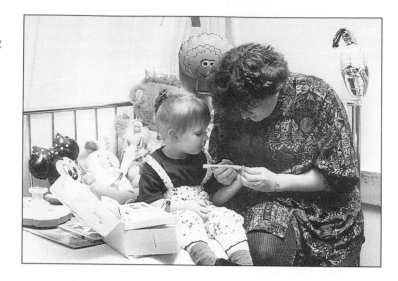

Parents are taught the techniques for blood sugar level monitoring.

Nursing staff provide various different models of glucometers for parents and their children to look at, handle and try out. All the machines vary slightly, so it is important that the family understand the differences. For example, a family with a young child may find it difficult to get their child to place the drop of blood needed onto the test strip when the strip is already in the glucometer. On the other hand the family with a teenager who usually self-tests may have no problem with this and will prefer a machine of this type, which has the advantage of being more compact, and reading the blood glucose level in only 20 seconds. All machines available in Australia comply with high standards and all should be accurate provided they are cleaned and checked regularly.

The families are also instructed on how to load and use an autolet and a pen-type pricking device; while the pen type devices are more popular, each family must have the option to choose the device most suited to their child's needs.

The areas on the fingers most suited to obtain blood are demonstrated and ways of obtaining a good-sized drop of blood are discussed. With tips such as 'ensuring the fingers are warm before pricking' and 'holding the fingers down lower than the child' and a little practice, the family usually have no difficulty in obtaining the required specimen.

Care of the fingers and appropriate areas in each finger to be used for specimen collection are discussed. It is recommended that the child use the top outer aspect of each side of the finger and rotate sites to include all fingers and each thumb in an effort to reduce callused finger tips.

Injection site and rotation

The goal of teaching is for the family to learn the locations of injection sites and the importance of site rotation.[3]

Nursing staff demonstrate injection sites with teaching aids, such as diagrams and a doll with the sites indicated. Injection sites are also shown to parents on their own child. It is recommended that the same site be used for one whole week and a different site is used each week. This strategy ensures each site has minimal chance of developing lipodystrophy.

*Parents are taught
how to administer
insulin.*

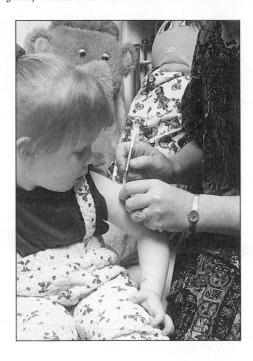

Lipodystrophy

Lipodystrophy is a reversible change in the amount of fat between the skin and the muscle. Atrophy, seen as pulling the skin or hypertrophy, where lumps or bumps in the skin appear are the result of lipodystrophy. Hypertrophy is the more common of the two. Lipodystrophy can be avoided by changing injection sites on a weekly basis and by keeping insulin at room temperature.

Urine testing

The goal of teaching is for the family to develop a clear understanding of the rationale and technique of urine testing.[3]

The family are taught that urine testing is important and should be undertaken at particular times: at least once a month for ketones, as a preventative measure; when the blood glucose level is above 15 mmol/L; and when the child is feeling unwell, irrespective of blood glucose level.

If ketones are present in the urine, the family is encouraged to contact the doctor as adjustments may need to be made to the insulin dose, in order to prevent ketoacidosis. The family is taught what ketones are, why they occur and their relationship to ketoacidosis. The technique of urine testing is taught stressing that good light and accurate timing of the dipstick will provide a true reading.

Record keeping

The goal of teaching is to provide the family with the skills needed to keep a clear and accurate record of daily blood glucose levels and treatment.[3]

The family is provided with a diabetic record booklet which will enable them to show the degree of control achieved, assist when making decisions about daily insulin doses and provide useful information for the doctor. They are taught how to record blood glucose levels numerically and to graph them. Daily insulin doses are also recorded by showing the amount of long-acting insulin first and the short-acting insulin second. Explanation of the insulin reactions of hypoglycaemia and hyperglycaemia are also provided, as are the reasons why they occur.

The parents are encouraged to document clearly and record the results of urine tests for ketones.

Daily living and management

The goal of this teaching is for the family to be able to deal appropriately with common management concerns of diabetes.

The family is given the opportunity to vent any fears or anxieties about previous teaching and discuss any issues that may have arisen throughout their admission to hospital. These are dealt with appropriately so that the family is able to leave hospital with confidence and a thorough understanding of diabetes.

Reinforcement of all teaching is included to enable the family to have an acceptable understanding of the relationships between blood glucose monitoring, insulin injections, diet and meal times by:

- stating the time at which blood glucose monitoring and insulin injections are required;
- explaining the ideal time delay between insulin injections and eating meals; and
- verbally planning a day's schedule.

Instructions are given to the family regarding the need for appropriate care and management of their equipment at home by explaining the following.

- The need for proper storage arrangements for insulin and suggesting possibilities such as a container in the fridge or a cool dark cupboard out of reach of young children.
- The importance of checking for contaminants.
- Describing suitable storage arrangements for blood and urine testing strips, possibly a bathroom cupboard.
- That it is safe to use a syringe twice and monolets up to 9 times providing that they have not been touched by anything other than the child's cleaned skin.
- When and why there is a need to check expiry dates on insulin, urine test strips and blood test strips.
- Finally, an explanation is given on the safety aspects of equipment disposal such as sharps. This is also an appropriate time to discuss and plan for less common occasions like parties and holidays.

In a teaching program, it is essential that each family is taught the same technique for insulin injections, blood glucose monitoring and urine testing in order to maintain consistency and prevent conflicting information.

FURTHER COMPLICATIONS

The risk of chronic long-term complications of insulin dependent diabetes mellitus can be minimised if the patient complies with prescribed treatment and maintains acceptable blood glucose levels. The primary complication of IDDM is changes to the blood vessels and nerve endings, which can lead to visual changes such as retinopathy or decreased peripheral circulation (i.e., neuropathy). With regular consultation and with appropriate health care, these problems can be detected early and treated.

SPECIAL NEEDS OF THE CHILDREN, PARENTS AND FAMILIES

Each family will experience its individual needs and problems. Firstly, the parents and child have to come to accept the diagnosis of diabetes mellitus and go through an experience similar to the grieving process. They may experience feelings of guilt, shock, denial, self-blame and misconceptions about diabetes. They may ask questions such as 'why me?', 'will he or she die?', 'how will I cope?', 'what did I do wrong?' or 'is it my fault?'.

As well as these initial anxieties, parents may have difficulties associated with the age group of their child.

Infants

Parental adjustment is the main issue as the parents are the main caregivers.

Toddlers and preschoolers

Injection time can be traumatic and the child may interpret injections as a form of punishment. In such instances a reward after the child's injection may be helpful so long as the parents understand that the child will expect this to continue with each injection. Cuddles and stories are appropriate, but it should be remembered that lollies and chocolates are not suitable.

Children of this age group may be manipulative with their food. Nutritional finger foods are often the most appealing for these young children.

School-aged children

This age group relies on their parents for their meals and injections. Children in this category may not be able to fully understand the reasons behind their treatment, and can use their condition to manipulate their parents.

Early adolescence

At times adolescents can become rebellious as they encounter pubertal changes and problems. They may feel different from their peers, and being a teenager, they often become non-compliant in order to be 'normal'.

Late adolescence

Uncontrolled diabetes can be the result in this age group if they do not accept their condition. This may result when an adolescent wants to have total control of their diabetes and refuses to accept parental advice.

REFERENCES

1. Tortora GJ, Anagnostakos NJ. *Principles of anatomy and physiology.* 7th ed. New York: Harper and Row, 1993.

2. Hamilton HK. *Nurse's reference library, diseases.* Nursing Books 85. Pennsylvania: Springhouse, 1985.
3. Woods M, Williams R, Abdulai A, Donegan S, Bain L, Eason M. *Diabetic teaching manual for registered nurses.* Melbourne: Royal Children's Hospital, 1991

Disturbances in Growth

Irene Mitchelhill

Nursing the paediatric endocrine patient, from newborn to adolescence, requires knowledge of the complex mechanism of the neuroendocrine system. Dysfunctions of the endocrine system often involve lifelong treatment and follow-up. This may involve various investigations and treatment regimens which may change over time as new management techniques are developed through ongoing research. It is most important that adequate education and a support network is provided for children and their families as they learn to deal with the day-to-day aspects of their disorder and treatment regimens.

The endocrine nurse must be familiar with all aspects of patient care, enabling her to provide assistance as the need arises. Advocacy, autonomy, empathy and good communication skills are essential qualities in the nurse to develop a rapport with the child and family and to provide a continuity of care to these patients.

When conducting clinical investigations on any patient, the nurse must be familiar with the physiology of the disorder, the protocol for the investigation, including an understanding of how the results will be interpreted, and the action of various medications. It is essential that there is a knowledge of drug regimens, pharmacology, dosages, side effects and antidotes.

As all abnormalities of the endocrine system affect growth, a few general comments on growth are appropriate.

The accurate measuring of a child is one of the most important yet simplest and least invasive procedures for the assessment of a child's health and progress.[1] It is essential to measure a child in any clinical contact, as growth records frequently provide the first clue to an endocrine abnormality or other chronic illness, and will often eliminate the need for costly laboratory tests,[2] although it should be remembered that illness in a child may affect the accuracy of such measurements.

Disturbances in neuroendocrine function in the infant, child or adolescent will be reflected in altered growth and/or development patterns and metabolic function.[2,3] The neuroendocrine system controls the homeostatic environment of the body under the control of the hypothalamus. These are either neural or hormonal, and act as stimulatory and inhibitory factors. In response the hypothalamus manufactures and secretes releasing hormones as the need arises to stimulate the target glands to secrete specific hormones. The negative feedback mechanism is controlled by both neural impulses and adequate hormone levels in the blood.[4,5] This delicate balance may be affected by any chronic system disorder, or psychological trauma which upsets this delicate balance.

Growth is a complex interaction between genetic predisposition and the prevailing environment and is a sensitive indicator of a child's well-being or state of health.[2,6] Poor growth is often the first sign of a disease process and the impact of this on the normal growth regulatory process may have irreversible effects.

A distinction between short stature in a healthy child and growth failure, or tall stature in a healthy child and excessive growth is very important. Children should be referred for further assessment if they are short or tall for their age or family and have growth deviating from their normal percentile. It is necessary to distinguish between familial effects and a disease process which causes growth failure or excess.[2]

A low height velocity recorded throughout an entire year in any child should also prompt investigation for an underlying medical disorder long before their stature slips to below the third percentile. Similarly, children who are excessively tall for their family and have a period of rapid growth should also be assessed.

An assessment therefore should include the taking of an adequate history of the pregnancy, delivery, birthweight and length, head circumference, medical and family history, nutritional assessment and include psychosocial aspects.[2–7] Measurements taken should be plotted on relevant percentile charts so that an appropriate assessment can be made.[1] A bone age x-ray of the left hand and wrist will assess skeletal maturation and allow a possible height prediction to be calculated.[1,2] Any child with dysmorphic features and any girl with short stature should undergo chromosome assessment to rule out abnormalities such as Turner syndrome.[2]

SHORT STATURE

Idiopathic short stature is a state or a condition for which no cause can be found. These children have a steady but below average growth rate rather than a slowing of growth rate. In contrast, growth failure is a disease process. There is a below average growth rate compared to the family's growth pattern and children of the same age, sex, ethnic background, or a significantly slower growth rate compared to the child's own previous growth rate.

Growth failure

Growth failure may be congenital (e.g., absence of an endocrine gland, or a genetic, chromosomal or enzymatic defect which directly effects the endocrine system) or acquired. Acquired growth failure is often the result of a wide variety of disorders which have a secondary effect on endocrine function. Growth abnormalities are often described as primary or secondary, and are discussed under neuroendocrine dysfunction.[9,10]

A child's height percentile position must be evaluated in terms of genetic background, gestational and past medical history, environmental and social factors, physical findings, growth pattern since birth and the current growth rate or velocity.[2] Specific features of growth problems caused by neuroendocrine pathology are evident in altered body proportions with an abnormal relationship between height, weight and head circumference and in upper/lower segment and span-minus-height ratios.

A further evaluation of the specific organ systems should be carried out if the physical examination and history warrant it and may include haematological, gastrointestinal, renal, cardiac, neurological or locomotor evaluation.[2]

Irrespective of the cause of short stature and growth failure, children are likely to suffer the same degree of psychological problems and disadvantages because of the onlooker's attitude. This may contribute to problems such as poor social competence and underachievement at school. The cause of the short stature is irrelevant in defining the way in which people will relate to a short child or person.[11–15]

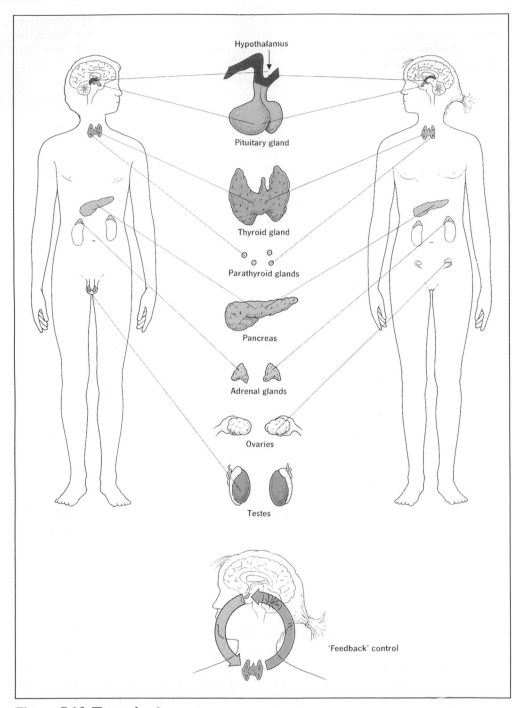

Figure 7.16 The endocrine system. (Reproduced with permission from KabiPharmacia, Sweden)

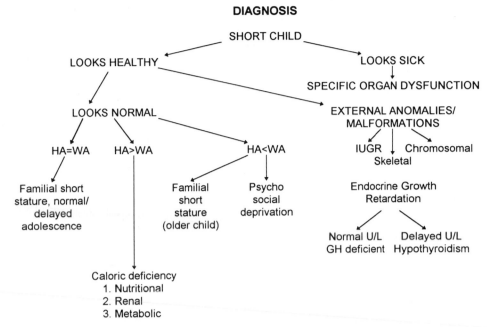

Figure 7.17 Assessment of a short child.

(Published with permission: Dr Gabriel Antony, Prince of Wales Children's Hospital, Sydney)

The management of short stature should include both medical and psychosocial intervention. It is now generally well recognised that because of the complexity in the regulation of growth hormone secretion, there is no satisfactory biochemical method or any combination of investigations which can be used to establish meaningful priorities in selecting patients for growth hormone treatment.[6,16–29]

The unlimited availability of biosynthetic growth hormone in recent years has created many major ethical and economic problems and guidelines have had to be formulated for selecting those children whose short stature may be modified on organic medical grounds against those whose short stature needs to be modified on the basis of psychosocial grounds.[6,16,18,19,22,24,28,29]

The overall aim of treatment is to improve height and promote normal psychosocial development. Children with growth hormone insufficiency have the physical disadvantages of a hormone deficiency in addition to the psychosocial disadvantages of short stature.

It is critical that any underlying disorder is treated before growth hormone therapy is considered. Once such a disorder is stabilised, growth hormone therapy may be considered if there has been no adequate improvement in the growth rate and the child is still considered to be short. The response of children with growth failure treated with growth hormone for reasons other than classical growth hormone deficiency is still under debate. Most children respond to therapy initially, but this effect appears to wane after the first year or two of treatment. Whether such treatment results in achievement of a greater final height is still unanswered and is being researched worldwide. Treatment appears to

Table 7.14 Causes of short stature and growth failure

Congenital	Acquired
Hypothalamic/pituitary hypofunction	Chronic systems disorders
Midline development defects	Malnutrition
Hypoplasia/aplasia of glands	Failure to thrive
Hypothyroidism — primary/secondary	IUGR — Russell Silver syndrome
Genetic X-linked autosomal recessive disorders	Head trauma — perinatal, fractures, child
Multiple pituitary deficiencies	abuse intraventricular haemorrhage,
Chromosomal abnormalities — Turner and	cranial irradiation brain tumours, cranial
Down syndromes, 13q deletion	surgery infection — meningitis,
Skeletal dysplasia- achrondroplasia,	encephalitis
hypochrondroplasia	Psychosocial deprivation
Tissue unresponsiveness to growth hormone &	Specific endocrine dysfunction-Cushings
its substrates	syndrome hypothyroidism,
	Pseudoparahypothyroidism,
	Prader Willi Labhart syndrome

Adapted from Berham et al 1987, Brook 1989[8], Kaplan 1990[10], Lifshitz 1986, Merenstein et al 1991[31], Styne 1988[1].

be benefical in the short term, enabling children to catch up to their peers in height, although still remaining at the lower end of the normal range of the percentile charts. It does not appear that it is possible to override genetic determination in the long term.

Adequate evaluation of the possible benefits of treatment or no treatment and of the physical and psychological aspects should be discussed with the parents and child. Expectations and duration of treatment, possible side effects and the considerable commitment which is required should be discussed at length.[6,16,18,19,22,24,28,29]

Evaluation of the treatment of growth disorders should follow the normal professional and ethical principles. No bias either on personal or economic grounds should influence the care given to patients because of the economic considerations of hormone replacement therapy. Decisions should not be made until all the relevant facts and existing knowledge are known and must be in the child's best interests.

TALL STATURE

Tall stature of a pathological cause will be evident in a rapid crossing of the percentile channels on the growth chart, and is often associated with abnormal body proportions and an advanced skeletal age. Causes include pituitary gigantism, precocious puberty, thyrotoxicosis, Marfan syndrome, chromosomal defects such as Klinefelter syndrome, maternal diabetes, Beta cell adenomas, and congenital adrenal hyperplasia.

Nursing assessment includes a detailed family and medical history, specialised measurements of the patient and family and a physical examination of the child. Any clinical findings of endocrinopathy and biochemistries such as abnormal thyroid function tests, increased insulin-like growth factor-1 (IGF-1), or gonadotropin levels are important for the diagnosis. Management of such disorders is discussed under the specific disorders.

Medical management includes treatment of the underlying disorder. Treatment of familial tall stature is controversial and is only undertaken after careful calculation of prediction height and evaluation of the psychological effects of excessive tallness. In children where the predicted height is considered excessive, treatment with oestrogen

Table 7.15 Causes of tall stature and growth excess

Congenital	Endocrine
Familial tall stature	Precocious puberty
Sotos syndrome	Growth hormone excess
Beckwith Weidman syndrome	Androgen excess (tall children, short adults)
Marfan syndrome	Androgen deficiency (short children, tall adults)
Klienfelter syndrome	Hyperthyroidism
	Hyperinsulinaemia (β cell adenoma)
	Obesity — increased insulin levels
	Growth hormone secreting adenomas
	Klinefelter syndrome
	McCune Albright syndrome

Adapted from Berham RE et al 1987, Brook CGD 1989, Hindmarsh PC et al 1991, Kaplan S 1990, Lifshitz F 1986, Merenstein GB et al 1991, Styne DM 1988

therapy in girls or testosterone therapy in boys may be used to accelerate fusion of the long bones and hence decrease final height.[1,2]

Nursing intervention includes undertaking accurate measurements, providing education and support during the treatment phase and monitoring for side effects. Nausea is common, but avoidable if oestrogen therapy is carefully managed and psychological support provided. A brief growth spurt may be observed initally, excessive weight gain and hypertension may be observed. Irregular menses may occur though the cyclic use of progestagens will prevent breakthrough bleeding.[2]

Frequent monitoring, usually every 3 months, of growth and development is required to evaluate the progress of treatment and allow for adjustments to medication doses. Reductions in height of between 1.8 and 3.6 cm with a bone age of 14 to 15.5 years, and 4.9 to 5.8 cm with a bone age of 10.5 to 13.0 years at the commencement of treatment are possible.[2] Frequent visits allow the nursing and medical staff to build up a rapport with the child and family and allows them to form a support network for the family.

Neuroendocrine Dysfunction

Neuroendocrine dysfunction is either primary, secondary or tertiary and manifests as either hypo or hyperfunctioning of the hypothalamus, pituitary or target glands (e.g., thyroid, gonads, adrenals) or failure of peripheral target tissues to respond to a stimulus. There may be aplasia, hypoplasia of any gland or a receptor or tissue enzyme defect which prevents the conversion of a hormone to its more active form.[2]

HYPOFUNCTIONING OF THE ANTERIOR PITUITARY GLAND

Hypothalamic hypopituitarism

Panhypopituitarism is the partial or complete absence of all six trophic hormones from the anterior pituitary. It is often the result of a midline developmental defect causing

Figure 7.18

DYSFUNCTION OF THE NEURO-ENDOCRINE SYSTEM

Disorders are either congenital or acquired, primary, secondary or tertiary.

NEURAL CONTROL

ENDOCRINE CONTROL

Receptors in CNS:
(visual, thermo, chemo, osmo)
relay messages by electrical
nerve impulses to hypothalamus

Stimuli are received from
chemical messengers (hormones)
circulating in the blood.

Positive and negative feedback systems regulate hormonal control.
Signals are either neuronal or hormonal.

ACQUIRED ABNORMALITIES	HYPOTHALAMUS		CONGENITAL ABNORMALITIES

Physical and psychological illness
"inhibits" hypothalamic regulation of the
endocrine system.
Chronic Systems Disorder:
malnutrition, FTT, IUGR
trauma and hypoxia,
IV Haemorrhage, infection,
tumours, cranial surgery
cranial irradiation.

Regulates:
Homeostasis
Metabolism
Growth
Reproduction

Secretes:
Regulatory
hormones

(a) Stimulatory   CRF
GHRF
TRF

(b) Inhibitory   SMSIH
GHIF

Midline Development Defects
Aplasia/hypoplasia of glands.
Genetic X linked autosomal recessive
causing multiple pituitary deficiency.
Chromosomal - Turner, Down
syndromes, 13q deletion.
Cell Receptor defects -
tissue unresponsiveness.
Enzyme defects.
Skeletal dysplasias.

Inhibit
function

Stimulates
pituitary

PITUITARY

Anterior Pituitary - secretes trophic hormones

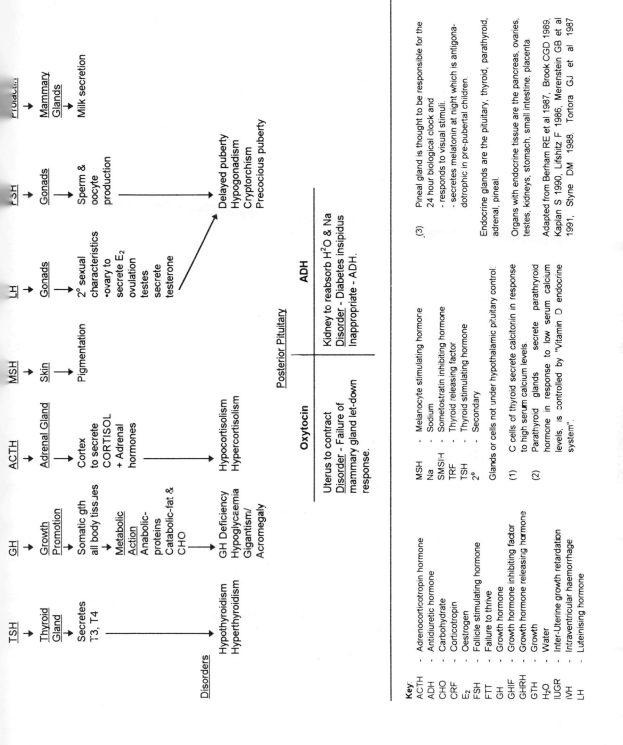

TSH → Thyroid Gland → Secretes T3, T4

GH → Growth Promotion → Somatic gth all body tissues → Metabolic Action: Anabolic-proteins, Catabolic-fat & CHO

ACTH → Adrenal Gland → Cortex to secrete CORTISOL + Adrenal hormones

MSH → Skin → Pigmentation

LH → Gonads → 2° sexual characteristics; •ovary to secrete E_2, ovulation, testes secrete testerone

FSH → Gonads → Sperm & oocyte production

Prolactin → Mammary Glands → Milk secretion

Delayed puberty
Hypogonadism
Cryptorchism
Precocious puberty

Disorders

Hypothyroidism / Hyperthyroidism

GH Deficiency
Hypoglycaemia
Gigantism /
Acromegaly

Hypocortisolism
Hypercortisolism

Posterior Pituitary

Oxytocin	ADH
Uterus to contract. Disorder - Failure of mammary gland let-down response.	Kidney to reabsorb H^2O & Na. Disorder - Diabetes insipidus. Inappropriate - ADH.

MSH   - Melanocyte stimulating hormone
Na   - Sodium
SMSIH - Sometostratin inhibiting hormone
TRF   - Thyroid releasing factor
TSH   - Thyroid stimulating hormone
2°   - Secondary

Glands or cells not under hypothalamic pituitary control:

(1)   C cells of thyroid secrete calcitonin in response to high serum calcium levels.

(2)   Parathyroid glands secrete parathyroid hormone in response to low serum calcium levels, is controlled by "Vitamin D endocrine system".

(3)   Pineal gland is thought to be responsible for the 24 hour biological clock and
      - responds to visual stimuli.
      - secretes melatonin at night which is antigonadotrophic in pre-pubertal children.

Endocrine glands are the pituitary, thyroid, parathyroid, adrenal, pineal.

Organs with endocrine tissue are the pancreas, ovaries, testes, kidneys, stomach, small intestine. placenta

Adapted from Berham RE et al 1987, Brook CGD 1989, Kaplan S 1990, Lifshitz F 1986, Merenstein GB et al 1991, Styne DM 1988. Tortora GJ et al 1987

Key:
ACTH - Adrenocorticotropin hormone
ADH   - Antidiuretic hormone
CHO   - Carbohydrate
CRF   - Corticotropin
E_2 - Oestrogen
FSH   - Follicle stimulating hormone
FTT   - Failure to thrive
GH   - Growth hormone
GHIF - Growth hormone inhibiting factor
GHRH - Growth hormone releasing hormone
GTH   - Growth
H_2O - Water
IUGR - Inter-Uterine growth retardation
IVH   - Intraventricular haemorrhage
LH   - Luteinising hormone

absence, aplasia or hypoplasia of the gland, trauma, infections or is iatrogenic.[30] The defect may occur either in the hypothalamus or the pituitary. The resulting metabolic disturbances include hypoglycaemia, hypoadrenalism, hypothyroidism, hypogonadism, diabetes insipidus, headache and visual disturbance and growth retardation. Prolonged hyperbilirubinaemia in the neonate may also be present. Diagnosis can be made on clinical grounds and is usually supported by biochemical and radiological data. Symptoms are often evident soon after birth, but may also develop slowly, and are usually evident by 6 months of age. Computed tomography (CT) or magnetic resonance imaging (MRI) of the pituitary fossa and clinical investigations for pituitary function will help confirm the diagnosis.[2]

Nursing assessment will identify signs of hypoglycaemia, hypoadrenalism, hypothryroidism and growth hormone deficiency leading to an alteration in metabolism, an impaired central nervous system function and a reduced ability to respond in stress due to adrenal insufficiency. There is impaired growth and development, hypogonadism, physical and emotional immaturity and developmental delay.

Psychosocial and emotional difficulties occur for the child and parents and are related to the chronic nature of the disorder, requiring invasive treatment routines and investigations.

Hypoadrenalism

Hypoadrenalism manifests as a deficiency in the production of glucocorticoids and mineralocorticoids from the adrenal cortex. It occurs secondary to hypothalamic hypopituitarism caused by a deficiency in the secretion of adrenocortical stimulating hormone (ACTH). A deficiency of glucocorticoids (cortisol), will have an effect on blood glucose homeostasis because of reduced gluconeogenesis and the body's inability to respond to stress. A deficiency of mineralocorticoids (aldosterone), will affect electrolyte and water metabolism, causing salt loss.[31] Signs and symptoms include weight loss, nausea, muscular weakness, diarrhoea, fever, hypoglycaemia, cyanosis and shock with hypotension, pallor, apnoea, deterioration in conscious level leading to an adrenal crisis if untreated.[1,3] An adrenal crisis is usually precipitated by infection, trauma, excess fatigue and drugs such as morphine, barbiturates and anaesthetic agents. Symptoms may be mild or severe and manifest abruptly or insidiously.[7]

Growth hormone insufficiency

Growth hormone insufficiency is manifested by persistent hypoglycaemia in infancy. It is caused by the loss of the glucoregulatory effects of growth hormone in conjunction with glucocorticoids.[1] Short stature (less than the 3rd percentile) with poor growth (less than 5 cm/year) and a delayed bone age are significant. The child will have normal body proportions and head circumference, but will appear immature for their age. In addition there is excess subcutaneous fat and increased skinfold thickness, poorly developed musculature, crowding of the midface, pseudofrontal bossing, a depressed nasal bridge and delayed and later crowded dentition. There may be a single central incisor, a high-pitched voice because of a small larynx, and a small phallus and scrotum.[2,3,7]

Hypothyroidism

In the neonate the following clinical manifestations may signify hypothyroidism: transient hypothermia; feeding difficulties; respiratory distress from reduced oxygen intake; lethargy;

hypotonia; bradycardia; pallor; mottling; a persistently enlarged posterior fontanelle; large anterior fontanelle; prolonged jaundice; and constipation.[1,3,30,31] The upper: lower segment ratio, growth and bone age are delayed with the weight age usually greater than the height age. The features of prolonged hypothyroidism are coarse facies, flattened nasal bridge, coarse cry, umbilical hernia and a protruding tongue. Myxoedema and pericardial oedema will develop from progressive accumulation of fluid in the tissues, with mental retardation occuring if the patient is left untreated.[30] In patients with hypothalamic and hypopituitary hypothyroidism, thyroid failure is secondary to a lack of thyroid stimulating hormone (TSH) from the pituitary gland, which normally stimulates the thyroid gland to release thyroxine. Laboratory testing will show an absence of normal levels of TSH, thyroxine (T4), and tri-iodothyronine (T3). In primary hypothyroidism, TSH levels will be raised.[1,3]

Hypogonadism

Hypogonadism is manifested by a micro penis (<2.5 cm) and small testes in the newborn or young infant, and a lack of secondary sexual development in the adolescent. The child has normal stature with eunuchoid proportions (long arms and legs). The growth of the lower segment is greater than the upper segment for age and there will be a delayed bone age. The gonadotrophin levels will be prepubertal. Some children may demonstrate hyponosmia or anosmia, a reduced or absent sense of smell. Kallman syndrome often manifests in this way and is always associated with anosmia.[1,7] The medical diagnosis is made on clinical assessment, biochemical data and diagnostic investigations such as a computed tomography (CT) or magnetic resonance imaging (MRI) of the pituitary fossa. The latter radiological examinations will determine a small sella turcica, absent or hypoplastic pituitary or hypothalamus. Blood tests will determine hormonal and biochemical status.[1,7,30]

Nursing intervention in the short term will involve instigation of emergency procedures in a crisis situation and the prevention of such situations. In the long term, nursing interventions aim to promote normal growth and development as the child recovers from any deficit.

The nurse must prevent prolonged periods of fasting and ensure adequate carbohydrate and fluid intake to prevent hypoglycaemia. Nursing actions include the monitoring of vital signs, observing for hypoglycaemia or hypoadrenalism (refer to endocrine emergencies), instigating intervention according to emergency protocols for these situations and immediately reporting any changes to the treating physician.

Replacement therapies are administered to prevent hypothyroidism, hypoglycaemia and adrenal crisis and are given on a specific time schedule in an attempt to mimic normal physiological production. The nurse provides a support network for the child and family and ensures that an after-hours telephone number is available in case of emergencies.

Education of the child and family is the responsibility of the nurse. It is essential that they are instructed in the pathophysiology of the disorder and its management, drug therapy and potential complications of illness, including how to administer intramuscular hydrocortisone in emergency situations of physiological and psychological stress to prevent adrenal crises. It is important that parents are told to notify the doctor when the child is not well, to obtain guidance in instigating possible emergency treatment. It is usual that the parents will be instructed to increase the daily dose of oral hydrocortisone prophylactically until the child is well again when the dose is returned to normal. If parents are unable to contact their doctor to check the seriousness of their child's illness, they are instructed to give hydrocortisone parenterally if in doubt, and then seek medical attention immediately.

A 'Medi Alert' identification bracelet or pendant which states the child's name, date of birth, hospital number, telephone number, CORTISOL DEFICIENT, give hydrocortisone 100 mg IMI stat in the case of illness, accident or operation should always be worn. A letter of instruction from the treating physician should also be carried along with hydrocortisone for administration in such cases of emergency.

The importance of regular follow-up for assessment of growth rate, health status and adjustment of medication dosage cannot be over-emphasised. The nurse must ensure that the child and family have a basic understanding of the disorder, its treatment and of the importance of follow-up assessments.

HYPOFUNCTIONING OF THE POSTERIOR PITUITARY GLAND

Diabetes insipidus

Diabetes insipidus (DI) is the inability of the distal tubules of the kidneys to reabsorb water and therefore concentrate the urine.[30] It is caused by either a deficiency in the secretion of antidiuretic hormone (ADH) from the posterior pituitary gland or failure of the kidneys to respond to ADH.[30,31]

Neurogenic or central diabetes insipidus is caused by posterior pituitary hypofunctioning or defective synthesis or deficiency of antidiuretic hormone produced by the supraoptic nuclei, or defects in hypothalamic osmoreceptors. This form of diabetes insipidus may also occur secondary to head injuries, or tumours of the pituitary fossa, namely craniopharyngioma in childhood.[1,30,31]

Nephrogenic diabetes insipidus is caused by renal tubule unresponsiveness to ADH.[2,7,30,31]

Psychogenic diabetes insipidus is the result of compulsive water ingestion and requires psychotherapy; these children can concentrate their urine if water deprived.[7,31]

Inappropriate ADH secretion is a transient condition causing a hypersecretion of antidiuretic hormone and is caused by infection (e.g., meningitis, encephalitis), subarachnoid haemorrhage, trauma from post-transphenoidal surgery, perinatal asphyxia, or drugs such as vincristine, vinblastine, chlorpropramide.[1,2,7,31] A sustained release of antidiuretic hormone leads to iatrogenic hyponatraemia and is treated with fluid restriction and replacement of fluid output.[1,2,7]

The nursing assessment will reveal polydypsia, urinary frequency, polyuria and nocturia, a low urinary specific gravity, poor weight gain, anorexia and constipation. If the condition has existed over some time, growth may be retarded.[1,7,30] As hypertonic dehydration becomes severe, vital signs will be altered, exhibited by tachycardia, hypotension from hypovolaemia, increased respiratory rate and fever. The skin will be dry and have poor turgor. In small children excessive crying and irritability are common if the thirst mechanism is impaired or oral fluids are withheld. If dehydration continues the neurological status will be altered with headache, irritability, apathy and general weakness with drowsiness. These effects suggest circulatory collapse and coma are imminent. Diagnosis is made by assessing the biochemical parameters of the blood and urine. A water deprivation test may be done. Urine osmolality will be low <280 mosm/L, serum osmolality will be high >305 mosm/L.[1]

Nursing intervention includes monitoring to detect any changes in vital signs and neurological status. Management of fluid replacement therapy until the fluid deficit is returned to normal, prevention of a further fluid deficit with the administration of intranasal or intramuscular vasopressin and observing for fluid retention is a vital part of the nursing role. A strict fluid balance must be recorded accurately and should include urinary specific gravity and electrolyte levels. A twice-daily weight recording allowing monitoring of excessive gain or loss, is a simple means of assessing the child's fluid status and is extremely important in the initial and long-term management of this disorder. As vascular equilibrium is restored to normal, there will be a return of all parameters to within normal limits, and with good metabolic control, normal growth and development will occur.

The nurse is responsible for educating the patient about the disorder in easy-to-understand terminology by explaining and demonstrating the basic concepts of the disease process and the management routines relating to treatment. Management incudes daily weighing, regulation of oral fluid intake and the administration of intranasal or intra-muscular vasopressin at home. Parents are taught to monitor for the signs of overhydration or dehydration and are provided with an emergency contact telephone number. Explaining the importance of regular follow-up and the reporting of any unusual or adverse conditions cannot be over-emphasised. Each child should wear a 'Medi Alert' bracelet or pendant with the details of the disorder.

Hypothalmic hyperpituitarism is exceptionally rare in children and is often associated with neoplasia of the pituitary, such as adenomas which secrete excess growth hormone, ACTH or prolactin, leading to pituitary gigantism, Sotos syndrome, and excess prolactin levels. Pituitary tumours may subsequently cause compression of pituitary tissue which eventually leads to hypopituitarism.[7]

Primary Endocrine Disorders

HYPOTHYROIDISM

Hypothyroidism is a deficiency in the secrction of thyroid hormone and is classified as primary, secondary, tertiary, transient or acquired.[1,2,7,30]

Primary hypothyroidism is caused by dysgenesis, agenesis or hypoplasia of the thyroid gland or inborn errors of thyroid hormone production. Blood tests will show raised levels of TSH, and low levels of T3 and T4.[1,7,31]

Secondary hypothyroidism is the result of a dysfunction of the hypothalamus or pituitary gland. There is a deficiency of thyroid stimulating hormone (TSH) and there will be low levels of TSH, tri-iodothyronine (T3) and thyroxine (T4) levels.[1,7,30]

Tertiary hypothyroidism is caused by abnormalities in thyroid binding proteins. It may be transient because of an immaturity in thyroid development as in prematurity, or an ectopic or hypoplastic gland that decompensates with time, giving blood levels of raised TSH and normal T4. Other causes are 'low T3 syndrome', which is evident either during an acute or chronic illness, high iodine uptake, or raised TSH levels.[1] Acquired hypothyroidism is caused by autoimmune lymphocytic thyroiditis, exposure to goitrogenic agents, absorption of iodine from topical iodine preparations in the neonate, dysgenesis of the thyroid gland. It may be transient following an acute illness.[1,2,7,31]

Neonatal screening is performed on all babies at 3 days as part of the newborn screening program. Blood is collected onto filter paper following a heel prick. Raised levels of TSH suggests primary hypothyroidism but TSH testing alone will miss hypothalamic/pituitary hypothyroidism. Babies may miss screening because of interhospital transfer, early discharge programs or home birth.

Nursing assessment will identify the following: hypothermia and bradycardia related to a decreased metabolic rate; lethargy; hypotonia; pallor and skin mottling related to a decreased metabolic rate; poor feeding because of lethargy and upper airway obstruction; and constipation because of decreased muscle tone and motility.

Nursing interventions aim to promote normal intellectual development and a euthyroid state by ensuring replacement therapy is given as prescribed. Oral thyroxine (T4) in an age adjusted dose dosage is the usual regimen.[32] Some physicians may still prefer to use tri-iodothyronine (T3). In treating primary hypothyroidism in the neonate, it should be noted that the TSH level is difficult to suppress with levels often staying elevated for months or even years because of a persistent negative feedback mechanism. The goal of therapy should be to maintain normal growth and development. Over-treatment may cause advancement of bone age and craniosynostosis.

Monitoring for over or under treatment includes recording growth and development, vital signs, hormonal levels and ensuring an adequate caloric and fluid intake. Promotion of a normal psychosocial environment for the child and family may be achievable by education of the family about disease and its treatment, correct administration of the medication, the importance of frequent assessment of growth and development and adjustment of replacement therapy as the child grows.

It is important to teach parents that when administering the medication they should not add the crushed tablets to the child's bottle as some of the drug will form a sediment on the bottom of the bottle and the full dose will not be received. The medication should be mixed with a teaspoon of pureed food such as strained apples or pears to ensure that the complete dose is received.

HYPERTHYROIDISM

Hyperthyroidism may be primary or secondary in origin and is caused by excessive thyroid hormone production[7,30] resulting in a hypermetabolic state. Primary hyperthyroidism may be the result of an overactive thyroid gland causing excessive thyroid hormone production, or be caused by an overingestion of thyroid hormone. Secondary hyperthyroidism is the result of excessive stimulation by thyroid stimulating hormone (TSH) produced by the pituitary gland resulting in hypertrophy and hyperplasia of the thyroid gland. Graves disease is the most common form of hyperthyroidism and results from an autoimmune defect of the T-lymphocytes.[1,30]

Congenital hyperthyroidism occurs in infants of thyrotoxic mothers. Initially the baby may be hypothyroid because of the suppressive effects of propylthirouracil (PTU) taken by the mother, with hyperthryoidism occurring between 3 and 6 days of age as the serum PTU level falls. A goitre will develop with or without exopthalmos, the result of the transplacental transfer of thyroid stimulating immunoglobulins (TSI). Clinical signs are tachycardia, fever, restlessness, irritability, hyperactivity and unusual alertness.[1,7] Both primary and secondary hyperthyroidism may result in premature fusing of the cranial sutures (craniosynostosis), minimal brain dysfunction, accelerated skeletal age and a goitre.

Nursing assessment reveals evidence of an increased metabolic rate with emotional disturbances, irritibility, excitability, restlessness, nervousness, emotional lability and poor concentration. Motor hyperactivity with tremor and brisk reflexes and muscle weakness is present, and the patient will have a flushed appearance with smooth sweaty skin, hyperthermia, heat aversion, sweaty palms, tachycardia, dyspnoea and palpitations. In severe cases an apical systolic murmur will be audible as the result of mitral regurgitation, an exophthalmos and lid retraction with stare will be present along with an enlarged goitre. Puberty will be delayed.

The patient will have an insatiable appetite, but have weight loss related to the increased metabolic rate. The appearance will be gaunt because of the weight loss and hyperdefaecation caused by an increased gut motility, which are associated with the increased metabolism. There will be a history of visual disturbances and reduced school performance.

Nursing intervention in the short term includes the maintenance of an appropriate environment. A quiet and restful environment is encouraged, with physical activity reduced to a minimum. Ensuring a diet high in calories, protein and vitamins which can meet the needs of an increased metabolism and the administration of medications as ordered is vital to the recovery of the child. Medications include tranquillisers to control nervousness and sympatholytic drugs such as propranolol, which decrease the peripheral conversion of T4-T3 and diminish cardiovascular and certain neurological symptoms. Antithyroid medications such as propylthirouracil and carbimazole, which totally suppress thyroid function, are commenced immediately. Total replacement therapy with thyroxine is given 1 to 2 weeks later, once suppression is achieved.[1,7,30]

In the long term, the nurse aims to provide emotional support for the child and family, providing ongoing education about the disease process, stressing the importance of compliance with the treatment regimen and frequent follow-up. This includes how to recognise the signs of a recurrence of the disease. Monitoring the physical signs and symptoms of the disease is an important function of the nursing role. Compliance with treatment will be evident with adequate control of the symptoms being achieved in 2 to 3 months. The outcome of normal growth and development of the child is the goal of treatment as the family comes to term with the disorder and its long-term management implications.

A goitre is an enlargement of the thyroid gland and may be euthyroid, hypothyroid or hyperthyroid. Goitres are rare in infancy and childhood. Most are the result of ingestion of goitrogens or an inborn error of thyroid biosynthesis. Acute thyroiditis produces an acute inflammatory goitre from a viral or bacterial infection. Hashimoto's (lymphocytic) thyroiditis, which causes hypothyroidism, is most prevalent in adults, but is occasionally seen in the pubertal child and may be associated with diabetes mellitus and Addison's disease. Lymphocytic thyroiditis clusters in families, and is more common in girls than boys. Goitres in children are rarely cancerous, and medical treatment should always be the first line of management. Surgery is not recommended in children.[1,7,30]

ADRENAL HYPOFUNCTION

Adrenal insufficiency in children is part of a global adrenal insufficiency or a selective defect.[2] It may be congenital or acquired and can be either a primary or secondary defect.[30,31] The critical factor in this disorder is that these patients have an inability to mount a stress response in situations of physical or emotional stress.

Addison's disease is primary adrenal insufficiency and is characterised by a decreased mineralocorticoid, glucocorticoid and androgen secretion from the adrenal gland. It may be caused by agenesis, aplasia or atrophy of the adrenal gland, an autoimmune response, tumours, haemorrhage, infection or irradiation of the adrenal gland.[1,7,8] Adrenalin hypofunction may also occur secondary to a defect in the pituitary or hypothalamus such as aplasia, hypoplasia, infection, head injury, tumours or irradiation of the head. It may be the result of an enzymatic defect in steroid production or by glucocorticoid therapy leading to cortical atrophy.[7,30]

Nursing assessment will reveal: failure to thrive; vomiting; lethargy; anorexia; dehydration; and pallor. Circulatory collapse leading to adrenal crisis is seen in infants.[7] If the disorder develops insidiously in older children there is muscular weakness, lassitude, anorexia, weight loss, generalised wasting and low blood pressure from decreased energy metabolism. Increased pigmentation of the skin, especially the face, hands, genitalia, axillae, nipples and joints, develops in severe, untreated cases from excess corticotropin releasing hormone (CRH) which stimulates adrenocorticotrophic hormone (ACTH) production.[7]

If an adrenal crisis is imminent there will be signs of vomiting, diarrhoea, weakness, fatigue, dehydration, fever, hypoglycaemia leading to cold clammy skin, rapid laboured respirations, pallor, cyanosis, a weak pulse, low blood pressure, circulatory collapse, convulsion and death.[7,31] The emergency treatment is discussed under endocrine emergencies.

Nursing intervention for the patient with adrenal insufficiency includes monitoring the administration of replacement hormones. Cortisol is given as hydrocortisone and aldosterone as fludrocortisone. Regular blood tests for hormone and electrolyte levels assist in the monitoring of compliance. Assessment of growth and development by undertaking routine measurements and correctly plotting them on percentile charts will reveal progress with the treatment.

Education of the child and family about the disease should include information about the importance of compliance with the treatment routine and the steps to be followed in an emergency, or if the child is unwell. The nurse is responsible for instructing the parent in the administration of intramuscular hydrocortisone, which is given in times of acute illness or accidents. It is important for parents ensure that their child receives hydrocortisone cover if surgery is undertaken.

ADRENAL HYPERFUNCTION

Congenital adrenal hyperplasia (CAH), also known as adrenogenital syndrome, is the most common disorder associated with hyperfunction of the adrenal gland. It is caused by an enzyme deficiency in the pathway of corticosteroid biosynthesis. Five enzymatic defects are known, with only some resulting in virilisation of the genitalia. With the lack of cortisol production there is an absence of the negative feedback mechanism to the hypothalamus which causes secretion of high levels of ACTH. This hypersecretion of ACTH causes adrenal hypertrophy, resulting in an excessive secretion of adrenal androgens (other than cortisol) and leads to virilisation and masculinisation of the genitalia.

Twenty-one hydroxylase (21OH) deficiency is the most common of these disorders (occurring in 95%). It is an inherited autosomal recessive trait that causes a deficiency of the enzyme 21OH. In utero, excess androgens have little effect on the male fetus. An increased phallus size and pigmentation of the scrotum are the only signs. The female fetus will develop ambiguous genitalia because of the virilising effect of the circulating androgens.[3] Serum adrenal androgens, 17-hyproxyprogesterone (17OHP) and urinary 17 ketosteroids (17 KOS) are elevated.[2,7] All CAH patients lose salt to some degree, but many are able to compensate until times of stress.[7]

Nursing assessment of babies born with congenital adrenal hyperplasia will take into account the critical situation regarding the parents not knowing the gender of their baby. The psychosocial aspects of this emergency are discussed in the section on endocrine emergencies.

Nursing intervention requires the infant to be closely monitored. Vital signs, blood pressure, fluid balance and biochemistries are evaluated for evidence of sodium loss, dehydration and adrenal crisis. Blood tests are required for urgent chromosomal and hormonal analysis with results available in 24 hours.

The medication routine is extremely important and includes such drugs as hydrocortisone, a glucocorticoid which is given orally to suppress the pituitary secretion of ACTH and achieve adrenal suppression. Ideally, the medication is given 3 times daily in order to mimic as closely as possible the diurnal rhythm of normal production of cortisol by the body. Half the daily dose is given at 8 am and a quarter at 12 noon and at quarter at 4 pm. The dose required to suppress adrenal hyperfunction is 20 to 25 mg/m^2/day for infants and 25 to 100 mg/m^2/day for older children.[10] Such doses provide a negative feedback mechanism and prevent excess ACTH production from the pituitary gland and subsequent virilisation. Adequate treatment should see normal linear growth and development.

In times of stress, the glucocorticoid dose should be increased 3 to 4 times during an acute illness but only under a doctor's instructions. If illness is severe and there is a change in the patient's alertness, an intramuscular injection of 100 mg hydrocortisone should be given immediately. Failure to respond indicates that the child is not having an adrenal crisis, and another diagnosis should be sought.[7] Stress doses should be 10 times the normal maintenance dose[33] given by intravenous infusion over 24 hours, for 3 to 4 days, after which the usual routine is generally resumed. This management is further discussed under endocrine emergencies. Other medications include mineralocorticoids (fludrocortisone) which are required by children who lose salt. Some will require additional sodium chloride.

Reconstructive surgery is required for children with ambigious genitalia. A partial clitoridectomy in females should be done as soon as possible after diagnosis. This procedure will preserve all the neural and vascular elements and be cosmetically acceptable. Correction of labial fusion and urogenital-sinus may require several operations and is undertaken when the child is older. Genital reconstruction allows for normal physiological functioning at puberty.

Genetic counselling is extremely important and is required to allow parents to come to terms with the cause of the disorder. Minimal staff should be involved, and discussions take place only when all the facts are available.[2] Follow-up is critical. Education of the parents and immediate family is extremely important for the child's future psychosocial development.

Failure to recognise the disorder or poor compliance with treatment will lead to the patients exhibiting signs of slow virilisation, marked skin pigmentation, delayed puberty, rapid growth and be susceptable to an adrenal crisis. Subsequently, these children are tall for their age, but short as adults following the early closure of the epiphyses of the long bones. Adequate treatment permits normal growth, sexual development and fertility. Female pseudohermaphrodites raised mistakenly as males may have serious psychological disturbances if the child's gender is reassigned later than 3 years of age, as imprinting of gender identity is then well established. Delayed gender assignment is usually the cause of great parental anxiety.

CUSHING SYNDROME

Cushing syndrome encompasses all pathological conditions secondary to chronic excessive production of glucocorticoids[30,31] and androgenic hormones, which lead to varying degrees of virilisation, hirsutism and abnormal carbohydrate, protein and fat metabolism.[7,31] The 3 main causes in children are: adrenal Cushing syndrome, where primary hypercortisolism is the result of a malignant or benign tumour of the adrenal gland; pituitary Cushing syndrome, which is secondary to excessive secretion of ACTH from the pituitary or CRF from the hypothalamus; and iatrogenic, following glucocorticoid treatment which leads to cortical atrophy and an inability of the gland to secrete cortisol.[30] The prognosis is poor if untreated because of the side effects of high glucocorticoid levels.

Nursing assessment determines an altered body image related to increased deposits of adipose tissue, hirsutism, acne, deepening of the voice, virilisation, pigmentation and menstrual irregularities. Psychological changes such as depression, euphoria, insomnia and fatigue may be present. Muscle weakness and atrophy related to the catabolic process of excess glucocorticoids, diminished immunity due to the immunosuppressive effect of excess glucocorticoids on lymphocytes and soft tissue injury such as bruising are common. Hypertension is present because of the increased circulating volume.

In the long term, osteoporosis will occur because of increased catabolism, and adrenal diabetes may eventuate from 'beta cell burnout' because of the increased secretion of glucoregulatory hormones.

Nursing intervention aims to promote a safe and quiet environment. As glucocorticoids can mask the symptoms of infection, monitoring vital signs is essential. Education of the child and parents about the disorder, stressing the importance of protection from injury and infection, is given. The child and family need to have an understanding of the disease, any procedures that may be necessary such as surgical removal of the adrenal gland, and the requirements for replacement therapy.

Malignant tumours cannot be distinguished from benign tumours and surgery is therefore indicated. The preoperative and postoperative care is the same as that for Cushing syndrome. While the signs and symptoms will regress following surgery, the pigmentation, pubic hair and deepening of the voice may persist.

HYPERALDOSTERONISM

Hyperaldosteronism is rare in children and is usually caused by tumours of the adrenal gland. Children present as an acute admission with hypertension, hypernatraemia, and hypokalaemia, excessive sweating, flushing, pallor, rash, polyuria, polydypsia.[7,30]

HYPOALDOSTERONISM

Hypoaldosteronism is seen mainly in children with CAH. Signs include hyponatraemia, hyperkalaemia, failure to thrive, vomiting, hypovolaemia, dehydration and circulatory collapse.[3]

Parathyroid Dysfunction and Calcium Metabolism

Calcium metabolism is significantly under the control of the vitamin D endocrine system. Low calcium levels stimulate the production of parathyroid hormone, which increases the conversion of 25 vitamin D to 1,25 vitamin D. Vitamin D increases calcium absorption in the gut, decreases calcium excretion via the kidney and stimulates bone resorption, freeing calcium from the bones. Calcitonin is produced by the C-cells of the thyroid and has the reverse effect.[1,4,7] Because weight-bearing exercise promotes bone formation, patients on prolonged bed rest have an increased risk of fractures and hypercalcaemia.

HYPOPARATHYROIDISM

Hypoparathyroidism is a cause of hypocalcaemia. It may be either idiopathic or transient, or result of an autoimmune response or a parathyroidectomy.[1] Pseudohypopara-thyroidism is an X-linked dominant disorder caused by end-organ (renal tubule) unresponsiveness.[1] Hypocalcaemia also occurs in the sick neonate when there is an inability to absorb calcium from the gut and when immaturity of the parathyroid glands prevents the mobilisation of calcium from the bones.[7,30]

Hyperparathyroidism is associated with multiple endocrine adenomas and causes high calcium levels.[1,7,30,31]

RICKETS

Rickets, a defect of calcification of the metaphyses of the long bones, is caused by a deficiency of vitamin D intake, malabsorption or a genetic defect in vitamin D metabolism.[1] In childhood it leads to hypocalcaemia and hypophosphataemia. It is manifested in soft bones in infants, cranial tabes (flat back of head), a prominent forehead, poor growth, failure to thrive, irritability, convulsions, hypotonia from poor muscle tone, delayed gross motor function and delayed dentition.

Once the child is weight bearing, genu varum (bowing of tibia) or valgum (knock knees), a protruding abdomen and a sway back become evident and pseudopapilloedema may be noted. Radiological findings show a widening of the metaphyses of the long bones. Treatment consists of small doses of vitamin D (100 IU daily) for rickets caused by a vitamin D deficiency. Phosphaturic rickets requires phosphate and large doses of calciferol (1000 to 10 000 U daily) or calcitriol to counterbalance the calcium lowering effect of phosphate.[1,7,30]

HYPOCALCAEMIA

Nursing assessment will find altered neuromuscular activity and fluid homeostasis in the child with hypocalcaemia. In acute conditions symptoms such as a high-pitched cry, jitteriness, irritability, muscle twitching, cramps, parasthesiae, weakness, lethargy, laryngospasm, tetany or convulsions will be evident.[1] A prolonged QT segment will be evident on electrocardiogram (ECG). A positive Chvostek sign (where a tap in the front of the ear produces spasm of facial muscles) and a positive Trousseau sign (where a prolonged compression of the upper arm produces carpopedal spasm) will be present. In prolonged cases, growth retardation, delayed dentition, blepharospasm and chronic conjunctivitis, cataracts, diarrhoea, photophobia, irritability, bizarre behaviour, skin rashes, ectodermal dysplasias, fungal infections and calcifications of the basal ganglia are present.[1,7,30,31]

Nursing intervention aims to manage an emergency situation by maintaining circulation and respiration, monitoring vital signs and administering medications as prescribed. Acute hypocalcaemia is treated with an infusion of calcium gluconate diluted in isotonic solution and given slowly over 2 hours to avoid bradycardia. The nurse must observe the cannula site as the hypertonic nature of the infusion will cause sloughing, necrosis and calcifications if the the fluid escapes into the tissues. Thiazide diuretics are given to stimulate urinary calcium resorption. Monitoring of vital signs, ECG monitoring and serum calcium level estimations are essential during treatment. Chronic hypocalcaemia is treated with oral calciferol, calcitriol and calcium.[1,7,30]

With effective treatment, serum calcium levels will be maintained in the normal range. Neuromuscular irritability will abate and vital signs will return to normal. Following educational sessions, the parents should demonstrate an understanding of the complexities of the disorder, be able to identify the signs and symptoms of hypocalcaemia, as well as hypercalcaemia, which may occur from over-replacement. It is important that the need for compliance with medications and a high-calcium diet with adequate phosphorus intake are understood.

HYPERCALCAEMIA

Hypercalcaemia is rare in children. Nursing assessment reveals lethargy, weakness, loss of concentration, depression, nausea, vomiting, anorexia, constipation and weight loss. Polyuria occurs in response to the high levels of circulating calcium, which prevent the renal distal tubule from responding to anti-diuretic hormone. This may lead to dehydration and renal calculi in the long term. An electrocardiogram will demonstrate a short QT interval.[1,7,30]

Nursing intervention aims to maintain good hydration to promote calcuria. Oral fluids are encouraged and intravenous saline is infused. The volume required is 1.5 to 2 times normal maintenance. Frusemide is also administered to increase urinary calcium excretion. Explanation of all procedures and education about the pathophysiology of the disorder in simple terminology to both the child and parents is extremely important for their acceptance of the disorder and its long-term management and positive outcome. Compliance with medication and regular long-term follow-up is required.

Table 7.16 Causes of Hypocalcaemia and Hypercalcaemia

Hypocalcaemia	Hypercalcaemia
Hypoparathyroidism	Adrenal insufficiency
Pseudohypoparathyroidism	Hyperparathyroidism/tumour/hyperplasia
Renal osteodystrophy	Hyperthyroidism
Calcium malabsorption	Familial hypocalcuric hypercalcaemia
Rickets, nutritional/Vit D deficiency	Thiazides, diuretics
Prematurity, neonatal illness	Hypervitaminosis- excess vitamin D
High phosphate intake	↑ sensitivity to activated vitamin D
Magnesium deficiency	Immobilisation
Anticonvulsants	Idiopathic
	Williams syndrome

Adapted from Berham RE et al 1987: p1208, Styne DM 1988: p 117, 119

Gonadal Dysfunction and Disorders

THE HORMONAL CONTROL OF PUBERTY

Puberty is the acquisition of secondary sexual characteristics and reproductive capability. The variation in pubertal development may often be considered abnormal by the individual concerned, peers, parents and medical advisers.[8] It is therefore important to understand pubertal development and its various influences.

Puberty brings about a change in body size, shape and strength as well as psychosocial maturation. The commencement and the span of puberty varies from child to child and is influenced by familial traits and other internal and external influences. Puberty spans anywhere from 1.5 to 6 years in girls, and 2 to 4.5 years in boys.[1]

The mechanism for the hormonal control of puberty is influenced by genetic, familial and environmental factors, the body mass index and normal psychological functioning in a happy environment.

The hypothalamic-pituitary-gonadal axis is influenced by a normal homeostasis. The hypothalamus, under the correct conditions, is stimulated by the neuroendocrine system and produces gonadotrophin releasing hormone. This in turn stimulates the pituitary to release luteinising hormone (LH) and follicle stimulating hormone (FSH) which stimulate the gonads (ovaries and testes) to produce the sex hormones, oestrogen and testosterone respectively. A critical factor in the hormonal control of puberty is the nocturnal pulsatile nature of the gonadotrophins. 'Gonadarche' is thought to be under the influence of the pineal gland which might control the biological clock. It is this pulsatility which stimulates the ovaries to produce oestrogen and the testes to produce testosterone.[1,4]

In boys, LH stimulates the Leydig cells imbedded between the seminiferous tubules to grow and produce testosterone, which influences development of the secondary sexual characteristics, testicular enlargement and penile growth. FSH influences the seminiferous tubules, which make up the bulk of the testes, to produce sperm. The sertoli cells, also imbedded between the seminiferous tubules, protect and nourish the sperm. FSH has little effect until spermarche, at approximately 16 years of age.[8]

In boys, the first sign of puberty is testicular growth, which is not associated with a growth spurt. Gonadotrophin releasing hormone (GNRH) from the hypothalamus stimulates the pituitary to release LH and FSH. LH stimulates the Leydig cells in the testes to secrete testosterone, and increase the size of the seminiferous tubules. Penile growth occurs first in length, followed by breadth and the development of the glans. FSH is primarily involved at spermache and occurs approximately one year after the beginning of penile growth.[8] Gynaecomastia is common in males in early adolescence due to high levels of circulating testosterone being converted to oestrogen, and usually subsides spontaneously within 6 to 18 months.[1]

In girls, menses occurs approximately 2 years after the first sign of breast development, with accelerated linear growth preceding signs of pubertal development. Ovulation occurs approximately 3 to 12 months after menarche has occurred. Gonadotrophin releasing factor is secreted by the hypothalamus to stimulate the secretion of LH and FSH from the pituitary. LH stimulates the development of ovarian follicles but has little effect until ovulation. FSH stimulates the initial development of the ovarian follicle, which secretes oestrogen.[8]

The hypothalamic pituitary gonadal axis is responsible for the hormonal control of pubertal development. Disorders affecting development of secondary sexual characteristics may be primary or secondary in origin.

DELAYED PUBERTY

Puberty is considered delayed if there has been no development of secondary sexual characteristics by the ages of 14 in boys and 13 in girls. It may be caused by a temporary delay in growth and puberty, chronic disorders, hypothalamic hypogonadism or primary hypofunction or damage to the gonads. In addition, a wide range of conditions already dealt with under hypogonadism may be implicated.[1,30] Delayed puberty may be categorised as hypogonadotrophic or hypergonadotrophic and be either congenital or acquired.[30]

Primary hypogonadism is caused by either a hormone excess *in utero*, infection, inflammation, trauma, tumours, irradiation, gonadal dysgenesis or surgical removal of the gonads and is hypergonadotrophic.[1,7,30] Seconary hypogonadism is caused by hypothalamic pituitary hypofunction, hypogonadotropism, hypothyroidism, tumours, cranial irradiation or excess androgen production as in adrenogenital syndrome. Temporary hypogonadism may result from strenuous exercise, chronic system disorders, malnutrition or anomalies of the reproductive tract.[1,7,30]

Nursing assessment will reveal small, underdeveloped genitalia in the newborn and failure of the development of secondary sexual characteristics in the pubertal-aged child. The growth pattern is usually normal but no pubertal growth spurt has occurred.

Gonadal dysgenesis

Gonadal dysgenesis is an example of hypergonadotrophic hypergonadism. It is characterised by the anatomical malformation of the gonads caused by sex chromosome abnormalities. Some 80% of these children have 45X0 chromosome determination, with no paternal X chromosome.[8] Other combinations may be quite varied with determination of XO/XX, XO/XY, 45X/46XY or 47XYYY.[2,7] These children have a male or female phenotype, but have abnormal dysgenetic gonads which are surgically removed prophylactically because of the risk of gonadoblastoma. Turner syndrome, a chromosomal disorder in girls, is synonymous with gonadal dysgensis and has an incidence of 1:2500 to 3000 female births.[1,7,30]

Nursing assessment reveals minor dysmorphic features such as low-set rotated ears, low hairline, webbed neck, ptosis, shield-shaped chest, puffy hands and feet (congenital lymphoedema), small nails partially covering the terminal phalanx of the finger, high arched palate, hyperflexible joints, short stature, failure to develop secondary sexual characteristics and infertility. Ear, eye, heart and kidney problems are also common.[2,7] These children are intellectually normal with good verbal skills, but may have some perceptive and visual spatial difficulties.

Nursing interventions will monitor growth and development and aim to promote normal psychosocial development by providing emotional support and information. The nurse provides education for the child and her parents about the pathophysiology of the disorder and the importance of compliance with hormonal replacement therapy and long-term follow-up.

Each child should be encouraged to be involved in her treatment routine, which is supervised by the parents. Instruction in the preparation and administration of their own growth hormone injections will enhance independence and normal psychosocial development. Frequent follow-up is required to ensure compliance and evaluate progress. Emotional support and adequate explanation is required when discussing issues relating to sexuality and infertility and the need for replacement therapy with oestrogen and progesterone.

Cryptorchidism

Cryptorchidism (uni/bilateral undescended testes) may be caused by the decreased secretion of gonadotrophin releasing hormone or structural lesions such as a short spermatic cord or short spermatic arteries or veins.[1,31,34] Cryptorchidism occurs in 30% of premature infants; 3% of all term male infants have one cryptorchid testes, 75% of which descend by the age of 1 year. The testes are histologically normal at birth. Failure to correct the anomaly at the appropriate age can lead to infertility, and in the 3rd or 4th decade, malignant testicular tumours.[2,7] Surgery is preferably carried out between 1 and 5 years of age, and should be completed before puberty.

Nursing assessment will reveal an empty scrotal sac and undescended testes. Interventions will include informing the parents about the procedures which will take place during hospitalisation for surgical correction and biopsy of the undescended testes and postoperative care.

Klinefelter syndrome

Klinefelter syndrome is a disorder in males and is characterised by the presence of two or more X chromosomes in the form of 47XXY, or 46XY/47XXY. It occurs in approximately 1:500 males and causes seminiferous tubule dysgenesis. Because the phenotype is male, the diagnosis is often not made until puberty.[1,7,30] Two per cent of the patients presenting for medical attention with an XXY karyotype have atrophic sclerosis of the seminiferous tubules of the testes, but have normal Leydig cell function and partial virilisation. Hypergonadotrophism is evident with partial hypogonadism and testosterone levels in the lower normal range.[1,7,30]

Nursing assessment reveals failure of pubertal progression, small genitalia, small firm testes, bilateral gynaecomastia, obesity and a eunuchoid appearance with long lower extremities. Emotional instability with personality disorders and difficulties with social adjustments are usually evident and are related to problems with gender identity.

Nursing interventions aim to be supportive and informative in helping the parents and child cope with social adjustment and integration during adolescence. No medical intervention is required until puberty. The nurse administers or teaches the parents to administer the testosterone injections which are given monthly or fortnightly. This treatment will help improve the overall physical, emotional and social functioning of the adolescent and will help in the attainment of normal sexual function as an adult.[1,34]

Routine physical examination should reveal normal progression of secondary sexual development. Improvements in emotional well-being and behaviour, either observed or reported, should be recorded.

The nurse provides long-term emotional support, acts as confidante and advocate for the child and family while supervising treatment and conducting education about the disorder. Formal psychological counselling is sought to assist the child and his family in adjusting to the emotional difficulties associated with the child's gender identity.

Sexual precocity

Sexual precocity is classified as being either central precocious puberty or pseudoprecocity and is defined as the onset of secondary sexual characteristics before the age of 8 years in girls, and 9.5 years in boys. Precocity is caused by the premature maturation of the hypothalamic pituitary axis.[1,7,31] Central precocious puberty is gonadotrophin dependent and is caused by the increased pulsatility of gonadotrophin releasing hormone (GNRH) stimulus from the hypothalamus. It may be idiopathic, familial, or caused by tumours, infection, trauma or insults to the central nervous system.[1,7,31] Pseudoprecocity, however, is not gonadotrophin dependent and is thought to be caused by ovarian cysts, adrenal, ovarian or testicular tumours or the use of exogenous steroids. Treatment is for the underlying disorder.

Disorders of puberty generate their own psychological and physiological needs. The onset of precocious puberty creates significant emotional difficulties for the parents as well as for the child. As early maturation stimulates rapid growth, these children are often taller than their peers, look more mature and are expected to act accordingly. Girls are embarrassed by breast development and pubic hair while boys are embarrassed by the enlargement of their phallus, scrotum and the development of pubic hair. As these children are often quite young it is difficult for them to understand why they are different from their friends. Some children, boys specifically, exhibit precocious behaviour which is extremely distressing for their parents and requires behaviour modification techniques. It is important to explain that the changes are normal but are occurring at an earlier age. Treatment may be instigated to temporarily delay puberty until a more appropriate psychological age, especially if there has been a progression in skeletal age which is jeopardising final stature.

Nursing assessment includes observation of an increased growth rate, the signs of secondary sexual development such as breast development and onset of menses in girls and phallic and scrotal enlargement in boys. These children are often emotionally immature. They will have an advanced skeletal age greater than their height age. Serum gonadotrophin, adrenal androgen and urinary gonadotrophin levels are elevated. In girls a pelvic ultrasound will reveal ovarian leuteal cysts and uterine enlargement. If there is no definable cause for the precocity, a CT scan of the brain and adrenal glands is undertaken. The underlying cause must be defined and treated.

Nursing interventions aim to assist the child and parents in understanding the pathophysiology of the disorder and subsequently coming to terms with it. Education is the primary role of the nurse, who provides an explanation of all procedures and treatment regimens. The nurse is responsible for conducting clinical investigations such as gondadotrophin releasing hormone (GNRH) stimulation tests, which will diagnose central precocity, and are used to assess the patient's response to treatment. Reassurance and a positive approach will enhance patient and parental acceptance of these procedures. The nurse will be required to teach the child and parents on how to administer the subcutaneous injections of LH-RH analogue used to treat central precocious puberty. These injections are given twice daily in order to inhibit the pulsatility of LH and FSH which stimulate the gonadal axis. Monthly depot preparations are now being used successfully.

Premature thelarche

It is important to distinguish the breast development of precocious puberty from premature thelarche, which commonly occurs around 1 and 2 years of age.

Premature thelarche is caused by an unusually high sensitivity to circulating oestrogen levels or the ingestion of exogenous oestrogen. The breast development is usually bilateral without nipple enlargement and may persist for some months. Rapid growth, bone age advancement and menses however, do not occur. Extensive investigations are not warranted and puberty occurs at the normal time. Parents are usually reassured when the details of premature thelarche are fully explained.[1,7,30,31]

Premature adrenarche

This is the premature development of pubic hair occurring in both sexes at any age prior to the onset of puberty. It is a common feature in one-third of organically brain-damaged children. This is thought to be caused by an increase in adrenal androgens in children who otherwise have normal biochemical parameters. True virilisation does not occur and the children are of normal stature with an appropriate bone age. It is important that the nurse reassure the family and explain the disorder to them.[1,7,30,31]

Metabolic Disorders

INBORN ERRORS

Metabolic acidosis is the excess accumulation of hydrogen ions and a deficit of base (bicarbonate).[4] In infancy, it may indicate one of the following inborn errors of metabolism: organic acidaemias of lipid or amino acid; lactic acidosis; glucogenesis; or gluconeogenic defects. These errors of metabolism are often lethal in the neonatal period. Inborn errors of metabolism are caused by disturbances in the complex biochemical pathways causing abnormal metabolites to accumulate in the blood, tissues or urine. The error is usually autosomal recessive and, less frequently, X-linked.[30]

Common disorders are defects in the urea cycle (hyperammonaemia), or in amino acid, carbohydrate and lipid metabolism and organic acidaemias which present with symptoms that are both acute and overwhelming. Inborn errors are diagnosed by finding increased levels of abnormal substrates (e.g., phenylalanine), or decreased levels of normal products in the blood and urine.[7] A family history of an unexplained death of a sibling or parental consanguinity should alert one to the possibility of a metabolic derangement. Early diagnosis is critical in preventing mental retardation from the accumulation of such toxic substrates.

Inborn errors are extremely rare. The most common ones seen are phenylketonuria, galactosaemia, methylmalonic aciduria, maple syrup urine disease, tyrosinaemia, acteyl-COa, multiple carboxylase deficiency and lysosomal enzyme deficiency.

Nursing assessment in severe cases will reveal a newborn with a history of poor feeding, irritability, Kussmaul respirations, vomiting and drowsiness. There will be an altered neurological status, hypotonia and apnoea with tachycardia related to the encephalopathy. Convulsions occur and there is often hypoglycaemia and hypocalcaemia. The signs are evident soon after birth and usually present following a period of normal behaviour and feeding.[7] Deterioration is rapid with the child appearing septic with persistent jaundice and dehydration. An abnormal urinary odour is a common feature and has been described as musty or mousy, or having the odour of maple syrup, sweaty feet, cabbage or rotting fish. If undiagnosed and untreated, these disorders can lead to coma and death. Older children will present with failure to thrive and physical, intellectual and developmental abnormalities.

Nursing intervention involves careful assessment of the clinical situation. Instigation of emergency measures such as maintenance of the airway, respirations and circulation are the immediate priorities of care. Fluid and electrolyte replacement, which will include intravenous glucose to maintain normoglycaemia, is commenced. If the child becomes comatosed the nurse assists with peritoneal dialysis or haemodialysis, which are used to decrease the level of toxic substrates in the body. Sodium bicarbonate is used to correct the metabolic acidosis. Treatment aims to alleviate substrate accumulation and replace missing substrates.[30]

Significant emotional support and explanation is required for the parents of such a child due to the nature of the disorder and its abrupt onset. Education of the parents about the proper dietary management is required.

OBESITY

Obesity is defined as a body weight at least 20% greater than the normal range for age.[1,4,30] It is said to be an imbalance between energy intake and energy expenditure, the individual's metabolic rate,[30,31] and frequently involves more than just overeating. Genetics determine the number of fat cells in the body.

Organic obesity is associated with specific endocrine conditions such as growth hormone deficiency, hypothyroidism, hypothalamic pituitary tumours, Cushing syndrome and pseudohypoparathyroidism. These conditions are associated with minor obesity and can be distinguished by their other characteristics. When associated with tall stature, obesity is often the result of hyperinsulinism or hypothalamic anomalies. Prader-Willi-Labhart syndrome is diagnosed by the presence of obesity, insatiable hunger, short stature, delayed puberty, hypotonia, mental retardation, almond-shaped eyes and small hands and feet with an advanced bone age. Psychotherapy and behaviour modification is the mode of treatment used in these cases.[30]

Exogenous obesity is associated with advanced skeletal maturation, early puberty and tall stature during childhood but with no increase in final stature. It relates to dietary intake and reduced activity levels with, for example: intake of foods high in refined sugar and fat content; parental anxiety and over-nurturing with over-feeding; and sedentary habits.[31] Lipomastia is a common feature in boys.[1] This form of obesity has associated medical risks such as the development of hypertension, hyperlipidaemia, cerebral vascular accidents, diabetes mellitus, slipped femoral epiphysis and distorted peer relations.[31] The prognosis for losing weight and maintaining a normal weight is poor. It has been shown that if an individual enters puberty obese, there is a 4:1 chance against achieving a weight within the normal range. If an individual leaves puberty obese, the chance is 28:1.[31]

Self-perception of bodyweight varies according to social class, educational level and ethnic group. Society as a whole is influenced by the media, which shapes our view of obesity. They portray obese people as lazy, untidy and intellectually impaired. Such images contribute to feelings of social isolation and poor self-image, and often predispose the child to depression.

Nursing assessment reveals a child overweight in appearance. Obesity is confirmed when the weight is compared with the population standards for age. The child may have difficulties undertaking physical acitivities and will often complain about being teased at school. A dietary history will detail the type and quantities of food and fluids consumed, although the quantities are often underestimated.

Nursing intervention will involve counselling as a first priority for dysfunctional families. Psychotherapy for the child and family is advised before attempts are made to encourage dietary restrictions and exercise. It is essential for the whole family to adhere to the dietary advice so that the child will not feel singled out. For a young child, parental supervision is essential. The nurse must reassure the child, encourage individuality, promote the child's positive aspects and praise achievements. Families may be referred to a dietitian for education about healthy foods and dietary tactics. Restricted access to school tuckshops may be of some help.

Endocrine Emergencies

Disorders with acute presentations will include hypoglycaemia, hyperglycaemia, hypoadrenal crisis, hypocalcaemia, hypercalcaemia, thyrotoxic crisis, ambiguous genitalia and metabolic disorders.

NURSING ASSESSMENT

The initial presentation in most children will be an altered neurological status. Drowsiness, lethargy, central nervous system or neuromuscular irritability, behaviour and visual disturbances in the older child, can progress to feeding difficulties, respiratory distress, apnoea, hypothermia or hyperthermia, bradycardia, tachycardia, fluid imbalance, hypoglycaemia, metabolic acidosis, seizures, coma and death.[31]

Emergency nursing interventions include the maintenance of airway and respirations, the management of convulsions and the monitoring of vital signs and hydration through careful observation of mucous membranes, skin turgor and fluid balance. It is vital that a blood sample be taken immediately before any biochemical treatment. This is essential in diagnosing the metabolic condition. The analysis will include blood sugar, biochemistry, a metabolic screen and adrenal hormones. The nurse will provide emotional support and explanation of all procedures as soon as possible to the child and parents.

HYPOGLYCAEMIA

Hypoglycaemia is the failure to maintain a blood glucose level greater than 3.5 mmol/L in a fasting state for prolonged periods of time. Altered metabolism, impaired neurological status and respiratory function occur with the presence of hypoglycaemia and metabolic acidosis. Hypoglycaemia may be caused by intrauterine growth retardation, sepsis, hypothermia, metabolic disorders, hypopituitarism, adrenocortical insufficiency, malnutrition and hyperinsulinism. Newborn babies of diabetic mothers are prone to rebound hypoglycaemia from hyperinsulinism which occurs because of exposure *in utero* to high levels of circulating glucose, which crosses the placenta and stimulates the fetal pancreas to excrete excessive amount of insulin. This often lasts for a few days after birth.[3,30,31,35]

Nursing assessment in the newborn will reveal drowsiness and seizures together with feeding difficulties, pallor, mottling, apnoea, and tachycardia. In children, behaviour disturbances and pallor are observed and can be followed by seizures. The adolescent will present with sweatiness, shakiness, tachycardia, visual disturbances and irritability.[2–4,7]

Persistent hypoglycaemia in the newborn may be a clinical manifestation of hypopituitarism. In the neonate, inborn errors of metabolism may cause hypoglycaemia and acidosis. As the pH falls there will be disturbances in vital signs with central nervous system depression and irritability occurring because of an inability of the lungs and kidneys to compensate for the accumulation of excess hydrogen ions in the body.[2–4,7]

Nursing interventions aim to contribute to the alleviation of neurological, respiratory and metabolic disturbances through the correction of hypoglycaemia and acidosis and the prevention of a seizure. Maintenance of an adequate caloric intake and avoiding long periods of fasting will prevent hypoglycaemia. Treatment for hypoglycaemia includes the oral administration of sweet liquids if the patient is conscious. The physician is notified to supervise further emergency interventions. In the extreme situation when there is no intravenous access and no medical support, 10 mL of 50% dextrose may be cautiously administered by dribbling small amounts onto the mucous membrane of the mouth in the unconscious patient, after first ensuring that the child is lying on their side. The nurse aims to prevent aspiration while achieving some absorption of necessary carbohydrate. The dextrose may also be administered via a nasogastric tube.

If a seizure is imminent, the maintenance of airway, the circulation and breathing are priorites. Cardiopulmonary resuscitation is commenced if required. Glucagon may be administered intramuscularly at a dose of 0.03 mg/kg[1] in patients who do not have an intravenous line but adequate glycogen stores. Ideally, 10% glucose should slowly be administered intravenously. A commonly used dose is 2 mL/kg of bodyweight.[7] Cannula patency must be ensured as the hypertonic nature of the infusion may cause an inflammatory response in the vein, and tissue damage if it extravasates. The child's vital signs

Table 7.17 Signs and symptoms of hypoglycaemia at different ages

Newborn	Infancy	Childhood
persistent hypoglycaemia apnoea/cyanosis drowsiness	apnoea cyanosis respiratory distress irritability drowsiness hypotonia poor feeding low temperature myoclonic jerks convulsions sweaty, clammy	inattention staring strabismus lethargy somnolence difficult behaviour ravenous appetite pallor fatigue

Adapted from Aynsely-Green in Brook 1989, Mott S et al 1990, Lavin N 1986, Merenstein GB 1991

and blood sugar levels must be frequently monitored. Following treatment, the blood sugar and vital signs will stabilise and return to normal. A complete assessment is carried out to determine the cause and a thorough explanation and reassurance to the parents is required. They need to be able to demonstrate an understanding of the cause of the hypoglycaemia in order to prevent its recurrence and carry out emergency management. **Hyperglycaemia** with development of ketoacidosis is associated with metabolic diseases, such as diabetes mellitus, and is discussed under that section.

HYPOADRENAL CRISIS

Hypoadrenal crisis is the inability of the body to respond to stressful situations (e.g., infection, surgical procedures, accidents or prolonged periods of fasting) due to impaired adrenal function and an inability to produce cortisol. Children with panhypopituitarism, congenital adrenal hyperplasia, and those who have adrenal suppression because of pharmacological doses of glucocorticoids are susceptible.[1-3,7,31]

Nursing assessment will reveal symptoms of hypoglycaemia, hypovolaemic shock, pallor, sweatiness, hypotension, irritability, tachycardia, hypotension leading to unconsciousness and coma. There is altered central nervous system function because of the altered metabolism of glucose and electrolytes. Hypoglycaemia and hypotension occur because of the low cortisol production.

Nursing intervention involves administering hydrocortisone 50 to 100 mg intramuscularly in acute situations.[1] An intravenous line must be inserted as soon as possible and immediate treatment of hypoglycaemia is achieved by administering 25% glucose intravenously, which is subsequently reduced to 5 to 10% for maintenance. An adequate fluid and electrolyte balance is maintained. Hydrocortisone is added to the intravenous infusion at a dose 10 times the maintenance dose, divided over a 24-hour period.[33] Hypovolaemic shock is treated with intravenous fluid and electrolyte replacement regimens.[31] Monitoring of vital signs for a fall in blood pressure and evidence of further hypoglycaemia is essential.

In the long term, intervention aims to prevent future adrenal crises by teaching parents how to predict, and for the most part prevent, situations which could lead to an adrenal crisis such as fevers, intercurrent illnesses, excessive periods of fasting, omitting or forgetting medications and stressful situations such as operative procedures and anaesthesia. Ensuring that medications are administered correctly according to the appropriate schedule is of prime importance. The nurse instructs the parents in the administration of intramuscular hydrocortisone to be given by them in emergency situations. They are instructed that if their child is unwell, and they are unable to reach their doctor, they should administer the dosage and take the child to hospital immediately. This is critical and may save the child's life.

It is important that the parents are able to demonstrate knowledge about the disorder and understand how essential it is to the child that extra hydrocortisone is administered during periods of illness. A 'Medi Alert' bracelet should always be worn inscribed with the following instructions: name; hospital; phone and ID number; adrenocortical insufficiency; hydrocortisone 100 mg by injection in emergency, accident or illness.

It is imperative that the nurse ensures that a child who suffers from adrenal insufficiency is carefully observed during stressful situations. Education of the parents about this factor is critical. If the child becomes unwell at home, the parents should report any condition which alters the child's usual state of health by contacting the doctor or nurse specialist who is familiar with the patient's care and know to give emergency treatment as required. Glucocorticoid therapy is not arbitrarily changed, however, the emergency dose is promptly given if there is doubt about the child's health status.

Children who have adrenocortical insufficiency who require anaesthesia and surgery should receive hydrocortisone cover between 3 and 10 times their normal maintenance dose. The daily dose is given in a continuous infusion over a 24-hour period in a dextrose and saline solution. This should commence with fasting and continue postoperatively until after the first oral dose of hydrocortisone and fluids are tolerated. Stress doses of hydrocortisone should be given for approximately 3 days after surgery.

AMBIGUOUS GENITALIA

A child born with ambigious genitalia creates a significant psychosocial emergency for the parents who are unable to distinguish the gender of their child by its appearance. This situation needs to be handled in a very sensitive manner and by experienced staff. Ambiguous genitalia are caused by an inborn error of steroidogenesis or sex chromosome disorder which has prevented sexual differentiation.[1]

Nursing assessment will immediately reveal ambigious genitalia, which creates an emotional crisis for the parents. An adrenal crisis may also develop within 5 to 7 days, because of an inability of the infant to produce adequate levels of cortisol and aldosterone.

Nursing interventions are directed toward the psychological and emotional distress of the parents in the delivery suite at the appearance of the ambiguous genitalia. These parents require special consideration. Immediate discussion with the parents is encouraged and explanations must be given about the disorder together with reassurance that the gender will be determined within the shortest possible time, hopefully within 24 hours as this is critical to parental acceptance of the baby. A blood test is taken for chromosome estimation, biochemical and hormonal screening. If there is a diagnosis of congenital adrenal hyperplasia, treatment must be instigated as soon as possible to prevent an adrenal crisis. Treatment is outlined under the section on adrenal hypofunction.

A physician with relevant expertise should make the gender assignment and this is done in conjunction with the parents. Once this is made, the nurse must evaluate whether there is parental acceptance. Encouraging the parents to air their feelings is important as they need to feel comfortable with the child's gender. Nursing interventions aim to see the parents demonstrating a loving and caring attitude to the baby before discharge, which is a positive indication that rearing will be appropriate for the assigned gender.

The nurse should listen to the needs of the parents. Reassurance that the gender assignment will allow for normal sexual function and fertility is extremely important, and that cosmetic reconstructive surgery will be undertaken as soon as possible. This includes a reduction of the clitoral size in girls. Surgical correction of labial fusion and urogenital-sinus may require several operations when the child is older. The nurse should clarify any concerns of the parents with the physician. Counselling is encouraged as it is critical for the parents to be absolutely happy with the gender assignment.

Prior to the gender assignment, the nurse will make sure that the child is called 'baby and surname' and discourage any attempts by the staff and parents to make a gender assignment on the appearance of the external genitalia. To prevent confusion for the parents, a limited number of staff should be allocated to care for the parents and child. A case conference is held and the staff agree on what is to be said to the parents. This allows for consistency of information and prevents confusion.

PHAEOCHROMOCYTOMA

Phaeochromocytoma is a tumour of the adrenal medulla and is extremely rare in children. It causes hyperfunctioning of the adrenal gland and excessive production of adrenaline and noradrenaline.

Nursing assessment reveals sudden episodes of anxiety with tachycardia, flushing, sweating and palpitations.[1] Other symtoms and signs include headaches, dizziness, nausea, dilated pupils and blurred vision, persistent hypertension, discomfort from heat, precordial and abdominal pain and weight loss. There is papilloedema, retinopathy, and cardiac enlargement due to the excessive secretion of adrenaline and/or noradrenaline. Investigative findings reveal raised serum and urinary catecholamines. The kidneys are displaced on radiological examination.[1,31]

Nursing intervention includes caring for these patients in a quiet and cool environment, monitoring vital signs, especially the blood pressure, in case of a hypertensive crisis, administering medications to reduce hypertension and providing explanation and support for the child and family. Surgical removal of the tumour is the treatment of choice once blood pressure can be controlled with alpha-adrenergic (phenoxybenzamine) and beta-adrenergic (propranalol) medications given consecutively.[1,31] These patients need close supervison before and after surgery.

THYROTOXIC CRISIS

Thyrotoxic crisis is extremely rare and occurs usually because of inadequate management and poor patient compliance. Precipitating factors other than poor compliance are infection, surgery, and diabetic ketoacidosis.

Nursing assessment reveals signs of fever, sweating, tachycardia, decreased mental functioning, confusion and coma.

Nursing intervention includes making the patient comfortable, monitoring vital signs and administering medications as prescibed. Medical treatment includes propranalol to control tachycardia, digoxin for heart failure, dexamethasone to reduce T3 levels, intravenous sodium iodide to decrease T4, and propylthiouracil (PTU) to block organ-ification of iodine.[1]

Clinical Investigations of Endocrine Function

Clinical investigation in children usually involves the collection of multiple blood samples for hormonal or biochemical parameters to assess either endocrine or metabolic function. Most of these tests are stimulation tests, whereby a drug is administered to stimulate a response from an endocrine gland. These tests can be technically difficult and should only be undertaken to provide information which is unobtainable through clinical assessment or baseline sampling. It is imperative that investigations be carried out by experienced paediatric staff skilled in such procedures. This will prevent the child from being subjected to repeated, unnecessary and unpleasant procedures.

Preparation of the patient and family is essential for the successful outcome of a procedure. The child should be in a normal state of health. The investigation should be postponed if the child is unwell or recovering from a recent illness. The nurse will enquire about regular medications such as anticonvulsants or thyroid hormone, or special diets which may interfere with the results of the investigations.

Children should fast overnight, unless there is a concern about dehydration or hypoglycaemia. Because of these factors the fasting period is reduced to between 4 and 6 hours in small infants. Fasting provides a status of equilibrium on which all tests can be compared.

Testing is commenced at a set time following an overnight fast. An intravenous cannula is inserted to allow blood to be taken. Some investigations require insertion of the cannula the evening before to prevent a stress response on the morning of the test. Stress may influence the normal physiological production of growth hormone and cortisol. Reliable intravenous access should be selected, usually the antecubital fossa. A 22-gauge cannula is inserted and connected to a Luer-lock short extension tube, 3-way tap and syringe for flushing between sampling. A solution of heparinised saline is commonly used to keep the vein patent. Intravenous dextrose is not used as it will distort the results. Fluid balance and vital signs should be strictly monitored.

For accurate results, preparation is essential so that samples are collected at the correct time intervals. Blood tubes should be labelled and request forms signed. Total circulating blood volumes should be calculated and the minimum volumes required for the tests established with the laboratory. This alerts the laboratory to take extra care in handling these small volumes. The sampling procedure should be painless for the child and blood easily obtained to prevent haemolysis of the sample. The heparinised saline used for flushing is cleared from the sampling line before the sample is taken and the line flushed immediately after sampling. No child should be subjected to unnecessary and repeated venepuncture for an investigation. Topical local anaesthetic cream (Emla) should be applied for 1 hour prior to the insertion of a cannula and left for the duration of any investigation requiring more than one sample. A haemoglobin level should be taken at the beginning and end of the procedure and result obtained before discharge.

Nursing interventions include explanation of all procedures to be undertaken. The nurse specialist will discuss with the parents the arrangements for the admission and supply a list of instructions on fasting times and information about the testing procedures. Such details are essential to the success of the procedure. The nurse specialist is responsible for calculating the blood volume, coordinating the procedure and instructing the laboratory accordingly. Vital signs must be monitored. The resuscitation equipment is checked and ready for any untoward reaction such as anaphalaxis, hypoglycaemia or accidental blood loss.

NURSING IMPLICATIONS

The nurse must remain impartial, understanding and provide advocacy in a firm and guiding manner. Informal interaction will be beneficial in the assessment of potential problems. It is important that the nurse specialist listens and understands the patient and the parents' feelings of anxiety about the long-term prospects of their child and his or her disease. It is particularly important that parents are involved in the long-term planning and management for their child. They are, of course, the ones who best know their child.

Adequate education and support by the nurse will alleviate parental anxiety and enhance parental understanding and acceptance of the disorder. This will in turn influence the child's perception of his or her disorder. Such understanding and acceptance facilitates compliance with the daily administration and taking of medications and promotes normal physical and psychological growth and development of the child.

Frequent visits to the doctor are necessary and mean that the school and home routines are disrupted. Adequate education and explanation about the reasons for the follow-up and about specific problems to both parents and teachers is important in achieving a positive outcome for these children.

Nursing an infant, child or adolescent with a neuroendocrine disorder can be extremely difficult. Many signs and symptoms exhibited could be mistaken for another disorder. The child with an endocrine disorder will require long-term therapy and follow-up. A patient in good control of his disorder will grow and develop normally. Poor or rapid growth is a critical indicator for the nurse or physician that the well-being of the child is threatened. The nurse is in the unique position to become a friend and confidant to the child and family and is therefore more able to assess, diagnose and evaluate treatment outcomes.

REFERENCES

1. Styne DM. *Pediatric endocrinology for the house officer*. Baltimore: Williams and Wilkins, 1988.
2. Wilson JD, Foster DW, eds. *Williams textbook of endocrinology*. 8th ed. Philadelphia: Saunders, 1992.
3. Mott SR, James SR, Sperhac AM. *Nursing care of children and their families*. 2nd ed. Menlo Park: Addison-Wesley, 1990.
4. Tortora GJ, Anagnostakos NJ. *Principles of anatomy and physiology*. 7th ed. New York: Harper and Row, 1993.
5. Wong DL. *Whaley and Wong's nursing care of infants and children*. 5th ed. St Louis: Mosby, 1995.
6. Hindmarsh PC, Bridges NA, Brook CDG. Wider indications for treatment with biosynthetic growth hormone in children. *Clin Endocrinol* 1991; 34: 417–427.

7.   Berham RE, Vaughan VC. *Nelson textbook of pediatrics*. 14th ed. Philadelphia: Saunders, 1992.

8.   Brook CDG. *Clinical paediatric endocrinology*. 2nd ed. Oxford: Blackwell Scientific, 1989.

9.   Lifshitz F, ed. *Pediatric endocrinology: a clinical guide*. 2nd ed. New York: Marcel Dekker, 1990.

10. Kaplan SA. *Clinical pediatric endocrinology*. Philadelphia: Saunders, 1990.

11. Gordon M, Crouthamel C, Post E, Richman R. Psychosocial aspects of constitutional short stature: social competence, behaviour problems, self-esteem, and family functioning. *J Pediatr* 1982; 101: 477–480.

12. Kelnar CJH. Pride and prejudice — stature in perspective. *Acta Paediatr Scand* 1990; 370 (Suppl): 5–15.

13. Law CM. The disability of short stature. *Arch Dis Childh* 1987; 62: 855–859.

14. Seigel PT, Clopper R, Stablier B. Psychological impact of short stature. *Acta Paediatr Scand* 1991; 377 (Suppl): 14–18.

15. Skuse D. Annotation. The psychological consequences of being small. *J Child Psychiat* 1987; 28: 641–650.

16. Allen DB, Fost NC. Growth hormone therapy for short stature: panacea or Pandora's box? *J Pediatr* 1990; 117: 1: 16–21.

17. Benjamin M, Muyskens J, Saenger P. Short children, anxious parents: is growth hormone the answer? *The Hastings Centre Report* 1984: 5–9.

18. Bischofberger E, Gunnar D. Ethical aspects of growth hormone therapy. *Acta Paediatr Scand* 1989 362 (Suppl): 14–17.

19. Brook CDG. 1992 Who's for growth hormone. *BMJ* 304: 131–132.

20. Brook CDG, Hindmarsch PC, Healy MJR. Biosynthetic growth hormone: whom to treat? *BMJ* 1986; 293: 1185–1186.

21. Burke CW. The pituitary megatest: outdated? *Clin Endocrinol* 1992; 36: 133–134.

22. Lantos J, Seigler M, Cuttler L. Ethical issues in growth hormone treatment. *JAMA* 1989; 261: 1020–1024.

23. Lippe B. How should we test for growth hormone deficiency, and whom should we treat? *J Pediatr* 1989; 115: 585–587.

24. Lippe B, Frasier D. The Rational Use of Growth Hormone in Childhood. Clincial review 11. *J Clin Endocrinol Metabolism* 1990; 71: 269–273.

25. Milner RDG. Which children should have growth hormone therapy? *Lancet* 1986; 1: 483–485.

26. Parvord SR, Girach A, Price DE, Absolom SR, Falconer-Smith J, Howlett TA. Retropsective audit of the combined pituitary function test, using the insulin stress test, TRH and GNRH in a district laboratory. *Clin Endocrinol* 1992; 36: 135–139.

27. Shah A, Stanhope R, Matthew D. Hazards of pharmacological tests of growth hormone secretion in childhood. *BMJ* 1992; 304: 173–174.

28. Underwood LE, Rieser PA. Is it ethical to treat healthy short children with growth hormone? *Acta Paediatr Scand* 1989; 362 (Suppl): 1–6.

29. Warne GL. Contemporary issues in the use of growth hormone. [Annotation] *J Paediatr Child Health* 1990; 26: 122–123.

30. Lavin N, ed. *Manual of endocrinology and metabolism*. Boston: Little Brown, 1986.

31. Merenstein GB, Kaplan DW, Rosenberg AA. *Silver Kempe Bruyn & Fulginiti's Handbook of paediatrics*. Connecticut: Appleton Lange, 1991.

32. Robinson MJ. *Practical paediatrics*. 2nd ed. Melbourne: Churchill Livingstone, 1990: 469.

33. Chrousos GP. Adrenal insufficiency. *In: A current review of pediatric endocrinology*. Proceedings, Lawson Wilkins Pediatric Endocrinology Society Conference, 28 April–2 May, Washington, 1993: 73–83.

34. Pediatric Endocrine Nurses Society. *Pediatric endocrinology nursing resource manual*. USA: Pediatric Endocrine Nurses Society, 1992.

35. Ansley-Green A. Hypoglycaema. *In:* Brook CDG. *Clinical paediatric endocrinology*. 2nd ed. Oxford: Blackwell Scientific, 1989.

BIBLIOGRAPHY

Anderson DC. Physiology of human fetal sex differentiation. *In:* Brook CDG. *Clinical paediatric endocrinology.* 2nd ed. Oxford: Blackwell Scientific, 1989.

Tortora GJ, Anagnostakos NJ. *Principles of anatomy and physiology.* 5th ed. New York: Harper and Row, 1987.

Hamilton HK. *Nurse's reference library, diseases.* Nursing Books 85. Pennsylvania: Springhouse, 1985.

Emans SJH, Goldstein DP. *Pediatric and adolescent gynaecology.* Boston: Little Brown, 1990.

Hinwood BG. *Science for the health team.* Australia: Croom Helm, 1987.

Hurwitz LS. Nursing implications of selected pediatric endocrine problems. *Nursing Clin North Am* 1980; 15: 525– 534.

James SR, Mott SR. *Child health nursing. Essential Care for children and families.* Addison-Wesley: California, 1988.

Sanford SJ. Dysfunction of the adrenal gland: physiologic considerations and nursing problems. *Nursing Clin North Am* 1980; 15: 481– 498.

Savage MO. Clinical aspects of intersex. *In:* Brook CDG. *Clinical paediatric endocrinology.* 2nd ed. Oxford: Blackwell Scientific, 1989.

Shearman RP. *Clinical reproductive endocinology.* Edinburgh: Churchill Livingstone, 1985.

Solomon BL. The hypothalamus and the pituitary gland: an overview. *Nursing Clin North Am* 1980; 15: 435– 451.

Styne DM. The testes: disorders of sexual differention and puberty. *In:* Brook CDG. *Clinical paediatric endocrinology.* 2nd ed. Oxford: Blackwell Scientific, 1989: 367 397.

Underwood LE, Van Wyk JJ. Normal and aberrant growth. *In:* Wilson JD, Foster DW, eds. *Williams textbook of endocrinology.* 8th ed. Philadelphia: Saunders, 1992: 1079–1138.

Wake MM, Brensinger JF. The nurse's role in hypothyroidism. *Nursing Clin North Am* 1980; 15: 453–467.

Disturbances in Muscular Function

Robyn Pedersen

Duchenne Muscular Dystrophy

Muscular dystrophy is a general term used for a group of chronic, hereditary diseases that are characterised by progressive degeneration and weakness of voluntary muscles. The different types of muscular dystrophy vary in the age when muscle wasting becomes apparent and in the muscle groups first affected.[1] Duchenne muscular dystrophy is the most common form seen in childhood and only occurs in boys.

Duchenne muscular dystrophy is an X-linked recessive hereditary disease. There is a gradual deterioration of all skeletal muscles due to the lack of the protein, dystrophin, in the muscles. At this stage there is no cure and quality of life is an important issue. An electric wheelchair is required for mobility between the ages of 8 and 12 years. From the age of 12 most of the boys need assistance with daily living activities, progressing to total dependence on carers. The most common cause of death is by respiratory failure at an average age of 20 years.

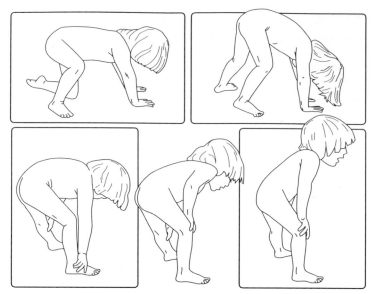

Figure 7.19 Gower's sign. This method of getting off the floor is an important diagnostic tool. (Medical Illustrations, Prince of Wales Hospital, Sydney)

The nursing role during the progression of the disease consists largely of supporting parents and meeting the needs of the affected boys. The nurse needs to be aware of the difficulties faced by the parents and child when a child has a long-term degenerative hereditary disease. Some of these difficulties are viewed differently by the boy and his parents. This factor needs to be considered by the nurse in the supporting role, and respect for both views acknowledged. The parents and child have different issues to confront as the boy progresses through his lifespan development.

INITIAL PRESENTATION

Assessment

The child is most likely to present for assessment at approximately 3 to 4 years of age. The child with Duchenne muscular dystrophy has a wide-based, waddling gait, is unable to hop or run and has difficulty with stairs. He has difficulty getting up from the floor and does so by climbing up his legs. This is known as Gower's sign (**Figure 7.19**). The child falls more than expected and, in comparison with boys of the same age, physical activity is impaired. He has prominent calves and possible stiffness at the ankle joints due to tight Achilles tendons (**Table 7.18**). These signs may be subtle at an early age.

Diagnostic assessment

Blood is taken for a serum creatine kinase (CK) level estimation (this enzyme is a product of muscle breakdown) and to screen for a deletion in the dystrophin gene. The child is admitted to hospital for a muscle biopsy in order to measure the dystrophin level in the muscle. The nurse needs to be supportive of the parents at the time of diagnosis because usually they are extremely anxious. All boys not walking by 18 months, and/or those who

Table 7.18 Duchenne muscular dystrophy. A comparison of motor and musculosk
function by age of boys with Duchenne muscular dystrophy

Nursing assessment	Age	Motor	Musculoskeletal
Presentation	Generally 3–4 years	• wide based waddling gait • unable to hop • does not run • difficulty in getting off the floor — uses a Gower's sign • where the child climbs up his legs to get up (Fig 7.19) • diffculty with steps • falling more than expected • impaired physical activity compared to boys of the same age.	• prominent calves • possible stiffness at ankle joints due to tight Achilles tendons
From presentation to use of wheelchair	Ability to walk is lost between 8–12 years	• increasing weakness of all muscles, especially weight bearing muscles • centre of gravity changing producing an unsteady gait as he walk more on his toes with increasing lordosis • easily knocked over in the school playground due to the shift in his centre of gravity • the ability to walk is lost between 8–12 years	• increasing tightness of Achilles tendons
Adolescence	13 years and upwards	• increasing weakness of all skeletal muscles including those in his arms • lose fine motor movements as well • help required for all activities of daily living — including hygiene, eating and drinking, moving in bed or wheelchair	• downward, inverted positions of feel • scoliosis may be a problem during growth spurt • weak respiratory muscles • possible cardiac problems • constipation may be a problem

have developmental delay of undetermined cause, should have a serum creatine kinase estimation.

Special needs of the parents and child

Genetic counselling is a must for the nuclear and the extended family. Because Duchenne muscular dystrophy is an X-linked recessive disease, healthy carrier females are at risk of having affected boys. Female siblings need special attention for genetic counselling, including testing for carrier status, especially in their middle teens when they are beginning to think about their prospects for marriage and a family. Parents are introduced to the support group run by the Muscular Dystrophy Association and/or another family who has a son with Duchenne muscular dystrophy.

Maintenance of activity is extremely important for the affected boy, as prolonged bedrest tends to exacerbate weakness. Contractures become a problem so physiotherapy is given to maintain flexibility. Stretching the Achilles tendons is particularly important.

THE CHILD WITH DUCHENNE MUSCULAR DYSTROPHY

Assessment

The boy experiences increasing weakness of all muscles, especially the weight-bearing muscles. He walks more on his toes with increasing lordosis and, due to the shift in his centre of gravity, he is easily knocked over in the school playground. He will experience increasing tightness of his Achilles tendons. The ability to walk is lost between 8 and 12 years of age.

Special needs of the child

The child must be informed about the disease at a level appropriate to his age. Information is provided either by his parents or the clinician, or both.

A specialist school counsellor is involved for correct educational placement for both physical access and intellectual ability. Approximately 20% of the boys have an intellectual disability. Intellectual capacity, however, does not alter during the disease process.[2] Learning to use a computer at this time is desirable as the boy will become slower at writing over time. There can be behavioural problems at school at this time as the boy proceeds to full use of a wheelchair.

Initially, a manual wheelchair is used for excursions at school or on family outings. The boy gradually progresses to full use of an electric wheelchair. The electric wheelchair is constructed to fit the individual boy and to negotiate the terrain that he usually uses. It may have central controls to maintain an erect posture in an attempt to prevent scoliosis for as long as possible. An electric wheelchair promotes independence and helps the boy to keep up with his peers. The use of a standing frame helps to maintain correct posture once a boy is using a wheelchair continuously. Some boys like to stand in a standing frame for short periods each day using straps across the chest and legs to prevent them from falling. A table is attached so that the boy can stand in class and still do his school work or, if at home, can watch television, play games or do his homework.

Lifting a boy with Duchenne muscular dystrophy is not like lifting other patients. If a child with Duchenne muscular dystrophy is lifted in the usual manner for a child (i.e., by placing the lifter's hands under the axilla) he will slip through the lifter's hands and he is likely to be dropped. This is due to poor muscle tone. The best way to lift a patient with Duchenne muscular dystrophy is to cross his arms across his chest and thread your arms under his shoulders and over his forearms (**Figure 7.20**).

Physiotherapy

The use of stretching exercises and activities to maintain muscle length and flexibility are continued as before, but with an increased focus on wrists and finger joints. Sometimes orthoses are used if the boy wishes. The boy uses an electric wheelchair so he can keep

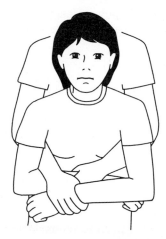

Figure 7.20 Method best used to lift boys with Duchenne muscular dystrophy.
(Medical Illustrations, Prince of Wales Hospital, Sydney)

up with his peers and to maintain independence in mobility. Quality of life and independence are the main issues. Learning to play a wind instrument may help with respiratory function.

Occupational therapy

The occupational therapist assesses the home and school and advises on appropriate equipment such as electric wheelchair, shower chair, hoists and ramps. Advice is also provided on the best way to transport the boy and wheelchair in a van, including the use of hoists, ramps and wheelchair restraints. An occupational therapist advises parents, teachers and peers about expectations and appropriate ways of helping. This promotes understanding of the disease process for all those who are involved with the child's everyday activities.

Special needs of parents

Often it is more difficult for the parents than the child to accept a wheelchair as the wheelchair is a reminder that the child's condition is deteriorating. Counselling helps the parents express their grief for the child's further loss of function. Assistance to the parents and siblings by appropriate professionals should be available on an ongoing basis. A parent support group is offered by the Muscular Dystrophy Association.

THE ADOLESCENT WITH DUCHENNE MUSCULAR DYSTROPHY

Assessment

All skeletal muscles, including arm muscles, become progressively weaker during adolescence. Fine motor movements also deteriorate. The child will require help for all activities of daily living including hygiene, eating and drinking, moving in bed or in the wheelchair. His feet develop a downward, inverted position. Scoliosis may be a problem during the growth spurt. As mobility and muscle power decrease, constipation may become a problem. Respiratory muscles become weaker and cardiac problems may develop.

Special needs of the adolescent

Appropriate schooling at this time is important for future employment. As the ability to write quickly, and therefore to keep pace, decreases it becomes important for the boy to have access to a computer, both at home and at school. As peers are generally more active and have no barriers to their movements a boy with Duchenne muscular dystrophy may find he is left out of their activities. He may feel rejected and alone. Support and counselling regarding body image, sexuality and peer interaction may be needed. Issues relating to employment and access to the workplace are important. Allowing the boy his independence and the freedom to make his own decisions is important, but often difficult for parents. Adolescence is the time when most boys start to ask questions about their lifespan and death, so arrangements need to be made so he can talk to the appropriate professionals and have ongoing counselling if required.

Nursing

It may be necessary for the boy to have surgery to straighten his feet. Surgery may also be necessary to correct scoliosis. Because scoliosis can compromise respiratory function it is corrected by spinal fusion. Rods are inserted to immobilise the spine while it fuses. During hospitalisation the boy needs to maintain control over his life, regardless of his age, by being part of the decision making for his care.

Postoperative care

The assistance that is required to help the boy maintain control needs to be discussed with him on admission. He is unable to move, to pull sheets or blankets up, to turn in bed, or even to scratch his nose. He has to ask for everything to be done for him. The boy must be turned several times during the night and frequent change of position is required during the day as he is unable to move any part of himself to relieve pressure. He is able to feel pain and discomfort as normal. He requires help to drink or eat as he cannot move his arms. Help is needed with all aspects of hygiene including teeth cleaning. Constipation can be a problem requiring nightly aperients.

The safest way for both the patient and the nurse to lift an adolescent with Duchenne muscular dystrophy is to use a hoist. If a hoist is not available then at least 2 people are required for the lift. Reduced muscle strength and tone is such that he is unable to assist, consequently it is like lifting a rag doll.

Respiratory support

Attention to respiratory function is important and may require the use of nocturnal ventilation at home. This becomes necessary because of poor gaseous exchange during REM sleep. Progression to 24 hour ventilation occurs when the boy is unable to maintain his respiratory function unassisted during the day. The parents, assisted by a community nurse or the Home Care Service, usually care for the boy at home while he is on the ventilator.

Physiotherapy

The physiotherapist determines ventilator requirements by progressive lung function assessment. Physiotherapy to wrists and finger joints keeps them as flexible as possible and aims to prevent contractures. If contractures of the wrist or fingers develop, the boy can no longer grip adequately.

Occupational therapy

It is important that the boy be kept as comfortable as possible. Occupational therapists give advice on a suitable bed and/or mattress and various mechanical lifting devices. Wheelchair comfort, including seating, mouldings and head rest, is considered. Advice on access to the place of employment and the need for special equipment may be necessary. Information about wheelchair sports is also given.

Special needs of parents

Most families suffer from chronic grief as they watch their son and brother gradually deteriorate physically, so continued support of parents and siblings is necessary. This is usually provided by support groups, counsellors, nurses, allied health and medical staff.

REFERENCES

1. Dubowitz V. *A colour atlas of muscle disorders in childhood.* London: Wolfe Medical, 1989.
2. Emery AEH. *Duchenne muscular dystrophy.* 2nd ed. Oxford: Oxford University Press, 1993.

Disturbances in Gastrointestinal Function

Coeliac Disease

Trish Comerford and Margaret Yates

Coeliac disease is commonly referred to as a malabsorption syndrome It is characterised by abnormal intestinal mucosa resulting in a permanent intolerance of gluten. The removal of wheat, rye, barley and oats from the diet will allow regeneration of the intestinal mucosa to normal. Coeliac disease is a life-long disease which may present at any age from infancy to old age. The disease will not occur unless gluten is in the diet. Children with coeliac disease will remain sensitive to gluten throughout their life, but with the elimination of gluten from their diet, normal health can be enjoyed. Research indicates that the disease is almost exclusive to children of European ethnic origin. The disease is found in Australia, Britain, Europe and North America.[1]

NURSING ASSESSMENT

The child with coeliac disease who is admitted to hospital will often present with failure to thrive or, depending on the age of the child, a history of weight loss. The symptoms of the disease will not manifest until the child is at an age where gluten-containing solids are a regular component of the diet.

The nurse, on assessment, may find the child miserable, fretful, clingy, irritable and uncooperative. The child may be pale, malnourished, abdominally distended and have buttock and leg muscle wasting. This is due to the lack of absorption of nutrients and fats. The parents will give a history of chronic diarrhoea with stools which are characteristically pale, loose and very offensive. They may report anorexia or alternatively an enormous appetite in the child. Episodes of abdominal pain may also be a feature.

In some instances, a young child may present in coeliac crisis. The manifestations are an acute, severe episode of profuse watery diarrhoea and vomiting. This may be precipitated by a gastrointestinal infection. A protracted episode will lead to fluid depletion and electrolyte imbalance requiring fluid replacement.

MEDICAL MANAGEMENT AND INVESTIGATION

Diagnosis is dependent on demonstrating damage to the bowel lining. This is unlikely to occur after a gluten-free diet has been implemented.

Medical diagnosis is made on the results of small intestinal biopsy. There are two methods for biopsy:

- Endoscopy, where a gastroscope with a standard cup biopsy forcep, is used to obtain a sample of duodenal mucosa.
- A small capsule attached to a fine plastic tube is swallowed and passed into the small bowel. The position of the tube is monitored by low intensive organ imaging. Suction is applied to the tube gently to extract a small piece of bowel lining for biopsy.

Once a gluten-free diet has been instituted, a progress small bowel biopsy should be taken to exclude other diseases which cause damage to the lining of the bowel. Absolute assurance of the diagnosis requires proof that the recovered small bowel will again deteriorate when gluten is reintroduced to the diet. Proof of the disease by a gluten challenge biopsy will give certainty as to whether or not a gluten-free diet is a life-long necessity.

Stool collection for faecal fat may be undertaken. The withdrawal of gluten from the child's diet, a subsequent weight gain and relief of symptoms is, however, the most reliable diagnostic outcome.[1]

NURSING INTERVENTION

Measurement of height and weight and plotting on a percentile chart on admission, will give a baseline on which to gauge the relatively rapid improvement in growth once gluten is removed from the diet. In the interim, hyperalimentation may be necessary to alleviate the immediate malnourishment.

During the initial phase of dietary alteration, replacement of deficient vitamins and minerals may be necessary. Iron, folic acid, and the fat-soluble vitamins A, D, E and K are administered orally.

The family and child will need preparation for life-long dietary modification and restriction. Adjustment to and education regarding a gluten-free diet should begin early in the child's hospital stay in consultation with the dietitian. The parents and child need clear guidelines on what food is nutritious and gluten free and how to prepare and make the food appetising for the child. The extent of food restriction will depend on the degree of bowel inflammation.

Some children develop a concurrent lactose intolerance which requires the additional elimination of foods containing milk, gas-producing vegetables, raw fruits and nuts until the inflammation abates. Difficulties may arise at a later stage when the child is asymptomatic and feels well. The children find it hard to continue on a selective diet which, in many instances, is different from that of their peers. This is particularly demanding for older children and adolescents. It is not uncommon for children or adolescents who waver from their diet to suffer relapse.

Parents and older children will benefit from a list of free foods and recipes in order to provide variety in meals. The parents will require guidelines for the signs and symptoms which indicate a relapse because of dietary indiscretions.

Once a gluten-free diet is implemented, behaviours such as irritability and clinginess will be alleviated, thus reducing the family's anxiety levels. Long-term manipulative behaviour which affects family dynamics may, however, need ongoing family therapy.

REFERENCE

1. Walker W, Durie P, Hamilton J, Walker-Smith J, Watkins J. *Paediatric gastrointestinal disease, pathophysiology, diagnosis and management.* Toronto: Decker, 1991.

Meckel's Diverticulum

Trish Comerford and Margaret Yates

Meckel's diverticulum originates during development of the embryo when the vitelline duct which connects the intestine to the yolk sac fails to completely obliterate. If the fetal gut does not separate from the yolk sac it will continue to herniate through the umbilical ring. By the 10th week of gestation the mid-gut normally returns to the abdominal cavity. The vitelline duct subsequently stops growing. If the duct continues to grow at the intestinal wall, a Meckel's diverticulum will result.[1]

Meckel's diverticulum usually occurs as an outpouching of ileum proximal to the ileocecal valve and is considered the most common congenital abnormality of the gastrointestinal tract.[2]

NURSING ASSESSMENT

The diverticular sac invariably contains gastric mucosa which produces hydrochloric acid and pepsin. The presence of acid irritates and erodes the bowel lining, which leads to bleeding and potential perforation.

The child will present with a history of bright red or dark red rectal bleeding and may exhibit intermittent central abdominal pain which is similar to that experienced with appendicitis. The child will often be anaemic from haemorrhage. The nurse should record baseline vital signs including blood pressure and continue to monitor the child for shock. The immediate care involves bed rest, stool chart and fluid balance maintenance.[2]

Additional nursing care is consistent with the child undergoing abdominal surgery (**see Chapter 6**).

MEDICAL DIAGNOSIS

A Meckel's scan will confirm the diagnosis. In addition, a rectosigmoidoscopy and barium enema may be performed to eliminate other diagnostic possibilities, e.g., polyps or intussusception.[2] The medical management is surgical removal of the diverticulum.

REFERENCES

1. Hutson JM, Beasley SW. *The surgical examination of children.* Oxford: Heinemann Medical Books, 1988.
2. Wong D. *Whaley and Wong's nursing care of infants and children.* 5th ed. St Louis: Mosby, 1995.

Hirschsprung's Disease

Trish Comerford and Margaret Yates

Hirschsprung's disease is also known as congenital aganglionic megacolon. Most infants are diagnosed within the first 12 months of life with only a small percentage not recognised until 3 to 12 years of age. There is a higher incidence of Hirschsprung's disease in male infants and it is frequently associated with Down syndrome.[1]

NURSING ASSESSMENT

Nursing considerations for a child with Hirschsprung's disease undergoing surgical correction will depend on the age at diagnosis. If the diagnosis is made during the neonatal period, a major focus will be to help parents adjust to and accept a congenital defect in their infant. Parents will need preparation for medical and surgical interventions and instruction regarding colostomy care for when they take the infant home. In the older child, existing signs and symptoms of a dysfunctional bowel can be established by listening to the child's history as furnished by the parents. It is important to establish the onset and pattern of constipation, a description of the consistency and odour of the stools and the frequency of bowel motions.

In addition, indicators such as poor eating habits, irritability, distended abdomen, signs of malnutrition, poor weight gain, pallor and fatigue are noted.[2]

MEDICAL DIAGNOSIS

Diagnosis may involve a series of procedures. A barium enema is the standard method for pinpointing the transition zone between the aganglionic segment and the dilated normal bowel. Anorectal manometry is useful in assessing innervation of the internal anal sphincter. It involves placing a balloon past the external sphincter, and another at the internal sphincter. When the balloons are inflated the response should resemble the presence of stool within the rectum. Children with Hirschsprung's disease, however, demonstrate contraction of the external sphincter without relaxation of the internal sphincter.[3] A rectal biopsy is performed to obtain a full-thickness specimen to establish histologically aganglionic cells. Histochemical stains of the biopsy to detect increased amounts of the enzyme acetylcholinesterase is a more reliable diagnostic method.[1,2]

MEDICAL MANAGEMENT

Rarely are children with Hirschsprung's disease managed without surgical intervention. Medical management is designed to stabilise the child with enterocolitis through a regimen of enemas, stool softeners and low-residue diets designed to evacuate the colon.[1]

Surgical correction is performed in three stages:

- *Step one:* The dysfunctional aganglionic section of bowel is removed. A temporary colostomy is performed in a section of bowel with normal innervation in either the sigmoid or transverse colon. This affords the rectal bowel time to rest, heal and recover normal tonicity.
- *Step two:* A 'pullthrough' reanastomosis is carried out which involves pulling the intact healthy bowel down and rejoining it at a point near the rectum.
- *Step three:* The colostomy is closed. In total, the correction is accomplished over a period of 3 months or more depending on the initial severity of the disease and the child's capacity for recovery.

PATHOPHYSIOLOGY

Hirschsprung's disease results from a deficiency of parasympathetic ganglion nerve cells within the submucosal and muscular layers of the colon.[3] The segment of colon affected varies, but the most common site is that which extends from the anus proximally as far as the rectosigmoid junction. The ganglion cells are responsible for the coordination of peristalsis, hence without them the bowel becomes functionally obstructed with secondary proximal dilatation. If the bowel remains obstructed, overgrowth of pathogenic organisms within the bowel will occur, resulting in enterocolitis which, if untreated, will progress to generalised sepsis and death.[4]

NURSING INTERVENTION

An assessment of nutritional status, state of hydration and electrolyte balance is carried out initially so that preparation for surgery can begin. The child may be admitted 48 hours before surgery and clear oral fluids commenced. Infants continue to breast feed. In addition, intravenous fluids are usually instituted preoperatively in preparation for postoperative fasting.

Preoperative bowel preparation involves administering normal saline enemas to cleanse the bowel. An enema stimulates peristalsis, which assists faeces higher in the colon to move down in order to be evacuated. The enema solution must be isotonic, hence the use of normal saline. Hypertonic or hypotonic solutions can cause osmotic fluid shifts resulting in hypervolaemia or hypovolaemia and electrolyte disturbances. Documentation of fluid balance is therefore vital.[3]

Table 7.19 Suggested enema volume in accordance with age[3]

Age	Volume
Infant/small baby (0–18 months)	50–200 ml
Toddler/preschooler (1.5–5 years)	200–300 ml
School age (5–12 years)	300–500 ml
Adolescent (12 years and older)	500–800 ml

PSYCHOLOGICAL PREPARATION AND FAMILY EDUCATION

The age of the child will determine the approach taken to explain colostomy care. Where possible, a stoma therapist will be involved. A stoma can be demonstrated in an illustration or with a doll for a child. Drawing a stoma on the doll and explaining that it is a different site for bowel motions, and attaching a bag will reassure the child as to the disposal of faeces. Since the child will have an abdominal suture line, this too can be drawn on the doll. Putting a dressing over the suture line will further help the child's understanding as bandaids or bandages are closely related to injury and healing in the young child's mind. This preparation should be as gradual as possible to give the child time to integrate the information and not become too anxious. Parents will need supportive preparation as well.

A colostomy represents a change in the child's body function and image. It is important to ascertain the parents' previous knowledge of colostomy. The parents' anxiety levels may be increased by a lack of understanding that Hirschsprungs disease is correctable and that a colostomy is temporary. Using the doll is equally as beneficial for parents.

The parents need to be aware of the 3 stages of surgery and the time treatment will take. There will be predictable disruptions to family life and routine. With forewarning parents may be able to arrange support from family and friends. Given the child will have had chronic feeding and possibly associated behaviour problems, the parents need to be prepared that these patterns can continue regardless of the defect being corrected. It will take time and patience for an improvement in feeding and behaviour. The stoma therapist will be engaged in teaching the parents and older child stoma care from admission to discharge, thus giving them adequate time to feel comfortable with the management of the stoma before having to give total care at home.[2]

POSTOPERATIVE CARE

In addition to routine postoperative care the child may have a nasogastric tube and will be nil by mouth for a minimum of 24 hours. Close observation of the stoma is imperative. The stoma should remain pink and moist, indicating adequate blood supply. Because the stoma will be oedematous immediately after surgery, a stoma appliance and bag should not be applied until the oedema has subsided. Application of vaseline gauze and a pad over the stoma will protect it and absorb any discharge in the immediate postoperative period.

When the parents are initially confronted with their child postoperatively they may have some difficulty coping with the reality of their child being attached to infusion pumps and having an abdominal wound and stoma. The nurse should ensure that everything is explained in terms which are understandable and emphasise their benefits for the child's recovery.

Closure of the colostomy is usually achieved within 12 months of the 'pullthrough' procedure. Nursing considerations during this period include the maintenance of skin integrity around the child's anus, remembering there has been no bowel motion passed for a prolonged period of time. The use of a protective ointment around the anus (e.g., zinc and castor oil) may be sufficient. It may be necessary, however, to seal around the anus with protective artificial skin as an optimum preventative shield.

The management of diet, eating habits, meal times and elimination will be different for the child. A re-education program about food and eating, especially for the older child, should be implemented in consultation with the dietitian and family. Toilet training may also be necessary. In cases where the child finds it difficult to comply to new eating habits, a behaviour modification program may be necessary.

REFERENCES

1. Kirschner B. *In:* Walker W, Durie P, Hamilton J, Walker-Smith J, Watkins J. *Paediatric gastrointestinal disease. Pathophysiology, diagnosis and management.* Toronto: Decker, 1991.
2. Wong DL. *Whaley and Wong's nursing care of infants and children.* 5th ed. St Louis: Mosby, 1995.
3. Mott SR, James SR, Sperhac AM. *Nursing care of children and families.* 2nd ed. Menlo Park CA: Addison-Wesley, 1990.
4. Hutson JM, Beasley SW. *The surgical examination of children.* Heinemann Medical Books, 1988.

Total Parenteral Nutrition

Victoria Cullens

WHAT IS PARENTERAL NUTRITION AND WHO NEEDS IT?

Since the late 1960s advances in parenteral nutrition (PN) have seen this form of nutritional support used increasingly in paediatrics and neonatology. This has led to increased survival rates for those children whose recovery would otherwise have been compromised by malnutrition.[1] The concept of PN involves the provision of intravenous macro and micro nutrients sufficient to ensure normal growth and development when the gastrointestinal tract (GIT) cannot be used. When enteral feeding is completely contraindicated, PN can comprise the entire nutrient intake, i.e., total parenteral nutrition (TPN). If some nutrients are provided via the enteral route, PN can be used to supplement these feeds to provide the total daily requirements.

Possible indications for PN include:[1]

- Neonatal — necrotising enterocolitis, exomphalos or gastroschisis, low birthweight infants, after gut surgery, short gut syndrome, congenital villous atrophy.
- Paediatric — intractable diarrhoeal syndromes, after gut surgery, ischaemic small bowel resection (e.g., volvulus), inflammatory bowel disease, pancreatitis, intestinal pseudo-obstruction, immunodeficency syndromes, bone marrow transplantation, malignancies, burns, intensive care patients.

NURSING ASSESSMENT

The health status of children on PN support will vary considerably. Some will require intensive care following such incidents as major trauma, surgery or burns, and their assessment will include some of the parameters necessary for the intensive care patient. Others will be relatively well and ambulant. Observation of the appearance and activity levels of these patients will give the nurse an indication of their health status. The alert, active infant who plays with toys and responds to caregivers and parents, is more likely to be thriving. Conversely, a child who is withdrawn and unresponsive may be in pain, be septic or suffering from some metabolic imbalance. Parents will also provide valuable information as to what is normal behaviour for their child.

HYDRATION

Accurate monitoring and recording of fluid input (including enteral feeds) and output is essential for all children receiving PN. Imbalances in hydration can occur through inappropriate prescribing or changes in treatment, e.g., the initiation of phototherapy. An imbalance can also occur through an alteration in a child's condition, such as the development of congestive cardiac failure. Close observation of the clinical signs of over or under hydration is therefore required.

Dehydrated patients present with slack tissue turgor, dry mucous membrane and thirst. In infants under 18 months the anterior fontanelle is sunken. Urine output is decreased. Output is measured for those patients whose fluid balance is critical and should be 2 to 4 mL/kg/hour. In the neonate and infant, urine collection can be difficult. An alternative method to bag collection is to weigh urine-soaked nappies or absorbent pads (1 g weight equals 1 mL of urine). The normal specific gravity is 1005 to 1015 and measurement every 6 hours is recommended in the initial 48 hours of PN support. Once stabilised, evaluation every 12 hours is sufficient.[2]

Patients who are overhydrated may develop oedema. This may be evidenced by inappropriate rapid weight gain, swelling of the extremities and periorbital oedema. A moist cough will be heard if there is pulmonary involvement. If fluid restriction is necessary, an increase in dextrose concentration of the PN solution will ensure adequate calorie intake.[3]

TOLERANCE OF LIPID INTAKE

Lipid overload occurs when the rate of infusion exceeds the body's ability to metabolise the lipid. Nursing staff can use a simple method to assess a child's tolerance to the lipid load by observing for plasma turbidity. The lipidity test is performed once a day, usually after pausing the infusion for 5 hours. The technique involves collection of a small amount of blood in a capillary tube following either a heel or finger prick. The sample is left strapped to a vertical surface, such as the side of a burette, until the plasma and formed elements separate. This process takes about 20 minutes. The plasma settles over the formed elements and, when inspected, should have a clear, straw-coloured appearance. A cloudy appearance of the plasma may indicate either an excessive lipid intake or sepsis. It should be emphasised, however, that this method provides uncertain correlations with serum lipid concentrations and preferably nephelometry should be used if available.[4] Nephelometry is a process for ascertaining the turbidity of a fluid by measuring the intensity of light scattered against a standard scale.

TOLERANCE OF DEXTROSE INTAKE

An adequate intake of calories is essential for normal growth and to avoid catabolism of body protein. With the right rates of dextrose infusion, hyperglycaemia may occur. Measurements of blood sugar level are taken every 6 hours while PN is being introduced, and every 12 hours once the regimen is established. Ideally, the blood sugar level should be maintained between 4 and 6 mmol/L.[2] A persistently low blood sugar level may indicate the need for an increased dextrose concentration in the PN solution. If PN is stopped abruptly, profound hypoglycaemia can occur as a result of hyperinsulinemia. If the PN flask is completed before another is available a 10% dextrose solution is used to cover the gap. Urinalysis is performed at the same time intervals as BSL. The presence of ketones may also indicate an inadequate intake of dextrose. At the other extreme, glycosuria may appear if a child is receiving a very high concentration of dextrose and the renal threshold is surpassed. Premature infants are particularly at risk of this problem. Glycosuria and hyperglycaemia may indicate the presence of sepsis and the child should be evaluated accordingly.

GROWTH

One of the aims of PN is to provide sufficient nutrients for growth. The easiest way to measure growth is by regular weighing of the infant or child. Children on PN support are weighed daily, ideally at the same time of day and on the same scales to ensure consistency. Infants should be weighed naked. The weight of attachments such as electrocardiograph dots and intravenous arm boards is deducted from the gross weight. Older children can be weighed in light clothing and without shoes. Weight is plotted on a chart with expected growth curves or percentiles. This additional information will help to assess if weight gain is appropriate.

Poor weight gain may be related to inadequate calorie intake. Excessive gain can be associated with oedema and may give a false impression of the child's progress. Excessive gains may also occur if the PN regimen is not adjusted as enteral feeds are introduced.

Other important indicators of growth are height and head circumference. Height is relevant for children on long-term PN and should be measured by a stadiometer. Head circumference is of particular importance in the neonatal period as it indicates brain growth. Mid-arm circumference and triceps skin fold can also be measured.[5]

COMPONENTS OF PARENTERAL NUTRITION

Parenteral nutrition is a complex combination of nutrients designed to meet the requirements of individual children. The solutions are prepared daily by pharmacists under sterile conditions, using a laminar flow hood.

Macronutrients

Amino acids are the building blocks for the formulation of proteins and are required for normal growth and development. There are 21 amino acids, 8 of which cannot be synthesised by the body and therefore are considered essential and must be supplied as part of the nutrient intake. Research suggests that the amino acids cysteine, taurine, tyrosine and histidine are essential in the neonate and should be included in PN solutions. Several new commercial solutions have been developed to meet the needs of premature neonates. Initial trials using these solutions indicate improved growth rates.[6-8]

Proteins have an energy value of 17 kJ (4 kcal) per gram. The body, however, seldom uses proteins as an energy source, unless energy intake is inadequate or stores are depleted. To ensure efficient use of protein as a building block rather than as an energy source, 150 to 200 non-protein calories are required per gram of nitrogen.

There are several amino acid solutions available. Vamin is commonly used for neonates and Synthamin for older children. Various techniques are used for commencing PN. Most start at 0.5 to 1 g/kg/day, increasing until the following requirements are met:[2,9]

- Premature neonate: 3 g/kg/day.
- Neonate: 2.2 g/kg/day.
- Child: 1.5 g/kg/day.
- Adolescent: 1.0 to 1.5 g/kg/day.

Carbohydrate is provided in the form of the monosaccharide dextrose and is the main source of energy in PN. Dextrose has an energy value of 17 kJ (4 kcal) per gram. Dextrose concentrations of 10% (10 g/100 mL) or above can lead to phlebitis and such concentrations should therefore only be given via central venous lines. Even using central venous lines, concentrations should rarely exceed 15%. Lower concentrations can be given by peripheral vein, although the child should be observed closely for extravasation, phlebitis and sepsis. Energy requirements vary according to the age and size of the child on PN. Energy requirements for body maintenance and growth are as follows:[9,10]

- Premature neonate: 510–640 KJ/kg/day (120–159 Kcal).
- Neonate: 470–510 KJ/kg/day (110–120 Kcal).
- Child: 250–290 KJ/kg/day (60–70 Kcal).
- Adolescent: 128–255 KJ/kg/day (30–60 Kcal).

Energy requirements will increase with fever, surgery, burns, sepsis and cardiac failure.[3] For balanced PN, the energy will be provided as 30% to 40% lipid and 60% to 70% carbohydrate.

Lipids are supplied as an isotonic emulsion of soybean or safflower oil, egg yolk phospholipid and glycerol. Concentrations available vary from 10% to 20% (10 to 20 g/100 mL). The role of lipids in parenteral nutrition is to provide a secondary energy source (42 kJ/g or 10.5 kcal/g) and to prevent essential fatty acid deficiency by providing linoleic and linolenic acid. Essential fatty acid deficiency results in scaly dermatitis, alopecia, hepatomegaly, thrombocytopenia and growth retardation.[11]

Lipid is introduced slowly to a PN regimen, increasing to a daily intake of 1 to 4 g/kg/day. It is administered at a slow rate over at least 15 hours to minimise the occurrence of adverse effects. These effects include fat deposition or emboli in the pulmonary microcirculation, which can cause an associated decrease in oxygenation. Lipids have the potential to displace bilirubin from binding sites on albumin. In premature infants at risk of kernicterus, dangerously high levels of unconjugated bilirubin could be produced. There is controversy about whether lipids cause depressant effect on the immune system, although it is known that lipid is cleared from the blood less effectively in children with sepsis.[4,6] Monitoring the child's tolerance by visual estimations of plasma turbidity,

Table 7.20 Electrolyte and mineral requirements in neonates and children[2]

	Children	Neonates
Sodium	2–3 mmol/kg/day	3–6 mmol/kg/day
Potassium	2–3 mmol/kg/day	
Calcium	0.5 mmol/kg/day	up to 2.0 mmol/kg/day
Magnesium	0.15 mmol/kg/day	
Phosphorus	0.5 mmol/kg/day	0.8–91.2 mmol/kg/day
Zinc	0.6 µmol/kg/day	up to 7.5 µmol/kg/day

Table 7.21 Average daily maintenance water requirements according to age[2]

Age	mL/kg/day
Day 1	60
Day 2	90
Day 3	120
Day 4	150
Up to 9 months	120–140
2 years	80–90
4 years	70–80
8 years	60–70
12 years	50–60

nephelometry or serum triglycerides level estimation will identify those children receiving an excessive amount of lipid.[11]

Carnitine is a peptide which facilitates the transport of lipid across the mitochondrial membrane where it can be metabolised for energy. Children, particularly premature infants, have a limited ability to synthesise carnitine. It has been suggested, therefore, that low birthweight infants receiving PN should receive supplements of carnitine.[4,12]

Micronutrients

Vitamins are organic nutrients essential for growth and normal development. The 9 water-soluble and 4 fat-soluble vitamins are provided in PN solutions to prevent vitamin deficiencies. It should be noted that some vitamins, especially riboflavin, are destroyed by light. Vitamin A is lost through adherence to the delivery tubing.[2,9]

Electrolytes and minerals are inorganic substances which help to regulate body processes. The daily maintenance requirements for infants and children receiving PN are given in **Table 7.20**. Requirements may need to be adjusted to suit individual children, e.g., a child losing large amounts of gastric aspirate will need sodium supplements.[3]

Trace elements are present in the body in very small amounts, but are necessary for many body processes. They are an important component in PN. Requirements are listed in **Table 7.20**. Iron is not routinely added because of the possibility of incompatibility.[9]

Water is included to increase the volume of PN solution and to meet the daily fluid requirements, according to age and weight of the child (**Table 7.21**).

Heparin is added to prevent blockage of catheters used to administer PN. The usual dose is 1 U/mL of solution.[8]

PERIPHERAL VEINS

The peripheral venous route is suitable for short-term (less than 2 weeks) PN support in children. Parenteral nutrition solutions can be very irritating to veins, especially if high concentrations of dextrose are used, and thus hourly observation of peripheral lines is required to detect extravasation. Should this be observed, the infusion should be stopped and the cannula resited immediately.[1]

CENTRAL VENOUS LINES

Central venous lines ensure venous access for long-term PN support. Delivery of PN solution to a high-flow central vessel ensures rapid mixing with the circulation and distribution of high concentrations of dextrose.

Cuffed catheters

These catheters are surgically introduced via a large vein such as the subclavian vein, into the superior vena cava. The entry point between skin and vein is separated by a subcutaneous tunnel of 10 to 15 cm, which reduces the risk of sepsis. A dacron cuff under the skin surface allows fibrous adhesions to develop, which helps secure the catheter against dislodgment.[2,10] Examples of this type of catheter in common use are Broviac, Cook (double lumen) and Hickman.

Percutaneous silastic central lines

The use of this type of central venous line has become popular in neonates. An extremely fine (2 French gauge) silastic catheter is inserted via a butterfly needle in a distal vein. The median basilic, scalp or femoral veins have been used. The silastic line is threaded into the superior or inferior vena cava, and the proximal end threaded onto a 25-gauge butterfly needle to enable connection to a giving line. The position of the silastic line top is checked by x-ray. Contrast medium may be needed if the silastic catheter is not radio-opaque. Any catheter not situated in a central vein should be removed.[13,14]

COMPLICATIONS

Sepsis

Sepsis is the most serious complication associated with PN and intravascular catheters. The most common infecting organisms are the *Staphylococcus*, *Pseudomonas* and *Klebsiella* species, *Candida albicans* and *Escherichia coli*.[8,13] In children, a core temperature above 38°C should be reported promptly so sepsis can be investigated. Sepsis can also present in neonates with hypothermia, lethargy and apnoea. Peripheral blood is taken for culture and sensitivity, additional blood is also taken from a central venous line, if one is in place. The PN solution should be cultured to rule out bacterial contamination. The catheter insertion site is examined for inflammation or pus formation. If the CVL is infected, it should be removed.[14]

Metabolic complications

The most common metabolic complications related to the administration of PN are:[5,10,15]

- hypoglycaemia/hyperglycaemia;
- electrolyte imbalance;
- trace element deficiency, e.g., zinc, copper, chromium;
- vitamin deficiency, e.g., biotin, vitamin D;
- liver dysfunction; and
- fat intolerance.

Catheter-related problems

A number of catheter-related problems have been described. Air emboli or haemorrhage will occur when cuffed catheters are inappropriately clamped or inadvertent disconnection occurs. Catheter-induced thrombosis of the superior vena cava results from stasis, endothelial disruption and injury secondary to hyperosmolar solutions. Clinical signs in children include swelling of the head, neck and chest with venous distension, cardiac murmurs and respiratory distress. Resistance to flushing and an inability to withdraw blood from the catheter will also be observed and the line must be removed.

Cardiac arrhythmia, e.g., supraventricular tachycardia, can occur if the catheter extends beyond the superior vena cava into the right atrium.[16]

NURSING MANAGEMENT

Successful PN support requires the close communication and cooperation of a multidisciplinary team of physicians, surgeons, pharmacists, pathologists and nurses. Skilled nursing care will ensure appropriate delivery of PN solution, prevent and detect complications and assess the child's and family's progress.

Delivery of parenteral nutrition

Parenteral nutrition solutions are refrigerated until an hour before administration. The flasks or packs are inspected for cracks, turbidity or precipitation prior to use. Other chemicals or drugs should not be added to the flask or 'piggybacked' to the line, as there is a risk of bacterial contamination or incompatibility and precipitation with the PN solution. Precipitate appears as a white, chalk-like substance that will not disperse. If precipitation is seen the infusion should be stopped immediately and returned to pharmacy for analysis.

A double giving line or 2 lines which can be joined at a side port are used to deliver the PN solution via the same route. A 0.22 micron in line filter can be included in the PN solution line to remove impurities. Lipid molecules are larger and would block the filter.[10] Some hospitals protect the PN solution from light with an opaque shield, such as foil, to prevent photodegradation of vitamins.[5]

Accurate rates of infusion are facilitated by the use of electronic infusion pumps which deliver a set amount of fluid per hour. Many have an alarm system which will alert to problems such as occlusions. The use of these pumps is mandatory in many hospitals and recommended for all children receiving PN.[2,10] The PN flasks and lines are changed every 24 hours at a time to suit ward routine. The procedure is performed with meticulous attention to avoid contamination of the solution or catheter. If PN is infused via a central vessel, a sterile technique requiring the nurse to scrub and use gown and gloves is recommended.[5,8]

Care of peripheral venous cannulae

Peripheral cannulae should be taped securely and the cannula protected from dislodgment. Very active neonates may need to have limb movement restricted, e.g., by pinning an arm board to the nappy. Tape should not cover the skin directly distal to the cannula insertion site. The site is inspected hourly for signs of infiltration (swelling, phlebitis or discolouration) and the infusion promptly suspended if these signs occur. This will avoid chemical burns from extravasated PN solution. If infiltration does occur, the cannula is removed and the affected limb is immobilised and elevated.

Care of central venous lines

The insertion site of a percutaneous silastic central line (PCSCL) is covered with semipermeable transparent dressing. This secures the silastic catheter and allows easy inspection. The dressing is changed every 7 days or if it is damp or lifting, to reduce the chance of infection and check for pressure areas under the dressing. Many hospitals use an antibiotic ointment at the insertion site.[2,13]

A minimum rate of 1 mL/hour is necessary to maintain patency of these lines. Interruption of the infusion, even for short periods, must be avoided as PCSCLs block quickly.

Cuffed catheters may be dressed as described above or with a non-adherent dry dressing. Three weeks following insertion, cuffed catheters may be left without a dressing as adequate scarring around the cuff will have occurred by this time. If a skin suture is in place, it is removed after 10 days. When disconnecting a cuffed catheter, it is essential to avoid air embolism by clamping the catheter. If the catheter does not have a clamp provided by the manufacturer, specially guarded forceps can be used. It is important to clamp over the reinforced area of the catheter to prevent trauma and eventual breakage. Clamps should be in close proximity to the child at all times.[5]

A cuffed catheter has the advantage that it can be 'capped' by flushing the line with heparin. PN can be infused intermittently and may be paused for up to a week depending on the strength of heparin used. Heparinised saline (50 U in 5 mL normal saline) will maintain the catheter's patency for up to 12 hours. For longer periods, heparin sodium 1000 U/mL is necessary. The volume of the flush depends on the dead space within the catheter.[2]

Oral hygiene

Children on TPN support receive no oral intake. Attention to oral hygiene is extremely important as their mucous membranes become dry and ulcerations can occur. Oral mucous membranes are therefore inspected every 8 hours. Oral hygiene is performed every 2 to 4 hours using a mouth rinse or teeth brushing for older children. Infant's teeth, gums and tongue are gently wiped with a glycerine-based mouthwash.

Infants receiving PN are at risk of oral colonisation with *Candida albicans*. Prophylactic use of oral antifungal agents, such as amphotericin, will help reduce the occurrence of this problem.[8]

Supporting children and their families

Eating is a necessary activity to meet the body's nutritional needs and provides a time for social interaction. Children and their parents may be confused and anxious as to why they cannot be fed. Nursing staff should look for opportunities to teach the child and their family about PN and the care of associated equipment. This may include repetition and reinforcement of the physician's explanations. Parents should clearly understand why their child needs nutritional support. Empathetic and supportive listening on the nurse's part will encourage parents to ask questions and express their feelings. Encouraging parents to participate in the physical care of their child, even if critically ill, may help them to feel they are making a positive contribution to their child's care.

Meal times can be a focus of family and ward routine. The child on PN support must not be made to feel isolated from these occasions. If the child can tolerate small amounts of enteral feeds these should be scheduled during meal times. This oral feeding may also help to avoid the development of behaviour problems such as choking and the spitting out of food once feeds are reintroduced. Non-nutritive sucking is important for the developing oral musculature necessary for the establishment of oral feeds in the neonate. Sucking on a 'dummy' also helps to soothe and settle an agitated, hungry baby. Infants should not miss out on the physical contact that occurs during breast or bottle feeding. Frequent cuddles are important for comfort and social development.[8]

HOME TOTAL PARENTERAL NUTRITION

Increased knowledge and experience with PN and the development of silastic catheters have enabled children to receive long-term PN in the home. Children with conditions such as short gut syndrome, Crohn's disease and intractable diarrhoea may benefit from such a program. To be suitable, the child's condition must be stable and the parents motivated and committed.[9]

Once the decision has been made a detailed education program for the parents and child is initiated. Parents must be competent and confident in the care of their child before discharge. Nursing staff are often the coordinators of such an education program. Issues to be covered include knowledge of PN, use of infusion pumps, care of the CVL catheter and sterile techniques, and the procedures required if problems or emergencies occur. Parents need to be able to deal with problems such as pump alarms or leakage from catheters and identify signs and symptoms of sepsis.

Other health professionals may need to be involved. If the child is receiving some enteral feeds, a dietitian will teach parents the preparation of special formulas. Additionally, physiotherapists can teach parents skills to facilitate their child's motor development.[17] Once the child is discharged home, regular follow-up visits to the hospital are arranged. It is essential that parents receive the support required from a specialised community nurse and know where they can get help 24 hours a day. Community organisations may provide additional support.

REFERENCES

1. Jakobowski DS. Nutritional support of the critically ill child. *In:* Bloedel-Smith J, ed. *Paediatric critical care*. New York: John Wiley & Sons, 1983: 466–521.
2. Royal Alexandra Hospital for Children. *Guidelines for intravenous nutrition*. Sydney: RAHC, 1986.
3. Arnold WC. Parenteral nutrition, and fluid and electrolyte therapy. *Paediatr Clin North Am* 1990; 37: 449–461.
4. Ballabriga A. Some aspects of the use of fats in enteral and parenteral nutrition in infancy. *Ann Nestles* 1988; 46 (2): 94–106.

5. Hass-Beckert B. Removing the mysteries of parenteral nutrition. *Paediatr Nursing* 1987; 13: 37–41.
6. Lemons JA, Neal P, Ernst J. Nitrogen sources for parenteral nutrition in the newborn infant. *Clin Perinatol* 1986; 13: 91–109.
7. Helms RA, Christensen ML, Mauer EC, Storm MC. Comparison of a paediatric versus standard amino acid formulation in preterm neonates requiring parenteral nutrition. *J Paediatr* 1987; 110: 466–469.
8. Moore MC. Total parenteral nutrition for infants. *Neonatal Network* 1987; 6 (2): 33–40.
9. Zlotkin SH, Stallings VA, Pencharz PB. Total parenteral nutrition in children. *Pediatr Clin North Am* 1985; 32: 381–400.
10. Ricour C. Total parenteral nutrition in children. *Ann Nestle* 1988; 46: 61–72.
11. Stahl GE, Spear ML, Hamosh M. Intravenous administration of lipid emulsions to premature infants. *Pediatr Clin North Am* 1986; 13: 133–162.
12. Helms RA. Intravenous carnitine during parenteral nutrition in neonates. *J Parenteral Enteral Nutr* 1987; 11: 98.
13. Abdulla F, Dietrich KA, Pramanik AK. Percutaneous femoral venous catheterisation in preterm neonates. *J Paediatr* 1990; 117: 788–791.
14. Leick-Rude MK. Use of percutaneous silastic intravascular catheters in high-risk neonates. *Neonatal Network* 1990; 9 (1): 17–25.
15. Bell RL, Ferry GD, Smith EO, Shulman RJ, Christensen BL, Labarte DR, Willis CA. Total parenteral nutrition — related cholestasis in infants. *J Parenteral Enteral Nutr* 1986; 10: 356–359.
16. Carey BE. Major complications of central lines in neonates. *Neonatal Network* 1989; 7 (6): 17–28.
17. Cady C, Yoshioka RA. Using a learning contract to successfully discharge an infant on home total parenteral nutrition. *Paediatr Nursing* 1991; 17: 67–71.

Intraosseous Infusion

Isobel Taylor

RATIONALE FOR USE

The rapid establishment of venous access may be the deciding factor in the outcome of resuscitative measures where peripheral or central venous access may not be feasible due to burns, cardiopulmonary arrest or peripheral circulatory collapse. The intraosseous route allows large-bore vascular access until intravenous access can be obtained. The intraosseous route may be the only viable solution to accomplishing the required volume replacement and drug administration in cases of severe trauma or cardiac arrest, by providing a virtually non-collapsable venous access within a bony cavity.

Peck and Altieri describe the procedure as safe, fast and effective and state that it can be performed by paramedics and emergency nurses as well as physicians.[1] The concept is not new. Intraosseous infusion was considered viable as early as 1922, when research into the circulation of the sternum indicated that there was a potential for using the sternum as a route for transfusions. In 1940, Tocantins' research formed the foundation for clinical application of the procedure using tibial access in rabbits.[2] Subsequent work by Tocantins and O'Neill led to refinement and more widespread use of the technique.[3]

By the late 1950s, intraosseous infusion had fallen into disuse. This was partly due to the development of plastic catheters and the relative ease of venous cannulation.[1]

INSERTION SITES

Potential sites of intraosseous infusion are the iliac crest, femur, distal tibia and proximal tibia. The sternum is not used in children as it is too thin and too poorly developed to ensure safe placement of the line.[4] Because the supine position is necessary for resuscitation, the anteromedial surface of the proximal tibia, one finger breadth below the tibial tubercle, is commonly used.

PROCEDURE

Local anaesthesia is necessary for pain control during insertion if the patient is conscious.

The skin over the insertion site is cleaned with an antiseptic solution and a needle is inserted at a 30° angle with the point directed towards the foot and away from the epiphyseal plate. A short, large-bore bone marrow needle or an 18-gauge needle with a stylet is used. The stylet avoids occlusion of the needle by bone plugs.[4]

To position the needle in the marrow cavity, a twisting or boring motion is needed to overcome the resistance of the bony cortex. The needle will then advance easily into the marrow cavity. The stylet is removed and a saline-filled syringe is used to aspirate the marrow. Saline is then injected into the needle to verify placement and clear the needle of any clots. Any standard IV tubing is then attached and the infusion of the liquid is commenced.[5] Following insertion, the tip of the needle lies in the medullary cavity of a long bone where marrow sinusoids drain into large medullary venous channels. The channels empty into nutrient and emissary veins and from there into the systemic circulation. Fluid infused by this route has an equivalent passage into the systemic circulation as the intravenous route in terms of rate of absorption.

Areas of cellulitis and infected burns should be avoided to reduce the risk of osteomyelitis. Recently fractured bones should not be used because of the risk of infection or of interfering with healing. Fragile bones, as in osteoporosis or osteogenesis imperfecta, are not suitable due to the abnormal architecture of the bone.

COMPLICATIONS

Various complications have been reported, and others have been suggested as potential problems. Those that have been reported include penetration of the bone through both cortices, osteomyelitis, subperiosteal or subcutaneous infiltration, and growth plate injury. Incorrect placement of the needle could result in damage to the growth plate with limb length discrepancy leading to a deformity. The damage may occur directly to the plate itself or through pressure leading to necrosis due to periosteal placement. The damage may not be apparent until later when the child grows and the discrepancy is revealed. The incidence of embolism has not been reported but must be borne in mind as a potential complication.[5]

Currently, intraosseous infusions are recommended for emergency short-term use only. When an alternative form of venous access can be established the intraosseous line can be discontinued and the site covered by a sterile dressing. The nursing focus is directed to the maintenance of the site, application of a sterile dressing and the immobilisation of the extremity. Monitoring the rate of the flow and the patients' response to treatment is the same as for IV infusion.

Appropriate education and practice is an essential prerequisite for health professionals whose work situation warrants this procedure. The protocols for the procedure need to be strictly adhered to for safe practice as well as meeting legal requirements related to standards of care.

REFERENCES

1. Peck KR, Altieri M. Intraosseous infusions: an old technique with modern applications. *Orthopedic Nursing* 1989; 8: 46–48.
2. Tocantins LM. Rapid absorption of substances injected into the bone marrow. *Proc Soc Exper Biol Med* 1940; 45: 292–296.
3. Tocantins LM, O'Neill J. Infusion of blood and other fluids into the circulation via the bone marrow. *Proc Soc Exper Biol Med* 1940; 45: 782–783.
4. Parrish GA, Turkewitz D, Skiendziewski JJ. Intraosseous infusions in the emergency department. *Am J Community Med* 1986; 4: 59–63.
5. Rosetti VA, Thompson BM, Millar J, Mateer JR, Aprahamian C. Intraosseous infusions: an alternative route of pediatric vascular access. *Ann Emergency Med* 1985; 14: 103–109.

Disturbances in Genitourinary Function

Jill Farquhar

Acute Renal Failure

Acute renal failure is a sudden deterioration of kidney function related to a decrease in glomerular filtration rate. Interruption to kidney function results in retention of nitrogenous waste products[1] and an inability to maintain homeostasis. Oliguria is a feature of acute renal failure.

Acute renal failure has a variety of aetiologies. The condition is classified into 3 diagnostic groups: prerenal failure, postrenal failure and intrinsic renal failure.[2] When planning the nursing and medical care of children with acute renal failure it is important to know which type of acute renal failure the child has, because appropriate intervention depends on the cause of renal failure.

NURSING ASSESSMENT

General appearance

The nurse caring for the child should observe the colour of the child's skin. The child's parents may comment that the child looks pale, or the skin may have a sallow appearance. Pallor occurs in acute renal failure as a result of anaemia caused by decreased erythropoietin production. Oedema, caused by a reduced urine output, may make the child's body appear swollen.

The child should be observed for bruising and petechiae. Petechiae are observed in children with haemolytic uraemic syndrome and Henoch–Schonlein purpura. Acute renal failure causes inefficient platelet activity, resulting in an increased risk of bruising and haemorrhage.

Vital signs

Elevation of blood pressure, bodyweight, heart rate and respiratory rate may occur. These abnormal observations indicate fluid volume overload.

Urine

If the child has a urine output, urine should be analysed at least once daily. Prerenal failure reveals an elevated urinary specific gravity. Intrinsic renal failure reveals a fixed specific gravity. Urine should be tested for the presence of blood and protein, which would indicate intrinsic diseases such as glomerulonephritis.

A urine culture may be collected to rule out infective causes of renal failure.

A reduced *urine volume* (oliguria), or reduced number of wet nappies, is often the first indication that a child has acute renal failure. Oliguria is defined as a drop in the hourly urine output to less than 0.5 mL/kg/hour.[3] Nurses caring for infants and children with acute renal failure must observe the child's urine output closely. It is difficult to measure the urine output of infants unless they are catheterised or have an adhesive urine collection bag applied. This is not usually desirable, so an accurate bare weight is an extremely important observation to assess the child's fluid status, and should be attended to twice daily.

A poor *urinary stream* or dribbling urine is an important observation because this is indicative of postrenal causes of renal failure.

A history of fever, or abnormal coloured or smelly urine is indicative of *urinary tract infection*. This symptom may indicate urinary reflux or some other urological disorder.

A recent chest, skin or throat infection is suggestive of acute poststreptococcal glomerulonephritis.

The child's parents should be questioned about any recent episodes of diarrhoea or vomiting. Diarrhoea and vomiting can result in dehydration and prerenal failure, or could be a prelude to haemolytic uraemic syndrome.[4]

Neurological status should be checked. Irritability, drowsiness, confusion or seizures indicate an elevated level of urea in the blood as a result of renal failure.

PATHOPHYSIOLOGY

Prerenal failure

Under normal circumstances the kidneys receive 25% of the cardiac output. If the renal perfusion drops for some reason, glomerular filtration diminishes, leading to acute renal failure. Causes of reduced renal blood flow are: a fall in cardiac output, extracellular fluid deficit, or decreased intravascular fluid volume.[5]

Renal tissue is not damaged in cases of prerenal failure, and the condition is rapidly reversible with fluid replacement therapy. However, if hypovolaemia is not corrected, renal perfusion will remain poor and renal tissue will suffer ischaemic damage.

Causes of prerenal failure in children are:

- Maternal blood loss and dehydration (newborns).
- Vasodilation (sepsis, anaphylaxis, drug induced).[2]
- Dehydration from causes such as gastroenteritis, salt wasting nephropathies, overuse of diuretics.
- Renal vein or artery thrombosis.
- Haemorrhage.
- Third space fluid losses, e.g., burns.
- Congestive cardiac failure and congenital heart disease.
- Severe respiratory distress.
- Increased intra-abdominal pressure.

Postrenal failure

This type of renal failure occurs as a result of an obstruction to urinary flow. The obstruction may occur anywhere in the urinary tract. Obstruction to urine flow results in an increased hydrostatic pressure within the kidney which damages tubular cells and glomeruli. Glomerular filtration decreases when there is raised hydrostatic pressure in the glomerular capsule.

Surgical correction of the obstruction usually corrects post-acute renal failure, however varying degrees of damage to the renal parenchyma may occur. The longer the duration of raised pressure in the kidney, the greater the potential for damage to renal tissue.

Urinary tract obstruction in children is usually congenital and is most common in infants less than 1 year of age.

Causes of postrenal failure in children are:

- Posterior urethral valves.
- Hydronephrosis.
- Renal calculi.
- Thrombosis.
- Pelvo-ureteric junction obstruction.
- Bladder neck obstruction.

Intrinsic renal failure

Intrinsic acute renal failure results from damage to the nephron by toxic agents or disease processes. In some instances, the kidney tubules suffer temporary, acute ischaemic damage. This condition is called acute tubular necrosis (ATN).

Causes of intrinsic renal failure in children are:

- Allergic reaction to certain drugs, dyes or chemicals.
- Haemolytic uraemic syndrome.
- Glomerulonephritis.
- Henoch–Schonlein purpura.
- Systemic lupus erythematosis.
- Tumours.
- Congenital abnormalities.

Acute intrinsic renal failure follows a course involving 3 phases.

1. *Oliguria/anuria*: This initial phase presents with a decreased urine output. Urine output is less than 500 mL/1.73 m^2/24 hours in older children, or less than 0.5 mL/kg/hour

in infants.[3] This phase persists for between 7 and 21 days in adolescents and older children, and is usually shorter (3 to 5 days) in infants and young children. Oliguria is accompanied by a rapid rise of serum urea and creatinine levels, anaemia, calcium and phosphate disturbances and interruption to electrolyte and acid-base balance.

Although oliguria is usually a feature of acute renal failure it is not always present. In some cases a small number of nephrons remain undamaged and continue to produce large quantities of dilute urine. These children present with a sudden rise in urea and creatinine and abnormal serum biochemistry levels.

2. *The diuretic phase*: The second phase may last up to several weeks. During the diuretic phase the kidneys begin to produce small amounts of urine. Urine output tends to double in volume each day for about 4 to 7 days. This phase is followed by a more gradual return to a normal diuresis.

It is unusual for children to become dehydrated during this phase despite the increased urine output, because the high urine output is usually in response to the fluid retained during the oliguric phase of renal failure. However, excessive urinary electrolyte and water losses does occur occasionally; therefore, close attention to hydration and serum electrolyte levels is necessary during this phase.

Initially in the diuretic phase, serum urea levels continue to rise and then plateau.[6]

3. *The recovery phase*: During the recovery phase, there is a gradual recovery of renal tubular function. It may take several months for complete recovery and a return to normal biochemical levels.

Unfortunately, a small number of children suffer irreversible renal damage which leads to chronic or end-stage renal failure.

NURSING CARE OF CHILDREN WITH ACUTE RENAL FAILURE

Children suffering from acute renal failure are critically ill and require intensive nursing care. Medical and surgical interventions are aimed at correction of the underlying cause of acute renal failure, therefore it is important for nurses to know the type of acute renal failure that the child has to enable them to plan appropriate nursing care.

Hydration

If prerenal failure is suspected, attempts to restore fluid volume with intravenous infusion of isotonic saline, or colloids (20 mL/kg for children, and 20 to 40 mL/kg for neonates) are made.[4] Some children require a central venous pressure line to monitor their hydration status. Twice daily observation of bodyweight and hourly measurement of blood pressure, fluid intake and output are essential.

Fluid challenge

If prerenal failure is suspected, attempts to reverse the situation by rapid infusion of intravenous fluids are made as discussed above. If there is no urine output within 2 hours of the fluid administration, a diuretic such as frusemide may be administered in an attempt to produce a diuresis. Nurses must observe the child closely during these interventions by frequent monitoring of pulse, respiratory rate, blood pressure and central venous pressure. If there is no response to diuretics, other strategies such as renal replacement therapy are indicated to support the child throughout the course of their acute renal failure.

Fluid restriction

Nurses must ensure that if a fluid restriction is necessary, it is strictly adhered to. To allow for insensible fluid loss, the child's fluid restriction will be calculated according to body surface area (300 mL/m^2), and urine output from the previous day.

Nutrition

Children with acute renal failure may develop a nutritional deficit due to poor intake and increased metabolic processes, leading to protein catabolism.[7] Supplementary feeding by nasogastric tube or total parenteral nutrition may be indicated. When selecting a formula for supplementary feeding, consideration must be given to the electrolyte content and fluid volume of the feeding. A restricted sodium and potassium diet is usually indicated.

MEDICAL INTERVENTION

Relief of obstruction

Surgical intervention to relieve obstruction is indicated in post-acute renal failure.

Vasoactive agent such as dopamine, a pharmacological agent that causes an increase in renal blood flow, glomerular filtration and sodium excretion, may be given. Dosages used in acute renal failure commence at 2.5 mg/kg/minute.[3] (See chronic renal failure for strategies for caring for children with the following complications of renal failure.)

- Altered serum sodium levels — hyponatraemia and hypernatraemia.
- Hypokalaemia.
- Hyperkalaemia.
- Alteration to body fluid status — potential for body fluid volume excess.
- Hypertension.
- Metabolic acidosis.
- Uraemia.
- Anaemia.
- Calcium and phosphate imbalance.
- Modification of drug dosages.
- Poor nutritional status.

RENAL REPLACEMENT THERAPY

Renal replacement therapy may be necessary to support the child during the course of acute renal failure.

INVESTIGATIONS

Daily or more frequent blood sampling is required for urea, electrolyte and creatinine levels, haemoglobin, white cell and platelet counts. Blood gases, and specific investigations to establish the cause of renal failure are attended as indicated.[8]

Investigation of the kidneys and urinary tract

Renal ultrasound is used to determine kidney size and check for obstruction and hydronephrosis. If hydronephrosis or obstruction are present, a micturating cystogram may be performed. Renal scan (DTPA) is used to demonstrate renal perfusion.

A renal biopsy may be performed to assist in diagnosis and treatment of the underlying cause of acute renal failure.

OUTCOME

The mortality of acute renal failure in children (<20%) is much lower than in adults. Many children recover completely, but a small number have permanent renal impairment varying from mild impairment to end-stage renal failure. Death from acute renal failure is predominantly caused by sepsis, respiratory and cardiac failure.

HAEMOLYTIC URAEMIC SYNDROME

Haemolytic uraemic syndrome (HUS) is an uncommon disease, but is the most common cause of acute renal failure in children. The disease has 3 characteristic symptoms: microangiopathic anaemia; thrombocytopenia; acute renal failure.[9]

HUS may be separated into 2 subgroups. The 1st group of children presents after a prodromal illness of diarrhoea (often with bloody stools); it is common for this group of children to present in the summer months, and to have a good recovery rate. The 2nd group of children does not have a prodromal illness. This group has a poorer prognosis, with 70% of the children having a relapsing form of the disease and progressing to chronic renal failure.[10]

Children with HUS typically present with a history of abdominal pain and diarrhoea, or an upper respiratory tract infection. Mini epidemics have been reported following *Escherichia coli* gut infections in children who have consumed contaminated meat products (e.g., hamburger mince, salami[11]). Children presenting with HUS have a pale, sometimes yellow, appearance due to the anaemia and retention of uraemic toxins. As acute renal failure develops they become anuric, irritable, and possibly fluid overloaded. Thrombocytopenia may cause a purpuric rash. A few children display abnormalities of the central nervous system such as seizures, coma or hemiparesis. The neurological dysfunction may be caused by uraemia, hypertensive encephalopathy or by cerebrovascular microvascular emboli.

Pathophysiology

Until recently the cause of HUS was not known but was suspected to have an infectious or immunological aetiology. It has recently been suggested that there is a strong association between HUS and intestinal infection with verocytotoxin-producing *Escherichia coli*.[12] Verocytotoxin has been shown to cause damage to endothelial cells.[9] There is damage to the epithelial lining of blood vessels which causes platelet and fibrin deposits and a decrease in the number of circulating thrombocytes (thrombocytopenia).[6]

Anaemia is believed to be caused by damage and fragmentation of red blood cells as they pass through the damaged glomeruli, which are occluded by fibrin strands. The damaged red blood cells are removed by the liver and spleen.[13]

Acute renal failure may develop because of injury to the glomerular capillary endothelial cells.

Management

The nursing management of HUS is as for the care of any child with acute renal failure: careful control of fluid and electrolyte balance; blood pressure control; renal replacement therapy if indicated.

REFERENCES

1. Brenner BM, Lazarus JM. *Acute renal failure.* Philadelphia: Saunders, 1983.
2. Gallego N, Gallego A, Pascal S, Liano F, Eslepa R, Orturia J. Prognosis of children with acute renal failure: a study of 138 cases. *Nephron* 1992; 64: 399–404.
3. Rogers MC. *Textbook of pediatric intensive care.* Vol. 2. Baltimore: Williams & Wilkins, 1987.
4. Holliday MA, Barratt TM, Vernier RL, eds. Pediatric nephrology. 2nd ed. Baltimore: Williams & Wilkins.
5. Oh TE. *Intensive care manual.* 3rd ed. Sydney: Butterworths, 1990.
6. Mott SR, James SR, Sperhac AM. *Nursing care of children and families.* 2nd ed. Menlo Park CA: Addison-Wesley, 1990.
7. Schafer P, Kelly MK, Lehr J, Scracco J. *Nursing care plans for the child. A nursing diagnosis approach.* Connecticut: Appleton & Lange, 1988.
8. Wong DL. *Whaley and Wong's nursing care of infants and children.* 5th ed. St Louis: Mosby, 1995.
9. Milford DV, Taylor CM. New insights into the haemolytic uraemic syndrome. *Arch Dis Childh* 1990; 65: 713–715.
10. Robson WLM, Leung AKC. The successful treatment of atypical hemolytic uremic syndrome with plasmapharesis. *Clin Nephrol* 1991; 35 (3): 119–122.
11. Brandt JR, Fraser KS, Watkins SL, Zelskwic I, Tarr PI, Nazar-Stewart V, Aurer EP. *Escherichia coli* 0157:H7-associated hemolytic uremic syndrome after ingestion of contaminated hamburgers. *J Pediatr* 1994; 125: 519–526.
12. Coad NAG, Marshall T, Rowe B, Taylor CM. Changes in postenteropathic form of the hemolytic uremic syndrome in children. *Clin Nephrol* 1991; 33 (1); 10–16.
13. Zimmerman SS, Gilder JH. *Critical care pediatrics.* Philadelphia: Saunders, 1985.

Chronic Renal Failure

Caring for children with chronic or end-stage renal failure presents a nursing challenge. Children with chronic renal failure undergo a wide variety of medical, dietary and surgical interventions to maintain life. These interventions are often unpleasant and sometimes painful. Due to the varying aetiologies and different stages of renal failure, intervention is highly individualised with no 2 children requiring the same nursing or medical care. Treatments require constant revision and will change frequently.

Chronic renal failure describes a disease process that over a period of time destroys the kidneys.

GLOMERULAR FILTRATION RATE

Estimation of the rate at which the glomerulus filters substances from the plasma is a useful test of kidney function. The kidneys receive 20% of the cardiac output. In adults, 125 mL of this blood is filtered across the glomerulus into the urinary space within the glomerular capsule every minute.[1]

The normal glomerular filtration rate is related to body size. In adults and children the normal glomerular filtration rate is expressed in mL/min/1.73 m^2 (the average adult body surface area).[1] Children over the age of 2 years have the same rate of glomerular filtration as adults, allowing for the difference in body size. The glomerular filtration rate in children under 2 years of age is still maturing, and consideration must be given to this when assessing glomerular filtration rate in this age group.

Measuring glomerular filtration rate assesses the progression of chronic renal failure. This is most accurately measured by performing a nuclear scan which assesses how well the kidney is able to clear the radioactive compound 99^{TC}m DTPA from the blood. The traditional method of measurement is to determine the amount of creatinine cleared in the urine during a 24-hour period, but this test may be difficult to perform in children who are not toilet trained.

PATHOPHYSIOLOGY

A reduction in glomerular filtration is responsible for many of the symptoms which become evident in chronic renal failure. Substances which under normal circumstances are filtered by the glomerulus accumulate in the circulation, imposing toxic effects upon the child.

It is usually not until the glomerular filtration rate is reduced to 25% to 50% of normal that children begin to show clinical evidence of the kidneys' inefficient control of homeostasis.

Signs and symptoms of chronic renal failure vary depending on the underlying disease process. Renal dysfunctions which initially damage the kidney tubules result in a tendency to excrete large quantities of sodium, bicarbonate and water. This occurs because the tubules lose the ability to reabsorb solutes. In contrast, diseases originating in the glomerulus initiate retention of sodium and water as a result of reduced glomerular filtration.[2]

Kidney damage continues over a period of months or years until eventually the kidney function remaining is insufficient to maintain life without the support of dialysis or a renal transplant. At this stage the child is said to have reached end-stage renal failure (ESRF).

Chronic renal failure may be divided into 4 phases.

Diminished renal reserve

In the early stages of chronic renal failure the child will show little evidence of renal impairment because the remaining, undamaged nephrons hypertrophy and compensate by filtering an increased solute load. Although glomerular filtration rate is reduced to approximately 50% to 60% of normal there is no disruption to homeostasis. At this stage the child has normal serum electrolyte levels, although urea and creatinine levels will be slightly increased. However, should the child be subjected to stressful complications such as infection, dehydration or haemorrhage, there will be an acute disruption to homeostasis which will present as increased serum urea and abnormal serum biochemistry levels. These symptoms will persist until the acute condition is treated. The child with diminished renal reserve related to reflux nephropathy or glomerulonephritis may be hypertensive.

Impaired renal function

The child is asymptomatic but displays elevated serum urea and creatinine levels. Glomerular filtration rate is less than 50% of normal. Blood biochemistry is abnormal (e.g., low calcium, high phosphorus, high potassium and low bicarbonate levels) and may require medical or dietary intervention. The child has an increased susceptibility to stressful events such as viral infections or dehydration, which may cause severe biochemical imbalances. These imbalances are reversible with medical intervention.[3]

Severe renal impairment

Five to 15% of renal function remains and the child will have permanently elevated blood urea and creatinine levels as well as fluid and electrolyte disturbances. The child will begin to display symptoms of uraemia.

End-stage renal failure

Less than 5% of renal function remains. Uraemia, abnormal biochemical and fluid status are life threatening at this stage. The child will require some form of renal replacement therapy to sustain life.

CLINICAL FEATURES

Kidney failure creates a disruption to homeostasis. Damaged kidneys fail to control fluid and electrolyte levels within normal limits and are unable to rid the body of the waste products of metabolism. Excess levels of waste products such as urea have toxic effects on the body.

Conditions occurring as a result of kidney failure are: electrolyte imbalance; fluid balance disturbances; metabolic acidosis; uraemia; anaemia; calcium and phosphate imbalance; growth failure; delayed puberty; developmental delay in infants; and anorexia resulting in poor nutritional status.

NURSING ASSESSMENT

The initial nursing assessment of the child with chronic renal failure will be quite extensive because of the adverse effects of renal disease on all body systems.

General appearance

Take note of the child's general appearance and behaviour. The child's skin colour is noted. Children with advanced renal failure may have a sallow complexion indicating anaemia and uraemia. Observe the child for signs of oedema, such as puffy eyes, face, hands, feet or buttocks. Ask the child or the parents about general physical activities and school attendance. As renal failure progresses, children tire easily and school attendance and performance diminish.[4]

Bodyweight

An accurate bare weight is taken on admission and compared with a recent weight if available. Bodyweight is a useful tool in assessing the child's fluid and nutritional status.

Vital signs

As with any nursing assessment temperature, pulse and respirations are recorded. An increased respiratory rate, shallow breathing or respiratory effort should be reported because it may indicate pulmonary oedema or metabolic acidosis.

An accurate blood pressure recording must be obtained, with an appropriately sized cuff. The cuff must encircle the child's arm completely and cover 75% of the upper arm. Using a cuff which is too small will result in overestimation of the child's blood pressure.

Height/length

The child's height is an important observation because it reflects the degree of renal failure. Children begin to grow poorly when renal function diminishes. Poor growth is a particular problem with renal failure in infancy and in children undergoing dialysis.

Elimination pattern

Ask the child or the parents how often the child passes urine and whether the child voids a small or large amount each time. It is important to know whether the child has an excessively high urine output or if the child is oliguric, so that fluid intake can be planned accordingly. A sample of urine should be obtained and tested for specific gravity, pH level, blood and protein.

Enquire as to whether the child passes urine normally or has a urinary diversion such as a ureterostomy. Some children with chronic renal failure require intermittent clean catheterisation.

Dietary history

Ascertain how good the child's appetite is and whether the child has any special dietary needs or restrictions.

STRATEGIES FOR CARING FOR CHILDREN WITH CHRONIC RENAL FAILURE

Medical and nursing interventions vary according to the cause of the child's renal failure, and the degree of renal function remaining.

Treatment in the early stages of chronic renal failure is aimed towards preservation of the remaining nephrons by dietary control of protein, phosphate and solute load and the prevention of further renal damage from hypertension, urinary tract infection or urinary tract obstruction.

The following problems present in children with chronic renal failure.

Abnormal serum electrolyte levels

Altered ability to conserve salt and water

In the early stages of chronic renal failure, the kidneys may fail to conserve adequate quantities of sodium due to an inability of the kidney tubules to reabsorb solutes efficiently. At this stage the kidneys are unable to concentrate urine during times of fluid deprivation.

Usually, sodium and water losses are balanced so that the serum sodium concentration in the extracellular fluid will remain normal. Some children, however, lose more salt than water and their serum sodium levels fall. Rarely, water losses exceed salt losses and serum sodium levels rise.

Infants and children with salt-wasting renal diseases require close observation of their hydration status. It is a nursing responsibility to ensure children are bare weighed daily on the same set of scales, and that any alterations in weight are reported to the medical staff. Blood pressure must be recorded every 4 hours. An accurate intake and output chart is maintained. If there is a reduction in the child's urine output, or the child's urine output is in excess of fluid intake, dehydration should be suspected and the child referred to medical staff for intervention. Some children require salt replacement in their diet or formula.

As chronic renal failure progresses the glomeruli fail to filter sodium and water efficiently. Sodium and water retention result in hypertension and oedema. A diet with no added salt may be implemented and antihypertensive medications are sometimes prescribed.

The best guide to salt and water retention is measurement of the child's weight and blood pressure. These will increase long before the child appears oedematous. If a child with end-stage renal failure drinks too much water, the serum sodium level will fall due to dilution.

Hypokalaemia

In the early stages of chronic renal failure some children excrete excessive amounts of potassium in their urine which leads to hypokalaemia. This condition is caused by a defect in the renal tubules causing them to be inefficient in their resorption capacity. Hypokalaemia may cause cardiac arrythmias, muscle weakness, hypotonicity, ileus and ventilatory failure.[5] Intravenous replacement is required if the child is acutely unwell. If hypokalaemia is a chronic condition, oral replacement may be required. Children who are well enough should be encouraged to eat potassium-rich foods such as bananas and stone fruit.

Hyperkalaemia

When glomerular filtration falls to approximately 10% of normal the damaged glomeruli do not filter potassium and the distal tubules do not secrete potassium adequately from the blood. These abnormalities result in high serum potassium levels.

It is important to maintain the intracellar and extracellular potassium level within normal limits in order to regulate the cardiac action potential. Hyperkalaemia is extremely dangerous because it disturbs that balance. Elevated serum potassium levels cause cardiac arrhythmia and asystole. Cardiac arrest may occur if hyperkalaemia is not treated promptly, and may be the first sign of unsuspected hyperkalaemia.

If a child with renal failure has blood collected for an urgent potassium measurement, the nurse caring for the child should make sure that the specimen is delivered to the laboratory immediately and that the result is phoned back to the ward within 30 minutes.

Nurses caring for children with chronic renal failure should have a knowledge of normal serum electrolyte levels because they are often the person who receives the telephone call from the laboratory reporting abnormal results. Potassium levels over 5.5 mmol/L must be reported to the medical staff immediately. Children with hyperkalaemia should be placed on a cardiac monitor and observed for widening of QRS complexes and tenting of T waves.[6]

In an emergency, the following treatment methods are implemented to reduce the serum potassium level rapidly.

- When the child is acidotic, intravenous sodium bicarbonate is administered to shift potassium back into the cells. This occurs as a result of hydrogen ions exchanging for potassium ions, as the blood pH is corrected. The nurse caring for a child with a diminished urine output receiving intravenous sodium bicarbonate must monitor the child for signs of intravascular fluid volume excess resulting from intravenous sodium administration.
- Intravenous glucose and insulin may be administered. Glucose stimulates insulin release, which facilitates movement of potassium into the cell.[7] Insulin facilitates the cellular uptake of potassium. Children should have hourly blood sugar measurements for 4 hours following this treatment.
- Intravenous salbutamol is gaining popularity as the treatment of choice for children with severe hyperuricaemia. Salbutamol binds to beta$_2$ adrenergic receptors in the liver and muscle cell membranes, which stimulates an enzyme reaction on the sodium–potassium ATPase pump, facilitating movement of potassium into the intracellular compartment.[8]

The above treatments have a rapid but short-acting effect. They are a temporary treatment measure until a longer acting therapy can be implemented.

A cation exchange resin such as calcium resonium or sodium resonium A is a longer lasting treatment method. Exchange resins exchange either sodium or calcium for potassium in the gut. Resonium is effective within 1 to 2 hours of administration.

Resonium is a powder that has to be mixed with water and made into a paste of a suitable consistency to either swallow or administer as a retention enema. It is best to add the water a little at a time and stir it well. If the mixture is to be taken orally, sugar or honey may be added to make the mixture more palatable. Oral administration is usually attempted first, however, the mixture has a rather unpleasant taste and many children either spit it out or refuse to swallow. If the child is extremely distressed or nauseated it is best to administer resonium rectally so as to avoid vomiting and inhalation.

Resonium is sometimes ordered as an ongoing, daily treatment for certain children. Nurses should discuss the most appropriate method of administration with the child and his or her parents prior to discharge home. Resonium may cause severe constipation so it is important to ensure that children have regular bowel actions.

Sodium resonium should be avoided in children who are oliguric or hypertensive because the increased sodium load may cause fluid retention and increased hypertension. The use of calcium resonium should be avoided in children with hypercalcaemia.

Occasionally, resonium is administered mixed with sorbitol. This mixture induces an osmotic diarrhoea and assists in fluid and potassium removal.

Dialysis removes potassium from the child's bloodstream by diffusion across a semipermeable membrane.

Alterations to body fluid status

Volume deficit

Initially, the child with chronic renal failure may lose excessive amounts of water via the kidneys due to an inability to reabsorb sufficient water to meet the body requirements. These children, therefore, excrete large volumes of dilute urine and have an increased thirst. To compensate for this they are encouraged to drink extra fluids. During this polyuric phase of chronic renal failure, children are unable to tolerate periods of fluid deprivation. Should this occur, e.g., when fasting for procedures, the progression of chronic renal failure towards end-stage renal failure may be accelerated. Children at this stage of renal failure should receive intravenous fluid replacement if they are unable to maintain their fluid intake orally.

Volume excess

As chronic renal failure progresses and glomerular filtration rate diminishes, the kidneys do not filter water adequately. Fluid retention occurs, and becomes evident as oedema and hypertension. Fluid retention may lead to hypertensive encephalopathy and seizures, breathlessness caused by pulmonary oedema, and congestive cardiac failure.

Medical intervention

In advanced renal failure, there is a reduction in the glomerular filtration rate resulting in salt and water retention. A diuretic such as frusemide may be administered or an oral fluid restriction may be implemented.

Assessment of body fluid status

Clinical signs indicating fluid depletion are:

- Sudden weight loss.
- Low blood pressure, and postural drop in blood pressure.
- Dry mouth and tongue.
- Decreased urine output in a child with a high or normal urine output. (Some children continue to have a normal urine output despite fluid depletion because their kidneys cannot reduce their urine output appropriately because of renal damage).
- Eyes appear sunken.
- Decreased skin turgor.
- Thirst.
- Increased biochemical levels such as urea, haemoglobin and creatinine (haemo-concentration).
- Sunken fontanelles in infants.
- Lethargy.

Clinical signs indicating fluid volume excess are:

- Weight gain.
- High blood pressure, headaches, seizures.
- Oedema.
- Jugular vein appears enlarged and may be pulsating.
- Moist tongue and mucous membranes.

- Tachypnoea, dyspnoea, child unable to tolerate lying down.
- Decreased blood sodium level caused by a dilutional effect.
- Moist cough with white frothy sputum.

Nursing intervention

Intravascular fluid volume excess

Children who are either anuric or oliguric require fluid restriction to prevent fluid volume excess. The daily fluid allowance will be ordered according to the child's residual urine output and insensible losses. Insensible losses are calculated as 300 mL/m^2 of body surface area. In cases of severe volume excess, fluids may have to be withheld until excess fluid is removed either by diuretics or dialysis.

If a child is placed on a fluid restriction all the fluid given must be measured and recorded, including fluids given with medications. Ice blocks, jellies and milk on cereal are fluids that caregivers sometimes neglect to record. It is important to include them in the calculations for a child's fluid restriction.

Adherence to a fluid restriction can be one of the most difficult aspects of caring for children with chronic renal failure. Children feel thirsty because of high serum osmolality related to the increased level of retained solutes in their blood, especially urea. Younger children become quite distressed and constantly request or cry for fluids. Older children frequently help themselves to drinks at times when they are away from adult supervision. Diversional activities in the form of play therapy can be implemented to distract the child.

There is a reasonably high incidence of non-compliance with fluid restrictions. Nurses must be firm with children and their parents. 'Just a little bit of extra fluid' will harm, particularly if there are several people involved in giving just a little extra.

Children and their families should be involved in planning for the even distribution of fluids throughout the day. Children should not be given a large volume of fluid early in the day because they will feel very thirsty later in the day if they have used up their restriction before dinner time. It is better to give a quarter, or half a cup of fluid more regularly.

High blood pressure

High blood pressure is related to sodium and water retention, or to a disruption to the renin–angiotensin system. When children with renal failure require hospital admission they should have their blood pressure recorded every 4 hours. Acceptable limits should be obtained from the child's physician and recorded on the nursing care plan. Any recordings outside of these limits must be reported to attending medical staff immediately.

Normal blood pressure relates to the age and size of the child and most paediatric textbooks contain normal percentile charts for blood pressure. **Table 7.22** lists average resting blood pressure readings for children. (See section on Glomerulonephritis for further details).

Medical intervention

Hypertension is controlled with dietary sodium and fluid restriction, and antihypertensive medications such as nifedipine, clonidine and enalapril.

Table 7.22 Normal and abnormal blood pressure recordings for children

Age	Systolic	Pressure (mmHg) Diastolic	Hypertension
neonate	70–90	50–70	95/70
1–2 years	80–110	50–70	115/75
2–5 years	85–110	50–75	120/80
5–10 years	90–115	50–80	125/85
10–15 years	100–120	55–80	130/85
15–18 years	100–130	60–85	140/90

Metabolic acidosis

Factors contributing to metabolic acidosis in chronic renal failure are:

- Diseased kidneys which are unable to excrete hydrogen ions and produce ammonia.
- Bicarbonate buffers which are excreted in the urine because damaged proximal tubules fail to reabsorb them.[9]
- Retention of acid end products of metabolism.[10]

Acidosis in chronic renal failure contributes to renal osteodystrophy because the body resorts to using other buffering systems such as bone salts to buffer acids.[10]

Metabolic acidosis aggravates hyperkalaemia because intracellular potassium ions move out of cells and into the extracellular compartment to be exchanged with extracellular hydrogen ions in an attempt to correct acidosis.

Nursing intervention

Nursing responsibilities include close observation of the child's respiratory status. Increased rate and depth of respirations is an indication of acidosis. Other clinical indications of acidosis include anorexia, nausea and abdominal pain, and a decreased level of consciousness. The nurse must monitor the rate of sodium bicarbonate infusion closely, because a too rapid infusion may result in complications from high serum sodium levels and fluid retention.

Medical intervention

Children may require oral bicarbonate supplements to correct and prevent acidosis. Oral supplements are usually withdrawn once the child starts dialysis because efficient dialysis corrects acidosis. If the child is acutely acidotic, intravenous sodium bicarbonate may be administered.

Uraemia

Urea is the end product of protein metabolism. Under normal circumstances excess urea is filtered from the blood and eliminated from the body by the kidneys. When kidneys fail, urea is no longer filtered and accumulates in the bloodstream. The build-up of excess urea in the blood is referred to as uraemia. Uraemia has a toxic effect on the body. The effects of uraemia are as follows:

- Neurological symptoms such as confusion, irritability, seizures, muscular cramps and twitching. In rare cases, uraemic encephalopathy leads to coma.

- Impairment of platelet activity causing bleeding of the gums and epistaxis, bruising, and prolonged bleeding times.
- Gastrointestinal symptoms: hiccoughs: build-up of excess salivary urea is converted to ammonia and causes a metallic taste in the mouth and bad breath (uraemic fetor); and nausea and anorexia causing poor nutrition and failure to thrive.
- The skin becomes dry and itchy and has a yellow tinge.
- The toxic effects of high levels of urea in infants cause developmental delay both in physical and mental ability.
- Uraemic pericarditis. Uraemic toxins irritate the pericardial membrane.[11]

Nursing intervention

The uraemic child requires a number of nursing interventions.

Nurses should be aware of the child's increased *bleeding tendencies* and aim to prevent blood loss. Children should be advised to use a soft toothbrush so as to avoid bleeding gums. Regular oral hygiene should be attended to reduce the unpleasant taste in the child's mouth and prevent mouth ulcers. If children require surgical procedures (e.g., creation of vascular access for haemodialysis or insertion of a peritoneal dialysis catheter) they will require close observation of the wound for signs of bleeding postoperatively.

Small, frequent *meals* should be offered. If the child is not eating, nurses should express their concern to the child's physician so that consideration may be given to nutritional support therapy.

Moisturisers should be applied to the child's *skin* to prevent the skin from becoming dry and itchy.

Medical intervention

Dietary protein restriction is sometimes implemented in an attempt to reduce the workload of the remaining nephrons, and prolong the progression to end stage renal failure. Dietary protein restriction in young children may not be appropriate because severe dietary restrictions impair growth.

Dialysis removes excess urea from the blood and is introduced when the child is exhibiting symptoms of uraemia such as poor progress at school, delayed milestones, linear growth failure, anorexia and malnutrition.

Anaemia

As chronic renal failure progresses, the kidneys become deficient in their ability to secrete erythropoietin. Reduced erythropoietin levels result in impaired red blood cell production which causes anaemia.[12]

Medical intervention

Recombinant human erythropoietin is a therapy that aims to replace the deficient erythropoietin production and reverse the anaemia of chronic renal failure. The drug is administered by intravenous infusion at the completion of a haemodialysis session, or by subcutaneous injection for children who are undergoing peritoneal dialysis. Some centres administer erythropoietin in peritoneal dialysis fluid, but this route is not common.[13,14] Subcutaneous injection of erythropoietin is quite painful. This discomfort may be alleviated to some degree by removing the drug from the refrigerator approximately 30 minutes before injecting. The frequency of administration of erythropoietin depends on the child's response and in most cases twice-weekly administration is required.

If the child is severely anaemic then he or she will require a blood transfusion. If the child is oliguric, precautions must be taken to prevent intravascular fluid excess and hypertension. Children who are dialysis dependent should only receive blood transfusions during dialysis. Transfusions must be administered slowly over 4 to 6 hours. Hourly blood pressure recording should be attended to during the blood transfusion and for several hours after completion. Children often become hypertensive during blood transfusion and elevated blood pressure must be reported immediately.

Children with end-stage renal failure who are potential renal transplant recipients should have their blood transfusion administered via a leucocyte filter in an attempt to prevent antibody formation.

Calcium and phosphate imbalance

Chronic renal failure causes alteration to calcium and phosphate homeostasis. Calcium and phosphate imbalance is difficult to control, has a dramatic effect on growth, and contributes towards the short stature, bone pain, rickets and bony deformities which are common features of children with renal failure.

Damaged kidneys do not produce activated Vitamin D which is responsible for stimulating calcium absorption from the gut. A decreased serum calcium level results, which in turn stimulates the parathyroid glands to release parathyroid hormone. Parathyroid hormone causes resorption of calcium salts from the bone in order to raise serum calcium levels. If this situation continues over a long period, as in chronic renal failure, bones become depleted of calcium and cavities form in the bones. Calcium is also required for neuromuscular activity.[14]

When the glomerular filtration rate is severely reduced, phosphorus and hydrogen ions are retained. Serum phosphorus is bound to calcium, and the two have an inverse relationship. If phosphorus is high, serum calcium level will be depressed to maintain the balance. The normal product of serum calcium and phosphorus should be under 4.0 mmol/L.

Elevated serum phosphorus levels also stimulate the parathyroid glands to secrete parathyroid hormone.[3] If the parathyroid hormones are stimulated by a high serum phosphate level for a prolonged period, they become overactive, resulting in extensive leaching of calcium from bones and the calcium deposits in blood vessels, eyes and joints.

Disturbance of calcium and phosphate balance causes bone demineralisation, and may result in the condition known as renal osteodystrophy. This situation is aggravated further by hydrogen ion retention resulting in acidosis which leads to alkaline bone salts being removed from the bone to neutralise the hydrogen ions.

Nursing intervention

It is a nursing responsibility to ensure that phosphate binding medication is administered at the correct times. Phosphate binders must be administered with meals so that the phosphate contained in food is removed from the gut. It is of no value to administer phosphate binders at any time other than meal times. Children and their parents require education and regular reinforcement about the importance of phosphate binders. Unfortunately, there is a high incidence of non-compliance with these drugs because of the monotony of taking tablets and the interruption they cause to meals and because taking tablets makes children feel different to other children.

Medical intervention

Prevention of renal osteodystrophy is attempted by removal of excess phosphate from the gut by the administration of phosphate binding medication, such as calcium carbonate or aluminium hydroxide. Aluminium-containing phosphate binders are rarely used to treat children because large quantities of the drug are required to control phosphate levels adequately. Excessive aluminium levels have a toxic effect on the central nervous system, resulting in brain degeneration and dementia.[15]

Vitamin D supplements such as ergocalciferol and calcitriol may be administered.

Some children require surgical correction of bony deformities caused by renal osteodystrophy. After a number of years children may require surgical removal of the parathyroid glands.

Growth failure

Most children with chronic renal failure grow poorly. The earlier the onset of chronic renal failure the more poorly the child grows. Most children with early onset of renal disease are below the 3rd percentile for height and weight. Growth failure is poorly understood, but there are a number of contributing factors:

- Calcium and phosphate disturbances causing renal osteodystrophy.
- Reduction in nutritional intake related to anorexia and/or dietary restrictions.
- Anaemia.
- Metabolic acidosis.
- Uraemia and other biochemical disturbances.[16]
- Prior to advanced renal failure many children have renal diseases that cause sodium and water wastage. Salt wasting and dehydration results in poor growth.
- Resistance to the effects of growth hormone because of the presence of uraemic toxins.

Growth failure is a major contributor to psychological maladjustments in children with chronic renal failure. Because of their short stature, frequent hospitalisation and the dependent nature of treatment strategies for chronic and end-stage renal failure, children with chronic renal failure are restricted not only in their linear growth but in the growth and development of their self-esteem and social skills. Parents and families of children with chronic renal failure tend to be very protective, making it difficult for children to achieve independence.

Nursing intervention

It is a nursing responsibility to ensure that accurate measurements of height are taken every time the child requires hospital admission.

Medical intervention

Recombinant human growth hormone therapy has recently been introduced in an attempt to achieve linear growth in children with chronic renal failure. It is reported to be effective in large doses.[17] Nutritional status should be optimised beforte instituting growth hormone therapy.

Delayed puberty

Adolescents with chronic and end-stage renal failure are noticeably delayed in pubertal development. Uraemic adolescent girls do not usually menstruate, and if they do, menstruation is irregular.

Adolescents and adults with end-stage renal failure are usually infertile, have a decreased libido and many males are impotent.[18] Uraemic toxins depress ovulation and sperm production. Sexually active females, however, should be advised to seek contraceptive advice because on rare occasions pregnancy may occur. Uraemia has an adverse effect on the fetus.[9]

Poor nutritional status

Providing adequate caloric and protein intake for growth in children with chronic renal failure presents a major challenge. Uraemic children have extremely poor appetites. Many children fail to thrive and their weight is often below the 3rd percentile for age.

Diet

Providing adequate nutrition while avoiding foods which will have an adverse effect on the child's remaining kidney function or exacerbate uraemic symptoms in children with renal failure is extremely demanding. The child's diet requires constant review and adjustments have to be made according to serum biochemistry results and the child's overall state of nutrition.

Serum urea levels may be controlled by dietary *protein restriction*. Occasionally, this strategy is implemented in older children in an attempt to prolong the life of the remaining nephrons and avoid the need for early initiation of dialysis. However, the advantage of this has to be weighed up against the effect of protein restriction on growth.[19]

Infant formulas should have a low *phosphate* and solute content. Breast milk contains less phosphate than cows' milk or commercially available formulas.[20]

Potassium restriction is usually only required for children with end-stage renal failure. A list of foods that are high in potassium should be available in wards caring for children with renal disease. Parents and children require regular reinforcement and information about which foods to avoid. Some examples of foods that are high in potassium are chocolate, bananas, stone fruit, dried fruit and nuts.

Salt restriction is required for children that have a low or no urine output, so that fluid retention and hypertension may be avoided. Children are advised not to add salt to their food and that they must not eat foods which are obviously high in sodium content. Examples are potato crisps, Twisties, Cheesels, Vegemite, peanut butter, tomato sauce, soy sauce, bacon, ham and processed meats. Parents must be advised against purchasing salt substitutes to achieve a salty flavour because these products contain potassium chloride, which may also be restricted.

Children with renal failure are usually anorexic and it is extremely difficult to achieve adequate caloric intake. For some children, anorexia and malnutrition may become life threatening. Because of this, dietary restriction is only ever introduced when there is no other alternative.

Children are encouraged to eat foods which are high in fat and carbohydrates to provide calories. Supplements such as Polyjuole provide extra calories and may be added to drinks, infant formulas or sprinkled on food.

Gastrostomy or nasogastric tube feeding may be introduced if nutrition is poor or if children are not growing. Tube feeding provides the best means for improved growth to infants 2 years and under. This period is normally a period of rapid growth and nutritional demands are high.[21]

Providing supplementary calories and protein by tube feeding may be hindered by the need for fluid restriction. This problem can be overcome by adding MCT oil, corn oil and Polyjoule to the feed.[22]

Modification of drug doses

Children with advanced renal failure require modifications in the dosage of those drugs which are excreted by the kidneys in order to prevent toxicity. A list of these drugs should be available in wards that routinely care for children with chronic renal failure. A common example is gentamycin, which is frequently used to treat urinary tract infections. Gentamycin can be ototoxic or nephrotoxic and lead to a further deterioration of the child's renal function if the dosage is not adjusted and blood levels monitored.

SURGICAL INTERVENTION

Urology surgery

Children with obstructive uropathy and reflux nephropathy require surgical interventions such as reimplantation of ureters or urinary diversion methods such as ureterostomy, vesicostomy, nephrostomy or ileal conduit. These procedures facilitate the free drainage of urine and prevent further renal damage and scarring from refluxing urine.

Dialysis access surgery

As older children and adolescents approach end-stage renal failure, vascular access may be created in preparation for haemodialysis. Most commonly a radiocephalic arteriovenous fistula is surgically created in the non-dominant wrist.

Preservation of blood vessels for arteriovenous fistula formation

Children with chronic and end-stage renal failure require frequent blood tests and intravenous cannulation for a variety of reasons. The cephalic vein should not be used as a site for intravenous cannula insertion. This vessel must be preserved because it will most likely be required for creation of vascular access for haemodialysis later. Unfortunately, this vein is often the easiest vein to access, and the temptation to use it is strong. Nurses, as the patient's advocate, must advise against this and insist that the child's consulting physician be notified before a decision is made to use this vessel. Likewise, the radial artery should not be used for blood gas analysis.

INVESTIGATIONS

Blood samples

Children with chronic renal failure undergo frequent venipunctures for blood analysis. This is extremely distressing for both the child and their parents. Only experienced staff should collect the blood, so as to avoid failed attempts at venipuncture. A local anaesthetic cream (Emla) may be beneficial for use in children who become extremely distressed about venepuncture, parents can be taught to apply the cream 1 hour before the blood is to be collected.

Blood should never be collected from an existing fistula arm, and the non-dominant arm should be avoided because the blood vessels on this arm may be required for future haemodialysis access.

Blood is collected for urea, electrolytes, calcium, phosphate and creatinine levels. Creatinine is the end product of muscle metabolism and is removed from the bloodstream by the kidneys. Unlike urea, it is little affected by the child's diet, so it provides a good indication of renal function. Elevated creatinine levels are indicative of renal failure. Elevated serum urea levels may also indicate renal failure, but urea may also be elevated in dehydration or following a gastrointestinal bleed when excess protein is absorbed following blood breakdown.

Urine

Urine collection may be required for a number investigations. Urine tests provide information about the kidneys' concentrating and diluting ability as well as the kidneys' ability to clear substances from the bloodstream. Paediatric urine specimen collection bags may be used to collect specimens from infants.

24-hour urine collections

A 24-hour urine collection may be requested for a quantitative assessment of the clearance of various solutes by the kidneys, such as creatinine, calcium and protein. All the urine that the kidneys produce in a 24-hour period is collected in a container. The first specimen is discarded and the time that the first specimen was voided must be recorded. All urine passed during the following 24 hours is placed into the container.

Some tests require a preservative to be added to the collection bottle and the nurse responsible for the collection should always enquire as to whether this is required.

Because 24-hour urine collections are extremely difficult to collect from young children and infants, they are not commonly requested. Unfortunately, collections are frequently spoiled by children forgetting about the urine collection or accidentally discarding the urine. Parents staying with their children in the hospital can assist in the collection. It is sometimes more successful for the 24-hour urine collection to be collected by the parents in their own home.

Investigation of the kidneys and urinary tract

See nursing care of the child with an infection of the urinary tract for a description of renal ultrasound, micturating cystogram, radionuclide scan and intravenous pyelogram.

Renal arteriogram

This test is used mostly in children with severe hypertension. Contrast medium is injected into the aorta or renal arteries via a femoral catheter in order to visualise the renal blood vessels, and therefore identify stenosis of the renal arteries, absent, extra or misplaced vessels. The child will be required to remain in bed for 24 hours after the investigation and pressure is applied to the catheter site in the groin. Close observation of circulation and peripheral pulses distal to the site is required following the arteriogram.

Renal biopsy

This diagnostic investigation involves the percutaneous needle aspiration of a minute specimen of renal tissue. The tissue is examined by electron microscopy to study the glomeruli and presence of disease processes. Immunofluorescence studies reveal immunological processes and deposits that may be occurring in the glomerulus. Renal tissue is also examined by light microscopy to look at the glomeruli and renal tubules. Electron microscopy provides information on basement membranes and the position of immune deposits.

CAUSES OF CHRONIC RENAL FAILURE IN CHILDREN

Glomerulonephritis

Glomerulonephritis of a variety of types accounts for about 40% of cases of chronic renal failure in children.

Congenital abnormalities

Renal agenesis

Renal agenesis may be unilateral or bilateral. The absence of one kidney may not cause any problems at all. Usually the single kidney hypertrophies to compensate for its increased workload.

Bilateral absence of kidneys (Potters syndrome) is a rare disorder which occurs in 1 in every 4000 births.[23] Affected infants characteristically have abnormal facies (wide-set eyes, parrot-beak nose, low-slung ears and receding chin), spade-like hands, dry wrinkled skin and pulmonary hypoplasia or dysplasia. About 40% of infants with Potters syndrome are still-born, and the remainder die of renal or respiratory failure shortly after birth.

Renal hypoplasia

This congenital abnormality results in a reduction in the amount of renal tissue formed. Affected infants have only 5 or less renal lobules. Although nephron formation is normal, if the condition is bilateral there is insufficient renal tissue available to maintain normal growth and development. Renal failure may present in infancy, however it may not become apparent until adulthood.[23]

Renal dysplasia

This condition occurs as a result of abnormal development of renal tissue. Kidneys are usually small and many children have associated urinary tract abnormalities.[3]

Renal dysplasia may be unilateral or bilateral. Children with bilateral dysplasia are usually recognised in infancy, particularly if they have associated urinary tract abnormalities such as obstructive uropathy or ureteric reflux. These children may also have bowel and genital abnormalities.

Children with renal dysplasia initially have an inability to concentrate their urine which causes increased sodium and water losses due to renal tubular dysplasia.

Triad syndrome (prune belly syndrome)

The prune belly syndrome is a congenital abnormality consisting of absence of abdominal musculature (which gives the abdomen a prune-like appearance), urinary tract anomalies and undescended testes. The syndrome occurs once in every 35 000 to 50 000 births and predominantly affects males.

Urinary tract anomalies usually consist of renal dysplasia or hypoplasia and enlarged and malfunctioning bladder and ureters. The enlarged bladder has minimal muscle tone, and urinary stasis and infection may be a complication. A few children with prune belly syndrome require urinary diversion measures to prevent further damage to the kidneys resulting from back pressure of poorly draining urine, and hence preserve renal function.

Surgical correction of cryptorchidism is undertaken early in life.

Affected children are usually fitted with a surgical corset for abdominal support and correction of posture.

Posterior urethral valves

This abnormality consists of valve-like folds of tissue in the posterior urethra in boys. The condition often causes urinary obstruction in early infancy and may be recognised by a distended bladder, and a weak, dribbling urinary stream.[23] Severe obstruction during foetal development may be suspected by the presence of enlarged fluid-filled spaces on antenatal ultrasound, and the presence of oligohydramnios.[24]

The newborn infant may present with failure to thrive, sepsis, renal failure and severe acidosis. The abnormal valves are obliterated surgically. In some children, even when posterior urethral valves have been treated at birth, end-stage renal failure may result around puberty. If valves are not detected until later in the child's life, the kidneys may have sustained irreversible damage from urinary reflux and kidney dysplasia.

Infantile polycystic disease

This is an autosomal recessively inherited disease which affects the liver and kidneys. Renal abnormalities present in early infancy prior to liver symptoms. Normal renal tissue is replaced by numerous cysts which cause the kidneys to become enlarged and have a spongy appearance. The renal tissue situated between the cysts consists of normal nephrons.

Infants present with hypertension, an abdominal mass and renal failure. Early presentation usually represents a higher incidence of cystic replacement of renal tissue. Cysts may become infected or bleed, causing anaemia and sepsis, however, this is less common than in the adult form of the disease. Older children may have liver involvement and sometimes present with portal hypertension and oesophageal varices.

There is an adult form of this disease. It is a dominantly inherited disease, and symptoms do not present until adulthood. Liver involvement is uncommon.

Medullary cystic disease (congenital nephronophthisis)

This disease is inherited and involves progressive sclerosis and scarring of glomerular and interstitial renal tissue and renal tubular atrophy. Cysts occur in the renal medulla. Children affected by the disease present with anaemia, sodium wasting and diminished renal concentrating ability. Children progress to end-stage renal failure between 8 to 10 years of age.

Cystinosis

Cystinosis is a rare metabolic disease, but a common cause of chronic renal failure in children. This disease is inherited by autosomal recessive inheritance. The disease involves excessive lysosomal storage of the amino acid cystine in a number of body organs. Accumulated cystine leads to crystal formation and cell death in various tissues.

Children present during their first year of life with failure to thrive, salt wasting, polyuria and polydipsia due to excessive renal tubular sodium losses. Affected children grow poorly and may develop rickets as a result of metabolic acidosis, hypophosphataemia and hypocalcaemia, which results from failure of the reabsorption capacity of the renal tubules.

Until recently, cystine crystal deposits destroyed the kidneys and end-stage renal failure usually occurred by age 10 years. Cystine depleting therapy (cysteamine) is now in use. Cysteamine enters the cells and reacts with cystine to form a compound which is able to leave the lysosome via a cellular transport mechanism. This mechanism does not require the cystine carrier, which is defective in cystinosis.[25] Cystine-depleting therapy must be introduced early in the child's life to be effective and must be administered regularly. As the medication is quite unpalatable, affected children and their parents require constant reinforcement and support to ensure compliance.

Oxalosis

Oxalosis is a rare, autosomal recessively inherited, metabolic disease in which there is an overproduction of oxalate resulting in its renal secretion. Calcium oxalate crystals are deposited throughout body tissues. Renal failure develops and is caused by stone formation and calcium oxalate deposits in the kidneys.[26]

Urinary reflux

Severe urinary reflux may cause damage and scarring of kidney tissue and result in chronic and end-stage renal failure. Urinary reflux does not usually cause end-stage renal failure until the child reaches late teens.

REFERENCES

1. Taylor C, Chapman S. *Handbook of renal investigations in children.* London: Wright Publishing Company, 1989.
2. Wong DL. *Whaley and Wong's nursing care of infants and children.* 5th ed. St Louis: Mosby, 1995.
3. Evans DB, Henderson RG. *Lecture notes on nephrology.* Oxford: Blackwell Scientific, 1985.
4. Zurzanello MH. Preventing acute renal failure in patients with chronic renal insufficiency: nursing implications. *Am Nephrol Nurses Assoc J* 1989; 16: 433–436.
5. Worthley LIG. Fluid and electrolyte therapy *In* Oh TE, ed. *Intensive care manual.* 3rd ed. Sydney: Butterworths, 1990.
6. Hamplas JR. *The ECG in practice.* 2nd ed. Edinburgh: Churchill Livingstone, 1992.
7. Schacht RG. Acute renal failure *In:* Zimmerman SS, Gildea JH. *Critical care pediatrics.* 1985 Philadelphia: WB Saunders.
8. Murdoch IA, Anjos RD, Haycock GB. Treatment of hyperkalaemia with intravenous salbutamol. *Arch Dis Childh* 1991; 66: 527–528.
9. Hamilton HK. *Renal disorders: nurses clinical library.* Pennsylvania: Springhouse Corporation, 1984.

10. Tortora GJ, Anagnostakos NP. *Principles of anatomy and physiology.* 7th ed. New York: Harper & Row, 1993.

11. Smith S. Uremic pericarditis in chronic renal failure: nursing implications. *Am Nephrol Nurses Assoc J* 1993; 20: 432–436.

12. York S. Current perspectives: iron management during therapy with recombinant human erythropoietin. *Am Nephrol Nurses Assoc J* 1993; 20: 645–650.

13. Muller-Wielel DE, Amon O. Use of human erythropoietin in children undergoing dialysis. *Sem Dialysis* 1994; 7: 413–420.

14. Pravant BF, Ryan LP, Satalavich RJ, Schmidt LM, Murray-Bell A, Kennedy JM, Baker BL. Effectiveness of a phosphorus education program for dialysis patients. *Am Nephrol Nurses Assoc J* 1989; 16: 353–357.

15. Ramirez JA, Goodman WG, Salusky IB. Optimal management of renal osteodystrophy in children treated with CAPD and CCPD. *Sem Dialysis* 1994; 7: 435–441.

16. Crittenden MR, Holiday B. Physical growth and behavioural adaptations of children with renal insufficiency. *Am Nephrol Nurses Assoc J* 1989; 16: 87–92.

17. Watkins SL. Use of recombinant human growth hormone in children undergoing dialysis. *Sem Dialysis* 1994; 7: 421–428.

18. Zarifian AA. Sexual dysfunction in the male end stage renal disease patient. *Am Nephrol Nurses Assoc J* 1992; 19: 527–532.

19. Stewart CL, Katz SP, Kaskel FJ. Unique aspects of the care of pediatric dialysis patients. *Sem Dialysis* 1988; 1 (3): 160–169.

20. Mott SR, James SR, Sperhac AM. *Nursing care of children and families.* 2nd ed. Menlo Park CA: Addison-Wesley, 1990.

21. Brewer ED. Supplemental enteral tube feeding in infants undergoing dialysis — indications and outcome. *Sem Dialysis* 1994; 7: 429–434.

22. Carreron RD. Children on dialysis: nutritional management an overview. *Dialysis and Transplant* 1991; 20 (6): 303–305.

23. Nelson WE, Behrmann RE, Vaughan VC. *Textbook of pediatrics.* 12th ed. Philadelphia: Saunders, 1983.

25. Adamson MD, Andersson HC, Gahl WA. Cystinosis. *Seminars in Nephrology* 1989; 9: 147–161.

26. Cameron S. *Kidney disease: the facts.* Oxford: Oxford University Press, 1985.

Disturbances in Haematopoietic and Immunological Function

Anaemia

David Sutton

Anaemia can be defined as a reduction in the haemoglobin level below that of normal for the patient's age.

At birth, haemoglobin levels range from 170 to 210 g/L and the red cells are macrocytic with a mean cell volume (MCV) of 119 fL. All values drop rapidly for about 2 months until mean haemoglobin is 110 g/L and MCV is 95 fL. Haemoglobin and MCV levels then rise slowly until adult levels are achieved by puberty. Generally speaking, anaemia can be said to be significant if the haemoglobin is below 100 g/L.

Table 7.23 Classification of anaemias

Anaemia caused by increased destruction of red blood cells (RBC)

acquired haemolytic anaemia
the thalassaemias
G6PD deficiency
sickle cell anaemia
blood loss anaemia

Anaemia caused by decreased production of RBCs

Blackfan-Diamond syndrome
aplastic anaemia
leukaemia
malignant disease

Anaemia caused by nutritional/metabolic disturbance of RBC production

iron (Fe) deficiency
folic acid deficiency
drug induced anaemia

Haemoglobin is a complex molecule, made up of 2 pairs of dissimilar globin chains; there are 4 important globin chains in humans, each given a letter of the Greek alphabet (alpha, beta, gamma and delta). These globin chains each have their own characteristic amino acid sequence, determined by their structural genes on chromosomes 11 and 16. To each chain is attached a haem group (an iron-porphyrin complex). Each chain is composed of about 150 amino acids. Haemoglobin contains about 65% of the body's iron stores and comprises about 99% of the red cell.

The bone marrow produces approximately 3 million red cells every second to replace those being destroyed at the end of their life cycle. The production of red cells is controlled by many factors. Abnormalities of red cell production from genetic, hormonal, nutritional or metabolic influences may result in decreased production leading to anaemia. In addition, anaemia may result from increased destruction or loss of red cells beyond the capacity of the bone marrow to replace loss. Grouping anaemias loosely according to these causative factors provides a convenient system of classification.

NURSING ASSESSMENT

Assessment of the child who presents with pallor, possibly due to anaemia, begins at the first meeting. The colour of the skin and mucous membranes can serve as a useful guide to the degree of anaemia present, once the other causes of pallor as outlined below have been excluded.

Fever

The pale, febrile child is often suffering from a severe infection, the source of which must be carefully ascertained by a thorough physical examination. Excluding disorders such as pneumonia, septicaemia and pyelonephritis is essential.

Acute blood loss

Apart from trauma, acute blood loss is not commonly seen in children. Overt bleeding is obvious to the parents of the child, however, damage to an organ resulting in haemorrhage into the bowel, or a haemothorax, is not. The parents may not know of an injury sustained by their child or they may have discounted an injury, such as a fall from playground equipment or bicycle, as being trivial. The occurrence of recent accidents such as these need to be excluded.

Pre-existing disease

Pallor may be present in children due to many and varied causes, such as chronic blood loss from an undiagnosed Meckel's diverticulum, renal or cardiac disease or hypoglycaemia. A family history of disorders such as thalassaemia, sickle cell disease, or G6PD deficiency (favism) serves as a firm pointer to the type of anaemia which may be present.

Anaemia cannot be diagnosed with any degree of certainty by a simple inspection of the skin and mucous membranes. These can, however, be used as a guide to the degree of haemoglobin drop that a child may have. Very severe anaemias may be present with few or no symptoms in the child if the anaemia has been of slow onset and is longstanding. An appreciation of the normal values of haemoglobin through infancy and childhood is of crucial importance in discerning true anaemia from a normal variation in haemoglobin.

While the reasons a child may present with pallor as outlined above are by no means exhaustive, it is essential to appreciate that obtaining a comprehensive nursing history from the parents of the child, at presentation, may facilitate early diagnosis and appropriate intervention.

DIAGNOSIS

Having established that the child is not suffering from another disorder, the type of anaemia present needs to be identified and the cause found. This involves a full paediatric history, relevant to the age of the child, a complete physical examination and appropriate investigations. The more important aspects of each are set out below.

History

Neonatal period

Premature infants and infants who are small for gestational age are at risk of iron deficiency anaemia. A history of jaundice, particularly when associated with blood transfusion or fetomaternal haemorrhage may indicate haemolytic anaemia in the infant. Infants born from a multiple pregnancy may have lower iron stores than normal, even though they may be full term.

Infancy

Diet is of the utmost importance in preventing anaemia at this stage of development. A diet rich in milk and cereals but poor in meat, green vegetables and other iron sources will result in iron deficiency. When obtaining a nursing history, enquiries should cover the total intake of milk and the time and type of solid foods that have been introduced. Prolonged breast feeding without a complementary solid diet will also result in the development of iron deficiency. Symptoms of iron deficiency become apparent in infants by about 4 months of age when iron stores are depleted. For premature infants, iron stores may have been incomplete at birth, as these iron stores are laid down in the fetus during the last weeks of pregnancy. Prematurity is almost always associated with iron deficiency and symptoms of anaemia may be apparent sooner.

Recent infections may be relevant to the development of anaemia with chronic infections almost certainly playing a significant role. For immigrant families, particularly from tropical climates, malaria may be a significant problem as may parasitic infections of the bowel (e.g., hookworm).

Bowel habits need to be ascertained as chronic diarrohea may be significant for the diagnosis. The character of stools should be noted as these may indicate the cause of the anaemia (e.g., coeliac disease, Meckel's diverticulum, or cow's milk allergy).

Childhood

Diet is again a significant factor in the development of anaemia as children may develop poor eating habits, particularly the eating of 'junk' food which has little or no nutritive value.

Infections of long duration, particularly bowel infections, will certainly be significant at this age. The development of anaemia following infectious hepatitis, although very rare, is of particular significance as this type of aplastic anaemia is associated with a very high mortality rate (60%).

Numerous drugs such as chloramphenicol, penicillin, phenytoin and phenylbutazone are known to induce or aggravate a haematological disturbance. The taking of such drugs by the child should be ascertained from the parents. Abnormal bleeding or bruising at any age may be significant in aiding diagnosis. The length of illness and its onset gives valuable clues to the nature of the anaemia. A long history indicates either a longstanding deficiency or a chronic haemolytic anaemia, whereas an acute onset suggests a systemic disorder or a haemolytic anaemia, especially if coupled with other symptoms (e.g., fever, pain, abdominal discomfort).

Lastly, the child's ethnic background may provide an indication as to which anaemia may be present (e.g., G6PD deficiency, thalassaemia, and sickle cell disease, which are more prevalent in persons of Mediterranean or South-East Asian origin).

Physical examination

A thorough physical examination is warranted with particular attention paid to:

- The skin and mucous membranes to determine the presence of pallor, bruising, telangectasias and petechiae.
- The conjuntiva to detect pallor and jaundice.
- The presence of splenomegaly, hepatomegaly and enlarged lymph nodes, which point to the possibility of a systemic disease (e.g., leukaemia).

Investigations

Relatively few investigations are needed to ascertain the type of anaemia.

Peripheral blood film

The peripheral blood film will reveal most information about the type of anaemia present and the processes that have occurred in its precipitation.

Table 7.24 Results of investigations in anaemia

Anaemia	MCV	WCC	Reticulocytes	Bilirubin
Fe deficiency	R	N	R	N
B12 deficiency	I	Slight R	R	N
Aplastic	N	Marked R	R	N
Blackfan-Diamond	N	N	A	N
Haemolytic	N	I	I	Marked I
G6PD deficiency	N	N	n/r	Marked I
Thalassaemia	R	N	n/r	Slight I
Blood loss	N	N	I	N

N = normal, R = reduced, I = increased, A = absent, n/r = not relevant

Haemoglobin level will be low with the MCV providing an indication of the type of anaemia (i.e., microcytic or macrocytic). The shape of the red cells is important as characteristic changes in shape occur in several anaemias. The white cell count (WCC) should also be noted, as a raised WCC will indicate a current or recent infection. In contrast, a substantially lower than normal WCC may indicate a developing aplastic anaemia, or bone marrow depression due to a viral infection, e.g., infectious mononucleosis or a developing malignancy, e.g., leukaemia. The reticulocyte count is also of importance as it provides a sensitive index to bone marrow performance. Normally, reticulocytes comprise 0.5 to 1.5% of all red cells, with a raised reticulocyte count indicating a marrow response to a drop in haemoglobin concentration, and a lowered reticulocyte count indicating poor red cell production.

Serum bilirubin

Measurement of serum bilirubin is useful as it provides a guide to the degree of haemolysis. Severe jaundice may make the observation of increasing pallor difficult.

Specific investigations for each anaemia

The following tests should be performed when a particular anaemia is suspected:

- Serum iron/ferritin, performed for suspected iron deficiency.
- Serum B_{12}, performed for suspected megaloblastic anaemia (pernicious anaemia).
- Bone marrow aspiration, for suspected aplastic anaemia, Blackfan-Diamond syndrome.
- Haemoglobin electrophoresis, for suspected thalassaemia.
- Coombs test, indirect antibody, plasma haemoglobin for suspected haemolytic anaemia.

Table 7.24 includes a summary of the results of investigations for the various anaemias of childhood.

TREATMENT

It must be remembered that anaemia is a symptom of a disorder and not a disease in itself. Due to the wide variety of causes of childhood anaemia there is no overall treatment approach, rather the treatment for each anaemia is quite specific. For all severe anaemias, blood transfusion is the primary treatment option, once investigations have ascertained the specific diagnosis. Dependent on the type of anaemia, the child may only require transfusion to a haemoglobin level that will reduce the risk of serious complications, and thus make the child feel more comfortable. Once this has been achieved treatment specific to the type of anaemia can then be instituted. Treatment of anaemia resulting from a nutritional deficiency would require correction of the deficiency together with an educational program for the child's parents that addresses correct nutrition practices. Management of anaemia resulting from a drug-induced metabolic disturbance requires alteration of the child's medication and elimination of the offending agent.

Management of anaemias resulting from either an increased destruction of red cells (e.g., haemolytic anaemia) or a decreased production of red cells, as occurs with a bone marrow defect, is much more complex and requires a complete understanding of the underlying cause. In these cicumstances treatment for one form of anaemia may be contraindicated in another. These treatment approaches are complex and beyond the scope of this text and can be found in more specialised texts on paediatric haematology.

NURSING CARE

When planning nursing care for children with anaemia, the nurse needs to take into account that most children with anaemia will have few symptoms attributed to the disorder, they may have compensated for even severe anaemias by altered activity patterns and even by physiological changes such as the development of cardiomegaly in an attempt to improve cardiac output.

If severe anaemia is present, the child will exhibit a very poor exercise tolerance. Nursing interventions undertaken to meet the child's needs, such as hygiene and toileting procedures, should be grouped together to alleviate exhaustion, allowing adequate time between procedures for the patient to recover before the next activity.

The anaemic patient may display poor tolerance to heat or cold and the ambient temperature should be set at the level of comfort. If the child is ambulant, warm clothing should be worn for outdoor activity.

Nursing measures should include appropriate interventions for the underlying cause (e.g., sickle cell crisis). The patient who is anaemic because of a sickle cell crisis will often have severe pain, usually in a limb or the lower back, due to infarction of areas beyond the location of the sickling. These children require adequate pain relief, which may include narcotics. Pain relief measures in these patients should be instituted early in a crisis as the child's pain will increase as sickling increases the area of infarction. Treatment is instituted early to reduce the amount of sickling. The infusion of copious intravenous fluids (3 L/m^2/day) with the addition of sodium bicarbonate 10 mmol/L, is indicated as this will decrease blood viscosity and counter acidosis in the areas of infarction. As poor oxygen saturation increases the amount of sickling, the child's oxygen saturation should be monitored and oxygen should be administered to keep the patient's saturation near to 100%.

The usual nursing management of patients receiving a blood transfusion should be followed. Some patients with an autoimmune haemolytic anaemia may be more prone than others to a severe reaction to the transfused blood due to the presence of antibodies in their serum that may react with surface antigen sites on the transfused red cells.

Nursing measures should include appropriate education for the child, parents and family and involvement of the appropriate personnel (e.g., dietician, social worker, maternal and child welfare nurse). This team approach should be initiated early after the diagnosis has been established to allow adequate time for learning to occur. Often, deeply ingrained cultural beliefs have to be overcome. This may occur with families whose understanding of English is poor. The use of professional interpreters who can use the family's own language to facilitate education will provide better results.

Families of patients who are anaemic due to a genetic cause (e.g., G6PD deficiency or thalassaemia) may feel guilt about their child's problem. Appropriate counselling for these parents is an essential component of the nursing role. Education is well facilitated by the nurse who is in the ideal position to reinforce and clarify information given by other health care professionals.

Lastly, children who are anaemic due to the much more sinister causes of aplasia or malignant disease, require a greater level of support. Due to the seriousness of the underlying disorder, their treatment is best undertaken in specialised haematology and oncology units. The nature of the information that needs to be given to patients and families about treatment options and outcomes for such disorders is highly specialised. The goal of health care providers should be to support the child and family as much as possible and to refrain from giving information that may be inaccurate, misleading or incomplete, hence referral to a specialised centre is essential to optimise care.

BIBLIOGRAPHY

Robinson MJ, ed. *Practical paediatrics*. 2nd ed. Edinburgh: Churchill Livingstone, 1990: 333–362.
Ekert H, ed. *Clinical paediatric haematology and oncology*. Melbourne: Blackwell Scientific, 1982: 80–160.
Hockenberry MJ. Evaluating anaemia in children. *J Pract Nursing* 1988; March: 46–50.
Willoughby MLN. *Paediatric haematology*. Edinburgh: Churchill Livinstone, 1977.

Clotting Disorders

David Sutton

Abnormal bleeding is one of the more distressing symptoms in childhood. Few people would not be alarmed by its presence. There are a very large number of causes of abnormal bleeding in childhood, but they can be reduced to disorders of one of the following:

- The blood vessels or their supporting tissue.
- The platelets.
- The coagulation system.

Following tissue injury, these 3 interact in a complex way to control bleeding.

Injury to a blood vessel causes damage to the endothelium and, in some cases, exposure of the collagen supporting matrix. Platelets then adhere to the exposed endothelium. This requires the presence of a factor of the coagulation system, von Willebrand's factor, part of a large protein complex known as factor VIII. Adhesion of platelets is closely followed by their aggregation to form a platelet plug. It has been well established that platelets contribute procoagulant activity which accelerates the process of coagulation at the surface of the platelet plug.

The coagulation process itself is a complex system in which each enzyme (factor) in turn activates an inert precursor form into its active form, in 2 pathways (intrinsic pathway and extrinsic pathway) which then combine into a common pathway, working like a cascade to amplify the response at each step. The system is controlled by a series of inhibiting and enhancing feedback loops. The end result of the process is the production of fibrin fibres that become cross-linked and enmeshed in the platelet plug, forming a network that then traps more platelets, red cells and white blood cells to form a clot. A more detailed descripion of the coagulation pathway is beyond the scope of this chapter, and can be found in haematology texts.

Using the 3 components of haemostasis as described above, one can classify the more common major disorders of bleeding in childhood as:

1. Disorders of haemostasis.

- Disorders due to vascular defects.
- Anaphylactoid purpura due to infective states.
- Congenital heart disease.
- Giant haemangiomas.
- Disorders of platelet function.
- Idiopathic thrombocytopenic purpura (ITP).
- Secondary thrombocytopenia.

2. Disorders of coagulation.

- Haemophilia A (classic).
- Haemophilia B (Christmas disease).
- von Willibrand's syndrome.

3. Disseminated intravascular coagulation (DIC).

NURSING ASSESSMENT

Assessment of the child with a suspected bleeding disorder, as with a child with suspected anaemia, should begin with the colour of the child. This serves as a guide to the degree of blood loss that the child may have experienced. The child's vital signs should be recorded. If the child has experienced an acute blood loss, pulse and respirations will be raised and blood pressure lowered. The child's conscious state should be evaluated; a sudden deterioration in conscious state may indicate a catastrophic haemorrhage, which may be only a small volume of blood if it occurs within the brain or other vital organ. If the blood loss is of a chronic nature, the vital signs may not be altered, but the child may still be agitated due to a low haemoglobin level.

Pain from a small haemorrhage into a joint, muscle or viscus may be severe and may alter vital signs. An examination of the child's skin for the presence of bruising and petechiae should be conducted. Spontaneous bruising due to a bleeding disorder is usually more pronounced on the limbs, the bruises are roundish in shape and are of varying age, unlike bruising due to trauma which assumes the shape of the object which caused it and is all of the one age. Petechiae, small spontaneous haemorrhages under the skin which look like multiple pinpricks, are easily observed. As with abnormal bruising, they are usually more prominent on the limbs but may be present in large numbers anywhere on the body. The stool should be collected and tested for the presence of occult blood;

frank blood and malaena should be obvious on visual examination. Routine urinalysis should be performed.

DIAGNOSIS

The search for a suspected bleeding disorder should include a search for underlying disorders that may be contributing. Fever can be used as a guide, as the child with a true bleeding disorder is rarely febrile due to the disorder, although infections may exacerbate their symptoms and may contribute to the disorder's presence in the first place (e.g., DIC). The presence of disorders such as systemic lupus erythematosus, liver disease, gross splenomegaly and malignant diseases should all be excluded by appropriate investigations.

Having established that the child is not suffering from another disorder, the exact nature of the bleeding disorder needs to be established. This involves a full paediatric history relevant to the child's age, a physical examination and appropriate investigations. The more important aspects of each are set out below.

The family history

Simple enquiry about bleeding within the family is insufficient to aid in diagnosis of a bleeding disorder. A proper family tree must be constructed. If the family tree shows that males were predominantly affected or that there were unexplained male infant deaths then a disorder with a sex-linked inheritance would be suggested.

Haemophilia and Christmas disease, the 2 most common disorders of haemostasis in childhood, are both transmitted in a sex-linked recessive manner. There may be generations in the family history that are skipped over by the disorder due to the birth of unaffected males.

Von Willebrand's disease is transmitted in an autosomal dominant manner with both sexes equally affected and frequently there are successive generations with a bleeding disorder.

A negative family history does not rule out these disorders, as new mutations of haemophilia and Christmas disease account for about one-third and one-fifth of new cases, respectively and in von Willebrand's disease symptoms may have been so slight as to escape detection.

A past history of easy bruising or bruising at abnormal sites, prolonged bleeding after minor trauma, surgery or dental extractions would warrant further investigation.

The dietary intake of vitamins is important to ascertain as vitamin C is essential to the correct formation of the intercellular matrix which supports blood vessels and a reduced intake of vitamin C leads to scurvy. Children who have poor dietary habits may be prone to this disease. Vitamin K is also of importance as low maternal vitamin K intake during pregnancy may lead to gastrointestinal bleeding in the neonatal period.

Several drugs may produce or exacerbate abnormal bleeding through irritation of the gastric mucosa (e.g., aspirin and non-steroid anti-inflamatory drugs), depression of clotting factors (e.g., warfarin and other anticoagulants) bone marrow suppression (e.g., chloramphenicol and cytotoxic drugs) or by direct inhibition of platelet action (e.g., aspirin). The child's parents should be asked about the taking of such drugs by the child.

In infants and very young children, the perinatal history should also be ascertained as fetomaternal haemorrage may result in the later formation of antibodies to platelets in the child.

Physical examination

The physical examination is of limited value in aiding diagnosis of a suspected true bleeding disorder, beyond the obvious such as bruising in abnormal places, and amount and presence of petechiae, pallor, swelling and pain due to haemorrage. However, it may be helpful in diagnosing underlying problems.

Specific investigations

A wide range of investigations is indicated in the establishment of the diagnosis, particularly if the bleeding disorder is secondary to another disease process. The following tests provide a logical starting point.

Activated partial thromboplastin time (APTT) and prothrombin time (PT) give an indication of an abnormality in the intrinsic or extrinsic pathway. Bleeding time (BT) is also a very useful test in aiding diagnosis.

If the intrinsic pathway is indicated, measurement of factor VIII level will indicate whether the child has haemophilia A. Measurement of factor IX level will indicate whether or not the child has Christmas disease.

Measurement of ristocetin cofactor (von Willebrand's), a function of the factor VIII complex, may be reduced even though the child has normal factor VIII levels. Reduction of the ristocetin factor indicates von Willebrand's disease. Platelet function studies performed after a finding of a prolonged BT will ascertain a platelet function defect. Full blood examination (FBE) will ascertain the platelet count. Bone marrow aspiration is carried out if a low platelet count is found on FBE, to look at levels of platelet production and to exclude such causes as malignancy and aplastic anaemia. Fibrin degradation products (FDPs/D Dimers) are used to look for their presence. FDPs are elevated in disseminated intravascular coagulation, a complication of many disease processes, in which there is activation of coagulation, followed by a depletion of procoagulant factors and generation of other factors which cause further tissue endothelial damage, vasodilation and shock. The end result of this is a bleeding disorder.

There are of course many other investigations that may need to be performed to obtain a diagnosis, but they are of a more generalised nature and are usually associated with other underlying disorders such as congenital heart disease, renal or hepatic diseases and infective states.

TREATMENT

Treatment of a bleeding disorder first requires the bleeding problem to be corrected. For bleeding due to abnormalties of clotting factors, tranfusion of missing or depleted coagulation factor(s) is necessary.

Not all coagulation factors are available as single products such as factor VIII at present, but many are available in combination such as in prothrombinex, a prothrombin complex concentrate, or fresh frozen plasma.

Factor VIII has a half-life of 8 to 12 hours and most soft tissue and joint bleeds in haemophilia A, can be controlled by a single infusion of factor VIII sufficient to raise factor VIII levels to 50% of normal using the formula that 1 unit of factor VIII/kg of bodyweight raises the factor VIII level by 2%. For bleeding at other sites (e.g., intracranial), higher levels of factor VIII may need to be maintained. The number of factor VIII infusions required to control bleeding and to permit return to normal activity is dependent

Table 7.25 Factor VIII infusions required for control of bleeding

Type of bleed	Number of infusions
Haemarthrosis	1–3
Muscle/soft tissue	1–2
Bleeding with nerve compression	3–6
Retroperitoneal haemorrhage	3–6
Oropharynx	3–6
Intracranial	7–14

on the site and severity of bleeding. **Table 7.25** provides a useful guide, but each patient and bleed should be treated individually.

Factor IX has a half-life of approximately 24 hours. The dose should be calculated as for factor VIII and increased by one-third. Subsequent infusions need only be given every 24 hours.

Other coagulation factors have differing half-lives and infusion requirements. There is a small number of patients who will develop antibodies to clotting factor replacement products. This is a severe setback to the efficacy of treatment for bleeding episodes as alternative products may need to be used to overcome the antibody problem, such as porcine factor VIII. There are several new products, such as activated factor VII, undergoing clinical trials that will help in the treatment of individuals with antibodies to conventional replacement clotting factors.

Von Willebrand's disease is best controlled by intravenous administration of the posterior pituitary hormone DDAVP, which will release the stored von Willebrand's factor (VWF) and provide haemostasis for about 4 hours. DDAVP is only useful in mild or moderate von Willebrand's disease. It can be repeated at 12 to 24 hour intervals, but not more frequently as synthesis of VWF takes around 12 hours. In severe von Willebrand's disease, factor VIII concentrates should be used and may not need repeating for 24 to 48 hours.

Transfusion of platelets is most effective in stopping bleeding if given at a rapid rate. As the volumes involved are small compared to the patient's total intravascular volume, this can usually be accomplished without fluid overload problems. However, the usual risks of transfusion reactions still exist and institutional practices regarding delivery and monitoring of transfusion of blood products should still apply.

The next step in the treatment process is relief of pain using appropriate analgesics for the degree of discomfort and splinting of the affected muscle or joint to reduce the prolongation of or the risk of recurrence of bleeding due to movement. For severe bleeding episodes into joints, surgical aspiration under general anaesthesia will provide excellent pain relief but it must be stressed that this technique should be reserved for severe bleeding episodes.

Treatment for underlying problems should be instituted concurrently with the above.

Inhibition of fibrinolysis has been shown to be useful in bleeding from the mouth and nose and in intracranial bleeds. There are two agents available, epsilon aminocaproic acid (Amicar, Ekaprol) 400 mg/kg/day and tranexamic acid (Cyclokapron) 2 to 4 g/day, both given in 6-hourly divided doses. Use of antifibrinolytic agents should be avoided in renal bleeds as they may give rise to clot retention.

In idiopathic cytopenic purpura (ITP) with an acute onset, strict rest in bed is usually

Table 7.26

Condition	Associated findings
Aplastic anaemia	Marrow hypoplasia
Leukaemia	Marrow replacement
Disseminated neoplasm	Marrow infiltration
Viral infections	Hepatosplenomegaly
CMV, EBV, Herpes simplex	Positive viral cultures

all that is needed to stop mucosal bleeding and bruising. Complete recovery occurrs in 75% of these cases within 12 weeks and a further 15% will have complete recovery within 26 weeks. The remaining 10% can be considered to have progressed to chronic ITP. For these children, treatment with prednisolone at a dose of 2 mg/kg for about 4 weeks with the dose tapered over a further 2 weeks will result in about a 70% recovery. For the remaining very few patients, splenectomy offers a greater than 90% chance of recovery. There is evidence that splenectomy raises the risk of serious bacterial infections, usually due to *Pneumococcus* or *Haemophilus influenzae*, and treatment should be instituted in such patients with an injection of Pneumovax (*Pneumococcus* vaccine) before surgery, and continued with the administration of oral pencillin twice daily for at least 2 years after splenectomy.

Thrombocytopenia may also be associated with other conditions, some of which are detailed in the **Table 7.26**. These conditions are self-explanatory and the treatment of them is beyond the scope of this work.

NURSING CARE

Each bleeding episode should be assessed and nursing measures should be planned on this assesment, with the aim of reducing or preventing further bleeding episodes. Clotting factor replacement should be given strictly on schedule as a delay may lead to lowered serum levels and further bleeding. Conversely, too short an interval between replacement doses may lead to clotting abnormalities of a different kind with the formation of venous thrombi due to raised serum levels of clotting factor(s) activating the clotting mechanism. Haemoglobin levels should be monitored and blood transfusion given as indicated. Even small bleeds such as tooth socket bleeds can lead to low haemoglobin levels if allowed to go on for a prolonged period.

Bleeding into muscles and/or joints requires splinting of the affected joint to prevent movement aggravating the bleeding problem, and also to reduce pain. Appropriate analgesia should be instituted early to aid immobilisation. The presence of nerve or blood vessel compression is a serious complication and nursing observations should be performed to check for signs of progression of this. The appropriate medical personnel should be informed if any progression is suspected, as permanent damage to the affected area could result if measures are not taken to limit compression.

For patients with bleeding due to platelet counts less than 20×10^9/L, physical activity should be severely curtailed to avoid the risk of accidental trauma exacerbating or causing further bleeding episodes.

Patients with mouth or oropharyngeal bleeds should have their diet altered to soft foods and extremes of temperature should be avoided. Removal of clots from the mouth, although tempting for aesthetic reasons, should be avoided until after clotting factor replacement has been instituted as removal will stimulate further bleeding. After clotting factor replacement has commenced, mouth washes may be instituted to gently remove clotted blood. Cleaning of teeth should be avoided until the bleeding episode has ceased.

Episodes of renal bleeding should be managed by strict resting in bed, and giving copious fluids (greater than twice maintenance). Patients who cannot tolerate oral fluids at this rate should have intravenous fluids instituted and monitoring of haematuria should be done by collection of serial samples for comparison.

For serious bleeds involving nerve or vessel compression and life-threatening bleeds such as an intracranial bleed, surgical measures can be taken under clotting factor replacement cover. However, the replacement program will need to be kept going for a prolonged period, often for around 2 weeks for an intracranial bleed, with no allowance for a delay in giving a dose of replacement factor. Good nursing care for such patients should take into account the extra workload involved in the administration of clotting factor replacement therapy.

Finally, minor bleeding episodes can be managed in small hospitals or even in some cases at home, but all bleeding episodes of a major or prolonged nature are best managed in a haematology unit set up specifically to deal with such problems.

BIBLIOGRAPHY

Robinson MJ, ed. *Practical paediatrics*. 2nd ed. Edinburgh: Churchill Livingstone, 1990.
Ekert H, ed. *Clinical paediatric haematology and oncology*. Melbourne: Blackwell Scientific, 1982.
Willoughby MLN. *Paediatric haematology*. Edinburgh: Churchill Livingstone, 1977.

AIDS

Marilyn Cruickshank

The acquired immunodeficiency syndrome (AIDS) was first described in 1981.[1] The illness is characterised by a cellular immune deficiency predominantly affecting the function of T-helper (CD4+) cells that makes the individual susceptible to certain opportunistic infections and malignancies.[1] The causative organism in AIDS is a retrovirus referred to as human immunodeficiency virus type 1 (HIV-1).

HIV is a lente or slow virus. Once inserted into the DNA of the host cell, the viral genes are there for life. All cells which posses the CD4+ receptor (T4 lymphocytes, B lymphocytes, macrophages, monocytes, brain and bowel cells) are susceptible to infection with HIV. HIV has a cytopathic effect on lymphocytes, leading to a depletion of these cells. Although other cells may have a relative resistance to HIV cytotoxicity, they may serve as a reservoir for the virus. The virus often lies dormant for several years, during which time the infected person may be unaware of the infection. Even so, secretions such as semen, vaginal fluids and blood are infectious and can transmit the virus. The virus appears capable of rapid genetic mutation, thus escaping the suppressive role of the body's immune system. HIV alters the genetic make up of CD4+ lymphocytes so that they reproduce HIV. The role of CD4+ lymphocytes is central to immune function (**Table 7.27**). Because B cell and monocyte function are affected by the activity of CD4+ lymphocytes,

Table 7.27 The role of CD4 lymphocytes

- Induction of cytotoxic T-cell function.
- Induction of natural killer cell function.
- Induction of suppressor cell function.
- Activation of macrophages.
- Induction of B-cell function.

---

further disruption of the immune system follows. The infected person is rendered immunodeficient and susceptible to a wide range of characteristic AIDS-linked disorders.

No cure for HIV infection has been discovered and the prognosis for long-term survival is poor. Lengths of survival vary depending upon general health, availability and promptness of treatment for specific conditions, the response to treatment and other factors.

EPIDEMIOLOGY OF HIV IN AUSTRALIA

Children have been infected by HIV through the infusion of infected blood or blood products,[2] implantation of infected organs[3] and by vertical transmission from an infected mother during pregnancy, childbirth or breastfeeding.[4] Since testing was introduced by the Blood Bank in April 1985, there have been no further infections through blood or blood products in Australia. As HIV continues to spread through the heterosexual population and the number of HIV-infected women of childbearing age increases, so too will the number of infected children. Australian statistics show that the incidence of perinatal HIV exposure in Australia remains low (less than 1:10 000) with 20 infants reported as born to seropositive women each year in Australia.[5] It is expected that new cases of paediatric HIV infection will be caused by vertical transmission.[6] To date, there have been no reported infections of HIV in children after sexual assault in Australia.[7]

HIV AND AIDS IN INFANCY

The first case of AIDS in a child was documented in 1982.[8] While the diagnosis of HIV in adults is readily established by the detection of antibodies to HIV, the situation is more complex in infants born to seropositive women since maternal antibodies are transferred across the placenta during pregnancy. In addition, the symptoms of HIV in infants may be similar to many common conditions found in that age group.[9] Although many seropositive adults are asymptomatic for many years before progressing to an AIDS diagnosis, clinical experience shows that some infants may have an AIDS diagnosis as early as 2 months of age.

AIDS DIAGNOSIS IN CHILDREN

About one-third of children with HIV infection will have an early onset of symptoms and rapidly progress to an AIDS diagnosis, while most will have later onset of severe symptoms and thus a better prognosis. An AIDS diagnosis is made in a child on the basis of a definitively diagnosed disease such as multiple bacterial infections, opportunistic infections, cancers, neurological manifestations and lymphoproliferative disease. Those diseases which indicate an AIDS diagnosis (according to Centers for Disease Control classification) are listed:[10]

- *Pneumocystis carinii* pneumonia;
- chronic cryptosporidiosis;
- disseminated toxoplasmosis;
- candidiasis (oesophageal/bronchial/pulmonary);
- extrapulmonary cryptococcus;
- disseminated histoplasmosis;
- mycobacterial infection;
- cytomegalovirus after one month of age;
- chronic or disseminated herpes simplex virus;
- recurrent serious bacterial infections (sepsis, meningitis, pneumonia, abscess of an internal organ, bone/joint infections).

The asymptomatic period tends to be shorter in children and infants than in adults.[11]

VERTICAL TRANSMISSION

Vertical transmission of HIV has been defined as the transmission of HIV from mother to infant during intrauterine, intrapartum or postpartum periods.[12] The rate of transmission from mother to child would appear to vary with the stage of the mother's illness — those in the later stages having a higher risk of transmission to their infant (that is, women with persistence of antigens in their blood being more likely to transmit the virus). Over all, the transmission rate would appear to be about 25%, with reports varying from 13% to 50%.[11,13] Australian data show that among Australian infants born between 1982 and 1994, and known to have been exposed to HIV *in utero* and/or during breastfeeding, there is a transmission rate of 23%.[14] Factors that may influence the risk of transmission are:[15,16]

- breastfeeding;
- symptomatic maternal infection;
- CD4+ lymphocyte depletion;
- reduced anti-gp 120 antibody levels;
- prior delivery of an HIV-infected child;
- presence of sexually transmitted diseases;
- maternal immune and clinical status;
- HIV inoculum and virulence;
- cofactors;
- mode of delivery;
- neutralising or specific protein antibodies;
- newborn passively acquired antibodies;
- maternal — fetal haemorrhage.

More recent Australian data have indicated a doubling of the vertical transmission rate in those infants who were breastfed.[17]

The timing of transmission from mother to infant is uncertain, but from clinical observation it would appear that infants may be infected either during pregnancy or delivery.[18] The fetus may be infected as early as 8[19] to 15[20] weeks' gestation. Infants thought to be infected earlier during the pregnancy may be symptomatic, have clinical signs such as lymphadenopathy and/or abnormal blood results soon after birth, and may have an

AIDS diagnosis within their first year of life. Transmission may also occur at delivery, and there is some evidence to suggest that caesarean delivery may reduce the transmission rate.[21] Infants infected late in the pregnancy or during delivery may have no signs of infection, either clinically or in virological tests, at birth but may develop symptoms and/ or abnormal blood results within the first months of life. It is thought that these children have a better prognosis and may not become severely symptomatic until the early school years or even later. HIV can also be transmitted postpartum through breastfeeding.

EFFECTS OF MATERNAL HIV INFECTION ON PREGNANCY OUTCOME

Initially, there were concerns that HIV infection would lead to higher rates of prematurity, low birthweight, premature rupture of membranes and other poor pregnancy outcomes. However, these reports involved small sample sizes and may have been described among women in the later stages of their illness. More recently, studies of asymptomatic, seropositive pregnant women and their infants demonstrated that the prevalence of premature delivery, small-for-gestational-age infants and neonatal disease was similar to that in a pregnant seronegative group of injecting drug using women (about twice that recorded in the general population).[22]

NEONATAL MALFORMATIONS AND HIV

Early reports of an embryopathy suggested craniofacial abnormalities, but there appears to be no evidence of an AIDS embryopathy.[23] Although the numbers are small, there have been no reported abnormalities in infants whose mothers were taking zidovudine during pregnancy.[24]

PRENATAL DIAGNOSIS

HIV cannot be diagnosed in the fetus during pregnancy for both technical and logistic reasons. The problems associated with prenatal diagnosis include:

- Maternal and fetal risks of the procedures.
- The potential to infect the foetus during the screening technique.
- The timing of transmission of HIV *in utero* is variable, therefore the foetus is vulnerable to HIV infection throughout gestation and during birth.
- The inability of tests accurately to diagnose HIV on the samples obtained. A diagnostic test must have a high degree of reliability to be useful.
- The risk of maternal contamination of foetal specimens is high.

DIAGNOSIS OF HIV IN THE NEWBORN

As passively transferred maternal IgG antibody can persist for up to 15 months, 2 definitions for HIV infection in children are required, one for infants up to the age of 15 months who have been exposed perinatally, and another for older children with perinatal infection and for infants and children of all ages acquiring HIV through other means. Infection in infants up to the age of 15 months who were exposed to infected mothers in the perinatal period may be defined by the following categories:

- Virus in blood or tissues, *or*
- HIV antibody, *and* evidence of cellular immune deficiency, *or*
- Symptoms meeting CDC case definition for AIDS.

HIV-infected children are classified into mutually exclusive categories according to three parameters: infection status, clinical status, and immunologic status.[25] Once classified, an HIV-infected child cannot be reclassified in a less severe category even if the child's clinical or immunologic status improves.

Clinical Categories

Children infected with HIV or perinatally exposed to HIV may be classified into one of four mutually exclusive clinical categories based on signs, symptoms, or diagnoses related to HIV infection. As with the immunologic categories, the clinical categories have been defined to provide staging classification (eg., the prognosis for children in the second category would be less favourable than for those in the first category).

Immunologic Categories

Three immunologic categories were established to categorise children by the severity of immunosuppression attributable to HIV infection.

The immunologic category classification is based on either the CD4+ T lymphocyte count or the CD4+ percent of total lymphocytes. If both the CD4+ count and the CD4+ percent indicate different classification categories, the child should be classified into the more severe category. Repeated or follow-up CD4+ values that result in a change in classification should be confirmed by a second determination. Values thought to be in error should not be used. A child should not be reclassified to a less severe category regardless of subsequent CD4+ determinations.

The diagnosis of HIV infection in the babies born to mothers who are themselves infected with the virus can be a difficult one. All babies receive antibodies from their mother during the latter part of pregnancy, therefore, all infants born to seropositive women will have passively acquired HIV antibodies regardless of whether or not they are actually infected with the virus. As tests routinely used to diagnose the presence of HIV rely on the presence of antibodies, these results will not determine whether an infant born to a positive mother is infected or not. The positive antibody result does not differentiate between maternal or infant antibody. Thus, uninfected infants will appear antibody positive until the maternal antibodies disappear.

However, other tests are available which although they do not give an HIV diagnosis on their own, when looked at together can help to determine if the baby has the virus. In the infants who are infected, most, if not all, of the following parameters will be abnormal, indicating HIV infection. There have, however, been some young children who have had some slightly abnormal results on 1 or 2 tests, but who clear the antibody and remain clinically well and are presumed uninfected. It has been suggested that these children may have actually been infected and cleared the virus from their system.

The tests that are used for diagnosis of HIV infection in infants born to seropositve women are as follows.

HIV antibody — ELISA or serodia and Western blot tests

Antibody tests determine maternal infection. The levels are high in newborns, reflecting the levels of their mothers, and begin to fall over the following weeks. Even in infected infants, the level falls initially and then start to climb again as infants make their own antibody to the virus from 3 to 6 months.[26] In infants who prove to be negative, or serorevert, the antibody levels continue to diminish till seronegative. This may take 12 to 15 months. Thus, all infants born to HIV-infected mothers are seropositive because of placental transfer of maternal IgG antibody or as a result of intrauterine infection. ELISA measures antibodies to HIV antigens within 4 to 6 weeks of infection; it is used as a screening test and if positive, requires verification with Western blot. Western blot measures antibody to viral proteins of HIV.

HIV antigens

HIV-associated antigens (core protein p24 and envelope proteins gp41 and gp120) can be measured in the blood and cerebrospinal fluid. Antigen levels tend to be higher soon after seroconversion and in the latter stages of the disease. The level of antigen is high when the infection is active. In infants who are positive for the virus, the antigen level is high soon after birth, and may be present in the cord blood sample. Quantitative viral titres are significantly higher for symptomatic HIV-infected patients, so that the degree of viraemia may have important implications for the clinical course of HIV infection and transmission of HIV. Some studies have indicated a higher transmission rate from mother to infant if the mother is antigenaemic.

HIV culture

Another test which may be done to determine diagnosis is to culture or grow the virus. If the virus is grown from the infant's blood, the diagnosis is positive. However, like most viruses, HIV is difficult to grow, so a negative culture is not always helpful. This test can take up to 4 weeks before the results are known. HIV can be identified in cultures from peripheral-blood mononuclear cells and plasma by assays for either reverse transcriptase or viral antigen. Although the tests are laborious, they are sensitive and specific. Viral culture is diagnostic for infants with perinatally acquired HIV.

Polymerase chain reaction (PCR)

A method called the 'polymerase chain reaction' is a very sensitive method that can be used to diagnose HIV infections quickly (within a week of the blood being taken). PCR uses DNA recombinant technology which amplifies HIV gene sequences within infected lymphocytes. PCR may detect HIV infection in the presence of a few infected cells so it is especially useful for testing young babies. From Australian experience, this technique, together with viral culture, may facilitate the early diagnosis of infection in infants of seropositive mothers in the first weeks of life.

CD4, CD8 percentage and enumeration

Human blood has different types of white cells. Each type of cell has a different function in the fight against disease. Monoclonal antibodies can be used to enumerate different cell types according to cell surface characteristics, e.g., the T-cell subsets defined by antibodies to CD4 and CD8 cells. CD4 cells are also called helper cells because they help other cells in the immune system to make antibodies. In a person with a healthy immune system, there are more CD4 cells than CD8 cells. However, in a person with HIV infection, as the CD4 cells are destroyed by the virus there are more CD8 (suppressor) cells than there are CD4 (helper) cells. This means that the body's defence against disease is

Table 7.28 Normal CD4 levels for young children

Age (years)	Cell $\times 10^9$	cells/mm^3
Less than 1 year	2.5–3.8	2500–3800
1–2 years	1.5–2.0	1500–2000
3–4 years	1.3–1.8	1300–1800
5–13 years	1.1	1100

weakened. When interpreting CD4 results, it is important to remember that the trend is more important than one result. This is because the number of T-cells can vary. At any time most of the body's T-cells are in the lymph nodes, spleen, the liver and other organs. Therefore, the number that are measured in the blood can vary without the total number of cells in the body changing. Other factors such as stress, drugs and infections can influence the number. Whereas the level for adults is around 900 cells/mm^3, for infants under the age of 1 year, the level is around 3200 cells/mm^3. It is not until the age of 5 years that the CD4 levels are similar to adult values. Normal CD4 levels for young children are shown in **Table 7.28**.[27]

CD4:CD8 ratio

The number of T4 cells are compared to the number of T8 cells. This is known as the T4:T8 ratio (ratio of helper-inducer T-cells to cytotoxic suppressor cells).

Immunoglobulin (IgG, IgM, IgA) levels

Rising levels usually mean that the virus is becoming more active. Raised IgG in response to an overstimulated immune system is a good indicator of HIV infection in children exposed to HIV. Rising IgG levels indicate progression of HIV and may be of concern in an infant of indeterminate category.

Beta 2 microglobulin

The outside of cells have markers that signal that the cell is part of the body and not foreign. The beta 2 microglobulin test measures part of that marker. The level rises due to the high turnover of white blood cells which occurs when the virus is active. The level may be a guide to the effectiveness of antiretroviral therapy. A high level may be an indication for commencement of antiretroviral therapy (e.g., zidovudine).

Total lymphocyte count

A comparative depletion of white cells may be present in infected infants.

Full blood count and differential

This may reveal anaemia, neutropenia, thrombocytopenia due to the effects of HIV infection. Anaemia may be due to side effects of antiretroviral medication.

CLINICAL ASPECTS OF PAEDIATRIC HIV INFECTION

The clinical presentation of HIV infection in children is variable. In comparison to adults infected with HIV, children are more likely to be symptomatic throughout the course of their disease. Clinical features of HIV usually present in infancy. Symptoms in early childhood may be non-specific and include lymph node enlargement, seborrhoeic dermatitis, fever, diarrhoea, failure to thrive as well as more obvious symptoms such as severe fungal infections (*Candida*) or *Pneumocystis* (PCP).

Blood is usually taken from the cord at birth or on Day 1 of life. This is followed by further samples taken at 1 week of age and then again at 6 weeks. We believe that babies infected during pregnancy will show positive results on these early tests. They are likely to do less well in terms of their HIV disease than are those infants infected just before birth or infected during the delivery. This second group of infants is likely to show definite positive results by the age of 6 months. Further tests will need to be done every few months throughout the infant's 1st year of life, depending on their health and well-being. By the age of 15 months, the maternal antibody should have cleared from uninfected children and a negative diagnosis can be confirmed. A final test is done at about 3 years of age in those infants whose tests have remained consistently negative.

Those infants who become seronegative, are virus-culture negative and continue to have no clinical or laboratory-confirmed abnormalities associated with HIV infection, are unlikely to be infected. However, they cannot be given a negative diagnosis until maternal antibodies have completely disappeared. These infants are then described as 'sero-reverters'. Early diagnosis of infants may be critical as prophylaxis against *Pneumocystis* (Bactrim, Septrim, Fansidar, Dapsone) can prevent significant morbidity and mortality in young, infected infants. Therefore, close monitoring and clinical evaluation are essential in these infants. The early administration of zidovudine for infants and children with symptomatic HIV (severe thrombocytopenia, decreased CD4+ cells, failure to thrive, encephalopathy) has been shown to improve clinical and neurological symptoms substantially.[28]

Intrapartum management[15,29]

Perinatal transmission of HIV may occur *in utero*, intrapartum or postpartum by breastfeeding. As infants born to seropositive women are more likely to be uninfected than infected, care should be taken during delivery to minimise exposure of the infant by promptly removing maternal blood and secretions from infants. Procedures that require piercing of the infant's skin should be delayed until maternal blood and secretions are removed. Routine infection measures should be adopted for all deliveries, not only for women for whom an HIV diagnosis is known. These procedures are outlined in **Table 7.29**. The management of the asymptomatic or mildly symptomatic woman otherwise does not need to differ from standard obstetric practice.[30] An interim analysis of seropositive women treated with zidovudine in the 2nd and 3rd trimester, throughout the intrapartum and to their infants for the first 6 weeks of life showed a substantial decrease in the rate of transmission from mother to infant from 24% to 8%.

Breastfeeding

The immunological and nutritional advantages of breastfeeding have been well described.[35] However, the transmission of HIV by breastfeeding may be an exceptional instance in which breastfeeding may pose real risks to the infant. The importance of breastfeeding in HIV transmission is of concern not only for infants born to seropositive women, but also for practices such as the pooling of breastmilk and wet-nursing. Breastfeeding has been known to be associated with the transmission of HIV, although the exact mechanism and risk of transmission are unknown.[31,32] Early reports from Australia, and later Rwanda, described HIV transmission to breastfed infants occurring at the time of the

Table 7.29 Intrapartum management of HIV infection

Avoid foetal exposure to maternal and blood products.	• Avoid use of scalp blood sampling for pH evaluation and scalp electrodes for heart monitoring. • Assess foetal well-being using non-invasive means • Frequent handwashing is essential.
Avoid contact with maternal vaginal secretions and blood and the infant.	• Intravenous access and intramuscular injections, eye prophylaxis to neonate should be avoided until maternal blood and secretions have been removed.
Reduce risk to Health Care Workers (HCW) by minimising direct contact with potentially infected blood and secretions from mother and infant.	• Use 'universal precautions' for handling blood and secretions of all patients as they may be infected. The use of protective barriers (gowns, eye protection, gloves) by all HCW undertaking procedures at risk of exposure to amniotic fluid where splashing is anticipated is advocated. • Water impermeable gowns or sleeves protection may be required for intra-uterine manipulation. Ensure proper handling of needles and scalpels. • Gloves are used by all HCW who come into contact with patient blood, body fluids, non-intact skin and mucous membrane (including handling new-born babies until blood has been removed or baby adequately wrapped). • The umbilical cord should be cut when pulsation has ceased and absorbent material should be placed over the site and cutting instrument to prevent spurting of blood.
Lessen the risk to HCW and to infant of oral exposure to infected secretions. Lessen risk of exposure to infants from infected maternal secretions.	• Avoid nasopharyngeal suctioning of the neonate using mouth suctioning devices. Bulb or wall suctioning (<140 mmHg) is used to avoid trauma to neonatal airway. Mechanical resuscitation equipment should be available to prevent to need for expired air resuscitation. • Avoid mouth-to-mouth exposure. • Baby should be washed as soon as possible with soap and water to eliminate surface secretions.
Be aware of exposure of infant to breastmilk.	• Breastmilk from an infected mother may be an added risk to the infant, but is negligible risk to HCWs if it contacts intact skin.
Restriction of blood spillage.	• Routine disposal of placenta using gown and gloves. • Gloves should be worn to clean up blood spillage using hypochlorite solution. • Hands should be washed immediately with soap and water if blood or secretions contact skin.
Promote, lessen anxiety of birth and possible transmission of HIV to infant.	• Diagnosis of infant may take some months during which time the parents are anxious. • Parents may also express guilt about their decision to have a child that may be infected.

Table 7.29 (*continued*)

Mode of delivery.	• Inconclusive evidence as to whether mode of delivery (vaginal or caesarean) influences transmission rate.[31]
	• Early onset of labour, lower birthweight[35] and less than 34 weeks gestation[34] may be associated with a higher rate of HIV infection.

mother's primary HIV infection.[36,37] The rate of transmission from mother to infant was about 30% in these circumstances.[38,39] The high rate of HIV transmission associated with primary maternal HIV infection may be attributable to the viraemia which accompanies HIV seroconversion. While the vertical transmission rate of HIV in Australia has been found to be around 30% in preliminary retrospective[17] and prospective studies,[26] breastfeeding was found to approximately double this figure.[34,38]

Although transmission of HIV via breast milk is not thought to be the principal mode of transmission of HIV from mother to infant, the World Health Organization has recommended that in countries where safe alternatives to breast milk exist, breastfeeding should not be advised for infants born to HIV seropositve mothers.[42] It is suggested that pending more definitive data, a working estimate for the impact of breastfeeding might be an increase in the transmission rate of more than 10%.

Diagnosis of HIV in older children

When HIV is suspected in a child, a careful history should be taken to elicit possible risk factors for the parents and the child. As the child may be the first person in such a family to become symptomatic, the parents, particularly the mother, should also be evaluated for HIV infection. If the mother does prove to be seropositive, other siblings should be evaluated. Infection within the family, other than perinatal or sexual modes of transmission, is highly unlikely.[43] Clinical features which may prompt assessment for HIV infection in infants and children are:

- Impaired growth or failure to thrive.
- Encephalopathy or developmental delay.
- Chronic interstitial pneumonia.
- Recurrent or persistent infection.
- Opportunistic infections.
- Hepatosplenomegaly or lymphadenopathy.
- Chronic parotitis.

Older children with perinatal infection and children with HIV infection acquired through other modes of transmission are diagnosed according to one of the 3 categories: virus in blood or tissues; *or* HIV antibody; *or* symptoms meeting CDC definition for AIDS. These categories apply to children under 13 years of age. Persons over the age of 13 should be classified according to the adult classification system. HIV infected children have an increased incidence of lymphoid interstitial pneumonitis (LIP) and bacterial infection compared to adults. Those children who acquired HIV infection vertically have a greater incidence of LIP and a shorter incubation period to an AIDS diagnosis that those children affected in the postnatal period.

Prognostic indicators

About one-third of seropositve infants develop severe symptoms of HIV in the 1st year of life. It is thought that these infants were infected early in the pregnancy, rather than during delivery. These children are likely to have a shortened lifespan of perhaps 4 or 5 years or even less. However, the remaining children appear to have a longer period to becoming symptomatic and are more like the adult picture of several years of well-being before becoming symptomatic. This bimodal picture has been described in Australia as well as overseas.[44-46] A number of laboratory markers may be useful to predict progression of HIV. These include a decrease in the number of CD4+ cells, elevated $beta_2$ microglobulin (a protein reflecting the rate of lymphocyte destruction), increased levels of neopterin (produced by macrophages) and the persistence of HIV antigen. Factors associated with a poor prognosis of HIV infection in children are:

- Young age at diagnosis.
- Young age at first opportunistic infection.
- *Pneumocystis carinii* pneumonia (PCP).
- Admission to intensive care for respiratory distress.
- Progressive encephalopathy.
- Raised tumour necrosis factor level.
- Impaired antigen-induced lymphocyte proliferation response.
- Absence of delayed hypersensitivity.
- Low immunoglobulin levels.
- Persistence of HIV antigens.
- Absence of specific neutralising antibodies.

Infection control[47-50]

In caring for children, infection control for the prevention of HIV requires good, basic hygiene. While the HIV-infected child does not require isolation *per se*, universal precautions regarding the body fluids of all children should be practised. A proportion of Australian children with HIV infection has been diagnosed as late as 4 or 5 years of age. These children have had the usual childhood experiences of attending preschool or school and some have had periods of hospitalisation for usual childhood complaints. Thus these guidelines should be followed for all children in the community and not just those known to be HIV positive. Many other diseases in our community are infectious and can be spread through contact with body secretions. The guidelines for infection control within community settings are:

- Teach children to wash their hands thoroughly before eating, after toileting, after playing with animals.
- Use gloves to change soiled nappies, especially if child has diarrhoea.
- Cover open wounds with an adhesive strip.
- Teach children not to touch other's blood and to allow only adults to clean up after a blood spill.
- Carers should wash their hands before preparing food, after toileting or changing nappies, wiping noses and between children.
- Use separate face cloths, towels, tissues or handkerchiefs for each child.

An outline of those guidelines for use within hospitals is given in **Table 7.30**.

Biting

Parents and caregivers often express concern with regard to biting as a possible source of infection in children. For HIV to be spread in this way, the biter would have to bite deep enough for blood to flow and this blood would then have to enter the bloodstream or be introduced into the skin, in order to pass on the virus. Rarely do children's bites break the skin and so they pose only a theoretical risk of transmission. It is, in fact, unlikely that this series of events would occur were an adult to intentionally bite another person.[51] The risk that an HIV seropositive child might transmit the virus by biting is negligible if there is no mixing of infectious body secretions.

NURSING MANAGEMENT OF HIV INFECTION IN CHILDREN

The nursing management of children with HIV infection is focused on maintaining health by early detection of infection and the promotion of growth and development. HIV infection can manifest itself in a wide spectrum of clinical symptoms including life-threatening opportunistic infections, neurological deterioration, failure to thrive, organomegaly, lethargy, malaise and lung pathology such as interstitial pneumonitis and PCP. The family caring for the infected child requires emotional and practical support to achieve a sense of normalcy and to be able to care for the child at home.

The management of HIV infection in children is based on:

- Prevention of transmission during pregnancy.
- Early diagnosis of HIV infection.
- Prophylaxis of opportunistic infections.
- Treatment with antiretrovirals.
- Attention to nutrition.
- Prevention of and early treatment of bacterial and viral infections.
- Immunisation.
- Palliation in the later stages.
- Family support services.
- Education of the family and reference groups within the wider community.

The management of these children involves a multidisciplinary approach with the nurse playing a unique role which encompasses all aspects of care. The nursing management of children infected with HIV thus covers a broad area, including clinical management, emotional support of families, liaison with nursing, medical and palliation services in the community, and the education of focus groups within the community to facilitate the integration of HIV positive children into schools and preschools. The management of children with HIV infection is largely done on an outpatient basis. The aim of nursing management is to keep the children well for as long as possible and to minimise their period of hospitalisation.

Nursing diagnosis

Actual and potential for infection related to immunosuppression.

Rationale

It is the destruction of the CD4+ cells by HIV that results in the profound immuno-suppression characteristic of AIDS. Because of the critical role of CD4+ cells in the

Table 7.30 Infection control management in hospitals

Situation	Nursing management	Rationale
Protection of existing wounds, skin lesions, conjunctivae and mucosal surfaces	• broken skin or open skin lesions should always be covered, for example, with a band aid dressing. Check skin integrity with an alcohol hand wash. Gloves should be worn if the care giver has cuts or breaks in the skin or where blood contact is likely.	Any blood which is removed or escapes from a patient's circulatory system may present a hazard. Occlusive dressings provide bacterial and viral barriers and are sterile.
Prevention of puncture wounds, cuts or abrasions	• all sharps should be disposed of by a method which reduces the amount of handling as much as possible.	The potential for transmission of HIV is greatest when needles, scalpels and other sharps are used.
Reporting of percutaneous/ mucosal exposure and critical risk assessment and management	• after a needlestick injury/exposure to blood, allow the wound to bleed, wash thoroughly with soap and water. If the source is known to be infected with HIV, report immediately for counselling, baseline blood tests and assessment for Zidovudine prophylaxis, and follow-up serological testing.	Workers seeking compensation for occupationally acquired HIV must prove infection occurred in the workplace rather than in activities undertaken outside of work. If not reported immediately, many accidental needlestick injuries will not be readily recalled or may not have been witnessed by others.
Protective barriers to avoid contamination and good basic hygiene practices which include regular hand washing	• gloves should be worn for direct contact with blood, blood-stained body fluids, mucous membranes or non-intact skin. If blood or other body fluids[1] splash onto skin, wash as soon as possible with soap and water.	Gloves can reduce the bioburden on the hands but do not prevent penetrating injuries.

Avoidance of sharps usage when possible but if use is essential then extreme care in handling sharps and disposal. Non disposable sharps should be placed in a puncture resistant container prior to decontamination	• used needles should not be recapped, removed from disposable syringes or purposefully bent, broken. • prompt disposal of sharps after use into puncture proof containers. • avoid overfilling containers.	Gowns, aprons and other protective apparel reduce the possibility of blood contamination of skin and soiling of clothing. Precautions should be taken to prevent injuries during procedures or disposal of used sharps.
Control of work surface contamination and decontamination maintenance of a safe hygienic environment by containment, cleaning and where necessary, disinfection	• body fluids should be cleaned up with detergent as soon as possible.	HIV is not stable in the external environment outside the body and no environmental mediated mode of transmission has been documented.
Safe disposal of biohazard waste contaminated with blood or body fluid	• soiled linen should be placed in bags that prevent leakage. • routine waste disposal practices apply.	Universal precautions apply to linen soiled with blood and body fluids.

[1] Body fluids include all fluids, secretions and excretions produced by the body. Not all these fluids are hazardous. Blood, tissue, cerebro spinal fluid, semen, vaginal fluid, and all serous exudates (pleural, pericardial, amniotic, synovial and peritoneal) are classed as hazardous for HIV. Any fluid containing a purulent or inflammatory exudate or serum is regarded as if it were blood-stained and therefore hazardous. In the context of occupational exposure to HIV, urine, faeces, sputum, breastmilk, vomitus, nasal secretions, sweat and saliva do not require universal precautions unless they contain visible blood. (Prince of Wales Children's Hospital Infection Manual. 1990.)

induction of immune responses, the elimination of this one subset of cells has devastating consequences. As the virus destroys the CD4+ cells, the immune system is unable to function and so the child becomes susceptible to infections and cancers.[52]

Nursing intervention

- Identification of infants who may be at risk for HIV infection by testing and close follow-up of infants born to seropositive women.
- Close monitoring of the child's health by regular checkups.
- Parental vigilance is important in recognising early signs of infection. Information as to when to seek medical advice should be given to parents.
- Minimise exposure of the immunosuppressed child to infections. Check immunisation status and measles antibody level after initial immunisation and annually. Passive immunisation with immunoglobulin should be considered for children exposed to measles.
- HIV positive children should receive all the routine immunisations. In symptomatic children (or those with symptomatic parents) and their siblings, inactivated Salk poliomyelitis vaccine (IPV) is recommended in preference to the oral Sabin vaccine (OPV) as the active virus may be excreted in the stool. It should be noted that the effect of vaccines may be reduced in the presence of HIV.
- Awareness of exposure to other infections (such as varicella). Zoster immunoglobulin is recommended for children exposed to varicella (chicken pox or shingles).[53]
- Prompt treatment of infections. Administer antimicrobial therapy as prescribed. Teach parents the importance of prophylactic therapy.
- Regular (monthly) gammaglobulin infusions have been found to prevent bacterial infections as HIV infected children also have a secondary B cell deficiency, but cotrimoxazole appears to be equally effective.[54]
- Teach the family and child the importance of hand washing before eating, preparing food, and after toileting and playing with animals.

Nursing diagnosis

Impaired gaseous exchange related to ineffective airway clearance, viscous secretions, fatigue and loss of functioning lung tissue.

Rationale

Respiratory disease is a leading cause of morbidity and mortality in children with AIDS. Lymphoid interstitial pneumonitis may lead to damage of lung tissue. PCP infection has a high morbidity and mortality.

Nursing intervention

- Assess respiratory status for signs of respiratory distress; perform oxymetry to assess oxygenation.
- Organise care to allow for maximum periods of rest and sleep.
- Provide postural drainage and percussion, evaluate breath sounds and observe for changes in respiratory pattern.
- Monitor measures used to provide optimum oxygenation (oxygen, suction, humidification).

- Educate parents/caregivers about the signs of changes in respiratory status that warrant reporting and checking.

Nursing diagnosis

Alteration in bowel function: diarrhoea related to bowel infection, medication and malabsorption.

Rationale

Diarrhoea may be caused by protozoan, viral and bacterial infections as well as antimicrobial drugs and high-osmolality feeding. Prolonged diarrhoea may result in fluid/electrolyte imbalance, acid-base imbalance and inadequate nutritional status. HIV enteropathy may be caused by the virus, resulting in a flattening of the villi causing malabsorption and diarrhoea.

Nursing intervention

- Monitor the child's general condition and assess for signs of dehydration. Document output and weight changes.
- Check fluid stools for reducing substances. Send specimen for culture and analysis.
- Change soiled nappies as soon as possible, clean perineal area thoroughly and check for secondary *Candida* infections. Wash hands thoroughly.
- Correct food preparation and storage should be discussed with parents to avoid food poisoning due to incorrect handling or preparing of food. This includes keeping food storage and preparation areas clean; cooking food rapidly and thoroughly to destroy bacteria; using serving utensils rather than handling food; and washing hands thoroughly before handling food or eating.

Nursing diagnosis

Alteration in nutritional status related to catabolic state, anorexia, nausea and vomiting, decreased oral intake due to difficulty in swallowing, pain, diarrhoea and malabsorption.

Rationale

Many children infected with HIV do not have a consistent growth rate. It is important to encourage children to eat foods which are high in calories. The child's height and weight should be monitored. If the child's weight develops a plateau or a fall across percentiles over several months, supplemental nasogastric or gastrostomy feeds may be indicated.[55] Children with AIDS develop a wasting syndrome which may make it difficult to gain or even maintain weight. Failure to thrive and growth failure have been shown to be strong prognosticators of the progression to AIDS.[56] The children tend to have little appetite and often prefer foods that are low in calories. Despite this, the children are usually active. Diarrhoea may develop as the result of a combination of factors. These include infection of the gut, HIV enteropathy or a side effect of medication. If the diarrhoea becomes chronic, nutritional problems may arise. Early attention to diet may help prevent weight loss and lessen the need for enteral and parenteral feeding.

Nursing intervention[57-62]

- Document weight and height, amount of vomiting or diarrhoea and intake patterns.
- Use creative and appropriate approaches to nutrition by offering small, frequent, attractive servings. Allow child to choose when appropriate to do so. Reward with stickers and special privileges for eating. Do not allow the child to feel failure by inability to regain weight.
- Administer vitamins and nutritional supplements as prescribed. Monitor laboratory tests (e.g., haemoglobin, protein levels) for signs of nutritional deficit.
- Implement frequent mouth care if child has oral lesions such as *Candida* or herpes.

Nursing diagnosis

Alteration in comfort related to pain.

Rationale

Pain is a common symptom in children with HIV infection and tends to increase as the disease progresses. The common sites and causes of pain in children with HIV infection are as follows.

The oropharynx

Oropharyngeal candidiasis is the most frequent cause of oral pain. Bacterial infections may cause necrotising gingivitis in spite of good oral hygiene. Dental abscesses are more common in persons with HIV infection than in the general population. Oral ulceration is common and may be caused by herpes simplex, cytomegalovirus (CMV), Epstein-Barr virus, mycobacterial infection, cryptococcal infection or histoplasmosis. Herpes simplex may be perioral or oral and may be severe, requiring long-term, systemic treatment.

The oesophagus

Oesophageal pain often causes anorexia and decreased food intake, thereby adding to the child's debilitated state. *Candida* is the most common cause of symptoms, but ulceration from CMV and herpes simplex may also occur. Reports of ulceration from zidovudine have also been made. In many cases, there are concurrent disorders contributing to oesophageal pain.

The abdomen

Abdominal pain may present difficulties in diagnosis and thus treatment. A variety of organisms may be responsible, such as *Cryptosporidium, Shigella, Salmonella, Campylobacter, Mycobacterium avium-intracellulare* (MAI) and CMV. Other abdominal pathology may also cause severe pain, such as perforation of the small or large intestine, intussusception of the small intestine and peritonitis.

Biliary tract and pancreas

Cholecystitis may occur as the result of gallstones or opportunistic infection. Acalculous cholecystitis may also present with right upper quadrant or epigastric pain. Pancreatitis is most commonly associated with either drug therapy, especially didanosine (ddI) and dideoxycytidine (ddC), or CMV infection.

Neurological pain

Headache and painful peripheral neuropathies may be the result of HIV or opportunistic infections or tumours. Headache may be due to HIV encephalitis, aseptic meningitis, bacterial meningitis, opportunistic infections (*Toxoplasmosis, Cryptococcus,* or *Mycobacterium*) or neoplasms. Other causes may be stress, anxiety, migraine or sinus infections. A variety of peripheral neuropathies has been described in HIV patients, involving both sensory and motor function.

Arthritis

Joint symptoms are frequently severe and may be unresponsive to non-steroidal anti-inflammatory drugs.

Myopathy and myositis

Myositis is thought to be a consequence of direct viral infection of the muscle cells. It has also been reported as the result of zidovudine therapy.

Nursing intervention

One of the concerns in the management of chronic illness such as HIV infection in children is that pain may be inadequately treated. One of the causes of undertreatment is inadequate assessment. The relief of painful symptoms may also be delayed until the diagnosis is made.

Pain may be alleviated by specific management of the cause, especially that caused by infection. The pain caused by oropharyngeal candidiasis, for example, will be relieved by the commencement of topical antifungal therapy. The symptoms of drug-induced pancreatitis (most notably, ddI or ddC) will usually resolve with the cessation of the drug. Acute herpetic infection will generally require systemic acyclovir treatment. The treatment of meningitis with the standard antibiotics or antifungals will also provide the relief of symptoms. Although the role of physiotherapy may be limited in acute rheumatological disorders, the use of heat and ice, together with rest and splinting, may supplement the treatment with non-steroidal anti-inflammatory drugs.

In combination with the treatment of the specific cause of the pain, standard pain management should also be commenced. The symptomatic management of chronic muscle, bone or joint pain involves a non-opioid drug such as paracetamol 20 mg/kg or NSAIDS (Aspirin 15 mg/kg/dose) given every 4 hours. The prolonged use of paracetamol, NSAIDS or morphine in patients receiving zidovudine, may lead to zidovudine toxicity as these medications may inhibit its metabolism.

If the pain is not contained, a weak opioid such as codeine or dextropropoxyphene should be added to the non-opioid. If pain still persists, a stronger opioid, such as morphine is indicated, at incremental doses until the control of pain is achieved. The side effects of opioids are constipation, drowsiness and nausea. Constipation is usually not a problem, as in late-stage HIV infection the child nearly always has diarrhoea.

The problems associated with pain relief in children with HIV infection are often associated with the delay in diagnosis which may involve invasive procedures such as endoscopy. A second problem is that some types of HIV pain, such as pain associated with peripheral neuropathy, headache, abdominal pain and pain from severe pressure sores, respond poorly to opioids. In these cases, adjunct analgesics, such as tricyclic depressants, anticonvulsants, anti-arrhythmics or steroids, together with non-drug measures have been used with success in adults with HIV infection.

For children in end-stage AIDS who are severely emaciated, the use of water or ripple mattresses, positioning and gentle massage may help to relieve skin pain.

Nursing diagnosis

Alteration to skin integrity related to immunosuppression and opportunistic infections.

Rationale

Skin integrity may be compromised by opportunistic infections such as herpes or *Candida*. Debilitation caused by AIDS can result in slow healing and skin breakdown. Night sweats and fever may also be experienced.

Nursing intervention

* Keep lesions clean and dry. Clean perineal area with warm soapy water after each nappy change. Apply water-occlusive ointment or anti-bacterial cream to buttocks or excoriated area.
* Reposition the child each 2 hours if she is unable to move herself. Gentle massage may promote comfort.
* Exematous rash associated with HIV infection may require the use of emollient oil for bathing. Psoriasis may require tar-based or steroidal treatment.

Nursing diagnosis

Potential for dental caries due to medications and oral infections.

Rationale

Children with HIV often require oral medications which are sucrose sweetened for prolonged periods of time and are thus at high risk for severe dental caries and periodontal disease.

Nursing intervention

Dental check-up every 3 months should be undertaken for assessment of dental caries and mouth ulcers. The application of preventative therapy can also be provided if required. A dental examination is the most thorough method of identifying opportunistic oral infection such as *Candida*.

Promote meticulous oral hygiene which is supervised by parent or caregiver. The teeth should be cleaned thoroughly at least once a day with a soft toothbrush.

Reduce the number of daily cariogenic exposures by planning medications at mealtime if possible; encourage children to drink, especially water, after oral medications to rinse the mouth; encourage a diet which restricts sweets and carbonated drinks.

Nursing diagnosis

Altered growth and development related to neurological changes associated with AIDS, psychosocial adjustments due to family separation, death or prolonged illness of other family members.

Rationale

Developmental delay may be due to HIV encephalopathy, an insult during pregnancy in drug-using women or poor stimulation and parenting skills. It is often difficult to ascertain which of these is the cause of the delay. It would be expected that HIV encephalopathy would be progressive and respond to zidovudine therapy. Early intervention services for infants delayed due to poor parenting or intrauterine insult should prove beneficial. Neurological function and dementia may result from progressive AIDS encephalopathy, resulting in delay in, or loss of milestones.

Nursing intervention

Care should be taken to isolate the child in hospital only when absolutely necessary, and not as a matter of routine.

Provide appropriate play therapy to maintain motor skills. Early intervention services may be required for infants and young children. Encourage school-aged children to attend school as frequently as possible.

During long-term admissions, develop a schedule that provides the child with routine and some control over their environment.

Nursing diagnosis

Grieving related to loss of a child, death of other family members; loss of body image, lifestyle; future.

Rationale

Australian children are affected by the AIDS epidemic in a variety of ways. A number will be orphaned or lose one parent to AIDS, others will lose a sibling or will themselves die from the disease. Some children will be the only survivor of their family. The challenge of providing services to families where several members may be infected with a terminal illness requires a multidisciplinary approach, involving both hospital and community services. The vertical transmission of HIV from mother to infant poses unique problems for the family. Not only is there a child with a chronic, terminal illness, but there is also a mother, whose health will deteriorate and who will most likely die while her child or children are young. The father may also be infected. Fortunately in Australia the number of children infected with HIV is low, due in the main to the relatively low rates of HIV infection among injecting drug users. However, the fear of social stigma and discrimination may initially prevent families from seeking services and/or family support.

Nursing intervention

Parents of children with HIV may have previously used or presently be using illicit drugs and experienced the deleterious consequences and association of doing so (i.e., poverty, prostitution, criminal activity, ill health). Thus they may feel dislocated and isolated from wider society, have difficulties establishing relationships with people they perceive to be in authority, including doctors, nurses and social workers. The diagnosis of an infected child may make a parent vulnerable to returning to, or increasing addictive behaviours in an effort to cope. A parent may feel guilty about their drug use and it being the 'cause' of their child's illness. Their own illness may be progressing to a point where they are less able to care for themselves or the child(ren). Other parents may be involved in a methadone program, finding some of the side effects of methadone difficult to deal with. It is imperative to provide non-judgmental support during the diagnostic period in an effort to discourage previous behaviours which may render a parent less able to care for an infected child. Specific drug and alcohol services should be consulted for advice on management.

STRESS FACTORS FOR FAMILIES AFFECTED BY HIV INFECTION

Any of the following factors is a major stressor for a family and its ability to function in a complex society. When these stressors are in combination the effect is very potent. All families with a child with HIV/AIDS will have a number of these stressors; some will have most.

One or both parents and other children may be infected, causing feelings of despair as well as practical difficulties.

Chronic illness limits the energy of ill parents to care for young children; they are often reluctant to place their children in respite or foster care as they realise the shortness of their time with their children. Children may experience unsatisfied emotional needs from parents who may be ill for many months before they eventually die.

Life-threatening illness creates an enforced need to make preparations for the future where child/ren may be orphaned. This confronts parents with their own death, and so they may delay making final plans, or committing them to paper.

Death. Families will suffer profound sadness and grief, especially when confronted by multiple deaths.

Psychiatric or personality disorder. Parents of infected children may have a pre-existing psychiatric or personality disorder which may be exacerbated by the child's positive diagnosis. This may be further complicated by illicit drug use. Some parents are very anxious about the situation in which they find themselves, projecting intense anger onto staff. Other parents may appear to be extremely disinterested and uncaring about the child's welfare, thereby alienating staff from the parent and child(ren). In some circumstances, it is extremely difficult for a working relationship to be maintained and it may be necessary for a psychiatrist to be consulted.

Previous or present addiction to alcohol, illicit drugs or nicotine. The indirect effects of drug use by parents will influence: standards of parental care and parenting skills; socioeconomic status of parents; nutrition; housing; medical attention; and social support systems.

Previous criminal activity/imprisonment. Parents of infected children may have previous/present experience with prison authorities. Case management plans should take into consideration the needs of incarcerated parents.

Arrangements for care of children. Parents who have HIV will need to arrange care for their child(ren) in the event of them becoming ill or dying. Extended family may be of assistance in the long term. However, some parents have difficult relationships with extended families, due to previous addictive behaviours, abuse during childhood, or psychiatric disorder. It may be necessary for these parents to be linked to an agency, for a respite/foster/adoption arrangement to be planned.

Ideally, children should be introduced to prospective adoptive parents and have short-term placements with them while the children's natural parents are still alive. This is beneficial in 2 ways — it gives the parents a chance to have a rest and gives the child a chance to become familiar with their prospective carers. This ideal arrangement may in reality be difficult to achieve. Parents, particularly mothers, find relinquishing the care of their child(ren) to fully functioning carers very threatening. It is usually accompanied by a sense of powerlessness that HIV disease is indeed progressing. Sensitivity and patience are required by workers trying to assist with these practical arrangements. Where possible, parents should be encouraged to have responsibility for manageable and achievable care of their children. Parents infected with HIV should be encouraged to make a will while they are relatively well.

It is a major commitment for a carer to agree to care for a child with HIV. The child's health professionals need to be mindful of the support and reassurance required by these carers. They also require relevant information about paediatric HIV disease and infection control. They may be unconfident initially and overly concerned about every ailment the child has. Alternatively, they may be blase about different illnesses and not seek appropriate medical care when necessary. With comprehensive education and support, these difficulties can be overcome.

Paternal bisexuality. A diagnosis of HIV infection in a child and mother may also indicate infection in the father. This may reveal past or present male-to-male sexual activity by the father, previously unknown to his partner. Depending on the partner's coping style, reaction to the news will vary between intense anger and bitterness to acceptance. It may be necessary to refer the couple for specific couple counselling or other services aimed at bisexual men and their partners.

Disturbed relationship with the family of origin. Relatives or guardians may also have problems accepting parental illness/death. The presence of an extended family is not always helpful — social stigma may also extend within the family and may be a reason for the child not being told of their diagnosis for fear that the child may inadvertently tell others. Previous sexual and/or physical abuse of parents in their family of origin may make contact and support from their family difficult, if not impossible.

Relationship difficulties with partner. Different patterns of dealing with illness and grief between family members may complicate relationships and cause tension and division.

Problematic encounters with authorities or bureaucracies. The need for privacy and confidentiality is often jeopardised when applying for emotional and practical support.

Employment. The ability of a parent(s) to work is lessened as HIV disease progresses in either the child or the parent. It is natural for parents who are employed to try to work for as long as possible. Deciding to give up employment is a difficult time for parents as it is an acknowledgment that HIV disease has progressed and is interfering in normal functioning. Self-esteem may suffer as a result of imposed retirement and may require special attention. Uninfected parents who are employed need to have a sympathetic employer as there may be ongoing disruptions to work. Assistance may be required to help a parent inform their employer about the special needs of the family, particularly when the child becomes ill. Income support or a carers' pension is available for parents where the breadwinner has given up paid employment to care for the child or the other parent.

Housing. A family's needs may be better served if it lives in an area with a wide range of local community services. Consideration may need to be given to changing locality to a better serviced area and/or a home that costs less to maintain. Families where parents have to give up paid employment to care for an ill child or because they are ill themselves, will suffer a substantial income loss. The public housing sector may need to be explored as a means of balancing the family's reduced budget. It is necessary for a family with a child with HIV to have ready access to a phone, especially for emergency purposes. It is also imperative that houses are hygienic and can be cooled in summer and warmed in winter. Appliances such as clothes dryers and microwave ovens enhance the quality of life for these families.

Transport. In addition to housing and utilities is the need to have access to either very reliable public transport, a well maintained car or other means of getting around, or volunteer transport available through major hospitals and AIDS councils. A person with HIV/AIDS requires regular medical care, particularly as the illness progresses. In a family where more than one member is infected, treatment will probably be at different centres, obviously made more difficult without good access to transport. For emergencies it is also preferable to have quick, reliable access to specialist treatment centres.

Domestic help. HIV in children results in a greater domestic work load. Drenching night sweats generate extra laundry; diarrhoea and vomiting necessitates more bathroom cleaning; preparation of food may be difficult for somebody who is continually feeling nauseous. The local community health service may need to be contacted for regular domestic assistance. Volunteer services are available through the AIDS Councils.

Nursing intervention

The psychological care of families with HIV requires an individual approach and awareness of the multiple problems. Although the families have many stresses in common (children suffering from a terminal illness, parent/s also infected and at times ill, constant visits to hospital, numerous hospitalisations, frequent blood tests and diagnostic procedures, uncertainty of the future), each family has different experiences and coping mechanisms.

Family counselling

Although the patient is the child, services must be directed to the entire family, taking into account the needs of the child, parents, siblings, extended family and significant social networks involved in the care of the child. This may include schools, playgroups, churches, neighbours and friends.

When a child is given a positive diagnosis it may be necessary to facilitate, with families, changes in some of these factors which impinge on the family's ability to cope. As it is highly likely that the child's mother will be similarly infected, all services must be delivered with this in mind. In addition to dealing with the chronic illness of a child, families must also be helped to cope in the presence of infection of one or both parents. A feeling of isolation is engendered by the need to maintain confidentiality and the frequent lack of accurate knowledge of HIV in their family, schools and community. Families require support and nurture to accept the diagnosis and the inevitable outcome. There are feelings of guilt, isolation, rejection, stigma, overwhelming sense of loss and grief, fear of themselves or others.

The family in the community

Children are legally required to attend school. It is also mandatory that state education department schools accept appropriate enrolment of children with HIV if requested. It is *not* mandatory for parents to inform schools of the child's health status. However, integration of children with HIV into schools, with full disclosure to the school community, has occurred successfully. The process involves a comprehensive education program for teachers, other staff, parents and children at the time of enrolment. Policies regarding infection control and supervision of children are then fully implemented by the school to reduce the risk of transmission to uninfected children and risk of other infections to the child with HIV. A team involving nurses and social workers should be involved in the process, not only to provide relevant information but to give back-up support to the school and reassurance to all concerned. The family benefits from the minimisation of the negative aspects of secrecy. The infected child receives acceptance and the opportunity to enjoy normal childhood experiences. Benefits to other children attending the school include an awareness of HIV/AIDS and the opportunity to discuss issues such as discrimination and perhaps even death. The school benefits by an increased sense of community.

MEDICAL MANAGEMENT OF HIV IN CHILDREN

Clinical aspects of paediatric HIV infection

The immunopathogenesis of HIV infection is based on the depletion of CD4+ lymphocytes. The clinical presentation of HIV infection in children whether acquired through perinatal transmission or from blood or blood products, is variable. In comparison to adults infected with HIV, children are more likely to be symptomatic throughout the course of their disease. Clinical features of paediatric acquired HIV usually present in infancy. As an effect of HIV, and consequent immune system failure, all body systems may be affected over time. The main manifestations of HIV infection in children are as follows:

Direct effects of HIV

- Seborrhoeic dermatitis.
- HIV enteropathy which may cause malabsorption, chronic diarrhoea, failure to thrive.
- Intermittent, unexplained fever for which there is often no focus of infection.
- Enlarged lymph nodes.
- Encephalopathy which may cause dementia, developmental delay.

Recurrent serious bacterial infections

Diagnosed by clinical manifestation and cultures, these are frequently caused by common childhood pathogens such as *Streptococcus*, *Haemophilis* and *Salmonella*.

Viral infections

It is difficult to differentiate asymptomatic from active disseminated cytomegalovirus (CMV). Gancyclovir controls CMV infection, which reactivates when the drug is stopped. Cytotoxic precautions are required for the administration, handling and disposal of gancyclovir. All staff should protect themselves from accidental exposure.

Herpes simplex may be diffuse and spread into the oropharynx and around the perineal area. Management may require acyclovir to be taken long term.

Opportunistic infections

The most serious opportunistic infection is *Pneumocystis carinii* pneumonia (PCP). PCP may resemble Lymphoid interstitial pneumonitis (LIP) on chest x-ray. PCP requires prophylaxis once CD4 cells fall to about 50% of normal for age. The exception is for infants under the age of 1 year in whom CD4 count does not appear to predict the incidence accurately.[63]

Fungal infections such as *Candida* may be present in the oesophagus, gut, perineum as well as the mouth. Long-term treatment with ketaconazole, amphotericin, flucytosine is usually required.

Cryptosporidium is a parasite which causes severe diarrhoea. It may be unresponsive to treatment or reactivate when treatment ceases. Enteral or parenteral feeding to maintain fluid and electrolyte balance and nutritional status may be required.

Cardiovascular

Cardiomyopathy and endocarditis may be detected initially on chest x-ray.

Other effects

Other effects include tumours for which there may be no effective treatment.

Diarrhoea may be chronic and lactose intolerance may be present in infants.

Lymphoid interstitial pneumonitis, a slowly developing, progressive interstitial lung disease, is often asymptomatic in the initial stages but progresses to shortness of breath and clubbing of fingers. Chest x-ray reveals diffuse, bilateral reticulonodular infiltrates and may allow a presumptive diagnosis. Definitive diagnosis of LIP is made by lung biopsy which shows interstitial infiltration of CD8 lymphocytes and plasma cells. LIP has a better prognosis than PCP. It is a histologically confirmed pneumonitis characterised by diffuse interstitial and peribronchiolar infiltration of lymphocytes and plasma cells, without identifiable pathogens.

Chronic parotitis is evident in many seropositive children. The discovery of chronic parotitis in an undiagnosed child should prompt investigation for HIV infection, as it is otherwise uncommon.

Failure to thrive may result from a combination of factors.

Treatment of children with HIV infection

Prophylaxis against pneumocystis

PCP is one of the most devastating opportunistic infections in children. It may present as the initial illness or as a later manifestation of HIV infection. Children who present with PCP have a high mortality rate and a short median survival time.[64] Early diagnosis of HIV is also important as a poor prognosis is associated with symptomatic PCP during the 1st year of life. PCP has been diagnosed in infants as young as 2 months.[65] CD4 counts in young children are much higher than in older children and adults. Whereas the lower range for adults is around 0.9×10^9/L, for infants in their 1st year of life the level is around 3.2×10^9/L. Prophylaxis against pneumocystis (oral, low dose co-trimoxazole) and the initiation of antiretroviral therapy (zidovudine) is advised at the CD4+ levels shown in **Table 7.31**.[66]

However, it would appear that some children are at risk of PCP infection above these CD4+ levels, so that recommendation is made to commence all infected children under the age of one year and those children born to mothers with CD4 counts less than 0.2×10^9/L on PCP prophylaxis.[67]

Table 7.31 CD4 level for commencement of PCP prophylaxis and zidovudine administration

Age (years)	PCP prophylaxis $\times 10^9$ (cells/mm^3)	Zidovudine administration $\times 10^9$ (cells/mm^3)
<1	1.5 (1500)	1.75 (1750)
2–6	0.5 (500)	0.75 (750)
>6	0.20 (200)	0.50 (500)

Antiretroviral therapy

Currently there are several antiretroviral agents available to treat children with HIV infection.

Zidovudine is the most extensively used and remains the drug of first line management. Use is indicated in children with symptomatic HIV disease or in asymptomatic HIV infection with evidence of declining immune function. Zidovudine is generally well tolerated in children, although the dose may need to be lowered and graded up to the usual dose if gastrointestinal or haematological toxicity side effects develop. Weight gains (standardised for age) when they occurred were found within 8 weeks of the commencement of therapy, suggesting that the drug was controlling direct viral effects (e.g., on gut mucosal function) rather than by preventing opportunistic infection, where the benefit would be expected to take longer to be evident.[28] While the advised dose has been 30 mg/kg/day or 720 mg/m^2 per day as 4 doses, the drug has usually been administered in 2 or 3 doses per day, with the total dose often being as low as half the dose with apparent preservation of benefit. Experience with *Didanosine (ddI)* in children in Australia remains limited at present. Recent marketing approval has allowed children to receive this drug simultaneously with adults for intolerance to or lack of benefit from zidovudine and a small number has received the drug in this way, a few more children had received the drug on a compassionate use basis before marketing approval. No serious toxicity has been reported though experience in these very ill children has been too limited to observe possible efficacy. As in adults, a neutral gastric pH is required. CSF penetration is poor but appears related to dose. Controlled studies of its use are still under way, but efficacy of ddI in children can be implied from the observations of rises in CD4 and falls in p24. Toxicity appears to be less problematic than with zidovudine. Pancreatitis has been observed at doses of 360 mg/m^2/day or greater and peripheral neuritis has not been reported. However about 7% of children receiving this drug may develop peripheral retinal atrophy so that regular ophthalmological review is required. Diarrhoea may occur if the gastric acid buffering is obtained with a magnesium compound.

Zalcitabine (ddC) is one of the more potent agents against HIV, but has less penetration of the CNS than other nucleosides. The dose-limiting toxicity for ddC is peripheral neuropathy. It is usually used in combination with zidovudine in children with disease progression. Although the long-term adverse effects in infants and children is unknown, the beneficial effects support their use.

Lamivudine (3TC) is in the same class of drugs as zidovudine, ddI and ddC. When given in combination with zidovudine, 3TC has been shown to produce significant and prolonged rises in CD4 counts and reduction in the amount of virus in the bloodstream. It would also appear to prevent resistance that occurs when zidovudine is used alone.

The size and duration of these effects is greater than would be expected by adding the effects of each drug used alone.

Combination therapy, alternating drug therapy of antiretrovirals or using lower doses in combination, reduces the toxicity associated with each drug alone while maintaining strong antiretroviral activity. Combination in either of these forms reduces the impact of drug resistance which develops after about 18 months of therapy.[68]

Corticosteroids may be used for specific indications such as immune thrombocytopenia and drug reactions and are of benefit in children with respiratory failure during episodes of PCP. Their use is recommended for children with lymphoid interstitial pneumonitis and hypoxaemia.

Neuropyschological assessment.[69] Many risk factors (premature birth, maternal drug use) place HIV-infected children at a higher risk for the occurrence of developmental disabilities. The detection of progressive abnormalities of muscle tone or reflex patterns, including the appearance of pathologic reflexes or the recurrence of primitive reflexes, may identify children with rapid central nervous system deterioration. HIV-infected children require frequent and on-going neurological and neurodevelopmental assessment. Children who present with neurological manifestation have a poor prognosis. HIV encephalopathy is the major cause of neurological impairment and consists of developmental delay, acquired microcephaly, pyramidal signs, ataxia, seizures and extrapyramidal signs.

ADOLESCENTS AND HIV INFECTION[70–77]

Although the number of adolescents infected with HIV tends to be less than adults, it is becoming increasingly obvious that many young adults were infected during their adolescence. This, together with the recognition that certain behavioural and psychological factors put adolescents at high risk, have increased the awareness that specialised prevention and treatment programs are required.

As the adolescent population is heterogeneous, the strategies for controlling HIV infection in this population must also be varied. While most adolescents live in the family home, many find that they are unable to do so, and become self-reliant at a young age.

Nursing diagnosis

Potential risk of infection during sexual activity related to knowledge deficit of risk behaviours.

Rationale

The transmission risks in adolescents are similar to those in adults (homosexuals and bisexuals, followed by injecting drug users). Concern exists that the number of adolescents infected may be high, partly because of the nature of adolescence itself. Development of a sexual identity and some degree of experimentation are normal during this time. Added to certain psychological factors, such as a sense of invulnerability, and the tendency to engage in high-risk behaviour, is cause for concern. Sexual activity is one high-risk behaviour; many adolescents have multiple partners, some of whom are homosexual or bisexual. The risk is compounded by the failure of adolescents to use contraception, especially condoms. That such unsafe sexual practices could contribute to the spread of HIV in the adolescent population is suggested by looking at the rates of other sexually transmitted diseases, such as syphilis and gonorrhoea. Male-to-male sex was the most common exposure category reported overall. In some studies of adolescents and HIV, it has been found that fewer than one-third of the infected patients had disclosed their HIV status to their sexual partners and very few reported consistent use of condoms. In a study of HIV-infected females, nearly all reported heterosexual intercourse as their only source of exposure and few knew of their partners' risk behaviours.

Drug-related behaviour is also of particular concern. Injection of drugs increases an adolescent's risk, but any drug use may cause an adolescent to participate in hazardous activity, such as trading sex for drugs and lessening their ability to negotiate safe sex.

Nursing intervention

Adolescents require accurate knowledge about 'safer' sex and the hazards of transmission of the virus during sexual activity.

Conflict between the parents' wishes that the child not be told of their diagnosis may present problems as the child reaches puberty.

Obtain a history of sexually transmitted diseases, including gonorrhoea, chlamydia, syphilis, genital herpes, and warts. Vaginal candidiasis and pelvic inflammatory disease may be manifestations of HIV infection in women. Adolescent females should be asked if they have ever had a pelvic examination and if they know their Pap smear results. In adolescence a high rate of abnormal cells is common. This high rate may be due to both behavioural and physiological factors. During early puberty, the columnar cells on the cervical surface (ectopy) may be more susceptible to infection than the squamous epithelial cells that later replace them. In addition, the more permeable cervical mucus present in adolescence may aid the transmission of infectious agents in the semen.

Obtain a menstrual and pregnancy history. If the adolescent has living children, note their ages, health, and care arrangements for purposes of follow-up. Both gay and straight females and males should be asked if they have borne or fathered any children. Contraception and condom use as well as intent to have children should be discussed.

HIV counselling and testing

When organising HIV testing services for adolescents, make pre-test and post-test counselling developmentally appropriate. Offer voluntary testing with informed consent. Assure confidentiality, particularly in settings such as foster care, residential institutions, or detention facilities. Try to arrange for a family member or adult to provide emotional support during the process. Because the adolescent may be overwhelmed by the diagnosis of HIV infection, ensure that testing programs provide appropriate follow-up with referral for care.

Since, unlike children, most adolescents are infected when the immune system has already developed, the natural history of HIV in post-pubertal adolescents will most likely resemble that seen in adults. However, studies of children, adolescents, and adults with haemophilia have shown that HIV-infected teenagers live longer than young children and appear to progress more slowly to AIDS than do adults.

Obtaining a sexual history

This can be done over the course of several initial visits. To understand the issues related to risk reduction for a particular adolescent, it is important to establish the age of first sexual intercourse, age and sex of initial and subsequent partners, sexual orientation, approximate number of sexual partners, history of sexual abuse, use of condoms or other contraceptives, and experience with 'survival sex' (the exchange of sex for money, drugs, food, or shelter).

Males who have intercourse with other males represent the leading exposure category for HIV infection among adolescents. These youths are at particular risk because of the higher prevalence of HIV infection among gay and bisexual adult men. Sexual behaviour is not the same as sexual identity; studies have shown that between 17% and 35% of males have had same-sex experiences to orgasm, frequently during adolescence, but that not all these adolescents identify themselves as gay or bisexual. For those youths who are gay, the development of an integrated gay identity is made more difficult by the tremendous social and family prejudices against homosexuality.

Despite safer sex programs in the adult gay community, the adolescent who is in the process of 'coming out' may not have access to this community or does not yet identify as gay. Conversely, safer sex programs for adolescents may not include explicit information for gay youths because it is deemed 'too controversial'. In addition, gay male and lesbian adolescents may engage in sex with heterosexual partners to hide their homosexuality from themselves and others, and this, of course, also carries a risk of HIV infection.

Adolescent females, unlike their adult counterparts, are more likely to become infected with HIV through sexual exposure than through injecting drug use. A program that follows a large cohort of HIV-infected adolescents found that although 85% of females contracted HIV infection through heterosexual intercourse, very few were aware that their male partners had HIV infection at the time of their exposure. Ongoing obstacles to safer sex included the need to convince male sexual partners to use condoms, fear that insisting on condom use would reveal HIV status, desire to have a baby, and lack of availability of female-controlled safer-sex methods.

Adolescents who engage in survival sex are at particularly high risk for HIV infection. Sexual abuse poses yet another risk for HIV transmission both directly from the abuser and indirectly, since previously abused children often have first intercourse at an earlier age, and demonstrate higher rates of other risk behaviours than their peers.

Obtaining a drug history

This should include the use of cigarettes, alcohol, marijuana, heroin, and other substances that can impair judgment. Determine the age at first use, periods of highest use, current use pattern, and history of needle use. Ten per cent of adolescents with AIDS in the US reported injecting drug use as their sole risk activity. A variety of drugs can be injected, including heroin, amphetamines, and anabolic steroids (by body builders).

Psychosocial evaluation

Obtain a history of living situation, education level, literacy, employment or other sources of income or support, and family and social supports. Include a history of psychological functioning, suicidal thoughts or attempts, depression, anxiety, psychosis, and psychiatric medications and hospitalisations.

Physical examination

Because adolescence is marked by changes in physical growth and intellectual function, assessments of HIV-infected youth should note the failure to progress as well as regression. A complete physical examination with special attention to vital signs and growth is necessary. Nutritional status should also be noted. Skin problems like acne can be confused with common HIV-related dermatological disorders such as folliculitis that may indicate disease progression. The lymph nodes should be examined as lymphadenopathy may indicate HIV infection. Examination for oral lesions (*Candida*, herpes), dental decay, and periodontal disease is essential. Sinusitis is also a relatively frequent symptom. Lung, heart, and abdominal examination should be performed as in adults.

Assessment of the genitalia should include the sexual maturity staging of Tanner and Whitehouse. This 5-part scale describes the development of pubic hair, breasts, and the male genitalia during puberty. For females who have had sexual intercourse, have unexplained pelvic pain, a yearly or twice yearly pelvic examination and Pap smear and an inspection for vaginal *Candida* is recommended. It is not known how HIV infection affects cognitive development in adolescents. Neuropsychological testing should also be performed if neurological involvement is suspected.

Medical treatment

Treatment for HIV infection and treatment and prophylaxis of opportunistic infections are generally similar to those in adults. Laboratory assessment in HIV-infected adolescents parallels that performed in adults, yet must take into account adolescent-specific normal values where these are available and differ from other age groups. CD4 cell counts remain the most useful measure of HIV disease progression. In post-pubertal adolescents, adult values apply. A complete blood count with differential should also be included in the laboratory assessment. During puberty, haemoglobin increases in males by 10 to 20 g/L to achieve adult levels of 130 to 180 g/L. Elevated alkaline phosphatase levels related to bone development occur during the adolescent growth spurt. Additional tests include a toxoplasmosis titre, hepatitis B serology and urinalysis. All sexually active adolescents should be screened for sexually transmitted pathogens, as asymptomatic infections are common. The STD screen includes tests for gonorrhoea (oral, genital, and anal cultures) and genital chlamydia. Also include a pap smear with colposcopy when indicated, as well as trichomonas and *Candida*. Pregnancy tests should be given when indicated.

Immunisation

Adolescents should receive age-appropriate vaccinations, such as CDT (diphtheria and tetanus) and MMR (measles, mumps, and rubella). Hepatitis B vaccine should be given to all adolescents who are not immune.

Conclusion

Health care for adolescents has frequently fallen between adult medicine and paediatrics without specific attention to the special needs of this age group. Different educational approaches are required, even among adolescents; e.g., sexually inactive school students require a different approach to sexually active or homeless adolescents. Issues that significantly influence the impact of HIV on teenagers include their coping strategies, and often, lack of social supports. Other issues which need to be addressed are legal and ethical issues such as parental notification, partner notification and disclosure.

Table 7.32 Diagnosis of HIV in adolescents

Test	Notes
ELISA	Identifies HIV antibodies. May give a false negative result if the test is performed early in the infection before sufficient antibodies have developed (4–6 weeks).
Western Blot	Differentiates antibodies. This test is used to confirm HIV diagnosis after a positive ELISA test.
T-cell subsets (CD3, CD4, CD8)	The number of lymphocytes decrease with disease progression. Antiretroviral medication and pneumocystis prophylaxis may be instituted as the level falls.
CD4+:CD8+ ratio	There is a decrease in the ratio with disease progression (usually 2:1).
IgG and IgA	Immunoglobulins are usually elevated as a result of activation of the immune system.
Platelets	HIV may cause thrombocytopenia.
ESR	May be elevated as the result of the infective process.
AST (SGOT)	May be elevated (associated with hepatitis).
Hepatitis screen	May be a carrier of hepatitis B or be hepatitis C positive especially if there is history of injecting drug use or homosexual activity.
Stool examination	May reveal parasite ova or infection, for example, cryptosporidium, salmonella.
Bronchoscopy/induced sputum/ bronchial lavage	For diagnosis of pneumocystis carinii pneumoniae.
Chest X ray	May reveal diffuse interstitial infiltrates (pneumocystis carinii pneumonia).
Open lung biopsy	May provide definitive diagnosis of kaposi sarcoma-related pulmonary symptoms or cytomegalovirus (CMV) infection.
Lesion cultures/biopsy	May reveal organisms such as candida.
Blood cultures	May reveal bacteraemia.
Lumbar puncture	May diagnose cryptococcus, HIV or CMV.
CT scan/MRI	May detect lymphoma, toxoplasmosis, or progressive leukoencephalopathy.

REFERENCES

1. Gottlieb MS, Schroff R, Schanker HM, et al. *Pneumocystis carinii* pneumonia and mucosal candidiasis in previously healthy homosexual men: evidence of a new acquired cellular immunodeficiency. *N Engl J Med* 1981; 305: 1425–1430.
2. Ammann AJ, Cowan MJ, Wara DW, et al. Acquired immunodeficiency in an infant: possible transmission by means of blood products. *Lancet* 1983; 1: 956–958.
3. Kumar P, Pearson JE, Martin DH, et al. Transmission of HIV by transplantation of a renal allograft, with development of AIDS. *Annals Intern Med* 1987; 106: 244–245.

4. Rubinstein A, Sicklick M, Gupta A, et al. Acquired immunodeficiency with reversed T4/T8 ratios in infants born to promiscuous and drug-addicted mothers. *JAMA* 1983; 249: 2350–2356.

5. McLaws ML, Brown ARD, Cunningham PH, Imrie AA, Wilcken B, Cooper DA. Prevalence of maternal HIV infection based on anonymous testing of neonates, Sydney 1989. *Med J Aust* 1990; 153: 383–386.

6. Ziegler JB. Vertical transmission of HIV in Australia. *Aust Paediatr J* 1994; Abst.

7. National Centre in HIV Epidemiology and Clinical Research. *Australian HIV Surveillance Report* 1995; 11 (3).

8. Centers for Disease Control. Unexplained immunodeficiency and opportunistic infections in infants — New York, New Jersey, California. *MMWR* 1982; 31: 665–667.

9. Oxtoby M. Perinatally acquired human immunodeficiency virus infection. *Pediatr Infect Dis J* 1990; 9: 609–619.

10. Centers for Disease Control. Classification system for human immunodeficiency virus (HIV) infection in children under 13 years of age. *MMWR* 1987; 36: 225–236.

11. European Collaborative Study. Children born to women with HIV-1 infection: natural history and risk of transmission. *Lancet* 1991; 337: 253–260.

12. Davis M. Vertical transmission of HIV. [Letter] *JAMA* 1988; 260: 29.

13. Centers for Disease Control. Recommendations for assisting in the prevention of perinatal transmission of human T-lymphotrophic virus, type III/lymphadenopathy-associated virus and acquired immunodeficiency syndrome. *MMWR* 1985; 34: 721–732.

14. Cruickshank M, Ziegler J, Palasanthiran P, Langdon P, Macdonald A, Kaldor J. Perinatal exposure to HIV in Australia, 1982 to 1993. *In:* Crowe S, Hoy J, eds. *Proceedings of the Vth Annual Conference of the Australasian Society for HIV Medicine.* Melbourne: ASHM, 1993.

15. MacGregor S. Human immunodeficiency virus in pregnancy. *Chemical Dependency and Pregnancy* 1991; 18: 33–50.

16. Nicholas S, Sondheimer D, et al. HIV infection in childhood, adolescence and pregnancy: a status report and national research agenda. *Pediatrics* 1989; 83: 293–308.

17. Cruickshank M. Risk of transmission of HIV through breastfeeding to infants of mothers with established HIV. *Pediatr AIDS HIV Infect* 1993; 4: 303.

18. Ehrnest A, Lindgren S, Dictor M, et al. HIV in pregnant women and their offspring: evidence for late transmission. *Lancet* 1991; 338: 203–207.

19. Lewis SH, Reynolds-Kohler C, Fox HE, Nelson JA. HIV-1 in trophoblastic and villous Hofbauer cells, and haematological precursors in eight-week fetuses. *Lancet* 1990; 335: 565–568.

20. Sprecher S, Soumenkoff G, Puissant F, Degueldre M. Vertical transmission of HIV in 15-week fetus. *Lancet* 1986; 2: 288–289.

21. European collaborative study group. Caesarian section and risk of vertical transmission of HIV-I infection. *Lancet* 1994; 343: 1464–1467.

22. Peckham CS, Senturia YD, Ades AE. Obstetric and perinatal consequences of human immunodeficiency virus (HIV) infection: a review. *Br J Obstet Gynaecol* 1987; 94: 403–407.

23. Embree J, Braddick M, et al. Lack of correlation of maternal HIV infection with neonatal malformations. *Pediatr Infect Dis J* 1989; 8: 700–704.

24. Sperling RS, Stratton P, O'Sullivan MJ, et al. A survey of zidovudine use in pregnant women with human immunodeficiency virus infection. *N Engl J Med* 1992; 326: 857–861.

25. Centers for Disease Control. Revised classification system for human immunodeficiency virus (HIV) infection in children under 13 years of age. *MMWR* 1994; 43 (3): 1–10.

26. Palasanthiran P, Ziegler JB, Cunningham A, Dwyer DE, Robertson P, Leigh D. Early diagnosis in a set of Australian infants at risk of perinatally acquired human immunodeficiency virus (HIV) infection. [Abstract] *Pediatr AIDS HIV Infect* 1993; 4: 315.

27. Erkeller-Yuksel FM, Deneys V, Yuksel B. Age-related changes in human blood lymphocyte subpopulations. *J Pedriatries* 1992; 120: 216–222.

28. Connor E. Antiretroviral treatment for children with human immunodeficiency virus infection. *Pediatrics* 1991; 88: 389–392.

29. Connor E, Bardeguez A, Apuzzio J. The intrapartum management of the HIV-infected mother and her infant. *Clin Perinatol* 1989; 16: 899–908.
30. Minkoff H. Care of pregnant women infected with human immunodeficiency virus. *JAMA* 1987; 258: 2714–2717.
31. Menez-Bautista R, Fikrig SM, Pahwa S, Sarangadharan M, Stoneburner RL. Monozygotic twins discordant for the acquired immunodeficiency syndrome. *Aust J Dis Child* 1986; 140: 678–679.
32. Thomas PA, Ralston SJ, Bernard M, Williams R, O'Donnell R. Pediatric acquired immunodeficiency syndrome: an unusually high incidence of twinning. *Pediatrics* 1990; 86: 774–777.
33. Hira S-K, Kamanga J, Mwale C. Perinatal transmission of HIV-1 in Zambia. *BMJ* 1989; 299: 1250–1257.
34. European Collaborative Study. Risk factors for mother-to-child transmission of HIV-1. *Lancet* 1992; 339: 1007–1012.
35. Sharpe AH, Hunter JJ, Ruprecht RM, Jaenisch R. Maternal transmission of retroviral disease and strategies for preventing infection of the neonate. *J Virology* 1989; 63: 1049–1053.
36. Ziegler JB, Cooper DA, Johnson RO, Gold J. Postnatal transmission of AIDS-associated retrovirus from mother to infant. *Lancet* 1985; 1: 896–898.
37. Van de Perre P, Simonon A, Msellati P, et al. Postnatal transmission of human immunodeficiency virus type 1 from mother to infant — A prospective cohort study in Kigali, Rwanda. *N Engl J Med* 1991; 325: 593–598.
38. Dunn DT, Newell ML, Ades AE, Peckham CS. Risk of human immunodeficiency virus type 1 transmission through breastfeeding. *Lancet* 1992; 340: 585–588.
39. Palasanthiran P, Ziegler JB, Stewart GJ, et al. Breast-feeding during primary maternal human immunodeficiency virus infection and risk of transmission from mother to infant. *J Infect Dis* 1993; 167: 441–444.
40. Kaldor J, McDonald A, Blumer C, et al. The acquired immunodeficiency syndrome in Australia: incidence 1982–1991. *Med J Aust* 1993; 158: 10–17.
41. Balis FM, Pizzo PA, Butler KM, et al. Clinical pharmacology of 2', 3'-dideoxyinosine in human immunodeficiency virus-infected children. *J Infect Dis* 1992; 165: 99–104.
42. World Health Organisation global program on AIDS. Consensus statement from WHO/UNICEF consultation on HIV transmission and breast feeding. *Weekly Epidemiological Record* 1992; 67 (24): 177–179.
43. White C, Saunders R, et al. Lack of transmission of HIV from infected children to their household contacts. *Pediatrics* 1990; 85 (2): 210–214.
44. Bryson YJ, Luzuriaga K, Wara DW. Proposed definition for in utero versus intrapartum transmission of HIV-1. *N Engl J Med* 1993; 327: 1246–1247.
45. Duliege AM, Messiah A, Blanche S, Tardieu M, Griscelli C, Spira A. Natural history of human immunodeficiency virus type 1 infection in children: prognostic value of laboratory tests on the bimodal progression of the disease. *Pediatr Infect Dis J* 1992; 11: 630–635.
46. Cruickshank M, Ziegler JB, Hughes C. Clinical manifestations of Australian children infected with HIV during the neonatal period. VI Annual ASHM Conference, Sydney. November, 1994.
47. Foy C, Gallagher M, et al. HIV and measures to control infection in general practice. *BMJ* 1990; 300: 1048–1049.
48. Foy C, Gallagher M, et al. Knowledge and attitudes of day care center parents and care providers regarding children infected with HIV. *Pediatrics* 1991; 87: 867–883.
49. Mendez H. Ambulatory care of HIV seropositive infants and children. *J Pediatrics* 1991; 119: 801–807.
50. Task Force on Pediatric AIDS. Pediatric guidelines for infection control of human immunodeficiency virus (acquired immunodeficiency virus) in hospitals, medical offices, schools, and other settings. *Pediatrics* 1988; 82: 801–807.
51. Shirley L, Steven A. Risk of transmission of human immunodeficiency virus by bite of an infected toddler. *J Pediatrics* 1990; 114 (3): 425–427.

52. Rosenberg Z, Fauci A. Immunopathology and pathogenesis of HIV infection. *In:* Pizzo P, Wilfert C, eds. *Pediatric AIDS: the challenge of HIV infection in infants, children and adolescents.* Baltimore: Williams & Wilkins, 1991.

53. NSW Department of Health. Vaccination of individuals with HIV infection. Sydney: The Department, 1991.

54. Williams P, Hahue R, Yap P, et al. Treatment of human immunodeficiency virus antibody children with intravenous immunoglobulin. *J Hosp Infect* 1988; 12: 67–73.

55. Editorial. Nutrition and HIV. *Lancet* 1991; 338: 86–87.

56. Brettler D, Forsberg A, et al. Growth failure as a prognostic indicator for progression to acquired immunodeficiency syndrome in children with haemophilia. *J Pediatrics* 1990; 117: 584–588.

57. Australian HIV and Nutrition Project. Positive eating for health and growth: a guide to nutrition for parents and carers of HIV positive children. Canberra: Commonwealth Department of Health, Housing, Local Government and Community Services, 1993.

58. Editorial. Malnutrition and weight loss in patients with AIDS. *Nutrition Rev* 1989; 47: 354–356.

59. Editorial. Refeeding and growth in children with AIDS. *J Am Dietetic Assoc* 1990; 11: 1620.

60. Holden C, Puntis J, et al. Nasogastric feeding at home: acceptability and safety. *Arch Dis Childh* 1991; 66: 148–151.

61. Laue L, Pizzo P, et al. Growth and neuroendocrine dysfunction in children with acquired immunodeficiency syndrome. *J Pediatrics* 1990; 117 (4): 541–545.

62. McLoughlin L, Nord K, et al. Severe gastrointestinal involvement in children with acquired immunodeficiency syndrome. *J Pediatr Gastroenterol Nutr* 1987; 6: 517–524.

63. European Collaborative Study Group. CD4 T cell count as predictor of *Pneumocystis carinii* pneumonia in children born to mothers infected with HIV. *BMJ* 1994; 308: 437–40.

64. Scott G, Hutto C, Makuch R, et al. Survival in children with perinatally acquired HIV type 1 infection. *N Engl J Med* 1989; 321: 1791–1796.

65. Bernstein LJ, Bye MR, Rubinstein A. Prognostic factors and life expectancy in children with acquired immunodeficiency syndrome and Pneumocystis carinii pneumonia. *Aust J Dis Child* 1989; 143: 775–778.

66. Pizzo PA, Wilfert CM. Antiretroviral therapy and medical management of the human immunodeficiency virus-infected child. *Pediatr Infect Dis J* 1993; 12: 513–522.

67. Ziegler JB. PCP prophylaxis in paediatric HIV. *HIV Journal Club* 1994; 3 (6): 46–47.

68. Skowron G, Bozzette SA, Lim L et al. Articles: alternating and intermittent regimens of zidovudine and dideoxycytidine in patients with AIDS or AIDS-related complex. *Ann Intern Med* 1993; 118: 321–330.

69. Butler K, Hilleman J, Hauger S. Approach to neurodevelopment and neurologic complications in pediatric HIV infection. *J Pediatrics* 1991; 119 (suppl. II): S41–S46.

70. Anonymous. Homeless youth and AIDS: knowledge, attitudes and behaviour. *Med J Aust* 1990; 153: 20–23.

71. Cochran S, Keidan J, Kalechstein A. Sexually transmitted diseases and AIDS. Changes in risk reduction behaviour among young adults. *Sexually Transmitted Dis* 1990; 17 (2): 80–86.

72. Hein K, Futterman D. Medical treatment in HIV-infected adolescents. *J Pediatrics* 1991; 119 (suppl. II): S18–S20.

73. Hingson R, Strunin L, Berlin B. Acquired immunodeficiency syndrome transmission: changes in knowledge and behaviours among teenagers, Massachusetts statewide surveys, 1986 to 1988. *Pediatrics* 1990; 85: 24–29.

74. Krasinski K, Borkowsky W, Holzman R. Prognosis of HIV infection in children and adolescents. *Pediatr Infect Dis J* 1989; 8: 216–220.

75. Krener P, Miller F. Psychiatric response to HIV spectrum disease in children and adolescents. *J Am Acad Child Adolescent Psychiatry* 1989; 28: 59–605.

76. Manoff S, Gayle H, et al. Acquired immunodeficiency syndrome in adolescents: epidemiology, prevention and public health issues. *Pediatr Infect Dis J* 1989; 8: 309–314.

77.   Vermund S, Hein K, et al. Acquired immunodeficiency syndrome among adolescents: case surveillance profiles in New York City and the rest of the Unites States. *Aust J Dis Child* 1989; 143: 1220–1225.

Cancer

Kim Burke

Cancer is the prominent cause of death in children aged between 0–14 years. This appears to be due largely to the progressive control that medical technology has gained over other childhood diseases.[1]

The major cancers are of the brain (such as astrocytomas, medulloblastoma, ependymoma and gliomas) and of the blood and bone marrow. The most common cancer affecting children is acute lymphoblastic leukaemia (ALL). Others cancers affecting children include neuroblastoma, Wilms' tumour, rhabdomyosarcoma, the bone tumours (Ewings sarcoma, osteogenic sarcoma), and the lymphomas (Hodgkin's and non-Hodgkin's lymphoma). The causes of childhood cancer remain unknown, but some cancers such as retinoblastoma have a genetic predisposition.[2]

When a child is initially diagnosed with cancer, the child and parents are involved in a crisis they find unfathomable. The initiation of a support program at such an early stage provides the foundations for the development of a trusting relationship between the family and the child and the staff members of the unit. Education of the family is an important part of this program, as it provides family members with an understanding of the disease, the treatment and the consequences of the treatment.

Most of the nursing interventions are focused upon caring for the side effects of the various treatment regimens and providing emotional support for families. Consequently, the following discussion is directed towards the treatment aspects of cancer nursing, rather than the disease process. The major forms of treatment are chemotherapy and radiotherapy.

CHEMOTHERAPY

Cancer cells increase without the inhibitory control that governs the normal tissue cells.[3] The principal effect of chemotherapy is to kill cancer cells by disrupting cell division. To effectively care for a patient receiving chemotherapy, it is necessary to understand the basis of the action of chemotherapy agents and their destructive effect on the cell cycle.[4,5] The importance of this cannot be overstated because, without a working knowledge of the cell cycle, it is difficult to comprehend how chemotherapy works and indeed why it has the potential to cause such debilitating side effects.

The cell cycle consists of the various phases which a cell undergoes from one division to the next. Chemotherapy affects only those cells that are in the process of division, so that cells in the 'resting phase' are protected from its effects.[6] Chemotherapy agents cannot differentiate between normal tissue cells and cancer cells. Consequently, fast-growing normal tissue cells are temporarily damaged. It is this damage that gives rise to the toxic side effects of chemotherapy.

The cycle plays a major role in the treatment of cancer because almost all chemotherapy agents exert their effect on some or all phases of cell division by affecting deoxyribonucleic acid (DNA) replication. Generally, chemotherapy agents interfere with the growth of a cell by inhibiting either DNA, protein synthesis or mitosis. Agents which act throughout the cell cycle are called 'cell cycle non-specific'. Other agents that act most effectively at a specific phase or phases are referred to as 'cell cycle specific'.

The treatment is calculated either by mg/kg or by mg/m^2 to ensure maximum drug concentration and effect on cancer cells. Chemotherapy is usually administered in blocks at regular intervals over a certain period of time (e.g., every 28 days over 2 years). This regimen allows normal tissue cells to regenerate and takes into account any cancer cells which may not have been eradicated during the initial phase of chemotherapy.[7]

Combination chemotherapy is now considered to be more effective than single-dose chemotherapy, for the very reason that combination chemotherapy achieves maximum cell kill, retards the development of new cancer cells and reduces the likelihood of resistance.[6] Depending on the patient's diagnosis, chemotherapy is administered intensely in the initial stage and gradually becomes less intensive as time progresses. The treatment regimen for acute leukaemia, for example, is divided into phases and enables maximum effect to take place close to the time of diagnosis.

RADIOTHERAPY

Radiotherapy is an important facet of cancer therapy because its purpose is either to destroy the cancer cells in a specific area or to irradiate the whole body as part of the conditioning regimen for a bone marrow transplant. The goal of the radiotherapy is to cause as much damage as possible to the cancer cells in order to prevent them from dividing, while at the same time causing minimal disruption to the division of normal cells.[8]

Radiotherapy is the emission of radiation energy in the form of waves or particles. Radiation energy is emitted as x-rays, gamma-rays or particle rays. In children the most common form of radiotherapy is an external beam that emits electromagnetic energy such as x-rays and gamma-rays.[8]

A unit of radiation is referred to as a Gray (Gy). A centiGray (cGy) is the amount of radiation that results in the absorption of 100 ergs of energy in 1 g of material. To ensure normal cell recovery, the radiotherapy doses are fractionated into a number of doses given over a specified time (e.g., 6 weeks). Fractionation of radiotherapy doses allows recovery of normal cells between doses. Like chemotherapy, radiotherapy also destroys fast-growing normal tissue cells as well as cancer cells, however, the side effects of radiotherapy depend upon the site being irradiated (**Figure 7.21**). Radiotherapy cannot be used for all cancer types because the required dose may be too toxic for the surrounding tissue.[8]

Diseases for which radiotherapy is used include acute lymphoblastic leukaemia, lymphomas, retinoblastoma, brain tumours (e.g., medulloblastoma), bone tumours (e.g., Ewings sarcoma), rhabdomyosarcoma (except for patients with localised disease), Wilms' tumour and non-Hodgkin's lymphoma (depending on the stage of the disease). It is also used as part of the conditioning regimen for bone marrow transplantation.

In order to assist the patient and family while the radiotherapy is being carried out, the nurse needs to be familiar with the radiotherapy procedure, the subsequent side effects and the types of diseases for which radiotherapy is used.

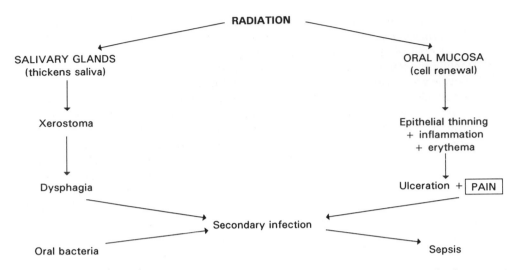

This figure demonstrates how a simple side-effect can escalate into a serious complication.

Figure 7.21 Side effects of radiotherapy.

Before radiotherapy begins, the child is required to go to the radiotherapy department for 'marking'. This is done to ensure that the required site is properly marked as well as serving as a guide for the radiotherapy staff administering the radiotherapy. Once the 'marking' has been carried out, the nursing staff should explain to parents that the ink is not to be washed off. In addition, the parents and the child should be informed that while the radiotherapy is being carried out, the child must remain absolutely still. Any child less than 3 years of age or who is unable to lie still will require sedation or anaesthesia. It should be explained to the child that heavy lead shields will be placed around surrounding vital organs. Children should also be informed that no-one can be in the room while the radiotherapy is carried out, but that their parents will be in the next room and will be able to communicate with them via an intercom.

NURSING MANAGEMENT OF THE CHILD WITH CANCER

The nursing care of a child receiving chemotherapy is directed towards the prevention or treatment of the side effects caused by the chemotherapy agents and to help the child and the family maintain a relatively normal lifestyle. These goals can be achieved by administering as much chemotherapy as possible on an outpatient basis, as well as providing an educational program to ensure the child and family understand both the treatment and its potential side effects.

Most children receiving chemotherapy have a central venous access device inserted to minimise the trauma of invasive techniques. Two types of devices are commonly used: the implantable device and the external line catheter (central venous line).

These devices have the advantage of providing venous access for fluids and medications without the pain and venous damage associated with repeated venipunctures. As the port of entry is either via the external catheter or at the hub of the catheter, their disadvantages include an increased potential for infections. Blockages may occur if these lines are not flushed adequately after the infusion of blood products, antibiotics and fluids that are incompatible with each other. External lines may split and in rare instances, accidental dislodgment of the line may occur. However, if these catheters are cared for appropriately few problems should occur.

The main nursing intervention required for an implantable device is to ensure that it is flushed regularly (e.g., monthly) with a heparin solution to prevent blockage. Access to the device is gained by inserting a Huber Point needle through the patient's skin and into the septum of the device. There is no other nursing intervention required, unless of course, the child is hospitalised and the device is accessed for a period of time. In such circumstances, the needle needs to be changed regularly to prevent infection. The frequency with which the needle is changed depends on hospital policy and may range from 4 to 7 days. The needle must be firmly secured to prevent accidental dislodgment.

Nursing interventions required for an externally placed catheter include cleaning the catheter exit site, ideally on a daily basis, with an antibacterial agent. Blockages may be prevented by regular flushing (e.g., weekly) with a heparin-based solution.

To ensure that the central venous line exit site and the oral mucosa do not become an avenue for infection, meticulous hygiene must be maintained. Cleaning of the central venous line exit site is a skilled procedure usually undertaken by nursing staff or by parents with the necessary knowledge and skills to do so. It is suggested that parents maintain this care when the child is admitted to hospital in order to decrease the number of people manipulating the central line and thus to decrease the incidence of cross-infection. It is usually recommended by oncology units that the cleaning of the exit site takes place after the child's bath in order to ensure maximum hygiene standards. The tubing needs to be changed on a regular basis.

Side effects

Chemotherapy agents and, to some extent, radiotherapy are myelosuppressive and immunosuppressive and the result may be a number of potentially toxic side effects (**Figure 7.22**). They include nausea and vomiting, neutropenia, thrombocytopenia, alopecia and mucositis. Pain may be a result of the disease process and/or of treatment.

Nausea and vomiting

Nausea and vomiting can be the most debilitating of all side effects for the child. They occur as a result of the effect of chemotherapy agents on the emetic centre in the brain. The emetic centre, which mediates vomiting, is located in the reticular area of the brainstem. It is excited by stimuli from sources such as the chemoreceptor trigger zone (CTZ) which is located on the floor of the 4th ventricle. It is believed that the CTZ is, in turn, excited by chemicals substances, such as chemotherapy agents.[9]

Nausea and vomiting may also be triggered by the damaging effect of chemotherapy agents on the gastrointestinal tract. Such damage stimulates a systemic release of serotonin, which, in turn, excites the serotonin receptor contained within the CTZ and thus activates the vomiting reflex.[9] Chemotherapy agents and radiotherapy, however, do not cause debilitating nausea and vomiting in all children.

In some instances, a psychological component can cause nausea and vomiting in children which also needs to be treated. This effect may occur once children come to associate a particular drug or the room in which they are frequently treated, with nausea and vomiting. The child will vomit on sight of the drugs or room. To overcome this

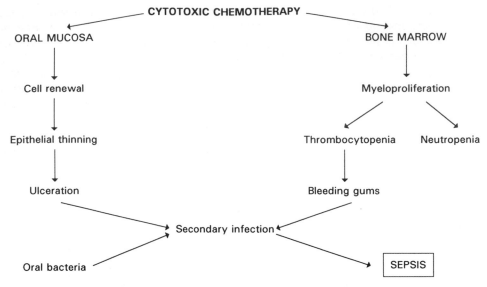

This figure demonstrates how quickly a less serious side-effect can progress to a serious complication.

Figure 7.22 Side effects of cytotoxic chemotherapy.

anticipatory type of vomiting, it is necessary to identify the stimulus that precipitates the vomiting. If anticipatory vomiting can be arrested as a result of some physical changes to the room or the manner in which the child is treated, the vomiting will usually subside for a period.

Anti-emetics are the treatment of choice for nausea and vomiting. Drugs such as those belonging to the phenothiazine group and the butrophenones are the most commonly used anti-emetics. These 2 groups of drugs suppress the CTZ and the emetic centre. The phenothiazines and butrophenones are not always effective for children receiving chemotherapy.[10] Unfortunately, both of these drug groups can cause side effects, such as, allergic reactions, insomnia, irritability and an overall feeling of disorientation which most children dislike intensely.

In addition to the phenothiazines and butrophenones, metoclopramide (Maxalon) is used. This drug acts by enhancing gastric emptying. In brief, it is thought to stimulate gastric mobility and dilation, thus inhibiting or partially inhibiting the vomiting reflex.[10] This drug also appears to exert its effect by blocking the dopamine receptors in the CTZ. Metoclopramide has side effects similar to the phenothiazines and butrophenones as well as increased drowsiness and a 'dystonic' reaction. This reaction is referred to as 'an extrapyramidal effect' and requires immediate reversal with benzotropine mesylate.

Since June 1991 oncology units within Australia began using a new anti-emetic, ondansetron. This drug, which has been trialled in both Europe and the United Kingdom, demonstrated a better control over nausea and vomiting than previous anti-emetics.[11] Ondansetron is a potent 5-hydroxytryptamine (5-HT3) antagonist. It is believed to act by inhibiting the activation of serotonin receptors in the chemoreceptor trigger zone and the gastrointestinal tract.[11]

The side effects of ondansetron appear to be minimal,[12] with episodes of headaches and constipation being the main effects reported.[11] Consequently, ondansetron has become the anti-emetic of choice when administering highly emetogenic agents. Despite the obvious advantage in using ondansetron, the other previously mentioned anti-emetics should not be discounted. Ondansetron is extremely expensive and the cost of purchasing the drug may well act as a deterrent for some units. The oncology nurse needs to note any unusual or unexplained adverse reactions when caring for the child who is receiving ondansetron. The oncology nurse also needs to have a comprehensive understanding of the anti-emetics being used and their side effects, so that optimal control of debilitating side effects can be obtained.

When a child is suffering from severe nausea and vomiting, dehydration and anorexia may develop. A strict fluid balance chart should be maintained and the child's electrolytes closely monitored to detect any imbalance in the early stage. The child may be tempted to eat if favourite foods are offered. If anorexia persists, the child's nutritional status will need to be carefully monitored and, if indicated, total parenteral nutrition (TPN) will be commenced.

Neutropenia

A transient and progressive fall in the number of neutrophils and platelets in the peripheral blood occurs within 7 to 10 days after the administration of certain chemotherapy agents. Different degrees of myelosuppression occur depending on the type and dose of chemotherapy administered, the lifespan of the cell and the number of cells undergoing division. Neutropenia tends to occur more frequently and more severely than thrombocytopenia because the lifespan of a granulocyte is approximately 6 to 12 hours, compared with 7 to 10 days for a thrombocyte.[13]

Neutropenia is usually the most serious side effect of chemotherapy. The severity of neutropenia will affect the seriousness of the infection. Neutropenia is defined as a neutrophil count of $<10 \times 10^9$/L. If the child is neutropenic and presents with an elevated temperature, (38°C or more), he or she will require admission to hospital for intravenous antibiotics. If the neutrophil count is reduced, but the child is asymptomatic, a 'wait-and-see' policy may be adopted. More often than not, however, the child will require admission to hospital for appropriate antibiotic treatment.

On admission to hospital blood cultures are taken, and any 'suspicious' portal of entry (e.g., a central venous line exit site) should be cultured as well as the usual urine, stool and sputum specimens. Most oncology centres now commence the child on broad-spectrum antibiotics until culture results return from pathology. Once the culture results are known, the antibiotics will be changed if indicated. While the child is undergoing antibiotic therapy, regular recordings of the child's temperature, blood pressure and pulse are necessary to evaluate sepsis.

Children usually remain neutropenic for approximately 7 to 10 days. If fever persists, a change in antibiotics may be indicated or it may be necessary to include antifungal agents in the regimen.

Thrombocytopenia

Thrombocytopenia often presents at the same time as neutropenia. The child with thrombocytopenia may present with an abnormal amount of bruising on the extremities or trunk or with a spontaneous nose bleed. Nose bleeds are treated by the application of manual pressure or cold packs to the nose.

The ordering and subsequent administration of platelets is paramount as no amount of pressure will be of benefit if there are insufficient platelets in circulation.

If the platelet count is greater than or equal to 20×10^9/L and the child is not bleeding, platelets may be withheld, but regular blood tests are carried out to detect a fall in the child's count. Once the platelet count drops below 20×10^9/L a platelet transfusion is usually ordered.

Alopecia

Alopecia occurs not only to the scalp, but to all body hair, including eyelashes, eyebrows and pubic hair. Because the eyelashes act as a filter to prevent dirt and grime from entering the eyes, nursing interventions are aimed at ensuring that the eyes remain well lubricated. The hair loss caused by the administration of certain chemotherapy agents and radiotherapy is reversible.

The reversibility of the hair loss may provide little comfort to the patient who feels vulnerable to ridicule or is deeply mindful of their own body image. Alopecia, therefore, has the potential to cause significant psychological effects in the child. The nurse should ensure that the child is informed about hair loss and take responsibility for ensuring the child is offered a wig in order to reduce these psychological problems. Not all children require one, but they should be offered the choice. Many children obtain a wig and never wear it. This remains their privilege.

Mucositis

Mucositis is the inflammation and ulceration of the oral mucosa and, in some circumstances, inflammation and ulceration of the stomach and bowel mucosa. Care involves the prophylactic administration of antibacterial and antifungal mouth washes on a regular basis, usually 4 times daily. This oral care should be carried out for the duration of the chemotherapy treatment program.

Most parents maintain a strict regimen both at home and when the child is in hospital. The required mouth wash can be kept by the bedside to enable the parents unrestricted access, and to maintain the normal home regimen.

The integrity of the oral mucosa needs to be examined frequently, especially when the child is neutropenic and receiving antibiotic therapy. While oral care does not prevent mucositis, it can minimise the severity of the inflammation and ulceration.[13] Thus, the goal of oral care is to maintain the integrity of the oral mucosa and to ensure the oral cavity is kept clean.

Pain

While chemotherapy does not cause pain, the side effects undoubtedly do. Pain is of a subjective nature and can only be described by the person suffering from it. Pain has been described by the International Association for the Study of Pain as an 'unpleasant sensory and emotional experience associated with actual or potential tissue damage or described in terms of such damage'.[14]

The oncology nurse's responsibility is to assess pain, bearing in mind its subjective nature, and to employ a variety of pain management strategies (**Figure 7.23**). Pain can be assessed using physiological and behavioural indicators or self-report scales and questionnaires.[15] There are also a number of self-report tools available for assessing paediatric

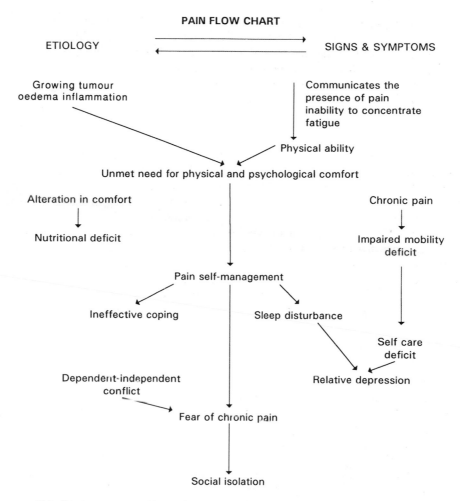

PAIN FLOW CHART

ETIOLOGY ⟶ ⟵ SIGNS & SYMPTOMS

Growing tumour
oedema inflammation

Communicates the
presence of pain
inability to concentrate
fatigue

Physical ability

Unmet need for physical and psychological comfort

Alteration in comfort

Chronic pain

Nutritional deficit

Impaired mobility
deficit

Pain self-management

Ineffective coping

Sleep disturbance

Self care
deficit

Dependent-independent
conflict

Relative depression

Fear of chronic pain

Social isolation

This figure represents the various mechanisms that are set in chain if a child
presents with untreated pain.

Figure 7.23 Pain flow chart.

pain, such as the Faces Scale,[16] Canada's Children's Hospital of Eastern Ontario Pain Scale,[17] and the Poker Chip Tool.

Acute pain may be experienced by patients who undergo invasive techniques, such as lumbar punctures, bone marrow aspirations and by children who have severe mucositis. To help overcome the fear and pain associated with invasive techniques, the application of a local topical anaesthetic cream (e.g., Emla cream) is useful. In addition, the inhalation of nitrous oxide for invasive techniques has been of enormous benefit to children in many units.

Further pain relief is, however, required for children suffering from severe mucositis or pain from the bone marrow harvest site. Any child suffering from this acute pain is given analgesics, usually a strong opioid such as morphine, either by mouth or intravenously with the dose being calculated according to bodyweight. Once the pain subsides the analgesia is titrated until it is no longer required. Collaboration between the nursing and medical staff as to the effective dosage required by the child, will achieve optimal dose levels.

When children are in the terminal phase of their disease, they may suffer chronic pain. This type of pain can envelop the child's whole life. It is multidimensional in that it can lead to lethargy, anger, anorexia and a change of behaviour or personality.[19] It is at this stage that the use of the 3-step analgesic ladder is of particular benefit. The 3-step 'analgesia ladder' has been suggested by Twycross[20] as an effective method in over-coming cancer pain. The 1st step commences with the administration of a non-opioid analgesic either with or without an adjuvant drug, which is commonly a corticosteroid. If the pain persists or increases, the 2nd step involves the administration of a weak opioid coupled with a non-opioid and in some instances an adjuvant drug. If the pain continues to persist the final step is taken by using a strong opioid as well as a non-opioid and an adjuvant drug. The combination of narcotic analgesia and adjuvant drugs, such as anti-inflammatory agents, antibiotics, diuretics or steroids is now the treatment of choice for patients suffering cancer pain.[21] Alternative strategies to help the child manage acute pain include play and thematic imagery (**see Chapter 9**).

ACKNOWLEDGMENT

Grateful acknowledgment is made to Libba O'Riordan who supplied information for this section of the chapter.

REFERENCES

1. Giles G. The descriptive epidemiology of cancer. *Cancer Forum* 1991; 15: 3–9.
2. Ekert H. *Clinical paediatric haematology and oncology.* Melbourne: Blackwall Scientific, 1982.
3. Hellman S, Devita VT. Principles of cancer biology. Kinetics of cellular proliferation. *In:* Devita VT, Hellman S, Rosenberg, SA, eds. *Cancer principles and practice of oncology.* 2nd ed. Philadelphia: Lippincott, 1982: 73–79.
4. Cain M, Tenni P. *Drug therapy in cancer. A practice guide for health professionals.* Sydney: Society of Hospital Pharmacists, 1992.
5. de Fraine AD, Diekman JL, Gaynor GM. *Clinical guidelines for the use of antineoplastic agents.* 3rd ed. Sydney: Editors Publication, 1990.
6. Devita VT. Principles of chemotherapy. *In:* Devita VT, Hellman S, Rosenberg SA, eds. *Cancer principles and practice of oncology.* 2nd ed. Philadelphia: Lippincott, 1982: 132–155.
7. Noyles NF. Chemotherapy. *In:* Hockenberry MJ, Coody DK, eds. *Paediatric oncology and hemotology. Perspectives on care.* Toronto: Mosby, 1986: 309–337.
8. Mooney KH. Aberrant cellular growth. Implications for the child and family. *In:* Mott SR, Fazekas NF, James SR, eds. *Nursing care of infants and families. A holistic approach.* California: Addison-Wesley, 1985: 1702–1704.
9. Jones AL, Cunningham D. Management of vomiting associated with cytotoxic therapy. *Br J Hosp Med* 1991; 45: 85–88.
10. Salva KM, Kuhn JG. Nausea and vomiting. *J Pract Nursing* 1986; 36: 22–27.
11. Dulfer S. New developments in anti-emetic therapy. International *Cancer Nursing News* 1990; 2: 3.
12. Ekert H. The paediatric experience: prevention of cyclophosphamide/cytarabine-induced emesis

in children with ondansetron, a 5-hy3 antagonist. 5-HT3 Antagonists and cancer therapy. A review of a series of symposia in Australia. *Exerpta Medica Australia* 1990; June: 9–11.

13. Goodman M. Managing the side effects of chemotherapy. *Sem Oncol Nursing* 1989; 5 (Suppl): 29–52.

14. International Association for the Study of Pain. Sub-Committee of the Taxonomy of Pain Terms. *Pain* 1979; 6: 249–252.

15. Algren CL, Algren JT. Pain management in children. *Plast Surg Nursing* 1994; 14: 65–70.

16. Wong DL, Baker CM. Pain in children: comparison of assessment tools. *Paediatr Nursing* 1988; 14: 9–17.

17. McGrath PJ, Johnson G, Goodman JT, Schillinger J, Dunn J, Chapman J. The CHEOPS: a behavioral scale to measure postoperative pain in children. *In:* Fields HL, Dubner R, Cervero F, eds. *Advances in pain research and therapy.* New York: Raven Press, 1985: 395–402.

18. Hester NK. The preoperational child's reaction to immunization. *Nursing Res* 1979; 28: 250–255.

19. Burke KE. Alteration in comfort-pain. *Proceedings 10th Annual National Conference.* Canberra 26–27 May, 1988.

20. Twycross RG. Opioid analgesics in cancer pain: Current practice and controversies. *Cancer Surv* 1988; 7: 30–53.

21. Twycross RG. *Symptom control for advanced cancer: pain relief.* London: Pitman, 1983.

Chapter 8

Care of the Infant, Child and Adolescent with Health Needs in the Community

Technology-dependent Children in the Community: Home Ventilation

Glenys Goodwin

Advances in medical technology over the last 2 decades have enabled the survival of infants and children with a variety of life-threatening diseases and, as a consequence, left them with the handicap of long-term technology dependence for their survival, e.g., ventilator dependence, oxygen dependence, parenteral nutrition and renal dialysis. Some of the advances responsible include improvements in resuscitation and stabilisation, particularly with the very low birthweight infant, safe and competent transfer of the critically ill newborn/child, state-of-the-art monitoring equipment, new modes of ventilation, advanced skills and procedures such as extracorporeal membrane oxygenation (ECMO), haemofiltration and diagnostic techniques and treatments.

The hospital environment, be it an intensive care unit or a special care unit set up to cater for special needs once intensive therapy is no longer required, has in many instances been the only home for these children. In North America, rehabilitation hospitals are gaining popularity for the management of these children, especially when they may not be suitable candidates for home care. It also enables expensive and usually fully occupied intensive care beds to be 'freed-up' for the acutely ill patient. Although this environment is geared towards the child's potential for growth and development, it still separates him from family, home and the community.

An increasingly popular and safe alternative is to provide the complex medical, nursing and technological care at home. Successful care for the ventilator-dependent child at home is being accomplished on a large scale all over the world. Goldberg et al. describe the successful discharge of 18 ventilator-dependent children from Illinois hospitals.[1] The discharge of 52 children from the Children's Hospital of Philadelphia, Pennsylvania, was described by Schreiner et al.[2] Donar highlights the statistics collected from a survey in 1987 by the US Congressional Office of Technology Assessment of ventilator-assisted children in Illinois, Louisiana and Maryland, describing patient enrolment in home care programs ranging between 15 and 75 children per year.[3] This number of children can easily be estimated to have at least doubled in 10 years. At the International Conference on

Pulmonary Rehabilitation and Home Ventilation in 1992, it was estimated by one speaker that more than 1000 individuals (adults) requiring long-term mechanical ventilation were being cared for in North America. The breakdown of these figures as to the number at home was not available and to date can only be estimated. Experience in Australia may seem minimal compared to the rest of the world, and the exact numbers are unknown because there is no central register; however, limited publications do exist.[4,5] Gillis et al. described 12 ventilator-dependent children in Victoria and New South Wales.[5]

The home environment has been shown to be a safer and more positive place for any child with a chronic illness than the hospital. There is no need to recreate an intensive care environment, just a harmonious family environment with trained family members and caregivers (if available). The management of these children in their homes and the community not only enhances their quality of life, but also helps to prevent costly and undesirable readmission to hospital. Readmission almost always results in the acquisition of an infection, which can be life-threatening in itself for this population. Experience in Australia and overseas[3] has shown that children usually experience fewer infections when cared for at home and if they do get infections, they are usually less severe than hospital-acquired infections.

Care at home also provides the child with normal cultural and spiritual socialisation, enhances growth and development of physiotherapy and occupational therapy programs in a less distracting environment, and thus enhances physical and cognitive development. Once home, some children improve to the point of no longer requiring technological support, seen especially in infants with chronic lung disease and oxygen dependency. This recovery has been shown to be quicker in the home environment than in the artificial and busy environment of the hospital, where continuity of care almost never exists.

Some personnel consider the home less safe with regard to lack of patient observation, equipment monitoring, ongoing technological support, electrical safety, lack of hands-on nursing, and accidental death. If this is considered to be true, then these issues must be weighed against the outstanding benefits.

Technological care in the home is not a new phenomenon. Experience has been gained from the need and expectations of the survivors of the polio epidemic of the mid 20th Century, who have permanent paralysis of the respiratory muscles. Many of these people have and still do live fulfilled and economically productive lives.

INDICATIONS FOR CHRONIC VENTILATOR SUPPORT

Chronic respiratory failure (CRF) is usually the result of an underlying respiratory disorder, perhaps slowly progressive, which causes respiratory insufficiency and thus hypoventilation or hypoxia. It may be caused by failure of one or more organs/systems.

Chronic respiratory failure is the main indication for long-term ventilator support, i.e, requiring a mechanical device to aid breathing and improve oxygenation for a minimum of 4 hours per day and for longer than 1 month.[1] The disease processes that result in CRF include the following:

- Direct injury or alteration to the respiratory system at any level, e.g., bronchopulmonary dysplasia or chronic lung disease, tracheo/bronchomalacia, tracheo-oesophageal fistula, sleep apnoea syndromes.
- Failure of neurologic control of ventilation, e.g., congenital or acquired central hypoventilation syndromes (Ondines curse).

- Ventilator muscle weakness, fatigue or failure, e.g., neuromuscular myopathies, phrenic nerve palsy, congenital abnormalities (spina bifida), high spinal cord injuries.

Dependence on ventilator support may be continuous and life long, as in high spinal cord injuries, intermittent as in sleep apnoea syndromes and/or short term as in chronic lung disease.

Long-term ventilation in the home should not normally be considered for children who are likely to die from a rapid progressive incurable disease. Long-term ventilation in the home should be undertaken with a positive rehabilitative approach, rather than as a means of delaying death.

GOALS OF VENTILATOR SUPPORT IN THE HOME

The goals of ventilator support in the home for children with chronic respiratory failure are quite different from the goals of assisted ventilation for children with acute respiratory failure in the intensive care unit. The goals of long-term ventilator support are to:

- Ensure safety of the child.
- Enhance and promote the quality of life.
- Facilitate and support re-integration into the home, school (if age-appropriate) and community.
- Enhance individual potential.
- Support and improve (if applicable) physical and physiologic function.
- Prevent costly hospital readmission.

In order to achieve these goals, diagnostic and management approaches, parental/caregiver training programs, acquisition of appropriate equipment, portability of ventilators and ongoing support, both nursing and technical, become important considerations and are essential.

DECISION TO INITIATE CHRONIC VENTILATOR SUPPORT

Usually, the decision to begin chronic ventilator support has been made non-electively. Typically, a child develops acute respiratory failure, is intubated and mechanical ventilation is initiated as a life-saving measure. Subsequently, it is not possible to wean the child from assisted mechanical ventilation. Because it is often emotionally and perhaps ethically difficult to stop mechanically assisted ventilation abruptly in an alert child who might experience severe distress without it, the transition to chronic ventilator support is made. Gillis et al.[6] refer to this sequence of events as the phenomenon of 'entrapment'. Thus the child, if developmentally able, and family do not have the opportunity to discuss this therapeutic option in advance.

More recently in North America, the trend has been to initiate chronic ventilator support electively in order to preserve physiologic function and to improve quality of life. Using this approach, the health care team begins the discussion of options for long-term care, including chronic ventilator support in those patients who can be expected to develop chronic respiratory failure. Discussions begin early, and well before the anticipated need. This allows the child and family ample time to investigate and evaluate the options thoroughly, discuss their feelings, preferably meet with other children and families who are well established in the home, and be able to reach a decision. Thus, the child and family have the opportunity to make a well informed decision about whether or not this form of treatment will suit their needs and demands.

SELECTION OF APPROPRIATE CANDIDATES

Successful home care for ventilator-assisted children requires careful selection of patients who are considered appropriate for safe, quality care in the home. The main focus is on rehabilitation and re-integration into the family unit and the community. Children should be assessed and evaluated at a tertiary paediatric centre.[2,7,34]

It should not be expected that all patients who require long-term chronic ventilator support will be candidates for home care. Criteria essential for successful home care include the following:

- A patient who has a disease leading to chronic respiratory failure.
- A patient whose condition must be compatible with a reasonable quality of life.
- A patient/parent who has a thorough understanding of their child's diagnosis and prognosis.
- A patient/parent who has given informed consent for treatment and understands the benefits, risks and problems associated.
- Physiological stability as indicated by a well established and stable airway, usually a tracheostomy in young children (i.e., those under 5 years of age).*
- A satisfactory pO_2 and pCO_2 on home ventilator settings, having been established no less than one month.
- No continued requirement for positive end-expiratory pressure (PEEP) and/or supplemental oxygen in the first instance.
- Stable metabolic status with blood electrolyte levels and other body chemistry within normal limits, or as normal as possible for the particular condition of the patient.
- An absence of acute infection.
- The ability to undertake an appropriate nutritional program which will facilitate growth and development.

Before the child is discharged, parents must be able to demonstrate:

- A willingness and motivation to care for their child at home.
- An understanding of the benefits, risks and potential problems associated with home care, noting the lack of government-funded nursing support to all patients and the lack of respite care facilities in this country at present for these patients.
- An ability to master the observational and technical skills necessary to care for their child.
- The provision of a safe and accommodating home environment.
- The provision of no less than 2 people living in the same home who are competent in caring for their child.

DISCHARGE PLANNING

Once the decision has been made to pursue ventilator support at home, the discharge team is consulted.

---

* More recently in Australia (1991), initiation of mask ventilation for intermittent positive pressure ventilation has been successful in children over 5 years of age.

Table 8.1 Discharge plan

	Name & Designation	Date
Written and submitted to team by:	....	....
Reviewed and signed by:		
Multidisciplinary team:	....	....
Parent/guardian:	....	....
Patient (if applicable):	....	....
Clinical case manager:	....	....
Primary physician:	....	....

Next review and revision of home management care plan:

The Home Management Care Plan should be revised according to the child's specific needs and reviewed six (6) monthly at case management meetings.

The discharge program requires coordination and management by the clinical case manager in consultation with the multidisciplinary team. Experience in Australia has shown that the position of clinical case manager is best suited to a nurse specialist with experience in respiratory nursing, intensive care and preferably community nursing. The ideal multidisciplinary team consists of doctors, nurses, technical support, social worker, allied health professionals such as physiotherapist and occupational therapist, and community supports. Some programs also involve the local doctor during the initial stages of discharge planning but, while recognising they are an important part of the team, we feel they are best used towards the time of actual discharge from hospital.

At this stage, the primary physician is identified. The primary physician is usually a respiratory physician who is experienced with prolonged mechanical ventilation of patients both in hospital and home. He or she is responsible for providing ongoing medical management, regular evaluation, emergency management, and will participate in case management meetings.

The clinical case manager is ultimately responsible for overall coordination of discharge with a particular focus on planning, assessing, implementing, coordinating and evaluating the home care plan, in consultation with the patient, the family unit and their primary physician. The clinical case manager and primary physician work closely together in the design, implementation and evaluation of the home care plan.

The responsibilities of the clinical case manager also include:

- Evaluation of suitable patients for home ventilator support.
- Development and coordination of a comprehensive, cost-effective training program for the patient, the family and potential caregivers (**Table 8.1**). This program is presented to a case management meeting before training begins.
- Realistic assessment of care requirements, and the family's ability to meet them, including nursing care.

- Provision of appropriate long-term follow-up and support, including regular home visits and telephone consultation.
- Provision of on-call emergency services.
- Educational liaison with community supports such as schools, paramedical personnel, respite care workers and early childhood centres to name a few.

EDUCATION PROGRAM

A thorough education of the patient, family and potential caregivers in observational techniques, activities of daily living, technical aspects of care, equipment operation and maintenance, maintenance of supplies and emergency planning is commenced as early as possible.

The education program must be consistent and appropriate to the level of understanding of each participant. It must clearly define its goals and objectives and monitor individual participation, evaluation and documentation of all outcomes, both satisfactory, and unsatisfactory.

The clinical case manager draws up a written plan which clearly outlines the skills and techniques which require mastery before discharge. A skills checklist for each procedure is made and kept as a record of mastery and used for ongoing review, suggested 6 monthly. Each procedure must be mastered no less than 10 times before competency is assumed. Skills and techniques should be individually tailored to meet the patient's specific needs and will include:

- Assessment of normal respiratory function.
- Assessment of abnormal respiratory function, its meaning and appropriate interventions.
- Activities of daily living.
- Taking clinical observations — temperature, pulse, respirations, general condition and recognising the abnormal with appropriate interventions.
- Tracheostomy care — skin care, changing the tube (routine and emergency), changing the tapes, suctioning.
- Physiotherapy.
- Independent management of ventilator.
- Independent management of other equipment, e.g., suction apparatus and demonstrate routine maintenance, storage and cleaning procedures.
- Medication administration — verbalise rationale for dosage and desired effects, administration time, side effects and storage.
- Cardiopulmonary resuscitation (CPR).
- Nutrition.
- Safety — environmental, transport.

Each teaching session should be no longer than 45 minutes in order to achieve maximum absorption of information. Each session requires both a theory and a practical component followed by demonstration of the skill by the teacher. The parent is then asked to repeat the demonstration. Sessions may need to be repeated until considered mastered and the parent is confident.

A predischarge home assessment is made by the clinical case manager with the parents. Guidance can be provided in environmental organisation and storage of equipment and supplies. Potential problems can be identified and resolved and thus help to minimise parental anxiety and stress. Specific facilities to be assessed during the predischarge home assessment are:

- Appropriate electrical wiring, electrical outlets and installation of dedicated power supply for safe operation of the ventilator and suction equipment. A dedicated power supply will prevent any power overload or failure on that circuit from faulty or over-used household appliances.
- Environmental modifications such as physical accessibility and organisation of the child's bedroom and general living space. There is no need to recreate an intensive care unit in the child's bedroom — doing so negates the goals of home management. The room can be organised to minimise the abnormal and create a warm, friendly and human environment.
- Call system for the child, e.g., a bell or intercom.
- Reliable telephone service, in an accessible location.
- Bathroom location and accessibility.
- Type of heating/cooling system — reverse cycle air conditioning has been found to be the most appropriate but can be expensive to install.
- Adequate and reliable vehicle transport, keeping in mind the amount of equipment and supplies required when going out.
- Accessibility of local medical supports: general practitioner; hospital/emergency department; ambulance service. Prior to discharge the family are advised to familiarise themselves with the quickest and most accessible route to the nearest and most appropriate hospital or emergency department both during and out of peak traffic periods.

EQUIPMENT AND SUPPLIES

Once an assessment of specific needs of the child is made, the clinical case manager meets with the inhalation therapist (respiratory technician) to compile the equipment list, including supplies that will be necessary for home care. This equipment is usually dispensed by the discharging hospital and arrangements are made for further supplies, depending on where the child lives in relation to the hospital. The equipment should be kept as simple as possible for ease of use, reliable performance and patient safety.

Based on ventilator assistance via tracheostomy, the minimum equipment and supplies required will include:

- 1, but preferably 2, portable mechanical ventilators, which must include internal battery, external battery adaptation, high and low pressure alarm limits, choice of modes of ventilation and availability of PEEP
  (a) 1 heated humidifier
  (b) sterile water
  (c) 2 complete delivery circuits with at least 1 external pressure relief valve, swivel adaptor and air filters
  (d) 2 self-inflating ambu bags — size according to patient — and appropriate-sized masks (for emergency use only).
- 1 electric suction unit
  (a) 1 portable suction unit with internal battery and battery recharger
  (b) connecting tubing

- (c) suction catheters of appropriate size, including a small supply of catheters 1 size smaller, for emergency use
- (d) rinsing solution
- (e) sterile water/saline solution.
- Tracheostomy supplies
  - (a) 2 complete tracheostomy tubes of appropriate size with appropriate connectors
  - (b) 1 complete set of tracheostomy tubes of one size smaller and one size larger (for emergency use)
  - (c) cotton tape
  - (d) sterile saline solution
  - (e) syringes
  - (f) heat and moisture exchanger (swedish nose)
  - (g) scissors
  - (h) non-adherent dressing (telfa)
  - (i) cotton tip applicators
  - (j) hydrogen peroxide for cleaning tubes
  - (k) sterile container
  - (l) cleaning agent.
- Stethoscope.
- Thermometer.
- Torch.
- Intercom system (optional).
- Alternative power source, e.g., battery with charger or generator.

Equipment such as ventilators and suction apparatus should be available to the discharging hospital for evaluation and used at least 1 month prior to discharge to ensure patient compatibility, performance and safety. It also allows the family to become competent in its use.

Before discharge, community, medical, paramedical and nursing supports are informed in writing about the ventilator-assisted child the proposed date of discharge. A case conference is usually arranged by the case co-ordinator with the appropriate support personnel to discuss special needs and management issues. These support personnel and services include:

- Local general practitioner.
- Local hospital emergency department (if applicable).
- Ambulance service.
- Physiotherapist, occupational and speech therapist.
- Technical suppliers.
- Community health centre.
- Early childhood centre (if appropriate).
- Local pharmacy.
- Respite care (if available).
- School and appropriate support aides.

EMERGENCY PLANNING

Emergency procedures — as per emergency care protocols developed in accordance with the patient and family — are identified, planned, implemented and evaluated with the assistance of the clinical case manager in the first instance and with the contribution of appropriate personnel.

Failure to plan for emergencies can lead to confusion, accidents and possibly death. Emergency conditions which require immediate action refer to health, equipment and/or environmental conditions. Potential emergency conditions and resolution thereof are identified, planned and simulated (where appropriate) before discharge and become part of the training program.

The family is trained to respond in common emergency health situations such as tracheostomy decannulation, inability to insert a catheter when suctioning, inability to insert the tracheostomy tube, equipment and electrical failure, and cardiopulmonary collapse. Training in cardiopulmonary resuscitation is recommended for all direct caregivers, including school personnel and appropriate others.

A list of supplies to be carried with the child at all times is prepared with the family and includes regular items such as ventilator and suction apparatus, other items required for routine and/or emergency care as well as back-up items in the event of a malfunction.

Equipment failures become medical emergencies, thus mechanical troubleshooting and problem solving are included in the training program. Equipment failures such as power/ventilator failure or delivery circuit disconnection are simulated during education sessions. Further, situations are created while parents sleep and their response is monitored and evaluated. Parents are expected to respond and correct the problem in a safe and timely manner. Further instruction is given if required. Discharge programs should provide 24-hour on-call personnel, familiar with the child and the family. The Australian experience has shown that this is best provided by the clinical case manager, program nurses or the respiratory technician. Alternatively, the equipment vendor is expected to be available within 2 hours to provide emergency equipment back-up.

External conditions such as power failure and telephone malfunction are included in the training program. Essential services such as electricity, gas and telephone companies are notified in writing by the clinical case co-ordinator that a child is on life support equipment in the home and the exact geographical location. These essential services must ensure priority service and restoration in the event of an interruption to service. In the event of a child returning to country areas, the police and fire department are also notified of a child in their area utilising electrically operated life support equipment. Also, the family are advised to purchase a generator in the case of power failure. The fire department is asked to visit the home and review home safety and planned response/evacuation procedures in the event of a fire. It also enables the fire department to know the exact location of the child and the equipment within the house. Parents have found this service to be beneficial in the past.

Available community resources are identified and listed for the family before discharge. The telephone resource list (**Table 8.2**) provides a practical reference list of contact personnel, and who to contact when; the list can be kept in a prominent position in the home, usually next to the telephone.

THE FAMILY

The stress faced by the family of a child with chronic illness, coupled with that of a ventilator-dependent child, is well documented.[8] Parents who choose to care for their child at home believe that being at home is better for their child and themselves than hospital care. Despite this positive decision, it remains a stressful and difficult experience

Table 8.2 Home resource telephone list

Planned for: NAME: .... DOB: ....

ADDRESS .... MRN: ....

....

TELEPHONE: ....

FOR ALL EMERGENCIES

1. Dial 000 for ambulance

2. Telephone the hospital on

    and ask for

3. Contact the 24 hour on call personnel on
    and state your name and the nature of the emergency.

OTHER NUMBERS	NAME	TELEPHONE
Primary Physician:	....	....
Specialists:	....	....
Clinical Case Manager:	....	....
Technical Support Personnel:	....	....
Home equipment supplier:	....	....
Telephone company:	....	....
Fire Department:	....	....
Police Department:	....	....
Local doctor:	....	....
Pharmacy:	....	....
School:	....	....
Other, e.g. Parent work:	....	....
Transport:	....	....

for the family. Changes in the family lifestyle may be overwhelming, despite their expectations. In Australia, the lack of external financial support is a major component of stress. Responsibility for the cost varies considerably for each case and depends on the underlying circumstances which led to long-term ventilator dependence. For example, patients who are quadriplegic following a motor vehicle accident will usually be covered by third party compensation, which covers the cost of equipment and the caregivers. Others rely on purchase or donation of equipment and the ongoing expenses, which are numerous, are the responsibility of the parent unless some respite funds can be accessed.

Every effort is made to support the family by providing them and other caregivers with easy access to health expertise, support groups, counselling and provision of respite care if available. At present in Australia, the only form of respite care is readmission to hospital. It is often the experience of clinical case managers that unless the child is unwell and requires readmission to hospital, patients and/or parents do not access this service, the reasons for which have been raised earlier.

Invasion of privacy can produce a significant stress on family life. Once the patient is discharged, the family home is 'invaded' by strangers including nurses, inhalation therapists and doctors, to name a few. It is important from the outset that trusting and professional relationships are formed with the family, especially by the clinical case coordinator, who will be having the most contact with the family unit in order to facilitate adaptation to the new, unique way of life.

CONCLUSION

Caring for technology-dependent children at home is in its infancy in Australia compared with other countries. We are learning by the experiences and expertise of other programs around the world and more recently by designated programs here in Australia. As the number of families increase, the advantages, disadvantages, benefits and risks will continue to be formally assessed, clinically monitored and evaluated.

It should be emphasised that the decision to transfer the care of the technology-dependent child to their home depends largely on the wishes and ability of the parents to assume the responsibility of the treatment and to make informed consent to continue such treatment. It should not be forgotten that the ultimate goal of sending ventilator-dependent children home is to enhance life, and not simply to prolong death.

REFERENCES

1. Goldberg AI. Faure AM, Vaughan CJ, Snarski R, Seleny RL. Home care for life-supported persons: an approach to program development. *J. Paed*: 1984; 104: 785–795.
2. Schreiner MS, Donar ME, Ketterick RG. Pediatric home mechanical ventilation. *Pediatr Clin North Am* 1987; 34: 47–60.
3. Donar ME. Community care: paediatric home mechanical ventilation. *Holistic Nurse Practice* 1988; 2 (2): 68–80.
4. NHMRC. *Report of the Health Care Committee, Expert Panel on Home Mechanical Ventilation in Children and Young Adults*. Canberra: AGPS, 1994.
5. Gillis J, Tibbals J, McEnierny J, Heavens J, Hutchins P, Kilham HA, Henning R. Ventilator dependent children. *The Medical Journal of Australia* 1989; 150: 10–14.
6. Gillis J, Kilham H. Entrapment. *Critical Care Med* 1990; 18 (8): 897.
7. O'Donahue W Jnr, Giovannoni RM, Goldberg AI, Keens TG, Make BJ, Plummer AL, Prentice WS.

Longterm mechanical ventilation: Guidelines for management in the home and at alternative community sites. *Chest* 1990; 1 Suppl 1s–37s.

8. Hamlett KW, Walker W, Evans A, Weise K. Psychological development of technology-dependent children. *Journal of Pediatric Psychology* 1994; 19: 493–503.

Sudden Infant Death Syndrome

Gill Patterson

In the early 1970s a definition of sudden infant death syndrome (cot death or crib death) was formulated. This definition, 'the sudden death of any infant or young child which is unexpected by history and in which a thorough post-mortem examination fails to demonstrate the adequate cause of death'[1] remains valid today, despite the time, money and effort spent in the search for a cause or causes of the enigmatic problem. Sudden infant death remains a major cause of death in infancy.

The search for a cause or causes of sudden infant death syndrome (SIDS) has gone on for many years, and involved innumerable possibilities. These possibilities range from cortical insufficiency, to electrolyte imbalance, bacterial infection, hyperactive dive reflex, nasal obstruction and infanticide.[2] During more recent times, researchers have investigated respiratory causes of SIDS including apnoea of prematurity, central apnoea and obstructive apnoea, but Rahilly[3] has demonstrated that pneumographic studies do not predict sudden infant deaths. Other avenues of investigation of possible causes have been the 'non-specific stress syndrome'. Stressors are said to involve gastro-oesophageal reflux, overheating, vaccination, and the use of inductions and painkillers at birth.[4] Dettman and Kalokerinos (quoted in[5]) have designated the cause of cot death as 'a multifactorial insult to the child's immune system' leading to depletion of vitamin C stores, and apnoea. They have labelled immunisation as the primary insult to the immune system, but this has never been proven.

Engelberts and de Jonge[6] have reviewed available data, and stated 'there is an association between sleeping prone and cot death', but were unable to prove a causal relationship. Overheating of infants (by overwrapping or artificial environmental heating) is also being investigated as a potential cause of, or contributor to, sudden infant death syndrome.

However, recent research in this area has focused on reducing the potential risks of cot death. The aim of the 'Reduce the Risks' campaign, which began in Victoria in 1990, was to alter infant care practices in the home. Parents were advised to avoid prone positioning of infants during sleep, overwrapping of infants, and maternal smoking. Through a public education campaign, efforts were also made to encourage breastfeeding.

The overall rate of SIDS deaths in Victoria was reduced by 50% following this campaign.

In Australia, the incidence of deaths attributed to SIDS is 1.9 to 3.7 deaths per 1000 live births; 80% of deaths occur before 5 months of age, with deaths occurring rarely before 1 month or after 1 year of age. Most deaths occur during sleep, with deaths occurring predominantly during the winter months.[7] Despite this, there is no proven association between respiratory illness, any particular viral agents and sudden infant death syndrome. Although there has been a general decline in infant mortality, the incidence of SIDS has remained constant.

The reaction of parents to the death of their baby from SIDS is one of shock. These parents exhibit behaviour which is not typical of their normal behaviour. They may seem unaffected, or show signs of aggression, hysteria, bewilderment and anger. The nurse can assume an important role at this time by supporting the family. There is no 'right' or 'correct' response to this overwhelming shock and the needs of parents at this time differ greatly. Some may wish to say goodbye to their baby, others may not.

It is imperative that parents are given privacy, support and time. The process should never be hurried. The immediate care provided for the family will make an enormous difference to the eventual resolution of their grief. Nurses, in their role as support persons, help by just being with the parents, allowing them to talk about their feelings, or by just sitting in silence with them. Referral to appropriate professionals, as well as to the Sudden Infant Death Association (SIDA) should be encouraged. SIDA offers support, comfort and information to parents and families and is made up of parents who have suffered a cot death within their family. Raising money to enable these services to be offered, as well as to facilitate the supply of home apnoea monitors to families who have had an infant die of cot death, and who have subsequent children, and funding research into sudden infant death syndrome are the primary roles of SIDA.

It is important to note that many parents are very fearful of having further children following the death of an infant, and need support through the subsequent pregnancy, birth and the first months of the infant's life.

ACUTE, LIFE-THREATENING EPISODES

An infant who is found to have stopped breathing for a long period (20 seconds or more) but who recovers, is said to have suffered an aborted cot death, near-miss SIDS, or an acute life-threatening episode. These infants are resuscitated, sometimes by parents, friends, sometimes by paramedical staff, and sometimes in accident and emergency departments, and are often admitted to hospital for investigations which attempt to find the cause, or causes, of the episode.

The management and assessment of these infants must start with a complete history and physical examination. In some cases a cause for the episode (e.g., sepsis, seizures, or gastro-oesophageal reflux) may be found and treated. In other cases where no cause is found, continuous apnoea monitoring may be advised in the hope that this monitoring will alert parents to any further episodes. During admission, these infants are usually continuously monitored on cardiorespiratory monitors, but other care remains the same as, or similar to, care at home prior to the episode.

Investigations to be undertaken depend on the history, and on the observation of the baby by nursing staff after admission.

Home monitoring may also be considered for siblings of SIDS victims, for infants with abnormal pneumographic studies (sleep studies recording heart rate, depth and frequency of respirations, and pulse oximetry), for preterm infants with a history of apnoea, and for some infants whose parents are over-anxious regarding sudden infant death. Monitors for home use vary greatly and include a simple mat-under-the-mattress monitor, which picks up movement (and is not effective if a patient has obstructive apnoea), a monitor which picks up both heartbeat and respirations and one which is a complex machine and is computerised to record one minute before and after any alarms. This monitor can be 'downloaded' by telephone to a master computer which then graphs these alarms.

The home monitoring field is one which is constantly growing. Home monitors are becoming smaller, more portable, complex and efficient. Monitoring is effective and can provide reassurance for parents if there are full counselling, support and technical services available.

These services include full instruction in the use and functioning of the monitor, in resuscitation techniques and the provision of, during and after hours, technical back-up should the monitor be found to be faulty or not functioning.

It is important that parents are made aware that a monitor is not a life-saving device and will not prevent all cot deaths.

Instruction in resuscitation techniques is carried out by a registered nurse and involves the use of a baby resuscitation model and simple instruction card. Having been instructed, parents are encouraged to practise with the model to enable them to feel a little more confident.

Despite all efforts, sudden infant death syndrome remains a mystery and research must continue if we are to solve or at least better understand this phenomenon.

The role of the nurse in caring for families affected by this enigmatic problem is a supportive and counselling one, and one which is, and will continue to be, ever-expanding to cope with advances in medical knowledge in this field.

REFERENCES

1. Bergman AB, Beckwith JB, Ray CG, eds. *Sudden infant death syndrome: proceedings of the Second International Conference on Causes of Sudden Death in Infants.* Seattle: University of Washington Press, 1970: 18.
2. Hyne J. What causes cot death? *Nursing Times* 1991; 87 (16): 70–71.
3. Rahilly P. Pneumographic studies: predictors of future apnoeas but not sudden infant death syndrome in asymptomatic infants. *Aust Paediatr J* 1989; 25: 211–214.
4. Scheibnerova V. Cot death as death due to exposure to non-specific stress or general adaptation syndrome; its mechanisms and prevention. Special Scientific Paper of the Association for Prevention of Cot Death, 1990.
5. SIDS lab research a scientific sham. *Med Dissent* The newsletter of the Health Care Reform Group 1991; Autumn-Winter: 2–3.
6. Engelberts AC, de Jonge GA. Choice of sleeping position for infants: possible association with cot death. *Arch Dis Childh* 1990, 65: 462–467.
7. Cot death: help pin down the causes. Fourth Annual Report 1990, Sudden Infant Death Association of NSW Inc. 1991.

Feeding Problems in Infancy

Gill Patterson

Feeding difficulties in infants can be devastating for parents, and can prove to be a multifaceted problem for health care providers.

Although there may be a number of reasons for an infant not feeding, or being difficult to feed, these usually fall into one of the following categories:

- A structural abnormality, e.g., cleft lip and/or palate, Pierre Robin sequence.
- Abnormal or incoordinate suck and swallow reflex.

- Abnormal tongue or mouth movements, e.g., tongue thrusting in infants suffering from cerebral palsy.
- An underlying condition which causes exhaustion with the effort of feeding, e.g., congenital heart disease.
- A medical or surgical condition which has necessitated being on long-term nil by mouth, particularly those infants who have never fed orally.
- Trauma, pain or unpleasant sensations which have been associated with feeding. For example, an infant with severe gastro-oesophageal reflux may scream with hunger but still refuse to feed or an infant who has been force-fed may refuse to eat.

When presented with an infant who is difficult to feed or who refuses to feed, the most important task for the nurse is taking a full and accurate history from the primary caregiver (usually the mother) regarding the infant, the feeding behaviour, and the circumstances surrounding the infant (family setup).

The nurse should note in the history any vomiting, spitting out of feeds, chewing or chomping of the teat or nipple rather than sucking, as well as noting who usually feeds the infant. Observing the infant and mother or caregiver during the feeding process may further help to assess the behaviour.

A full assessment of the nutritional status of the infant must be carried out. He or she should be weighed, have his or her length measured and have both weight and height recorded on percentile charts. Any other available measurements such as birthweight and length and the early childhood centre weight record should also be recorded to further determine the infant's progress. Failure to gain weight, to grow in length or poor weight gain are all good indicators of actual or potential problems.

It is necessary for the nurse to calculate the approximate amount of fluid required by the infant, based on 150 to 160 mL/kg/day, and to compare this with the infant's actual intake. With an infant who is bottle fed this process is quite simple, but it is more difficult with breast fed infants. Test weighing, the weighing of the clothed infant both before and after a breast feed to determine intake, can be of benefit, but only if it is carried out over at least a 24-hour period.

The infant's hydration and history of elimination also need to be accurately documented. An infant who is refusing to feed on a continual basis will become dehydrated. Frequent loose or fluid stools may cause an infant to fail to gain adequate weight or to actually lose weight, while an infant who is constipated may simply refuse to feed.

Medical diagnosis can play a major role in the assessment of problems associated with the feeding of infants, for example infants with some cardiac anomalies are too tired to suck. The diagnosis must obviously be considered when formulating a plan to deal with the infant's feeding problem.

TREATMENT

Infants with feeding difficulties which have not been overcome by the nurse after a period of observation and/or investigation, may be referred to a speech therapist, who is a specialist in this field. The therapist can demonstrate to parents and health care providers a range of oral stimulation exercises involving the muscles used for sucking and swallowing and for closing the lips around the teat or nipple. The suck/swallow mechanism and the movements of the lips, tongue and jaw are observed for difficulties (e.g., tongue thrusting, inadequate lip closure and lack of coordination). On some occasions the therapist may suggest a change in the bottle or teat, the feeding technique or in positioning during and after feeds.

Referral for some patients to paediatric occupational therapists or physiotherapists may be appropriate. These therapists work in a similar manner to the speech therapist and can be of particular benefit for the infant whose diagnosis may include a neurological abnormality, such as cerebral palsy.

If an infant has been admitted to hospital with feeding difficulty, it is imperative that nursing staff, medical and paramedical staff meet to discuss the plan of care for that infant. Parents must receive the same information and advice from all staff regarding their infant's feeding problem. Different advice from different professionals only further confuses and distresses parents.

To feed or not to feed! Scheduled feeds, demand feeds, feeds by the clock, modified demand or scheduled feeds; there is a confusing array of choices. The best method for determining the frequency of feeds is one which takes into account the infant's needs.

A small, frail or malnourished infant may require short, frequent feeds, or may need feeds to be given via a nasogastric or orogastric tube. As the infant grows, becomes stronger and gains weight, a change to a system of alternate tube and bottle or breast feeds, which progresses to all oral feeds, is recommended.

Other methods of feeding small infants or infants who only tolerate small volumes of feed include the use of a continuous milk drip via nasogastric tube for 24 hours per day, or for 12 hours overnight. If overnight milk drip feeds are given, the infant is usually offered oral feeds during the day. Lack of fluid intake during the day becomes less important using this system since increased volumes may be given at night.

The hospitalised infant with feeding difficulty should have a consistent caregiver. If the parent is unable to live in and care for the infant for the majority of the time, a primary nurse or a small core of nursing staff should care for the infant to establish consistency.

FEEDING EQUIPMENT

There is a huge array of bottles, teats and other forms of infant feeders available today, and by the time a mother seeks help for herself and her infant she has often spent large sums of money buying different devices.

Most teats and bottles are designed to perform in a similar way, and the constant changes only increase the infant's distress and confusion.

There are, however, bottles designed to assist the exhausted infant, or infants with a poor suck reflex. These are soft plastic, squeezable bottles where the person feeding gently squeezes milk into the infant's mouth. A Haberman feeder, using a feeding system with a non-return valve and variable controlled flow teat, may also be of assistance.

FORMULAE

A large number of formulae is available today, many of which have a similar composition. Often, well meaning friends, relatives or health professionals will advise formula changes in an effort to solve the infant's feeding problems. Unless there is evidence of feed intolerance with diarrhoea or vomiting, an infant's formula should not be changed. Lactose intolerance usually presents with watery diarrhoea, and may necessitate a change to a low lactose formula, while a cow's milk protein allergy, which may present with melaena, may indicate the need to change to a non-cow's milk based formula. Advice on infant formulae should be sought before making any changes.

The vomiting infant may benefit from having the formula thickened using one of the commercially available thickening agents or cornflour. Recipes for this thickening of formula are available from specialist dietitians.

For the infant who is failing to thrive when all possible causes have been investigated and no cause found, the addition of extra calories to the formula may be required. This should be done on the advice of a specialist dietitian. Calories may be increased using a number of products such as glucose polymers, long or medium chain triglycerides, and, in rare cases, by concentrating the formula. The dietitian will advise the most appropriate method and provide the recipe.

Infants must be handled and held gently but confidently. Anxiety in the caregiver is easily picked up by the infant, and will make the infant more distressed, fretful and irritable. During feeding, maintaining eye contact and speaking to the infant are vital. If the infant is feeding poorly when bottle fed, resting one finger under the infant's chin can stimulate sucking. Some infants require finger pressure on each cheek, as well as under the chin, in order to achieve a good seal of the mouth around the teat and to stimulate sucking. While this may sound difficult, it can be achieved, and just requires dexterity.

It is important to note that while perseverance with the feeding of difficult infants is paramount, the parent and health care provider should avoid tiring the infant, thus preventing a cycle of feeding difficulty where perseverance is followed by tiredness resulting in poor feeding.

A calm, quiet area in which the infant may be fed is essential, because some infants are very easily distracted. In the same way, the infant should be cared for by a core of people either at home or in hospital if hospitalisation should become necessary.

Further education of parents and of health care providers within the community must take place if these infants with feeding problems or difficulties and their families are to be assisted. Admission to hospital should be a last resort. Whether in the community or the hospital it is important that all those involved work together as a team in order to avoid further complicating the problem.

Genetic and Chromosomal Abnormalities

Robyn Pedersen

Genetic abnormalities, including chromosomal abnormalities, occur in 4% to 6% of newborn infants, accounting for 22% to 27% of admissions of children to hospital and 40% of deaths in children. Thus genetics and genetic counselling are important issues for nurses, whether in a hospital setting or in the community. Genetic diseases have a number of different causes, which are listed in **Table 8.3**.

Genes, chromosomal abnormalities, abnormalities due to a single gene defect, multifactorial inheritance, mitochondrial inheritance and other causes of birth defects

Table 8.3 Modes of inheritance and prevalence of genetic diseases and chromosomal abnormalities

Mode of inheritance	Defect type	Sub-groups	Example	Prevalence per 10 000 births
Chromosomal	chromosomal abnormalities	trisomy translocation deletion duplication inversion extra sex chromosomes less sex chromosomes mosaic (more than one cell line)	Down syndrome	60
Mendelian (also called monogenic or unifactorial)	defect in one gene pair	autosomal dominant autosomal recessive X-linked recessive X-linked dominant	achondroplasia cystic fibrosis Duchenne muscular dystrophy incontinentia pigmenti	100
Multifactorial	defect due to more than one gene plus non-genetic causes such as environment		Hirschsprung's disease pyloric stenosis neural tube defect	900
Mitochondrial	defect in mitochondrial DNA (in the cytoplasm of the cell)		mitochondrial myopathies	?

will be discussed. A discussion of the needs of the parents and child with a genetic disease will follow.

THE HUMAN GENOME

The nucleus of every cell in the body contains tiny, thread-like structures called chromosomes. Thousands of genes, which are responsible for a person's growth, development and characteristics, are arranged linearly along each chromosome. There are approximately 100 000 genes in the human genome. The genome is a term used to refer to all genes carried by a single gamete (egg or sperm).[1]

Genes have been defined as:

- A defined length of deoxyribonucleic acid (DNA) which encodes a protein.
- The smallest functional hereditary unit that occupies a specific position along the chromosome. That specific position on the chromosome is called a gene locus.
- A unit that has one or more specific effects upon the phenotype, which is the observable characteristics of a person.
- A unit that can mutate to various forms called alleles.

The genotype refers to those genes that are present whether or not they are expressed. The reasons for the variability of expression of features, especially within families, with some autosomal dominant disorders (e.g., neurofibromatosis) have not yet been determined.

With the exception of the gametes, each normal human cell contains 23 pairs of chromosomes, making 46 chromosomes in total. Those chromosomes numbered in decreasing size from 1 to 22 are called autosomes, of which there are 22 pairs. The other two chromosomes, making the 23 pair complement, are the sex chromosomes. In a female the pair is XX and in a male the pair is XY. The gametes contain 23 chromosomes comprising a single set (termed haploid). Thus, after fertilisation there is one full set of 23 pairs (termed diploid).

CHROMOSOMAL ABNORMALITIES

Some 15% of recognisable pregnancies, and about 40% of all conceptions, miscarry. About 60% of early spontaneous miscarried foetuses are chromosomally abnormal.[2] Chromosomal abnormalities result from an alteration in the number or the structure of the chromosomes. **Figure 8.1** contains a list of the different chromosomal abnormalities.

Abnormalities of number

Abnormalities of chromosome number occur when there are either too many or too few chromosomes in the cell (aneuploidy), usually the result of non-disjunction. Non-disjunction (the failure of chromosome pairs to migrate independently during meiosis) results in one daughter cell having no members of a pair and the other daughter cell having both members of a chromosomal pair. Thus when fertilisation occurs there is an abnormality of chromosomal number in the foetus (**Figure 8.2**). When there are 3 of the same chromosome rather than the normal pair (such as 3 of chromosome 21) the term used is trisomy (**Figure 8.3**). Other trisomies seen in liveborn infants are trisomy 13 and trisomy 18. Infants with trisomies have 47 chromosomes.

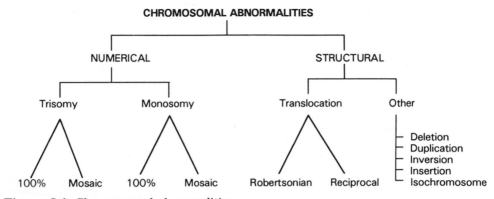

Figure 8.1 Chromosomal abnormalities.

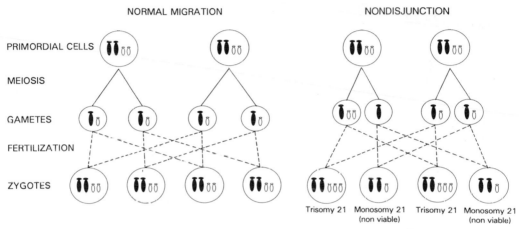

Figure 8.2 Normal migration is seen in the diagram on the left. The diagram on the right illustrates gamete and zygote (which grows into the foetus) formation where a chromosome 21 pair has failed to migrate during meiosis in the primordial cell on the left-hand side. The chromosome pair on the right has migrated normally. Two chromosome pairs only have been used as an example.

(S. Laing, Fragile-X programme, Prince of Wales Children's Hospital, Sydney)

Non-disjunction and the associated risk of abnormalities of chromosomal number increases with maternal age. **Table 8.4** exemplifies the increasing risk for Down syndrome as maternal age increases.

Sex chromosome abnormalities of number

The sex chromosomes can also be trisomic. Females can have 47, XXX, whereas males can have 47, XXY, known as Klinefelter syndrome, or 47, XYY.

Females can be monosomic for the X chromosome, which is written as 45, X and known as Turner syndrome. Most 45, X pregnancies, however, end in spontaneous miscarriage. Other chromosomal aneuploidies occur but are rare.

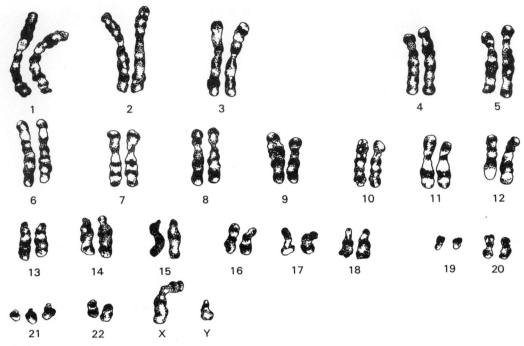

Figure 8.3 Karyotype of trisomy 21. The chromosomal complement (karyotype) of a boy with Down syndrome. Note the extra chromosome 21.

(Prepared by Cytogenetics Department, Prince of Wales Hospital, Sydney)

Table 8.4 Risk for Down syndrome in liveborn infants by maternal age

Maternal age at delivery (years)	Risk	Maternal age at delivery (years)	Risk
15	1:1578	33	1:574
16	1:1572	34	1:474
17	1:1565	35	1:384
18	1:1556	36	1:307
19	1:1544	37	1:242
20	1:1528	38	1:189
21	1:1507	39	1:146
22	1:1481	40	1:112
23	1:1447	41	1:85
24	1:1404	42	1:65
25	1:1351	43	1:49
26	1:1286	44	1:37
27	1:1208	45	1:28
28	1:1119	46	1:21
29	1:1018	47	1:15
30	1:909	48	1:11
31	1:796	49	1:8
32	1:683	50	1:6

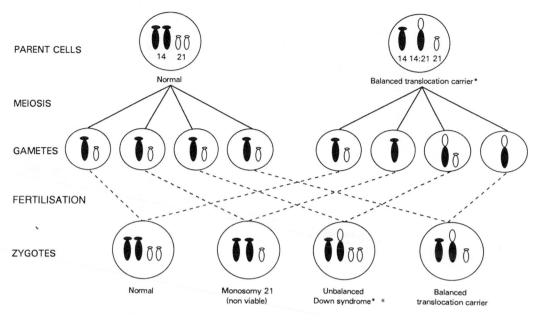

*Note normal chromosome count (46) in unbalanced state with Down syndrome, one less than normal (45) in balanced translocation carrier.

Figure 8.4 Transmission of a balanced 14:21 Robertsonian translocation.

(S. Laing, Fragile-X programme, Prince of Wales Children's Hospital, Sydney)

Abnormalities of structure

Abnormalities of chromosome structure are caused by 2 mechanisms, chromosomal breakage and unequal crossing over.

Chromosomal breakage and failure to rejoin the broken ends can result in loss (deletion) of chromosomal material causing abnormalities, or a rejoining of the broken piece to another chromosome (translocation) in such a way as to cause mispairing of the chromosome pair. When no genetic material is lost in the translocation, a balanced translocation results which is not usually associated with abnormality. However, during meiosis, balanced translocation carriers can produce unbalanced gametes which have either duplicated or deleted material and this alteration in genetic material results in foetal death or an abnormal child (**Figure 8.4**). If a couple have repeated miscarriages it is advisable for them to be tested as either partner may have a balanced translocation or some other balanced chromosomal rearrangements.

A special type of balanced translocation involving a fusion of the long arms of 2 acrocentric chromosomes which have no or almost no short arm (chromosomes 13,14,15,21,22) is called a Robertsonian translocation. The chromosome count in the balanced state is 45 (2 fused long arms make one 'combined' chromosome) (**Figure 8.5**).

Down syndrome is caused by an unbalanced Robertsonian translocation in approximately 5% of instances.[3] If Down syndrome is caused by a translocation the parents' blood should be examined for carrier status. If one of the parents is shown to be a carrier of a balanced translocation, there is a greater risk of recurrence in siblings than with Down syndrome caused by non-disjunction or a translocation occurring for the first time.

A chromosome can also break in 2 places, leading to an inversion of the gene sequence.

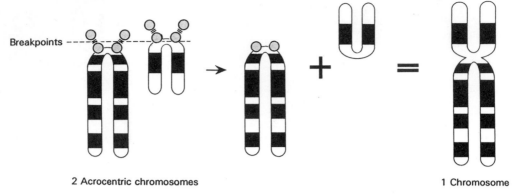

Breakpoints

2 Acrocentric chromosomes

1 Chromosome

Figure 8.5 A Robertsonian translocation.

(S. Laing, Fragile-X programme, Prince of Wales Children's Hospital, Sydney)

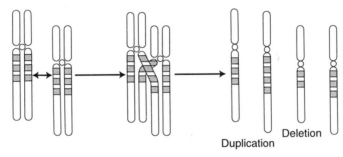

Duplication

Deletion

Figure 8.6 Unequal crossing over in meiosis, resulting in duplication of a chromosomal segment in one gamete and deletion of a segment in the other[2].

The chromosome segment is turned around completely so that the gene sequence for that segment is reversed. Such inversions are balanced rearrangements as no genetic material is gained or lost.

The second mechanism causing structural abnormality of chromosomes is unequal crossing over during meiosis. Unequal crossing over causes mispairing of chromatids resulting in deletions or duplications in segments of a chromosome pair (**Figure 8.6**). The deletion producing alpha-thalassaemia is due to this mechanism.

TESTING FOR CHROMOSOMAL ABNORMALITIES

It is generally accepted that women over 35 years should be offered prenatal diagnosis because chromosomal abnormalities of number in offspring increase with age. The tests offered are vaginal chorionic villus sampling (CVS) or abdominal CVS (**Figures 8.7, 8.8**) between 10 and 12 weeks' gestation or amniocentesis (**Figure 8.9**) between 14 and 18 weeks' gestation. These tests are also recommended to women of any age who have already had an offspring with a chromosomal abnormality or when the foetus is considered to be at risk for other reasons.

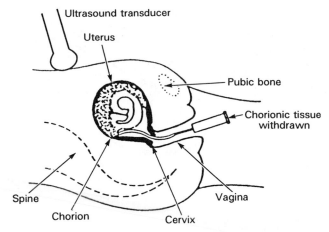

Figure 8.7 Chorionic villus sampling in which about 10–20 mg of chorionic villi are removed from the vagina and cervix usually during the 10th to 12th week of pregnancy. (Reproduced with permission[4])

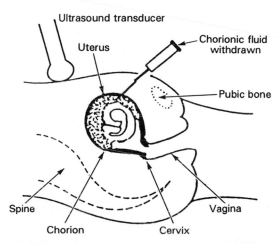

Figure 8.8 Chorionic villus sampling in which about 10–20 mg of chorionic villi are removed through the abdomen usually during the 10th to 12th week of pregnancy. (Reproduced with permission[4])

ABNORMALITY DUE TO A SINGLE GENE DEFECT

Information for normal development and function is provided by genes. The basic structure of genes can be altered by:

- one base in the DNA of the gene being replaced by another (point mutation)
- a piece missing (deletion)
- a piece rearranged in some way (inversion, insertion)
- a piece being duplicated (duplication).

The message for making the protein is then garbled and ineffectual.

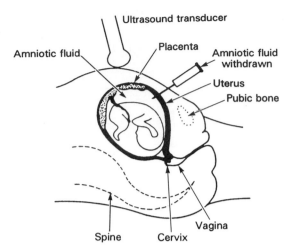

Figure 8.9 Amniocentesis in which amniotic fluid (containing foetal cells) is sampled during the 14th to 18th week of pregnancy. (Reproduced with permission[4])

Gene changes are referred to as mutations. A mutation in a single gene can be traced through families and may be inherited in an autosomal dominant, an autosomal recessive or an X-linked recessive pattern. These patterns of gene defects follow the rules of inheritance first recognised by Mendel. A family tree, or pedigree of a family may show a pattern seen in a particular type of inheritance. A pedigree is a valuable tool when assessing a family history and is drawn using the symbols shown in **Figure 8.10**.

Autosomal dominant inheritance

In an autosomal dominant disease only one member of the gene pair on an autosome is defective and this is sufficient to express the disease. The disease usually is passed from one affected parent to a child but, as it has to start somewhere in a family, the affected person could be a new mutation. Males and females transmit the gene to offspring of either sex. Where one parent is affected each child has a 1 in 2 chance of inheriting the defective gene. The expression of autosomal dominant diseases, and therefore the severity of symptoms, may vary widely even within the same family. Autosomal dominant diseases tend to occur in more than 1 generation and in more than 1 branch of the family of the affected person (**Figure 8.11**). Examples of diseases inherited in an autosomal dominant manner are Huntington disease, achondroplasia and myotonic dystrophy.

Autosomal recessive inheritance

In an autosomal recessive disease both members of a gene pair on a pair of autosomes are defective. It takes 2 defective genes at the same locus to express the disease. The person who expresses the disease is termed a homozygote. Diagnosis in a child establishes both parents as obligate carriers of a single copy of the mutation. In the heterozygote, such as in the parents, where the defective gene is paired with a normal gene, the individual is not affected. Although they do not have the disease they can still pass on the defective gene, and are carriers of the disease. There will be carriers in previous generations and other branches of the family. Once a couple has had an affected child there is

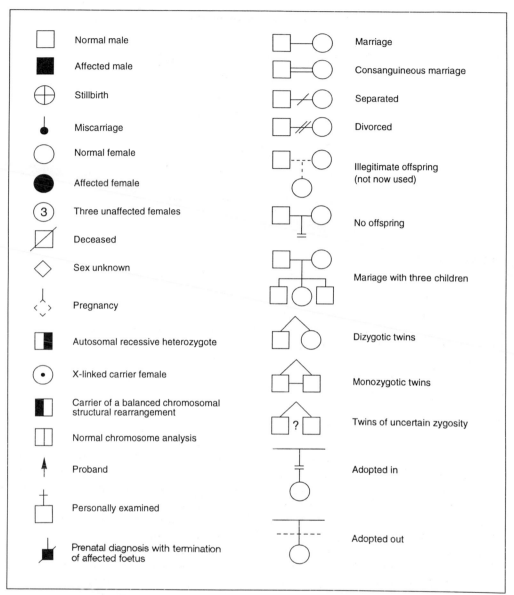

Figure 8.10 Symbols used to draw a family tree.

a 1 in 4 chance of having another affected child, a 2 in 4 chance of having an unaffected child who is a carrier, and a 1 in 4 chance of having a non-carrier, non-affected child (**Figure 8.12**).

Males and females transmit the gene to offspring of either sex. Autosomal recessive diseases tend to occur in one sibship (sisters and brothers of the same parents) of a family and rarely in other generations or branches of a family, except when explained by a marriage between relatives (consanguinity) (**Figure 8.13**). Examples of autosomal recessive diseases are phenylketonuria (PKU), cystic fibrosis and thalassaemia.

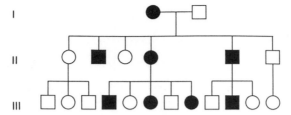

Figure 8.11 Pedigree to illustrate the inheritance of an autosomal dominant disease.

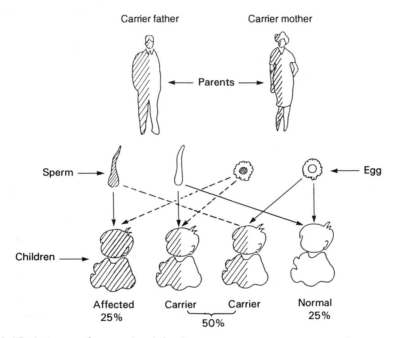

Figure 8.12 Autosomal recessive inheritance. (Reproduced with permission[5])

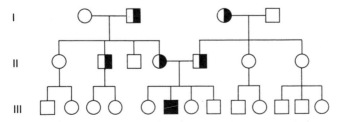

Figure 8.13 Pedigree to illustrate the inheritance of an autosomal recessive disease.

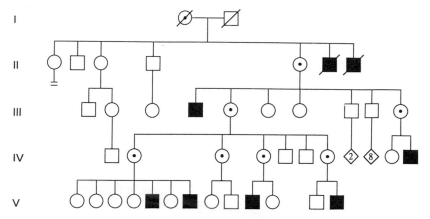

Figure 8.14 Pedigree illustrating the inheritance of an X-linked recessive disease.

X-linked recessive inheritance

In an X-linked recessive disease the defective gene is carried on the X chromosome. A female carrying a defective gene on one of her X chromosomes will not be affected, because her other X chromosome will produce the gene's message. There is no gene to compensate for the gene defect on the male's one X chromosome, so males are affected. Unaffected female carriers transmit the disease. When a female carrier has children, there is a 1 in 2 chance of her son being affected and a 1 in 2 chance of her daughter being a carrier (**Figure 8.14**). There is no male-to-male transmission in X-linked recessive diseases. All sons of an affected male, whose partner is not a carrier, are unaffected as they get his Y chromosome, and all his daughters are carriers as they get his X chromosome with the defective gene. In some X-linked recessive diseases, new mutations make up a high proportion of affected individuals (e.g., Duchenne muscular dystrophy). Examples of X-linked recessive disorders are Duchenne muscular dystrophy, haemophilia and colour blindness.

Multifactorial inheritance

Some conditions have complex inheritance where a combination of several genes and non-genetic causes give rise to the trait. This is known as multifactorial inheritance. Examples of conditions with a multifactorial inheritance pattern are diabetes mellitus, neural tube defects and Hirschsprung disease.

Mitochondrial inheritance

Although most DNA in a cell is present in the nucleus, mitochondria in the cell's cytoplasm have their own DNA. Sperm do not contribute mitochondria to the developing embryo, even though there is a small amount around the nucleus of the sperm. A small number of disorders are known to be due to mitochondrial DNA. These are transmitted to their children by females but not by males.[2] Maternally inherited myopathy and cardiomyopathy (MIMAC), and Kearns-Sayre syndrome are examples of diseases due to mitochondrial inheritance.

OTHER CAUSES OF BIRTH DEFECTS

Some other causes of birth defects include environmental agents, mechanical problems in the uterus and problems due to the failure of the cells to migrate to their predetermined location at the appropriate time in fetal development.

Teratogens are environmental agents that cause defects following exposure in pregnancy during the critical period of fetal development, e.g., alcohol, hydantoin, valproate, radiation, rubella, maternal hyperthermia.

Mechanical problems, such as a decrease in the available uterine space (bicornuate uterus, oligohydramnios) cause deformation sequences. The foetus has normal development, but due to prolonged pressure develops abnormalities (e.g., one cause of talipes, early amnion rupture sequence).

Failure of the cells to migrate at the appropriate time in fetal development has many causes and produces abnormalities in the foetus (e.g., cleft lip, with or without cleft palate, neural tube defect).

A sequence results when all the abnormalities in a child can be explained on the basis of a single event in the development of the foetus that leads to a number of subsequent defects[5] (e.g., DiGeorge sequence, anencephaly sequence).

A syndrome is a group of abnormalities that occur together more frequently than by chance (e.g., Marfan syndrome, Down syndrome). Recognition of a syndrome may give knowledge as to the cause, natural history and chance of recurrence. Syndromes can be chromosomal, autosomal dominant, multifactorial, or may result from an unknown cause.

NEEDS OF THE PARENTS AND CHILD

Most of a child's care is provided by the parents at home, but when a child with an hereditary disease is admitted to hospital, it is important for the nurse to be sensitive to both the child's and parents' needs. In some diseases there can be multiple admissions to hospital and the admission/treatment is just one more burden the child and the parents have to face. Liaison between the family and the medical team is also an important function for the nurse.

The implications of any disease affect the whole lifestyle of the individual and the family to which they belong. The parents, siblings and the child need to know how the disease is going to affect the child, and what treatment is available to help the condition. Sometimes the correct diagnosis may not always be obvious, and so repeated assessments will be necessary. The nurse needs to be aware of the need for genetic counselling and to know where that counselling is available. Referral to a genetics clinic is vital.

Genetic counselling

Parents need to understand the way heredity contributes to the disease and therefore counselling focuses initially on the way the disease is inherited in families. It may take several sessions before this information is fully understood, partly due to the complexity of the information. However, parents often hear very little after the diagnosis has been explained to them, as they are usually in shock. Some genetic disorders are not diagnosed until adulthood, (e.g., Huntington disease) and clients may reject the diagnosis and its consequences at the initial consultation.

Parents need to understand the risk of recurrence of the disease both in their immediate family and in other relatives. The risk will vary with the mode of inheritance, and therefore parents need to know the options for dealing with it. With accurate information available to them, parents can make informed decisions regarding future pregnancies that are in accordance with their values, goals and religious beliefs.

Prenatal diagnosis

Diagnostic tests for prenatal diagnosis that can be offered to parents include the following:

- An ultrasound examination which can detect certain abnormalities in the foetus (e.g., spina bifida).
- Examination of maternal blood can be used to screen for increased risk of Down syndrome and neural tube defects.
- Cord blood can be taken directly from the foetus at 18 weeks' gestation (cordocentesis) for examination. The risk of producing a miscarriage is approximately 1%.[2]
- Chorionic villus sampling between 10 and 12 weeks' gestation or amniocentesis between 14 and 16 weeks' gestation can be offered in diseases where the genetic defect is known or genetic markers can be traced through the family. Both techniques can test for chromosomal abnormalities, DNA studies and some biochemical assays. Amniocentesis can detect neural tube defects. The risk of producing a miscarriage is 1% to 2% for chorionic villus sampling and approximately 0.5% for amniocentesis.[4]

Other options for dealing with the risk of recurrence include having no further children, adoption, tubal ligation or vasectomy, artificial insemination with donor sperm or in-vitro fertilisation with donor ova. These options will depend on the way the disease is inherited and/or the sex of the affected parent. All are viable options and parents may need help in evaluating those that are acceptable to them. The aim is to support the parents in whatever decision they make.

Family dynamics

Attitudes of the family are important and these are interwoven with their own individual values, hopes, dreams, lifestyle and the expectation of the child and themselves. Some families are unable to accept any abnormality in their child, some can accept intellectual impairment but not physical disability, while others can accept physical but not intellectual disability.

Understanding the parents' and patient's reactions to the diagnosis is important. These reactions include grief, blame, guilt, anger, rejection of the extended family, denial and feelings about their own self-worth. Sometimes the extended family rejects a child with an abnormality, leaving the parents without family support. The realisation by the parents that the child may not be normal represents a painful loss of the desired 'normal child' and may precipitate grieving.[6] Grieving also occurs when the parents and/or child realise that the disorder significantly curtails the child's activities and/or shortens the child's life. Parents may experience feelings of loss and grief when significant life events, such as the child starting school, leaving home or marrying, are delayed or do not happen.

Many families experience chronic sorrow. Even after they have picked up the pieces of their lives they continue to feel sad over the child's situation and over the lifestyle adjustments they have had to make to accommodate the child within the family. They do not 'get over it' but may gradually adjust to problems as they arise.

The initial reaction to the diagnosis of a genetic disorder in a family is often for parents to blame themselves, and the children, if old enough, may blame the parents.

When the grandparents' reaction is, 'well it's not on our side', it tends to alienate the family just when they need the most support. In X-linked diseases especially, some husbands blame their wife for the condition of their son, and some mothers blame themselves for giving it to their sons. Some women believe they have failed as wife and mother, and as a person. They feel worthless and have a negative view of themselves because they see themselves as carrying a 'bad gene'. If the disease has been diagnosed later in life, the client may also develop feelings of worthlessness and may see themselves as being punished.

Family members may respond differently to genetic counselling and may not be in the same emotional space at the same time, because people grieve in different ways. A parent may not be able to live in the same house as their affected child, resulting in a break in the family. The parents may reject the child or, if the life expectancy is short, may resist becoming attached to the child. Parents may deny the existence of the disease, especially when the child looks unaffected at birth. It can be devastating for a family to know shortly after birth that their child has a genetic disorder, such as Duchenne muscular dystrophy, and to see no effect of it until the child is 3 or 4 years of age.

Education and ongoing counselling help to ameliorate some of the problems faced by the parents and child. As parents live with the condition of their child, they normally pass through 5 stages of reaction: shock, denial, sadness and anger, equilibrium, and reorganisation;[7] not dissimilar to the stages of bereavement. These stages overlap, and members of families do not necessarily progress at the same rate. Sometimes additional stresses on the family precipitate a crisis and the family members may regress to feelings belonging to an earlier stage. An example of such a crisis could be seen in a family where a boy with Duchenne muscular dystrophy requires an electric wheelchair permanently. The parents experience sadness and sometimes anger even though they had come to some equilibrium following the diagnosis.

Siblings go through the same stages as their parents. They may even blame themselves for their sister or brother having the disease. They worry about their own health, and whether they too will get the disease. They may go through a stage of 'why them and not me', especially if there is more than one sibling affected or if it is X-linked, and only boys are affected. Sometimes they do not want to get attached to the sister or brother in case they die. If the disease is X-linked, a sister may worry that she is a carrier of the defect and that she may eventually produce an affected child. Siblings of a person who is diagnosed later in life are faced with going through the tests to see if they have the disease. They may have already had their children and with an autosomal dominant condition each of those children have a 1 in 2 chance of having the disease. With most genetic disorders, carrier status cannot be definitely identified.

Friends and the extended family also go through a period of readjustment when they learn a child has a genetic condition. Many feel uncomfortable and stay away. Consequently, any support or help that would normally be available at the birth of a baby is not forthcoming. Sometimes the parents do not tell their friends and extended family or do not allow them to visit. Support for the family is very important. It can be provided by professionals, such as genetic counsellors, nurses, occupational therapists, social workers, physiotherapists, staff of a developmental disabilities unit, or by non-professionals such as individuals, families, or support groups pertaining to specific diseases. People who are in a similar situation are often in a better position to help the newly diagnosed family. Although each family is different, they know what it was like for them when they received the diagnosis and can often help with practical advice.

Ethical and privacy issues need to be addressed. An issue of privacy may arise when members of the extended family need to be tested to rule out either having the disease or being a carrier. Some families may have estranged members or do not wish other family members to know about the diagnosis. This is an ethical dilemma as the client has a right to privacy, but the members of the family have a right to genetic counselling.

SPECIAL NEEDS OF THE CHILD

The most important concern for health professionals is assisting the parents and child to maximise the child's potential through appropriate treatment, early intervention and school placement. Emotional support for the child and family is also important.

Treatment can range from diet control to ongoing physiotherapy, hospital admissions and occasional surgery for the remainder of the person's life. The aim of treatment is to prevent complications. Long-term care can be onerous for the carers when the treatment required is tedious or painful for the child. The necessity for care can be so constant that it places severe strain on family relationships. In some families, relationships break down.

A school must be found that is academically and physically suitable for the child. Some children with genetic diseases have an intellectual disability as well which imposes additional educational difficulties.

As the child grows, acceptance by their peers is an important issue. The child can feel isolated and rejected if peer interaction is missing. Adolescents face the usual problems of adolescence as well as those associated with their disease. Because their physical condition may make relationships more difficult than they might have otherwise been, sexuality and relationships need to be discussed.

Problems with employment may occur, as any physical limitation has to be taken into account. The person may need to work in a building with wheelchair access, extra office space may be required for turning and furniture may need to be of a particular height. Transport to and from the workplace may be difficult and expensive.

There may be financial difficulties because of ongoing medical problems and the cost of special equipment. The home might have to be altered to have ready access for a wheelchair and to make the nursing care easier for all concerned. If a child requires constant use of an electric wheelchair, some families purchase a van to transport the child while in the chair. This is easier for the carers and more acceptable to the person who would otherwise have to be lifted into a cramped space.

OVERVIEW

Parents and the extended family need information about the genetics of the disease, recurrence risks and the options for any future children. They need to understand their reactions to the diagnosis and to the child. The child may have special needs for daily living, education and, later, employment. The normal problems of adolescence need to be addressed.

The nurse in the community or hospital setting is in a special position to assist both the child and parents to maintain control over their own lives.

Genetic diseases have a number of different causes. Accurate diagnosis, effective genetic counselling and follow-up support for those families affected is essential. The nurse is an integral part of the supportive network available to the families.

REFERENCES

1. King RC, Stansfield WD. *A dictionary of genetics.* 3rd ed. New York: Oxford University Press, 1985.
2. Connor JM, Ferguson-Smith MA. Essential medical genetics. 3rd ed. Oxford: Blackwell Scientific Publications, 1991.
3. Harper PS. *Practical genetic counselling.* 4th ed. Oxford: Butterworth-Heinemann, 1993.
4. NSW Genetic Education Service. *Prenatal diagnosis, special tests for your baby during pregnancy.* Sydney: NSW Genetic Service, 1991.
5. Jones KL, ed. *Smith's recognizable patterns of human malformation.* 4th ed. Philadelphia: Saunders, 1988.
6. Williams JK. Genetic counselling in paediatric nursing. *Paediatric Nursing* 1986; 12: 287–289.
7. Hamilton AK, Noble DN. Assisting families through genetic counselling. *Social Casework: J Contemporary Soc Work* 1983; Jan: 18–25.

Chapter 9

Psychosocial Care of the Infant, Child and Adolescent with an Illness

Sue Nagy

Illness and disability during childhood place strain on all the family, and when the illness is severe or becomes a chronic problem, the associated stress is correspondingly greater.[1] Children with chronic illnesses are up to 3 times more likely than healthy peers to experience a major psychological or social problem.[2] Such problems are most likely to be manifested as behavioural and social problems.[3]

Over the last 20 years, however, research has shown that while long-term illness places great strains on children and their family members, most are able to make satisfactory emotional adjustments.[4-8] This is in direct contrast with the results of earlier research,[9-11] which presented a much more pessimistic picture. While some of the differences in these findings may be due to improved research techniques, they may also reflect improvements in the support services available to these children and their families. For such a trend to continue, it is vital that health care services are both extended and improved.

The purpose of this chapter is to help paediatric nurses firstly to recognise families who are finding it difficult to cope and secondly to implement nursing care that will facilitate emotional adjustment during the course of the illness, during hospitalisation and, if necessary, during the terminal stages of the illness. A supportive and constructive environment may, at best, help families to find positive features from the experience, and at the very least, reduce the negative effects.

The Effects of Long-term Illness on Family Members

Long-term illness imposes stresses on all those involved. Stress threatens to become overwhelming when people feel they have insufficient resources to manage the demands of the situation.[12] Extreme and persistent stress can have physical, emotional and social effects on the person. The ability to cope depends on a complex, interrelated set of factors which include the person's available economic, personal or social resources and their repertoire of coping strategies.[13]

Coping strategies can be categorised as either 'problem-focused' strategies (or 'direct coping'), and 'emotion-focused strategies' (or 'defensive coping').[12] Problem-focused strategies aim to reduce stress by attempting to change the situation, such as seeking information or seeking practical help. Emotion-focused strategies aim to reduce the negative emotions associated with stressful experiences. They are attempts to help the person feel better. Emotion-focused strategies include accepting the situation, focusing on positive aspects, or refusing to focus on the negative aspects.[14]

THE CHILD

Some children seem to find effective ways of managing the stresses imposed by protracted illness, while others appear to drift in and out of adaptive patterns of behaviour. Still others, unable to develop effective coping systems, may become caught up in cycles of maladaptive behaviours.

Mattsson studied children with long-term chronic illness.[15] He found that it was possible to identify 3 distinct behaviour patterns among those who had adjustment problems. The first pattern consisted of children who were highly anxious, and particularly dependent on their families, especially their mothers. They had generally passive attitudes to their environment and tended not to become involved in activities outside the family. The second pattern consisted of children who were aggressively independent. They insisted on demonstrating their independence by engaging in behaviours that were particularly risky for them because of their health status, such as diabetic children bingeing on fast foods and refusing to take their insulin. The third, but less common pattern, was that of shy, lonely and resentful children who seemed to have developed an image of themselves as 'defective outsiders', even within their own families.

During childhood, behaviour patterns are established that can affect, for better or worse, the course of future development. When children experience severe or protracted illness, they may be deprived of experiences and opportunities that are important for normal development.[16,17,18] For this reason, a sound knowledge of the process of normal development is fundamental for the assessment of the chronically ill child.[18]

As children are physically, economically and emotionally dependent on their families, assessment and management should be undertaken within the context of their family system. Children are likely to be affected by their parents' responses to stressful situations. Even infants respond to stress in their mothers by becoming increasingly tense and difficult to settle.

Toddlerhood is the time for developing a sense of autonomy by exploring the world and gaining an understanding of the extent and limitations of one's competence. Satisfactory development may be hampered in ill toddlers who have serious restrictions placed on their mobility.[17]

During middle childhood, elementary social and academic skills are established. Inadequate social or educational experiences may lead to greater feelings of inferiority. Children who have disabilities may be rejected by their peers,[19] even when their peers are as young as 3 years.[20] Children who are disfigured are more likely to be rejected by girls, whereas boys tend to be more intolerant of functional disabilities.[21]

Adolescence is a time for emancipation from the family. Long-term illness or disability is likely to delay the adolescent's achievement of physical and emotional independence. Reductions in educational opportunities affect the range of occupational choices, and extend the period of financial dependence on the family.

Peers play a particularly important role in adolescent social and psychological development. When periods of ill health restrict opportunities for peer interaction, adolescents are more likely to have difficulty learning the accepted modes of behaviour and becoming part of a supportive network of peers. Body image is constantly adjusted during adolescence in order to keep pace with rapid body changes. Adolescents develop a realistic body image by comparing their own body with those of same-sex peers. Disabled and ill adolescents are less likely to be comforted by such comparisons and may, therefore, need support to maintain a sense of self-esteem. Boys' self-esteem is more likely to be affected when illness or disability affects their body's physical ability, while girls have more difficulty when their physical appearance is affected. Low self-esteem may hamper the satisfactory development of relationships with the opposite sex, setting up a cycle of isolation and poor self-esteem.

There are a number of ways that children can be helped to manage the stress of illness. For example, stress management training has be shown to be effective with adolescents.[22] However, recent research suggests that one of the most important factors influencing children's adaptation to illness appears to be the support of their parents.[23-25] And the effectiveness of the way the family functions as a unit.[26]

PARENTS

Parents of children with long-term illness have to make especially significant adjustments. These adjustments may extend to every aspect of their lives, requiring changes in their economic[27] and domestic circumstances as well as affecting their physical and emotional well-being.[28-30] It is often necessary for them to carry out treatment for the child's illness at home, and to provide emotional support for the child.[31]

The major emotional crisis period, that frequently accompanies the diagnosis, seems to last about 1 year.[32] It is during this time that parents (especially mothers) are particularly vulnerable and in particular need of support.[31]

Some of the difficulties faced by parents occur in most illnesses, such as sadness at the loss of the healthy child, and the distress incurred during episodes of severe illness.[33,34] Others differ according to the characteristics of the illness or disability.[35,36] Parents of children with haemophilia, for example, have to respond to intermittent life-threatening crises when there are bleeding episodes, although outside these episodes the child may function normally.[37] While children are being treated for leukaemia, parents must support the child during painful and invasive treatment,[30] and learn to deal with feelings of helplessness while others do the treatment.[39] Conversely, parents of children with diabetes and cystic fibrosis take a major and continuing responsibility for implementing treatment and may worry about their competence.[31,40-42] These parents are often subject to anxiety and depression. When the prognosis is death, parents must begin to cope with their grief in anticipation of the child's eventual death.

Genetic disorders, such as cystic fibrosis or thalassaemia, impose their own stresses upon the parents. They may have periods of feeling guilty and 'responsible' for their child's genetic condition. They may also have to decide whether or not to have more children. If the disorder is not genetic, parents may engage in a great deal of soul searching about their role in the development of the child's illness, asking themselves: 'If I had only done . . . ?' or 'If I'd not done. . . . ?'.

Sometimes the effects of serious disorders, such as diabetes or cystic fibrosis, are not immediately obvious to people outside the family. The child may appear to be perfectly well, and friends and relatives can have difficulty in reconciling the diagnosis with an apparently healthy child. In such cases, friends and relatives may have no concept of the problems being faced by the family and support may not be offered. On the other hand, if the disorder is obvious, such as cerebral palsy, the child and family have to cope with the reactions of others. Disorders which are socially stigmatised, such as epilepsy, may result in the additional problem of social isolation of the child and family.

Factors such as income and education appear to affect parent's ability to cope.[43] Wealthy families are more likely to receive better health care services and to receive them sooner than poorer families. Persons with lower-status occupations may have less education and less control over their lives generally, which makes them more vulnerable to stress. Parents who are older, and who have been married longer than 4 years, seem to be able to manage the stress of chronic illness better than younger parents and those who have not had sufficient time to build a stable relationship.[44]

Social support is an important means of coping with stress.[45] There is compelling research evidence that when parents of chronically ill and disabled children are isolated and unsupported, they have greater difficulty in coping with the demands of a sick or disabled child.[26,46-49] Support may not always be offered by people in the parents' social network. Canam, for example, found that more than half the parents in her study did not talk to anybody about their feelings because they felt that no one was interested.[50]

Some parents find a strong source of social support in each other.[51] When the relationship between parents is good, they appear to make a more satisfactory adaptation to the crisis of having a sick child,[52,53] and to have families that function more effectively.[54]

While mothers often shoulder the major part of the burden of caring for ill children, support,[47] especially from fathers,[55] seems to be an important factor in helping them cope. Men can support their wives in a variety of ways; being involved in family life, helping with the children, providing emotional support.[27] or merely by indicating that they value the efforts of their wives in caring for the family in general, and for the ill child in particular.[55]

Coping is a skill that seems to improve with experience. Previous experience in coping with stressful situations appears to play a role in helping people to develop coping patterns that are effective in a variety of situations. Parents, for example, who have developed effective coping skills in previous times of stress have been found to cope better with a sick child.[56]

The support of health professionals is crucial for parents of ill children. When parents are able to cope they are able to provide better support for their children.[49] Nurses are particularly well placed to notice when parents are having difficulties, and to bring this to the attention of psychologists and social workers within the health care team. To do so nurses need to be observant and have the sensitivity to recognise cues that the family is having difficulty.

WELL SIBLINGS

Children spend a large amount of their time interacting with their siblings[57] and tend to exert strong socialising influences on each other. They are, therefore, highly likely to be affected emotionally when one of them has a protracted illness or disability.[58] Research into the nature of these effects, however, has lead to conflicting, and inconclusive findings. While some studies have found that such children learn to be more compassionate,[59] understanding and socially competent than their peers,[60,61] others have found evidence of psychological disturbance.[27,62–64] Increased demands are made on parents to attend to the needs of the ill child. Parents may reduce their expectations of the ill child's behaviour.[65] This may create conflict between ill children and their siblings.

The reaction of siblings may vary according to their developmental stage. Younger children may feel rejected and express it with regressive behaviour. Older children, who are more aware of the significance of the situation, may attempt to deal with their resentment and guilt by assuming greater domestic responsibilities.[63] Some well siblings find themselves assuming roles beyond those normally required of their age group, such as providing emotional support for their mothers when their fathers have failed to do so.[27] Lobato and co-workers found that some siblings seem to be more concerned by the effects on their parents and the sick child than on themselves.[62]

While it is clear that the factors that contribute to the satisfactory adjustment of siblings are highly complex and are not yet well understood, research has provided some guidelines for helping parents with their well children.

As parents try to manage the demands of the affected child, the needs of siblings may be overlooked and lead to feelings of resentment and jealousy.[62] Taylor found that the strongest feelings expressed by well siblings were those of isolation and deprivation of their parents' time and attention.[66] It is easy for parents who are preoccupied with their concerns for the ill child to fail to keep well siblings fully informed about the child's progress.[66] In such cases, siblings are more likely to feel left out of the dynamics between the parents and the ill child. Parents need to be encouraged to recognise their well children's need to be involved.[66]

Adjusting to Hospitalisation

Hospitals can be a frightening places for anyone, but especially so when the patient is a child. Indeed, hospital may be one of the most stressful experiences faced by most children. The lack of power and control that children have over their lives renders them particularly vulnerable to psychological trauma. Nursing and medical staff, on whom children are very dependent, may be relative strangers[67] and hospital routines may not be sufficiently flexible to cater for the needs of individual children. Pain, unfamiliar situations, separation from family and friends all have an impact. It remains for committed and understanding adults to help alleviate the stress associated with such experiences.

The intensity and duration of children's reactions may vary according to a number of factors, including the preparation that children receive before admission to hospital, the stressfulness of their actual experiences while in hospital, and the way that they understand or interpret their experiences while in hospital.

PREPARATION OF A CHILD FOR HOSPITAL

Children who have been given detailed preparation for the specific situations that they will encounter while in hospital, tend to be less anxious than those who are prepared with vague, non-specific information.[68] Some children arrive at hospital with at least some preparation, while others continue to be admitted with very little or even erroneous information, such as believing that they are going to have a holiday.

Many techniques can be used to prepare children, such as books, hospital visits, and films or videos of other children's experiences. Parents do not always know in advance that their children require hospitalisation and for this reason, many preschool programs include a hospital education segment. Parents can help their children become accustomed to temporary separations by arranging brief, but enjoyable, periods away from home.

THE CHILD'S EXPERIENCE OF HOSPITALISATION

As children react to the experience of hospital in many different ways, individual evaluation of each child is fundamental to their care. Assessment and intervention must take into account the developmental level of the child, their relationship with their caregivers, their understanding of their experiences, and the potential impact of the experience on their long-term development.

The effects of separation from parents

Children's relationship with their parents is critical for their long-term psychological health. As the infant's concept of object permanence develops, so do anxieties about being separated from caregivers and exposed to strangers. Hospitalisation has the potential to damage this relationship if parents are unable to give adequate support and children consequently feel abandoned. Paediatric nursing staff, who have a sound understanding of the psychology of the young child, are able to provide leadership and prevent or reduce the emotional damage caused by poorly managed hospitalisation.

Bowlby's stages of separation

Bowlby has described three stages that young children experience when separated from their caregivers.[69] The first stage is one of intense *protest*. The angry and crying child searches for her mother and screams loudly in an effort to get her to return. The attentions of other adults are frequently rejected. The child may continue in this state for hours and sometimes even for days. Some children protest continually while others do so intermittently.

At this stage, because of toddlers' need to develop a sense of autonomy, mobility may be an important coping strategy for them. It allows them actively to seek comfort from caregivers and assists them in working through emotional experiences. Most paediatric nurses have vivid images of small children crying and falling asleep while standing at the end of their cots and refusing to lie down. It is as if they need the comfort of at least being upright.

If the child's mother does not return, a feeling of *despair* may result. Crying becomes less furious and has a more despairing quality as if the child was giving up hope of having his mother return. She may even stop crying altogether. She is likely to withdraw from interaction with others, eat very little and lose interest in playing. Increased thumb-sucking, lying in a foetal position, or clinging to a security blanket may all be attempts to provide self-comfort. When the mother visits, the child may respond ambivalently, at times responding to her and ignoring her at others. Such behaviour may lead the inexperienced nurse to believe that the child is settling down and beginning to accept the situation. The keen observer, however, will note that the child looks sad and lonely.

In an effort to deal with the distress of separation, the child may begin the process of emotional *detachment* from her mother. She may begin to accept care from nurses, become more sociable and cooperative and recommence playing. When her mother returns, she may ignore or avoid her. Superficially, the child appears to be accepting of the separation, to be resuming her interest in her environment, and to be playing with other children and forming new relationships. Her behaviour, however, is not that of a happy, contented child, but rather that of one who is becoming resigned to the loss of her mother. Children do not always make their feelings obvious; it is, therefore, important to be especially attentive to the child's non-verbal behaviour.[70] It is easy to conclude that a cooperative child has made a satisfactory adjustment to hospital. The child, however, who is violently acting out his or her anxieties may be reacting in a healthier way than the child who is quiet, controlled and compliant.

Securely attached children, tend to cope better in the long term, although their protests at being left may be more vocal. Similarly, children whose family lives are relatively relaxed and stress-free tend to adjust to hospital with greater ease than those whose emotional resources are already severely strained.

If hospitalisation is sufficiently emotionally traumatic to impair the relationship between children and their parents, the parents may have difficulty controlling their children and behaviour problems may develop. There may also be long-term social effects as children who have lost trust in their relationship with their parents may have difficulty relating to other people. New relationships tend to be more shallow and the child's ability to form future, in-depth and trusting relationships may be damaged. The children who seem to be most affected by separation are those whose families do not have harmonious relationships and who are separated from both parents for a lengthy period of time. Children who have previously experienced short but enjoyable separations, such as visiting grandparents, appear to adjust better to longer, more stressful separations.[71]

Most children adjust to hospital more easily if at least one parent is able to stay most of the time. Parents seem to be able to help their children in a number of ways. They provide physical comfort,[72] they use diversionary strategies, act as advocates,[73] and provide information in a form which the child is able to assimilate.[74] Generally, they seem to be able help children to express their distress and cope more effectively with the stresses associated with hospitalisation.[75]

Some parents, however, are not always able, or willing to stay for long periods. They may be obliged to leave because of commitments to other children or to their jobs. It may be necessary for nurses to help parents to manage the situation so that the parent–child relationship can remain intact. Essentially, this means helping parents to minimise the child's distress and above all, to prevent the child from losing trust in his parents. Infants' and toddlers' attempts at self-comfort should be recognised for what they are. It is important that they are not obstructed from providing comfort for themselves or seeking it from others and that their mobility is not restricted any more than is absolutely necessary. Parents can be discouraged from leaving without saying goodbye, as children tend to adapt better to separation if parents tell their children why they are going,[76] and when they will be back. Leaving a small personal possession with the child to mind until they return, or leaving a good, clear photo of themselves can be helpful.[77] Familiar toys and objects from home may help the child feel less alienated.

Parents should be encouraged to visit, and made to feel welcome and needed. Nurses may not realise that many parents are intimidated by hospitals and hospital staff. Parents may take written instructions more literally than they are meant, such as the mother who would not cuddle her child on her lap because a sign on the cot said the child was to remain in bed, or the father who, after seeing the following sign on a cot 'Test stools for reducing substances' asked if it was alright to use the chair next to the child's bed. Parents may want to stay with the child but feel that they are in the way of important hospital work. They may not realise how important they are for their children's adjustment to the stress of hospital. Warm reassurances from nurses can do a great deal to relieve their uncertainties.

When parents cannot be at the hospital with their children, they can be encouraged to talk to them on the phone or to send tape recordings. Extended family members or family friends can be encouraged to visit if the parents cannot. Ward 'grandmothers' or other volunteers may also be helpful.

Nurses may find it necessary to fill in temporarily for absent parents. Nurses who have made friends with the child in his parents' presence will be in a better position to provide comfort when they have left. When parents leave, children should be allowed to express their anger and distress, but should be restrained from hurting themselves. It is better to avoid saying 'You are a good girl/boy not to cry!' or 'Aren't you brave!', but to let them cry and scream if it helps. Children tend to be more accepting of comfort if they have been allowed to express their anger. Nurses, however, can demonstrate their concern and sympathy by attending to the child and by providing comfort when the child is calmer.

Children's understanding of their hospital experiences

The child's understanding of their experiences is largely dependent on their level of cognitive development. Young infants in the sensorimotor stage of cognitive development tend to react mostly to input from their senses. Their very helplessness and their need to develop a sense of security means that the provision of comfort is an important way of helping them cope.[78] A distressed infant can sometimes be reassured by touch, such as wrapping him snugly in a bunny rug and patting him on the bottom until he is calmer. Self-comforting coping strategies, such as thumb sucking, are typical strategies of infants and toddlers.[73]

As children develop cognitively, their need to understand what is happening, or what might happen to them while in hospital, becomes more urgent. Explanations need to be tailored to the child's ability to understand.

Young children are particularly likely to be distressed by invasive procedures,[73] especially if the procedures are painful. Children need to know that nurses understand their anxiety about painful procedures.

Fernald and Corry compared the effectiveness of 2 explanations in helping children cope with an injection.[79] One group of children was prepared with the following 'empathic' explanation:

'I'm not doing this because you did anything wrong, but just to help you get well . . . In a minute, I'm going to stick you. You're probably feeling a little scared and its going to hurt a little bit, but it won't last long. And I don't mind if you cry because that's only natural.'

The other group was prepared with a more 'directive' explanation which was aimed at eliciting the child's cooperation, so that the procedure might be concluded promptly and with a minimum of fuss.

'In a minute, I'm going to stick you. I want you to stay still and not move because if you jerk your arm or flex, I may have to stick you again.'

Table 9.1 The child's response to pain

The following table illustrates some of the beliefs young children hold about injury. The second column lists some of the procedures which conflict with the child's belief, and the third column gives some of the typical responses directed at those carrying out the treatments.

Child's belief	Treatments and their reasons	Child's response
Healing and recovery are accomplished by resting the injured part and leaving it undisturbed.	Children are encouraged to move the injured part and dressings are changed daily.	Extreme resistance to weight bearing and any attempt to remove dressings.
Moving and touching sore parts causes pain.	Burnt areas are washed and limbs are exercised.	Screaming, kicking biting or pleading statements such as 'I can't move it — it's broken!'
Creams and bandages help wounds heal quickly. When they are taken off the wound should look better.	Removal of dressings often causes pain. Raw areas are exposed and often bleed during the bathing regimen. The appearance of the burn changes daily, and to the child and his parents, does not always appear to be healing.	Disbelief at the appearance of the wound. Comments such as 'You're skinning me';[6] 'Stop making it worse'; 'I'll be good if you stop'; 'You're trying to kill me'; and 'I want the other nurse'.

From Brodie L. Stop! You're hurting me. *Nursing in Australia* 1984; 2: 40–44.

Ten per cent of the children who were exposed to the empathic explanation cried, compared with 52 per cent of those who were given the directive explanation. The directive group exhibited more angry behaviour, were more likely to flinch and less likely to cooperate. Fassler found that children who were encouraged to express their fears and were given the opportunity to play with syringes and give dolls an injection were less anxious, cried less and were more cooperative than those who were given no interventions.[80]

A sound understanding of children's beliefs about the nature of pain, the causes of illness and how healing occurs can provide a good starting point from which to empathise with the child who is trying to cope with pain and with painful procedures. Brodie observed burned children's responses to treatment over several years and concluded that many of the beliefs that children have about pain and healing are in direct conflict with many treatment procedures (**Table 9.1**).[81]

Jerrett asked 5 to 9-year-old children what helped them feel better when they were in pain.[82] Their responses were classified into 3 categories: (1) direct action physical activities such as massaging, bathing or bandaging; (2) avoidance activities such as 'trying to think of other things' or reading; and (3) help-seeking activities such as seeking help from a parent or 'taking medicine'. Gonzalez, Routh and Armstrong trained mothers to distract their child during painful procedures.[83] Mothers talked to their children about events unrelated to the procedure (such as their pets at home). They found that this technique was more effective in relieving the child's distress than was mother's reassurances about the progress of the procedure (such as 'It's almost over!').

Young children have difficulty in differentiating between the structure and function of various body parts. As children mature, they begin to realise that organs have specific characteristics and functions, for example hearts must beat to keep people alive. The child, however, may have many misconceptions about the structure and functions of organs and how the various organs operate in relation to each other. For example some children believe that swallowing chewing gum is dangerous because it can wrap itself around the heart and make it stop beating. One child explained that the 'the appendix is just like Kleenex, made of tissue'.[84] A 6-year-old girl believed that a broken leg meant that the leg broke off, just like her doll's broken leg.

While the school-aged child has a limited understanding of the internal workings of her body, she is capable of understanding a great deal better if explanations include concrete representations such as models or drawings. With ingenuity and imagination, nurses can help children by making the more abstract and less obvious aspects of illness, more concrete so that the child can understand what has happened and how healing can be promoted. A tongue depressor, for example, wrapped in tissues and broken can simulate a fractured limb. Layers of tissues can become layers of skin to illustrate partial and full thickness burns.

During middle childhood, when a sense of mastery is critical for self-esteem, lack of privacy or threats to self-control may be of particular concern.[70] Strategies aimed at mastery and control are likely to predominate at this age.[78] For this reason, older children may benefit by being allowed to participate in decisions about their care.[70]

At this age, friends are important. A nurse, for example, could encourage a hospitalised 12 year old to write to his friends at school, and to request return letters. Parents can be encouraged to ask their child's special friend to visit. The child's teacher can be asked to arrange for the child's class to send him a get well card or write letters.

Hospital may be especially difficult for adolescents because of separation from friends and the loss of important social opportunities. Adolescents needed to be given direct information about their progress and to be fully consulted by health professionals when decisions are made about their treatment. Negative reactions may be exacerbated if they are treated like children by health professionals.

Understanding the way that a particular child interprets such experiences can form a sound basis from which to provide support. This seems to be equally true for adolescent patients. Favaloro and Touzel[86], for instance found that adolescents may not admit pain because they do not wish to be given an injection and that adolescent males were more likely to under-rate their pain than females. They also found that some adolescents felt that nurses knew when they were in pain and it was not, therefore, necessary to request pain relief medication.

Stevens identified 4 emotion-focused strategies and 2 problem-focused strategies which adolescents used to cope with the stress of hospitalisation.[86] The emotion-focused strategies were: (1) using distracting thoughts such as thinking about visiting Disneyland; (2) withdrawing from the situation by lying still or sleeping; (3) saving themselves from embarrassment by exercising control over their feelings; and (4) seeking support from their mothers, from nurses and from their friends. The 2 problem-focused strategies were: (1) yelling or crying during painful procedures; and (2) attempting to gain control such as demanding medication for pain relief.

Adolescents need to have explanations given to them directly, not via their parents. They need the opportunity to ask questions and to have them answered seriously and comprehensively. Many adolescents are not sufficiently assertive to deal with intimidating health professionals who have not recognised the need for information and reassurance.

THE EFFECTS OF HOSPITALISATION ON PARENTS

The hospitalisation of a child is stressful for parents and they also need support.[39,73] Children are likely to be affected by their parent's anxiety,[87] but parents cannot support their children adequately when their own physical and emotional resources are depleted. Perceptive and vigilant nurses will find many opportunities to reduce the impact.

Terry studied the needs of parents of hospitalised children.[88] She found that they were often feeling torn by the conflicting demands of the hospitalised child and the rest of the family.

To cope with the stress, parents also need to be able to preserve their own well-being. While information about the child's progress may be one of the parents' greatest needs,[89] they also need to feel that they are contributing to the child's care. Parents are more likely to take a short break from the hospital ward if they felt that the nurses were also concerned about the child's welfare. As many parents now stay in hospital with their children, it is increasingly becoming part of the nurses' role to provide support for parents, so that they may, in turn, continue to help their children. Nurses, for instance, can perform an important service to patients and to their parents by their willingness to keep a watchful eye on the child, while parents takes a well-needed break. Some parents feel unable to help their children and feel envious of nurses who have the skills to help the child medically.[39] Pointing out the special nature of the parents' role in helping the child cope with hospital can be helpful.

Helping the Child Manage the Stresses of Illness and Hospitalisation

THERAPEUTIC PLAY

Play is one of the most therapeutic strategies for helping children adjust to stressful situations. It can provide data on which to base more informed assessments of the child's thoughts and feelings and thus enable health professionals to reach a greater understanding of the child's point of view.[90] During play, for instance, a child may say that a doll had to have a needle because it was naughty.

During play children can be distracted from the more anxiety-provoking aspects of hospital and illness. Play can reduce the boredom of confinement.[91] It can promote social activity among the children and thereby enable them to support each other. It has been found to be an effective means of helping children express and deal with their fears of hospital and medical procedures.[67,91–93] Therapeutic play may also benefit siblings of children with long-term illnesses.[93]

When health care professionals spend time and effort to provide play opportunities, the child's sense of self-worth can be enhanced. Play can also help them improve their control of situations, changing them from being passive recipients of health care, to being active participants in the health care process. It can be a useful means of providing information to children about their illnesses, about hospitals and about nursing and medical procedures. Finally, it can be a very useful method of helping children to develop effective coping strategies.[91]

Play is most likely to be therapeutic when it takes place in a non-threatening and supportive environment. Children need to understand that no distressing procedures will

---

Box 9.1 Recipe for playdough

1 cup of salt
$1^1/_2$ cups plain flour
$^1/_2$ cup water
2 tablespoons of oil

Mix the ingredients to a firm, but pliable dough. It will keep for several weeks in a plastic container. Do not keep in a refrigerator as it will become too moist. Food colouring may be added.

---

be carried out in the playroom, so that while they are in there they can feel secure. Supervising adults should be warmly accepting and supportive of the children.

A variety of materials should be available for the child to use freely as a means of self-expression. Dolls can be easily made out of old socks by filling them with rags and tying them off at the neck. Flexible tubing can be wrapped around the body to add limbs. The child can be encouraged to draw in the facial features or any other part of the body.

A variety of drawing materials should be available, such as paints, marking pens, crayons and pencils. Hospital props can be added to the playroom so that the child can act out situations that are sources of anxiety and thus express his fears and aggressions. Tubing can be provided for simulating drips. A kit can be made up containing bandages, strapping, catheters, plaster to make casts, syringes (without needles), gauze and cotton swabs, bandaids, masks, wooden tongue depressors, medicine cups, and so on. When supervision is available, children may be allowed to use equipment such as stethoscopes, auriscopes, reflex hammers, sphygmomanometers and unbreakable thermometers.

Useful toys may be added; inflatable bobo dolls can be a useful method of relieving aggressions and anxieties. These are weighted at the base so that when pushed over, they automatically return to an upright position. Playdough can be used to encourage relaxing play (see **Box 9.1** for a recipe). Books about children's hospital experiences can provide information and correct misconceptions.

Care should be taken that playrooms and materials are safe and appropriate to the child's developmental stage. Toddlers need to have barricaded areas that are safe but sufficiently large for them to explore.

Children can be assisted to act out scenarios that may be causing them anxiety. Dolls or puppets dressed like nurses, doctors and patients can stimulate dramatic play. The dolls may be used as effigies of nurses and doctors and be operated upon or injected and become a tool for the expression of aggressive feelings. Alternatively, dolls may be used as patients and provide a means for the expression of the child's anxieties. A doll's house, or if possible, a cubby house, may be set up like a hospital. Puppets can be used to enact reassuring scenes, such as parents leaving a child in hospital and *returning*, or where a child is admitted to hospital, gets better and *is discharged*. Children's drawings can be useful sources of information and provide means for the expression of fears (**Figures 9.1, 9.2**).

Children should be allowed to participate in play in their own time. They may be more willing to join the other children if they are permitted to watch the others play while their

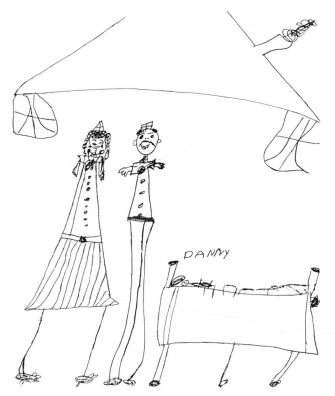

Figure 9.1 Drawing by Danny. Danny was a non-English-speaking child whose parents were unable to be in hospital with him. His drawing clearly shows his sense of being overwhelmed. He has drawn himself as disproportionately small and almost featureless. In contrast, the nurses are drawn larger than life and in great detail.

mother is present. Young children, who are anxious about being left, may be apprehensive of strangers and more clinging towards their mothers.

RELAXATION THERAPY

Relaxation is a useful form of stress management. It is based on the notion that tension and relaxation are incompatible states. Relaxation techniques take many forms ranging from isometric exercises to meditation.[94] Thematic imagery is a form of relaxation therapy that can be adapted for use with children.[95] It is a process of creating mental images centred around themes that promote relaxation.

In a paediatric setting, the most useful themes involve escaping to non-threatening, relaxing situations or places, achieving mastery over stressful situations, experiencing pleasurable and calming sensations. Basically, a child can be read to or told a story which develops any theme that is likely to promote relaxation and more effective management of stressful situations. It is not always easy to find an appropriate story, but with some initiative one can be devised. The main character in the story should be a child of the

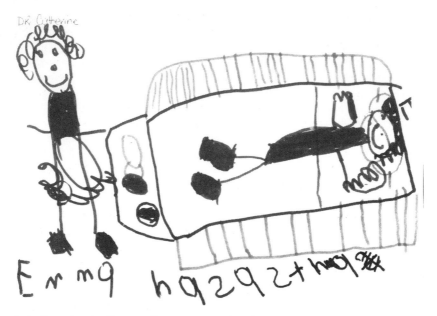

Figure 9.2 Drawing by Emma. Emma adapted to hospital well. Her family spend a large amount of time with her while she was in hospital and were very attentive to her needs. She has drawn herself as larger than 'Dr Catherine' and has depicted both in similar detail.

same sex, age and with the same disorder. Any characteristics can be included that help the child identify with the main character. The child's own name should not be used. The story should be woven around themes that will be soothing and *not exciting* to the child. The story should have a lead time into the theme, but, at the same time, the child's interest should be captured early in the story. The story should be told in a soft, flowing tone of voice, not in a staccato fashion. Below is an example of a script that may be used with children. It may be recorded onto a cassette tape so that a child can listen with earphones. The child should be in a comfortable position, either in a chair, in bed or on an adult's lap.

> Once upon a time there was a little boy called Athol. Athol was in hospital and he had his leg in plaster — just like you!
>
> One day Athol was sitting on the front doorstep of his house when a little pixie appeared in front of him and asked him what he was doing.
>
> Athol said to the pixie, 'I can't do anything because my leg is so heavy with this plaster on it.'
>
> The pixie said, 'Would you like to come with me to fairyland?'
>
> Athol said 'Yes, I'd like to do that.'
>
> 'Well,' said the pixie, 'come with me. It's a long way from here and you will have to come into the bush, but stand still while I sprinkle some magic silverdust on your foot so it won't be hard to walk.'
>
> The pixie pulled a little silver bag from his pocket and took out a pinch of some silverdust. He sprinkled it over Athol's foot, and it made a funny tinkling noise as it fell.

'Come on,' said the pixie, 'we have a long way to go.'

Athol got up off the step and was surprised to find that he could walk quite easily without getting tired or hurting his leg. He followed the pixie who walked slowly down the path to the bush that grew at the back of Athol's house.

They walked down a path that Athol had never seen before, even though he had played many times in the bush before. The path was brown dirt and part of it was covered with tiny little plants. Occasionally Athol could see little brown beetles slowly wandering along the path with the tiniest pieces of bark in their mouths. 'What are they doing?' he asked the pixie.

'They are taking bits of leaves and bark home to their nests to make soft beds for the baby beetles', said the pixie. 'They put them in a pile and the baby beetles lie on them and they feel lovely. Everything stops hurting the babies when they lie on these beds, because they are so soft.'

The path went on winding through the bush, and soon Athol and the pixie came to a small clearing. In the middle Athol could see a magic toadstool ring.

'Sit on one of the toadstools', said the pixie. Athol sat on one and as soon as he did he saw that there were many fairies standing in the middle of the toadstool ring. They were very beautiful, some had long golden hair and one had long brown hair which shone like it was made of silk. In the middle of the fairies Athol could see the loveliest of them all. She was dressed in the most beautiful golden dress, which had hundreds of tiny diamonds sewn on it. She was holding a wand which had a star on the end of it that sparkled like a sparkler.

'This', explained the pixie, 'is the fairy queen.' The fairy queen came up to Athol and said. 'Athol. I know you've been sick, but you're getting better now, and I'm so happy to see you.' She stroked him on his hand and Athol started to feel wonderful. He felt beautifully warm and his skin started to tingle. It was like having a little bit of pins and needles. The fairy queen told Athol to sit in one of the fairy's armchairs and watch the fairies dancing. Athol looked around and noticed rows of green, comfortable-looking armchairs around the toadstool ring. He sat in one of the them. Is was the most wonderfully comfortable seat he had ever sat in. It was made of a million soft pine needles, which were piled up in a mound and covered with moss that was as soft as velvet. When Athol sat in it, it felt very springy and he felt like he was floating. It also smelt wonderful, just as clean and fresh as a pine forest.

He sat in the sun and watched the fairies dancing. The wind swirled, rushed through reeds that were growing at the edge of the clearing, making musical sounds for the fairies to dance to. Athol could hear several birds adding their song to the wind's music. The fairies were very beautiful as they glided through their dance. Their silky flowing dresses drifted out behind them as they danced. The sun was warm on Athol's arms and he could feel a soft breeze that wafted gently over his face and brought with it the fragrance of the pine needles. Athol had never felt so wonderful before in his life. He felt completely contented. Gradually the fairies brought their dance to its close. The wind slowed down and the music grew quieter. The pixie who had brought Athol to fairyland came up to Athol and said softly, 'Athol it's time to go home now.' Athol rose from his seat and followed the fairy. He felt calm and didn't mind following the pixie to go home. They wandered back along the path until they came to Athol's place.

'Thank you, pixie', said Athol. 'I feel much better now. My leg doesn't hurt any more and it doesn't feel heavy. I wish I could go to fairyland every day.'

'But you can!' said the pixie.

'I couldn't find it', said Athol.

'You don't *find* fairyland, said the pixie, 'you just go there.'

'How?' asked Athol.

'You just think about it, that's the way to get to fairyland. You just have to remember what it's like and concentrate on it and you can go back there whenever you want to.'

'Can I watch the fairies dancing?'

'Of course', said the pixie.

'And sit in those wonderful fairy chairs?' asked Athol.

'Yes', said the pixie. 'All you have to do is remember it and you can go there as often as you wish. But if you forget what it is like, then you can't go there any more, unless someone from fairyland takes you there.'

'I won't forget it', said Athol. 'I'm going to go there every day.'

The pixie waved goodbye and Athol sat on the front doorstep of his house, but feeling so much better than he had before the pixie came.

Care of the Dying Infant, Child or Adolescent and their Families

In occupations such as nursing, where so many aspects of the work are psychologically demanding, caring for the dying child is one of the most difficult. In order to provide the best care, nurses need to communicate effectively and sensitively with both the child and the family.[96] Such communication requires a sound understanding of the ways in which people deal with major losses, together with insights into the ways that children of different ages understand the world. In addition, professionals working in this area need to be able to manage the impact of the work on their own mental health.

THEORIES OF GRIEF

Most of the theories developed to explain the processes of dying and bereavement describe a series of stages through which people progress.[69,97] The most well known of these theories is that of Elisabeth Kubler-Ross,[98] who outlined 5 stages. The 1st is a period of 'numbness' or denial which appears to be necessary for the person to have time to marshall resources before fully confronting their situation. Denial also allows the person to 'bring it out' when feeling more robust, and to 'put it away' when feeling more vulnerable. The 2nd stage begins when people initially confront the situation and grapple with their anger and with the question 'Why is this happening to me?'. At this time, anger may be displaced onto relatives or health professionals, for example a parent may 'unreasonably' complain of inattention from staff. The 3rd stage commences as the anger subsides and attempts are made to deal with feelings by bargaining. Bargaining may be expressed in the form of full compliance with treatment regimens, or seeking alternative cures, or prayer and so on. If the person becomes aware that these strategies are not working, then depression, the 4th stage, is a likely response. Eventually the dying person and family *may* come to terms with the situation with varying degrees of acceptance. This is the final stage. Progression through these stages is not necessarily sequential nor inevitable.

Conceptualising the bereavement process as a series of stages has its benefits. It facilitates understanding of the sometimes puzzling behaviours of people involved in a situation outside the experience of the nurse. Perhaps the major disadvantages to stage theories lie not so much with the theory but with the way it is interpreted. Health professionals may tend to regard Kubler-Ross's ideas as a *prescription* of how people ought to make sense of major losses rather than a description of how some people *actually cope*. In other words, the danger is that of making the person fit the theory, rather than the theory fit the person.

The stages concept may be applied too literally and the resultant pressure placed on people to conform is exemplified in such comments as 'You should be accepting this better than you are at this stage'; or, as a specialist physician told a patient 12 months after the death of her spouse, 'I think it's time you buried him'. Too rigid application of the concept to individuals may well be detrimental. All people do not proceed through the stages at the same rate, nor in the same order. At times the person may experience a confusing mixture of feelings from several stages. A further difficulty with the inflexible application of stage theories may be a feeling of failure on the part of those nurses who believe that their role is to 'get' a patient and family to the final stage prior to death.

A lesser known theoretical approach is that of Bugen.[99] Bugen claims that the more a grieving person believes that a death is preventable, the more *intense* the grief reaction. Grief is more *prolonged* when: (a) the bereaved feel a commitment to a deceased or dying person; (b) the deceased or dying person is seen as irreplaceable; and (c) when a close personal relationship exists. If any of these conditions are present, the relationship is described as 'central'. In the case of the sudden death of an infant, for example, since the relationship between parents and child is central, the parental grief process would be prolonged. Since they are likely to view the death as preventable, grieving is likely to be quite intense. Health professionals may regard the loss of a young patient from relatively minor surgery as preventable, and may thus be affected for a long time, although not as deeply as the child's parents.

COMMUNICATING EFFECTIVELY ABOUT DEATH AND DYING

There is much evidence in favour of frank and open discussion among all family members concerning the child's prognosis and its implications. Many studies have shown that children who are able to discuss their illness, treatment and prognosis with their parents in an open and honest way, adapt better than those whose parents 'protect' them.[100-102] There is also evidence that children who have survived a life-threatening illness, adjust better in the long term when they have been fully informed about the illness and its implications.[100]

A seminal study by Waechter in 1971 has convincingly illustrated the need of dying children to talk to adults about what is happening.[102] She measured the generalised anxiety levels of hospitalised children, some of whom had life-threatening illnesses and others who had chronic illnesses but favourable prognoses. The children were aged between 6 and 10 years. She found that the anxiety scores of the children with life-threatening illnesses were double those of the children with non-fatal prognoses. She then used pictures of children in hospital situations to elicit stories from the participants.

It was evident that the children identified with those in the pictures, especially in terms of symptoms and diagnoses. Even though most of the children with poor prognoses had not been told of their impending death, it was clear from the stories that all were aware of their prognoses. The stories of children who were not given opportunities to discuss their fears and prognoses tended to be imbued with feelings of isolation, alienation and a preoccupation with death.

The following passage comes from a story told by an 8-year-old girl with a recently diagnosed malignant tumour of the femur.

'She's in the hospital and the doctor is talking to her mother and father. She's sick — she's got cancer. She's very, very sick. She's thinking she wishes she could go home. She had an operation at the hospital but she didn't want it because she wanted to get out of hospital. This little girl dies — she doesn't get better. Poor little girl. This girl at the hospital, she has cancer. Her hip is swollen and her bone's broken. This little girl in the picture died and then they buried her. And then she went up to heaven. She didn't like it there because God wasn't there.'[102]

These results support the idea that children pick up cues from the changed behaviour of their parents. If their concerns are not addressed and their misconceptions remain uncorrected, anxiety can become overwhelming.

On the face of it, one might argue that there is little that one can do to relieve the anxiety of a child with a fatal prognosis. The fear of dying alone and unsupported, however, is undoubtedly worse than the fear of dying in the care of a loving family and concerned health professionals. The fear of living without being able to deal with one's anxieties may be worse than the fear of dying. Such feelings may unnecessarily disturb a child's last few months of life. The conclusion is clear. Children need honest and sensitive communication about their condition and prognosis from the time of diagnosis.

The benefits of such communication are not confined to the dying child. Memories of frank discussions with the child also appear to have long-term therapeutic effects for parents and for siblings.[103]

The failure of children to ask questions may be interpreted as a lack of concern. Indeed, adults may have an interest in interpreting the child's behaviour in this manner as it would relieve them of the difficulty of dealing with an enormously stressful situation. It is, however, more likely that such children are either unable adequately to articulate their concerns, or that the non-verbal messages from those around them are indicating that the subject is not open for discussion. In either case, the child and the family will benefit from help in opening up communication channels.

The research evidence clearly indicates the need for adults to communicate with children about death. The question remains 'How can we do it?' It is critically important that adults understand the meaning of the word 'death' to the child with whom they are trying to communicate.

The previous discussion demonstrates that effective communication about death and dying must not only be frank, it must also be consistent with the child's ability to understand the concept. Parents may need guidance from health professionals in beginning to discuss the situation openly with the child and other members of the family.

The development of the child's understanding of death must be considered when adapting information for children of different ages,[104–109] and has been described in detail in Part One of this book.

Information is better assimilated if it is given in manageable portions according to the child's attention span. For example, a healthy 4 year old may have an attention span of only a few minutes. Concentration of such a child may also be affected by both the disorder and its treatment. Selecting a time when the child is feeling sufficiently well to listen and when there will be a minimum of interruptions, may be fruitful.

Checking out the child's question will enable the person to answer the precise question the child is asking. For example, a child who asks 'When will I get better?' may mean 'Am I going to die?', or it could mean 'When will I stop feeling nauseated from chemotherapy?' In other words, it is important to check that you are answering the question actually being asked, not what you *think* is being asked.

Perhaps the most difficult question for adults to answer is 'Am I going to die?'. An open-ended reply such as 'It's difficult for me to know the answer to that question. Are you worried about dying?' will provide a starting point for discussion. Most children will appreciate the opportunity to express their feelings to a sympathetic and sincere adult.

COPING WITH DEATH

Children are frequently fascinated by the idea of death and it can permeate their games, their jokes and so on. Superstition is evident in their attempts to control death, such as the old ritual, 'Don't step on a crack or you'll break your mother's back', 'Hold your breath when you go past a graveyard or the ghosts will get you'.

Many adolescents seem to use a kind of denial as a defence, whereby they retain a lingering belief that death is something that happens to others and will not happen to them, or at least until they are much older. It is a kind of belief in one's own immortality.[110,111]

Parents reasonably expect their children to outlive them and the poignancy of the wasted potential affects everyone involved. When parents become aware that their child has a fatal prognosis, they may begin their 'grief work' before the child dies. Such a phenomenon is known as 'anticipatory grief'.[112] When parents are able to begin the grief process before the child's death, their sadness at the actual time of death may be modified by relief that the child is no longer suffering.[113,114] Knowing in advance, however, that the child's illness is terminal does not *necessarily* mean that parents will grieve in anticipation of the child's death or that such grieving will moderate their sorrow. Denial, for instance, may inhibit anticipatory grief.[112] When, however, the child outlives the prognosis and the dying process is more protracted than expected, anticipatory grief may outlive its usefulness.

Nevertheless, it is likely that parents who have time to prepare for the child's death, will cope better after the loss occurs than those who had little or no preparation time. Conversely, when a child takes longer to die than anticipated, parents may feel guilty that they have reached a stage where they have accepted the child's death while the child is still alive.[115] Nurses who understand the value of, and the problems surrounding anticipatory grief can facilitate the process. The role of parents is largely one of responsibility for the child's protection. In the normal course of events, parents are quite powerful in their ability to protect their children from both physical and emotional trauma, for example, the effectiveness of kissing the child better or applying a Bandaid. For many parents, when their child is terminally ill, the sense of being helpless is extremely difficult. The guilt associated with 'If only . . .' thoughts may be considerable and may be applied to one's self or to one's partner.

There is a great deal of variation in the ways that parents seek to cope with their feelings. Some need to gather as much information as possible to maximise their sense of control. Others rely more on the expertise of the health professionals. Fathers may grieve differently to mothers or parents may grieve differently to siblings. Misunderstandings may arise between family members who grieve in different ways. Counselling may identify these differences and enable family members to understand and accept them.

No matter what their preferred methods of coping, it is important that family members are aware of, and have access to as many resources as possible. It may be of use to help parents become aware of the resources available to them, and to encourage them to use, not only community resources, but practical help from neighbours, friends and family, sources of information, and sources of emotional, social, and financial help.

Sometimes it may help to act as a 'sounding board' to facilitate parent's clarification of their goals for the child's remaining life, such as filling their remaining lives with as many experiences as possible versus ensuring as normal a life as possible. It may be necessary to counsel parents that a radical change in lifestyle may be very disruptive to the child's denial. Familiarity and predicability interspersed with exciting events may be a better course.

All the family is under strain at this time and all need extra support.[116] The grief of fathers, for instance may not be acknowledged as well as that of mothers. A further problem is that dying children and their siblings most need enormous support from their parents at a time when parents may be least able to provide it. The demands on parents are immense, and they may feel pulled in many directions. Spinetta found that at times of disease exacerbation and when parents were preoccupied with the ill child, the maladaptive behaviour of siblings increased.[63] Parents may only be able to continue to meet such demands if they are well supported themselves.[45]

The Compassionate Friends is a group of parents who have suffered the loss of a child and have formed a support group. Based upon their experiences, they have developed a set of guidelines for nurses and doctors attending to the needs of parents of dying children. These guidelines are reprinted in **Box 9.2**.

The needs of siblings may be overlooked in the mistaken belief that they are not as affected as the ill child and the parents. They have, however, their own emotional ties to their brother or sister which must be dissolved.

Just as the dying child has a need for truthful and clear communication, so do siblings. Euphemistic explanations such as 'David has gone for a long sleep' may be confusing and frightening. Their belief in their own immortality may have been severely shaken. They may have faced extended absences of their parents during their brother's or sister's illness. It may have been necessary for them to stay in strange homes while their parents were preoccupied with the dying child.

Surviving siblings tend to adjust better to the loss if they are kept fully informed of the prognosis, have opportunities to be involved in caring for the dying child, if they are able to say goodbye both in the terminal phase and after death, if they attend the funeral, and if they are allowed to keep some of the dead child's possessions.[117] If a sibling wishes to see the body of the dead child, to say his own goodbye, he will manage better if he is fully and sympathetically prepared for what he will see, the appearance of the body, the look of the room and if the body is in a bed or a coffin.

It is important for children to be involved in the funeral because this allows them to participate in rituals that facilitate mourning. They should be able to express their feelings in the same way as adults around them. They should be prepared for the funeral by

Box 9.2 The Compassionate Friends: suggestions for doctors and nurses.

Prepare parents and siblings for what they will see before they see it. Explain beforehand the machines, tubes, needles etc.

Clean and bandage all you can before they come in.

If parents really want to watch, let them see what you are doing with their child. Let them lead in that decision. (They don't see the same things that you see.)

Anticipate their questions as much as possible. Avoid complicated terminology but don't talk down to families either.

ALWAYS TELL THE TRUTH. Tell them everything you know about their child's condition. Be honest in what you don't know. Tell them the numbers — blood pressure, temperature, pulse.

Let parents parent . . . they need to participate in the care of their sick child as much as possible. Later they need to be able to say 'I helped'.

Give parents permission to talk about their feelings, to be extremely tired, to CRY. Cry with them if you are truly sad.

Don't hide your feelings to protect them. You are in a position of authority and your permission (and modelling) gives their feelings validity.

Parents may not be accepting of bad news and cope by denial. Do be patient with parents as denial is a form of emotional protection and will disappear when an individual is ready. Everyone is on a different timetable. Recognise that sometimes there is a need to repeat explanations or information several times; parents in distress may absorb only a little of what you thought had been explained to them.

Reassure families that everything possible is being done. They won't systematically know or assume that. Keep on reassuring them that no method will be left untried in the attempt to save their child's life.

Take pictures of newborns who die and put them in the file in case parents want them in future weeks or months. (Many will.)

Make every effort to arrange for parents to be with the child at the moment of death if they want to be there. Please don't 'protect' parents from this opportunity. It will be extremely important in their later healing.

Refer to the child by name, especially after death.

Remember two things that concern parents most 'Will my child be in pain?' and 'Was my child afraid?' Be prepared to reassure as honestly as possible about these questions.

Try to treat parents equally in giving information and breaking news. Fathers need as much support as mothers.

Families judge you by your caring levels, as well as your medical skills. Convince them their child is special to you, that this is not 'just a job'.

Allow parent as much time as they need to be with their child (alone if they want) after death. This is vital for the healing process.

Box 9.2 (*continued*)

At the time of informing parents that their child has died, tell them what steps to take next. They are in shock (and disbelief) and will be confused and need direction and guidance. There is no such thing as 'expected death' when it happens.

Express your personal frustrations 'We try so hard, but sometimes nothing works', 'He was a wonderful child. It hurts us too that we couldn't save him.'

Touching is our most basic form of comfort and communication. Put your hand on their arms or your arm around their shoulders.

If possible, go to the visitation or funeral. It means more than you can imagine. Families will really appreciate your showing caring.

Most of the parents we've talked to have appreciated being asked about organ transplants. Parents who weren't asked felt left out or even insulted. However, parents need reassurances that their child's body will be treated with respect and dignity.

Don't expect the parents of a dying child to be logical or objective. Runaway emotions have left logic at the starting gate and it will take quite a while to catch up.

Don't 'hit and run'. If you must break sad news, don't rush away immediately. If you can't handle the situation sensitively, send or take along someone who can.

Care of parents whose child dies before reaching hospital

If a child is brought to hospital via ambulance DOA, please bring the child into the hospital setting to a suitable room where the parents may be given a humane leave-taking time.

Please understand that the surviving parents may have been involved in the same trauma or witnessed the event, or been told about it suddenly and will be in an extreme state of shock, fear, numbness or fright. Shock, trauma treatment or crisis therapy must be considered.

Do not allow a surviving bereaved parent to find his or her own way home.

Advise parents gently to see their own child. Call in a chaplain or a member of the Minister's Fraternal and allow the parents their own time for leave taking. Remember the child is still theirs although dead.

If one of the parents is injured and hospitalised consider the advisability of postponing the funeral until the parent can either see his dead child or is able to attend the funeral.

Ask if the parents wish to care for the dead child ... wash him or dress him or take a lock of hair.

Please don't destroy any of the dead child's clothing or belongings. Return them to the parents in a clean parcel, as if of great value. In most cases parents really want these and are most disturbed if they are not offered.

Do not expect the parents to make a decision to take a child off a life support system without a caring adviser being with them. (Parents have been sent to the car park or cafe to talk it over in the past.)

Box 9.2 (*continued*)

If an injured parent is in hospital for a long time, please allow privacy for the parent to grieve and for time alone with spouse and children. It may be necessary for crisis-care help for the surviving family.

Give parents information on the resources available for them in the community.

Send a social worker from the hospital to see how the family is coping and if they need further care.

Don't assume all anger is displaced, some of it is and needs to be ventilated and examined.

Don't give parents rationalisations about their child's death, such as 'Your child would have been a burden to you as he was.' Or, 'She just would have suffered if she had lived'. (This is the 'You're lucky he died routine'.)

Don't say 'You ought to be feeling better by now.' Nor anything else that implies a judgement about their feelings.

Don't point out they can always have another child or suggest they should be grateful for their other children. Children are not interchangeable; they cannot replace each other.

Don't suggest 'busy work' as grief therapy. Bereaved people know they need to have something to do, but they are extraordinarily tired for a long time, and whatever they do needs to have meaning and importance.

Don't be in a hurry to offer medication. There is a big difference between profound sadness and deep depression. Sad people are often medicated for depression unnecessarily.

REMEMBER: AS YOU TREAT THE PATIENT IN THE BED, YOU MUST BE CAREFUL NOT TO CREATE PATIENTS AROUND THE BED.

Reproduced with permission from The Compassionate Friends, Oak Brook, Illinois

simple, but complete, explanations of the service and the cemetery or crematorium procedure.

The way parents cope after the funeral may have consequences for siblings. For example, parental idealisation of the dead child may only promote guilt in remaining siblings that such a wonderful child died and they are still alive.

In summary, siblings are likely to adjust better to the loss of their brother or sister if they are fully involved in the family grieving process and rituals. When they are excluded they are denied the supports that are available to the adults in the family.

Child Abuse

Child abuse is usually categorised into 3 types: physical, emotional and sexual. There is, of course, difficulty in making sharp distinctions because all forms of abuse have emotional outcomes for the victim and sexual abuse has both physical and emotional elements. Sexual abuse is the involvement of children, who are too young to give informed consent, in inappropriate sexual activity. It may be violent or non-violent, committed by a stranger or a friend or family member. Most sexual abuses are committed by people who are known to the child.[118] The actual incidence of incest is difficult to estimate, because of reluctance by victims to report it and reluctance of adults to believe it.

Although it is possible only to speculate on the extent of child abuse, it seems that abuse is under-reported, particularly sexual abuse, with less than 10% of cases being notified.[119] The reasons for under-reporting are many. Sometimes the abuse is not evident, and at other times it is evident but denied. Recent media reports of prosecutions of innocent fathers for sexual abuse may have contributed to the reluctance of health professionals to report their suspicions, especially when the professionals are acutely aware that their feelings are *only* suspicions and may be based on incorrect assumptions. Other reasons for under-reporting include fears of media attention, of retribution, or of protracted and distressing court cases.

PSYCHOLOGICAL EFFECTS OF SEXUAL ABUSE

Children who are well supported by their families may recover without long-lasting effects. Incest tends to result in greater emotional harm than attacks by a stranger, because the harm is inflicted by those whom children normally expect will protect them.[120,121] Violent sexual abuse is more likely to result in serious emotional disturbance than non-violent abuse.[120]

Because father–son incest involves fears of homosexuality, it may be even more emotionally detrimental than father–daughter incest.[120] The boy develops a dislike and fear of his role model, which may turn into self-hatred. The situation for boys is exacerbated by male reluctance to identify themselves as victims and to discuss their feelings.

Incest which stops before adolescence seems to be less detrimental as guilt is more likely to be a problem in adolescence, when the child is more morally aware. The adolescent girl may be caught between fear of her father, and feelings of responsibility for keeping the family together.

RECOGNISING PARENTS AT RISK OF CHILD ABUSE

While there is no *typical* parent who is at risk of child abuse, there are some features that are more characteristic of abusing parents than others. It is also true, however, that many parents who possess these characteristics do not abuse their children. Assessment, therefore must be informed, judicious and sensitive.

Many parents who abuse their children, claim to have been abused by their parents[119,122,123] and to feel that they were deprived of love and affection during their childhood. Patterns of reacting to the stress of parenthood are often acquired from our parents and in the absence of appropriate models during childhood, it is more difficult to learn constructive coping patterns. The situation of such parents is exacerbated when, having been deprived of love and affection in childhood, they have unrealistic expectations of the ability of their own children to fulfil this need. The frustration and disappointment that comes from dealing with egocentric infants and children may be too much for the parent to accept. Scott (cited in Burns & Goodnow[124]) noted that an abusing father 'could not understand the child not wanting to play etc. not responding, not loving or understanding *me*'.

Oates reported research that suggests that abusing parents are more likely to have a lower self-esteem and more immature and impetuous personalities.[123] Immaturity tends to be expressed as self-centredness and a difficulty in understanding the needs of others. Such people are ill-equipped to cope with the exacting demands of child-rearing in modern society.

Abusing parents seem to lack effective parenting skills.[125] They tend to have poor knowledge of child development and therefore to have unrealistic expectations of the child's behaviour. They are more likely to threaten their children, to express disapproval of their behaviour, to use physical punishment and humiliation as disciplinary techniques, and to issue commands without explanation. Non-abusive mothers, on the other hand, are more likely to explain to their children why they should behave in certain ways, to seek their cooperation, to express approval of their behaviour, to demonstrate required behaviour and to laugh *with* their children rather than *at* them.[125]

Learning to be an effective parent is a complex process, and is easier if one has a strong support network. Many studies have found that abusing parents tend to have poorer social skills, to have minimal support from friends, family, the community in general or from their spouses and to be generally socially isolated.[124,126,127]

RECOGNISING THE ABUSED CHILD

There are certain children who are more likely to be abused than others. Research has shown that while 8% of the population was born prematurely, 24% to 40% of children who have been physically abused, were born prematurely.[128]

There are several reasons why this might be so. Early separation of infant and parents may have hindered the bonding process. Parents may find it more difficult to relate to the premature infant who is less physically attractive than a full-term infant and whose cries are sharper, more high-pitched and often more irritating.

Certain behaviour patterns in children seem to be associated with a history of abuse. The children tend to be excessively fearful, not turn to their parents for comfort when distressed, to be constantly watchful of adults and unusually compliant for their age group.[129]

Data from western countries on the characteristics of sexual abusers and their victims is generally consistent.[120] Studies show that, although children of all ages are sexually abused, victims are more likely to be female and to be aged between 11 and 14 years. Abusers are more likely to be male.[118] Most incest occurs between fathers and daughters, but also occurs between mother and son, father and son, mother and daughter, and brother and sister.[120] Most offences occur frequently and continue over a number of years.[120] The child is more likely to be coaxed into cooperation with threats or promises than to be forced to submit.

There are many physical and behavioural indicators that can raise suspicions in the mind of an observant adult. Children who present with trauma to the urinary, genital or rectal area or difficulty sitting or walking should be considered as possible victims of sexual abuse.[119,130] Unusually sophisticated sexual knowledge or complaints about sexual abuse should be attended to and acted upon. Perhaps the most reliable evidence of sexual assault is that the child tells you. Unfortunately, such children are often not believed. Many children will not tell an adult because they have been pressured, or even threatened, to keep the assault a secret.

REPORTING SUSPICIONS OF CHILD ABUSE

In most states of Australia, health personnel are legally required to report all known and suspected cases of sexual abuse. There are also moral reasons why it is important to report suspicions of child abuse. As victims tend to become psychiatric patients in adulthood, vital contributions to preventative psychiatry can be made by reporting cautiously acquired suspicions that are based on as much information as possible. Concerns about specific children can be aired with staff from the nearest sexual assault service. These services are located in public hospitals and community health centres in both urban and rural areas.

It is not unusual for parents to express fears that they may injure their children. Such fears should be responded to and counselling should be offered. Many abusing parents will be able to treat their children in more appropriate ways if they, themselves, are well supported.

Parents who abuse their children are also likely to be suffering difficulties and to have little help in dealing with them. If constructive work is to be done to rehabilitate them, it is crucial that health professionals avoid judgmental and aggressive attitudes towards them.

Summary

Paediatric nurses are well placed to identify families who are having difficulty coping with the stress of an ill child. They are also well placed to provide support for families and to act as a link between the families and other members of the health care team.

In order to do so effectively, nurses must be knowledgable about the kinds of stresses that illness imposes on families and must have an understanding of the ways that various members are likely to make sense of their experiences and react to stress.

There is a wealth of research literature that can form the basis for an understanding of the problems faced by families. The material in this chapter is intended to provide an overview of that literature. Nurses are likely to be most effective in creating a sensitive and supportive environment for families with sick children when knowledge, such as that outlined in this chapter, is combined with the wisdom acquired from the experience of working closely with families.

REFERENCES

1. Van Dongen-Melman, JEWM, Sanders-Woudstra JAR. Psychosocial aspects of childhood cancer: a review of the literature. *J Child Psychol Psychiatry* 1986; 27: 145–180.
2. Pless IB. Symposium on chronic disease in children: clinical assessment: physical and psychological functioning. *Pediatr Clin North Am* 1984; 31: 33–45.
3. MacLean WE, Perrin JM, Gortmaker S, Pierre CB. Psychological adjustment of children with asthma. Effects of illness severity and recent stressful life events. *J Pediatr Psychol* 1992; 17: 159–171.

4. Cowen L, Mok J, Corey M, Macmillen H, Simmons R, Levison H. Psychologic adjustment of the family with a member who has cystic fibrosis. *Pediatrics* 1986; 77: 745–753.

5. Drotar D, Doershuk CF, Stern RC, Boat CF, Boyer W, Matthews L. Psychosocial functioning of children with cystic fibrosis. *Pediatrics* 1981; 67: 338–343.

6. Johnson M, Muyskens M, Bryce M, Palmer J, Rodnan JA. Comparison of family adaptations to having a child with cystic fibrosis. *J Marital Family Ther* 1985; 11: 305–312.

7. Lemanek KL, Horwitz W, Ohene-Frempong K. A multiperspective investigation of social competence in children with sickle cell disease. *J Pediatr Psychol* 1994; 19: 443–456.

8. Lewis BL, Khaw K. Family functioning as a mediating variable affecting psycho-social adjustment of children with cystic fibrosis. *J Pediatr* 1982; 101: 636–640.

9. Lawler RH, Nakielny W, Wright N. Psychological implications of cystic fibrosis. *Can Med Assoc J* 1966; 94: 1043–1046.

10. McCollum A, Gibson L. Family adaptation to the child with cystic fibrosis. *J Pediatr* 1970; 77: 571–578.

11. Tropauer A, Franz MN, Dilgard VW. Psychological aspects of the care of children with cystic fibrosis. *In:* Moos RH, ed. *Coping with physical illness.* New York: Plenum, 1977.

12. Lazarus S, Folkman M. *Stress appraisal and coping.* New York: Springer-Verlag, 1984.

13. Lemanek KL. Research on pediatric chronic illness: new directions and recurrent confounds. [Editorial] *J Pediatr Psychol* 1994; 19: 143–148.

14. Barbarin OA, Chesler M. The medical context of parental coping with childhood cancer. *Am J Community Psychol* 1986; 14: 221–235.

15. Mattsson A. Long term physical illness in childhood: a challenge to psycho-social adaptation. *Pediatrics* 1972; 50: 801–811.

16. Blatti GM. Developmental aspects of childhood cancer. *Cancer Nursing* 1985; 8: 17–20.

17. Yoos L. Chronic childhood illnesses: developmental issues. *Pediatr Nursing* 1987; 13: 25–28.

18. Revell GM, Liptak GS. Understanding the child with special health care needs: a developmental perspective. *J Pediatr Nursing* 1991; 6: 258–268.

19. Santilli LE, Roberts MC. Children's perceptions of ill peers as a function of illness conceptualization and attributions of responsibility: AIDS as a paradigm. *J Pediatr Psychol* 1993; 18: 193–207.

20. Cohen R, Nabors L, Pierce K. Pre-schoolers' evaluations of physical disabilities: a consideration of attitudes and behaviour. *J Pediatr Psychol* 1994; 19: 103–112.

21. Harper DC, Wacker DP, Cobb LS. Children's social preferences towards peers with visible physical differences. *J Pediatr Psychol* 1986; 11: 323–342.

22. Boardway RH, Delamater AM, Tomakowsky J, Gutai JP. Stress management training for adolescents with diabetes. *J Pediatr Psychol* 1993; 18: 29–45.

23. Manne SL, Jacobsen PB, Gorfinkle K, Gerstein F, Redd WH. Treatment adherence difficulties among children with cancer: the role of parenting style. *J Pediatr Psychol* 1993; 18: 47–62.

24. Weist MD, Finney JW, Barnard MU, Davis CD, Ollendick TH. Empirical selection of psychosocial treatment targets for children and adolescents with diabetes. *J Pediatr Psychol* 1993; 18: 11–28.

25. Wysocki T. Associations among teen–parent relationships, metabolic control, and adjustments to diabetes in adolescents. *J Pediatr Psychol* 1993; 18: 441–452.

26. Hamlett KW, Pellegrini DS, Katz KS. Childhood chronic illness as a family stressor. *J Pediatr Psychol* 1992; 17: 33–47.

27. Allen J, Townley R, Phelan P. Family responses to cystic fibrosis. *Aust Paediatr J* 1974; 10: 136–146.

28. Burish TG, Bradley L, eds. *Coping with chronic disease. Research and applications.* New York: Academic Press, 1983.

29. Pless IB, Roghmann K, Haggerty RJ. Chronic illness, family functioning and psychological adjustment: a model for the allocation of preventative health services. *Int J Epidemiol* 1972; 1: 271–277.

30   Tew BJ, Laurance KM, Payne H, Rawnsley K. Marital stability following the birth of a child with spina bifida. *Br J Psychiatry* 1977; 131: 79–82.

31.   Quittner AL, DiGirolamo AM, Michel M, Eigen H. Parental response to cystic fibrosis: a contextual analysis of the diagnostic phase. *J Pediatr Psychol* 1992; 17: 683–704.

32.   Venters L. Familial coping with chronic and severe childhood illness: the case of cystic fibrosis. *Soc Sci Med* 1981; 15:287–289.

33.   Berenbaum J, Hatcher J. Emotional distress of mothers of hospitalised children. *J Paediatr Psychol* 1992; 17: 359–372.

34.   Haines C, Perger C, Nagy S. A comparison of the stressors experienced by parents of intubated and non-intubated children. *J Advanced Nursing* 1995; 21: 350–355.

35.   Holroyd J, Guthrie D. Family stress with chronic childhood illness: cystic fibrosis, neuromuscular disease and renal disease. *J Clin Psychol* 1986; 42: 552–561.

36.   Thompson RJ, Gil KM, Gustafson KE, George LK, Keith BP, Spock A, Kinney TR. Stability and change in the psychological adjustment of mothers of children and adolescents with cystic fibrosis and sickle cell disease. *J Pediatr Psychol* 1994; 19: 171–188.

37.   Markova I, Macdonald K, Forbes C. Impact of haemophilia on child-rearing practices and parental cooperation. *J Child Psychol Psychiatry* 1980; 21: 153–162.

38.   Koch A. 'If only it could be me': the families of paediatric cancer patients. *Family Relations* 1985; 34: 63–70.

39.   Able-Boone H, Dokecki PR, Smith MS. Parent and health care provider communication and decision-making in the intensive care nursery. *Children's Health Care* 1989; 18: 133–141.

40.   Cummings ST, Bayley HC, Rie HE. Effects of the child's deficiency on the mother: a study of mothers of mentally retarded, chronically ill and neurotic children. *Am J Orthopsychiatry* 1966; 36: 595–608.

41.   Cummings ST. The impact of the child's deficiency on the father: a study of fathers of mentally retarded and of chronically ill children. *Am J Orthopsychiatry* 1976; 46: 246–255.

42.   Kazak AE, Marvin RS. Differences, difficulties and adaptation: stress and social networks in families with a handicapped child. *Family Relations* 1984; 33: 67–77.

43.   Wyckoff PM, Erickson MT. Mediating factors of stress on mothers of seriously ill, hospitalised children. *Children's Health Care* 1987; 16: 4–12.

44.   Petrillo M, Sanger S. *Emotional care of the hospitalized child.* 2nd ed. Philadelphia: Lippincott, 1980.

45.   Cobb S. Social support as a moderator of life stress. *Psychosomatic Med* 1976; 38: 300–314.

46.   Kronenberger WG, Thompson RJ. The psychological adaptation of mothers of children with spina bifida: association with dimension of social relationships. *J Pediatr Psychol* 1992; 17: 1–14.

47.   Quittner AL, Glueckauf RL, Jackson DN. Chronic parenting stress: moderating versus mediating effects of social support. *J Personality Soc Psychol* 1990; 59: 1266–1278.

48.   Speechley KN, Noh S. Surviving childhood cancer, social support and parents' psychological adjustment. *J Pediatr Psychol* 1992; 17: 15–32.

49.   Thompson RJ, Gustafson KE, George LK, Spock A. Change over a 12-month period in the psychological adjustment of children and adolescents with cystic fibrosis. *J Pediatr Psychol* 1994; 19: 189–204.

50.   Canam C. Coping with feelings: chronically ill children and their families. *Nursing Papers* 1987; 19: 9–21.

51.   Hirose T, Ueda R. Longterm follow-up study of cerebral palsy children and coping behaviour of parents. *J Adv Nursing* 1990; 15: 762–770.

52.   Dahlquist LM, Czyzewski DI, Copeland KG, Jones CL, Taub E, Vaughan JK. Parents of children newly diagnosed with cancer: anxiety, coping and marital distress. *J Pediatr Psychol* 1993; 18: 365–376.

53.   Kupst M, Schulman J, Honig G, Maurer H, Morgan E, Fuchtman D. Family coping with childhood leukemia: one year after diagnosis. *J Pediatr Psychol* 1982; 7: 157–174.

54. Saddler AL, Hillman SB, Benjamins D. The influence of disabling condition visibility on family functioning. *J Pediatr Psychol* 1993; 18: 425–440.
55. Nagy S, Ungerer J. The adaptation of mothers and fathers to cystic fibrosis: a comparison. *Children's Health Care* 1990; 19: 147–154.
56. Kupst M, Schulman J, Honig G, Maurer H, Morgan E, Fuchtman D. Family coping with childhood leukemia: a two year follow-up. *J Pediatr Psychol* 1982; 7: 174–184.
57. Abramovitch R, Pepler D, Corter C. Patterns of sibling interaction among preschool-age children. *In:* Lamb ME, Sutton-Smith B, eds. *Sibling relationships.* New Jersey: Erlbaum, 1982.
58. Eiser C. *The psychology of childhood illness.* New York: Springer-Verlag, 1985.
59. Faux SA. Sibling relationships in families with congenitally impaired children. *J Pediatr Nursing* 1991; 6: 175–184.
60. Grossman FK. *Brothers and sisters of retarded children.* New York: Syracuse University Press, 1972.
61. Ferrari M. Chronic illness: Psychosocial effects on siblings — 1. Chronically ill boys. *J Child Psychol Psychiatry* 1984; 25: 459–476.
62. Lobato D, Faust D, Spirito A. Examining the effects of chronic disease and disability on children's sibling relationships. *J Pediatr Psychol* 1988; 13: 389–407.
63. Spinetta JJ. The sibling of the child with cancer. *In:* Spinetta JJ, Deasy-Spinetta P, eds. *Living with childhood cancer.* St Louis: Mosby, 1981.
64. Tritt SG, Esses LM. Psychosocial adaptation of siblings of children with chronic medical illnesses. *Am J Orthopsychiatry* 1988; 58: 211–220.
65. Ievers CE, Drotar D, Dahms WT, Doershuck CF, Stern RC. Maternal child-rearing behaviour in three groups: cystic fibrosis, insulin-dependent diabetes mellitus and healthy children. *J Pediatr Psychol* 1994; 19: 681–687.
66. Taylor SC. The effect of chronic childhood illnesses upon well siblings. *Maternal-Child Nursing J* 1980; 2: 109–116.
67. Rae WA, Worchel FF, Upchurch J, Sanner JH, Daniel CA. The psychosocial impact of play on hospitalised children. *J Pediatr Psychol* 1989; 14: 617–627.
68. Edwinson M, Arnbjörnsson E, Ekman R. Psychologic preparation program for children undergoing acute appendectomy. *Pediatrics* 1988; 82: 30–36.
69. Bowlby J. *Loss, sadness and depression. Attachment and loss.* Vol. 3. London: Hogarth Press, 1980.
70. May BK, Sparks M. School-age children: are their needs recognised and met in the hospital setting? *Children's Health Care* 1983; 11: 118–121.
71. Jacobson JL, Wille DE. Influence of attachment and separation experience on separation distress at 18 months. *Dev Psychol* 1984; 20: 477–84.
72. Savedra M. Parental responses to a painful procedure performed on their child. *In:* Azarnoff P, Hardgrove C, eds. *The family in child health care.* New York: Wiley & Sons, 1981.
73. Caty S, Ritchie JA, Ellerton ML. Helping hospitalized preschoolers manage stressful situations: the mother's role. *Children's Health Care* 1989; 18: 202–209.
74. Peterson L, Shigetomi C. One year follow-up of elective surgery child patients receiving preoperative preparation. *J Pediatr Psychol* 1982; 7: 143–148.
75. Gonzalez JC, Routh DK, Saab PG, Armstrong FD, Shifman L, Guerra E, Fawcett N. Effects of parent presence on children's reaction to injections: behavioural, physiological and subjective aspects. *J Pediatr Psychol* 1989; 14: 449–462.
76. Adams RE, Passman RH. The effects of preparing two-year olds for brief separations from their mothers. *Child Dev* 1981; 52: 1068–1070.
77. Passman RH, Longeway KP. The role of vision in maternal attachment: giving 2-year olds a photo of their mother during separation. *Dev Psychol* 1982; 18: 22–29.
78. Caty S, Ellerton ML, Ritchie JA. Coping in hospitalised children: an analysis of published case studies. *Nursing Res* 1984; 33: 277–282.

79. Fernald CD, Corry JJ. Empathic versus directive preparation of children for needles. *Children's Health Care* 1981; 10: 44–47.
80. Fassler D. The fear of needles in children. *Am J Orthopsychiatry* 1985; 53: 371–377.
81. Brodie L. Stop! You're hurting me. *Nursing in Aust* 1984; 2: 40–44.
82. Jerret M. Children and their pain experience *Children's Health Care* 1985; 14: 83–89.
83. Gonzalez JC, Routh DK, Armstrong FD. Effects of maternal distraction versus reassurance on children's reactions to injections. *J Pediatr Psychol* 1993; 18: 593–604.
84. Gellert E. Children's conceptions of the content and function of the human body. *Genetic Psychology Monograph 65* 1962: 293–450.
85. Favoloro R, Touzel B. A comparison of adolescents' and nurses' post-operative pain ratings and perceptions. *J Pediatr Nursing* 1990; 16: 414–416.
86. Stevens M. Coping strategies of hospitalised adolescents. *Children's Health Care* 1989; 18: 163–169.
87. Teichman Y, Rafael MB, Lerman M. Anxiety reaction of hospitalised children. *Br J Med Psychol* 1986; 59: 375–382.
88. Terry DG. The needs of parents of hospitalised children. *Children's Health Care* 1987; 16: 18–20.
89. McKay M, Hensey O. From the other side: parents' views of their early contact with health professionals. *Child: Care, Health Dev* 1990; 16: 372–381.
90. Gibbons MB, Boren H. Stress reduction. A spectrum of strategies in pediatric oncology nursing. *Nursing Clin North Am* 1985; 20: 83–103.
91. Gillis AJ. The effect of play on immobilised children in hospital. *Int J Nursing Stud* 1989; 26: 261–269.
92. Ellerton M, Caty S, Ritchie J. Helping young children master intrusive procedures through play. *Children's Health Care* 1985; 13: 167–173.
93. McEvoy M, Duchon D, Schaefer DS. Therapeutic play group for patients and siblings in a pediatric oncology ambulatory care unit. *Topics Clin Nursing* 1985; April: 10–18.
94. Smith JC. *Relaxation dynamics. Nine world approaches to self-relaxation.* Champaign, Ill: Research Press, 1985.
95. Lamontagne LL, Mason KR, Hepworth JT. Effects of relaxation on anxiety in children: implications for coping with stress. *Nursing Res* 1985; 34: 289–292.
96. Pantell RH, Lewis CC. Communicating with children in hospital. *In:* Thornton S, Frankenburg W, eds. *Child health care communication.* New York: Johnson & Johnson, 1983.
97. Kavanaugh R. *Facing death.* Baltimore: Penguin Books, 1972.
98. Kubler-Ross E. *On death and dying.* Macmillan: New York, 1969.
99. Bugen L. Human Grief: a model for prediction and intervention. *J Orthopsychiatry* 1977; 47: 196–206.
100. Carr-Greg M, White L. The child with cancer: a psychological overview. *Med J Aust* 1985; 143: 503-508.
101. Spinetta JJ. Adjustment and adaptation in the child with cancer: a 3-year study. *In:* Spinetta JJ, Deasy-Spinetta P, eds. *Living with childhood cancer.* St Louis: Mosby, 1981.
102. Waechter E. Children's awareness of fatal illness. *Am J Nursing* 1971; 6: 1168–1172.
103. Spinetta JJ, Deasy-Spinetta P, eds. *Living with childhood cancer.* St Louis: Mosby, 1981.
104. Anthony S. *The discovery of death in childhood.* New York: Basic Books, 1972.
105. Bluebond-Langer M. *The private worlds of dying children.* New Jersey: Princeton University Press, 1978.
106. Johnson-Soderberg S. The development of a child's concept of death. *Oncology Nursing Forum* 1981; 8: 23–26.
107. Lansdown R, Benjamin G. The development of the concept of death in children aged 5–9 years. *Child: Care, Health Dev* 1985; 11: 13–20.
108. Lonetto R. *Children's conceptions of death.* New York: Springer, 1980.
109. Nagy M. The child's theory concerning death. *J Genetics Psychol* 1948; 73: 3–27.

110. Freiburg KL. *Human development: a life span approach.* Boston: Jones & Bartlett, 1987.
111. Raphael B. *Anatomy of bereavement.* London: Hutchinson, 1984.
112. Sweeting HN, Gilhooley MLM. Anticipatory grief: a review. *Soc Sci Med* 1990; 30: 1073–1080.
113. Binger CM, Ablin AR, Feurstein MD, Kushner JH, Zoger S, Middelsen C. Childhood leukaemia: emotional impact on child and family. *N Engl J Med* 1969; 280: 414–418.
114. Natterson JM, Knudson AG. Observations concerning fear of death in fatally ill children and their mothers. *Psychosomatic Med* 1960; 22: 456–465.
115. Buckman R. *I don't know what to say.* London: Macmillan, 1988.
116. McCown DE. Concepts of loss and grieving. *In:* Schuster C, Ashburn S. *The process of human development.* 2nd ed. Boston: Little Brown, 1986.
117. Pettle SAM, Landsdown RG. Adjustment to the death of a sibling. *Arch Dis Childh* 1986; 61: 278–283.
118. Goldman RJ, Goldman DG. The prevalence and nature of child sexual abuse in Australia. *Aust J Sex, Marriage Family* 1988; 9: 94–106.
119. Powell MB. Investigating and reporting child sexual abuse: Review and recommendations for clinical practice. *Aust Psychologist* 1991; 26: 77–83.
120. Heilpern S. Paper on sexual abuse of children and incest. Child protection services. Department of Youth and Community Services, 1981.
121. Wagner WG. Brief-term psychological adjustment of sexually abused children. *Child Study J* 1991; 21: 263–276.
122. Martin HP. Abused children — what happens eventually. *In:* Oates K. *Child abuse: a community concern.* London: Butterworths, 1982.
123. Oates K. Parents who physically abuse their children. *Aust NZ J Med* 1984; 14: 291–296.
124. Burns A, Goodnow J. *Children and families in Australia.* Sydney: George Allen & Unwin, 1979.
125. Oldershaw L, Walters GC, Hall DC. Control strategies and noncompliance in abusive mother–child dyads. *Child Dev* 1986; 57: 722–732.
126. Rew N. Child abuse: a social or mental disease. *Aust J Early Childh* 1979; 4 June: 41–44.
127. Springthorpe BJ. A profile of child abuse in children attending a Sydney paediatric casualty — a controlled study. *In:* The battered child. Proceedings of the First National Australian Conference. Perth: Department of Community Welfare, 1975.
128. James D. Bonding: mothering magic or pseudo science. Selected Paper no. 40. Kensington: Foundation for Child and Youth Studies, 1985.
129. McRae KN, Longestaff SE. The behaviour of battered children — an aid to diagnosis and management. *In:* Oates K. *Child abuse: a community concern.* London: Butterworths, 1982.
130. Fore CV, Holmes SS. Sexual abuse of children. *Nursing Clin North Am* 1984; 19: 329–340.

Appendix A Percentile Growth Charts

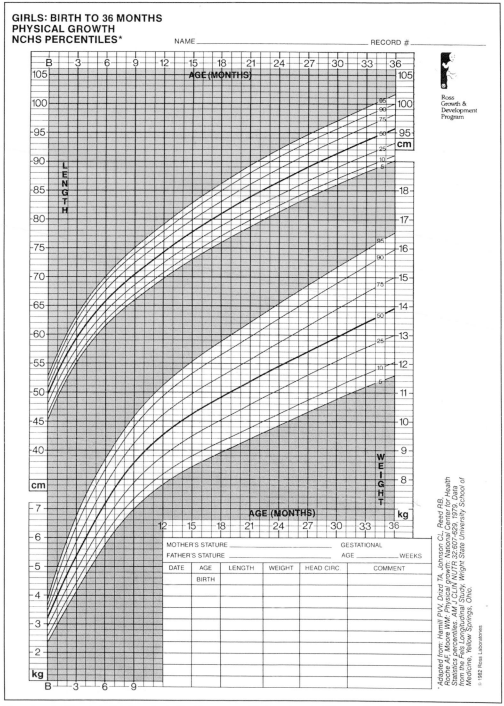

GIRLS: BIRTH TO 36 MONTHS
PHYSICAL GROWTH
NCHS PERCENTILES*

NAME _____ RECORD # _____

Ross
Growth &
Development
Program

* Adapted from: Hamill PVV, Drizd TA, Johnson CL, Reed RB, Roche AF, Moore WM: Physical growth: National Center for Health Statistics percentiles. AM J CLIN NUTR 32:607-629, 1979. Data from the Fels Longitudinal Study, Wright State University School of Medicine, Yellow Springs, Ohio.

© 1982 Ross Laboratories

Reproduced with permission from Australian Commonwealth Department of Human Services and Health.

Percentile Growth Charts — *continued*

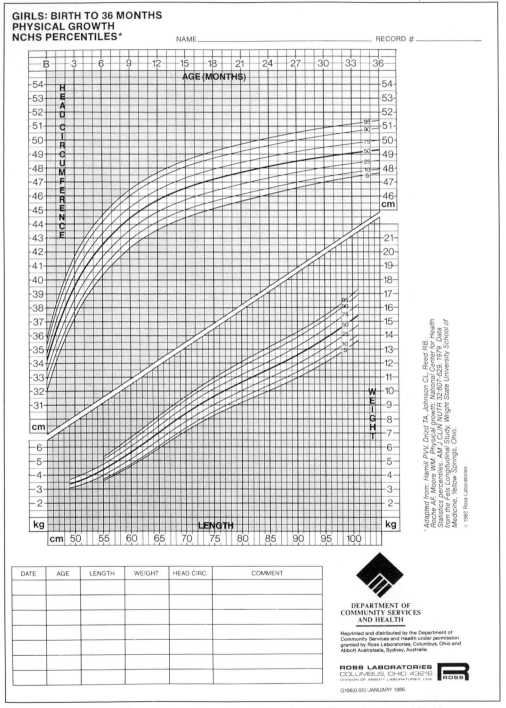

GIRLS: BIRTH TO 36 MONTHS PHYSICAL GROWTH NCHS PERCENTILES*

NAME _____ RECORD # _____

Reproduced with permission from Australian Commonwealth Department of Human Services and Health.

Percentile Growth Charts — *continued*

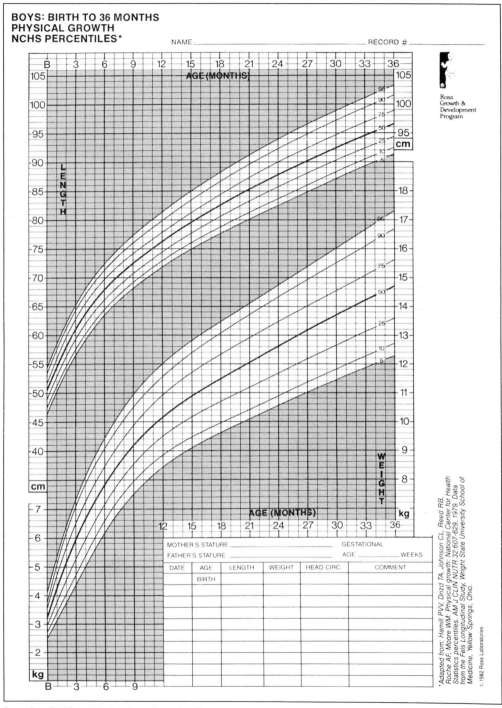

**BOYS: BIRTH TO 36 MONTHS
PHYSICAL GROWTH
NCHS PERCENTILES***

Reproduced with permission from Australian Commonwealth Department of Human Services and Health.

Percentile Growth Charts — *continued*

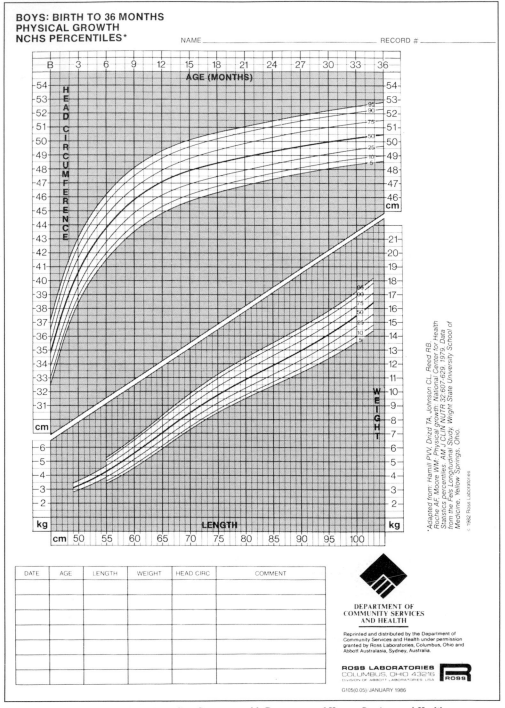

Reproduced with permission from Australian Commonwealth Department of Human Services and Health.

Percentile Growth Charts — *continued*

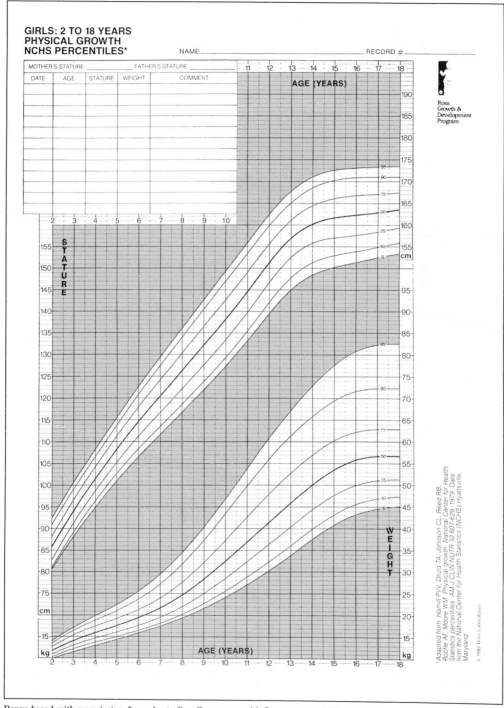

GIRLS: 2 TO 18 YEARS
PHYSICAL GROWTH
NCHS PERCENTILES*

Reproduced with permission from Australian Commonwealth Department of Human Services and Health.

Percentile Growth Charts — *continued*

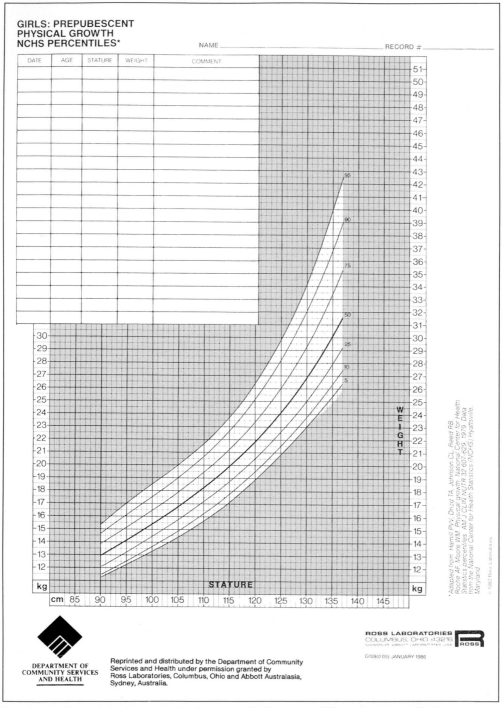

GIRLS: PREPUBESCENT
PHYSICAL GROWTH
NCHS PERCENTILES*

Reproduced with permission from Australian Commonwealth Department of Human Services and Health.

Percentile Growth Charts — *continued*

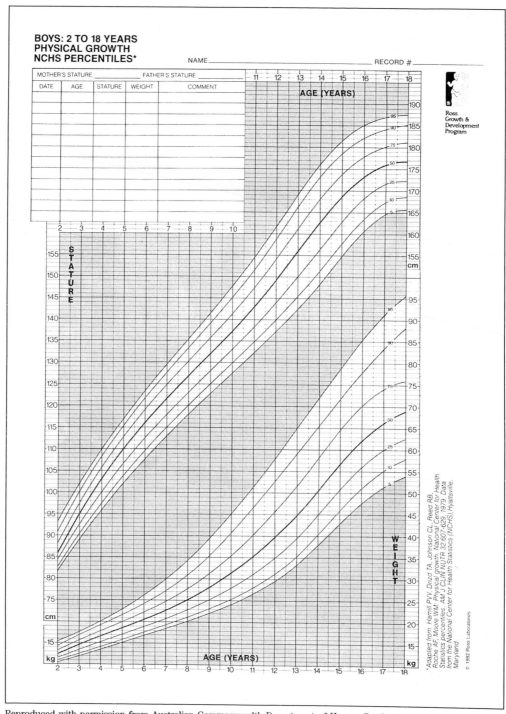

BOYS: 2 TO 18 YEARS
PHYSICAL GROWTH
NCHS PERCENTILES*

Ross
Growth &
Development
Program

© 1982 Ross Laboratories

Reproduced with permission from Australian Commonwealth Department of Human Services and Health.

Percentile Growth Charts — *continued*

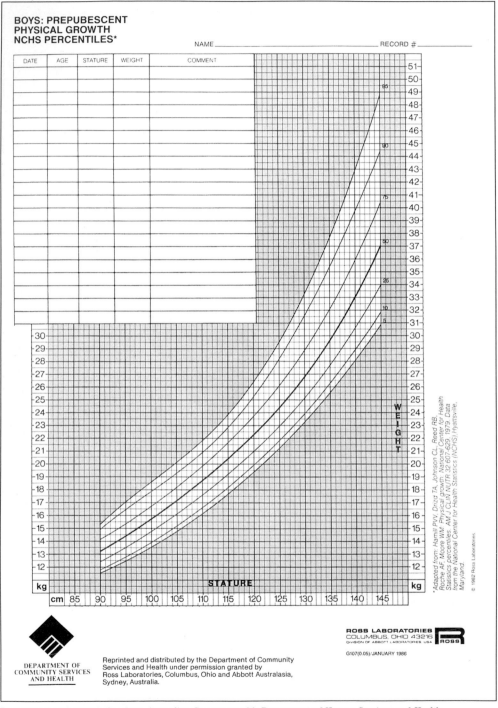

Reproduced with permission from Australian Commonwealth Department of Human Services and Health.

Appendix B   Neurological Observation Charts
Glasgow Coma Chart (Modified)

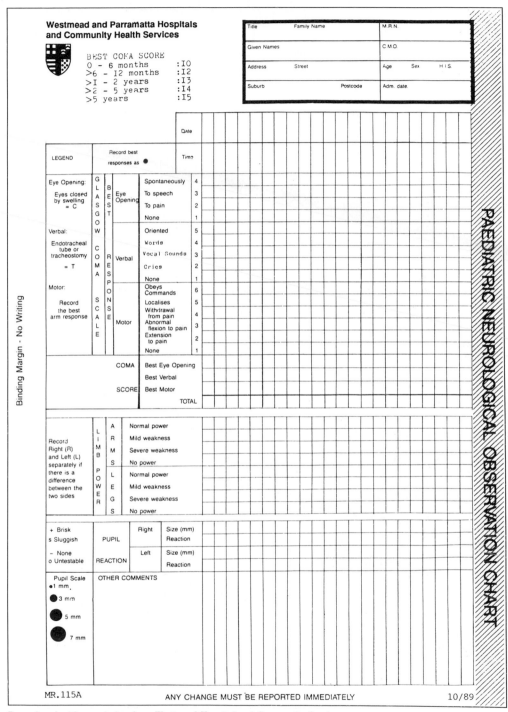

9

Neurological Observation Charts — *continued*

THE ADELAIDE PAEDIATRIC COMA SCALE
— EXPECTED NORMAL SCORES —

			BIRTH	>6 MONTHS	>12 MONTHS	>2 YEARS	>5 YEARS
Eyes Open	4	Spontaneous					
	3	To Speech					
	2	To Pain					
	1	None					
Best Verbal Response	5	Orientated					
	4	Words					
	3	Vocal Sounds					
	2	Cries					
	1	None					
Best Motor Response	6	Obeys Commands					
	5	Localises					
	4	Withdrawal from pain					
	3	Abnormal flexion to pain					
	2	Extension to Pain					
	1	None					
		TOTALS					

The above chart shows the expected normal scores for different age groups, as follows:

Eye Opening
No modification of the adult scale was needed in this category. The normal score, for all age groups, is 4.

Best Verbal Response
We assume that during the first 6 months of life the normally conscious infant will cry or grunt spontaneously or when disturbed; the expected normal score is therefore 2.

Between 6 and 12 months, the normal infant babbles and begins to vocalise; the expected normal score is 3.

After 12 months, recognisable and relevant words are expected, and the normal score is 4.

By 5 years, orientation, defined as awareness of being in hospital, or ability to give his/her name, is expected; the normal score is 5.

Best Motor Response
Motor responses are recorded in a 6 point scale.
However, the paediatric scale recognises that before the age of 6 months, the best normal response is withdrawal from pain; this scores 4.

In the period 6 months to 2 years, it is assumed that the normal infant will localise pain but will not obey commands; the normal score is 5.

Beyond 2 years, the normal score is 6.

Thus the normal aggregate scores at different ages are as follows:

Birth - 6 months	: 10
>6 - 12 months	: 12
>1 - 2 years	: 13
>2 - 5 years	: 14
>5 years	: 15

Reproduced with permission from Women's and Children's Hospital, Adelaide.

Appendix C   Vaccination Schedule

NHMRC Standard Childhood Vaccination Schedule
(August 1994)

AGE	DISEASE	VACCINE
2 months	Diphtheria, tetanus and pertussis	DTP - Triple antigen
	Poliomyelitis	OPV - Sabin vaccine
	Haemophilus influenzae type b (Hib) (Schedule 1 or 2)**	Hib vaccine (a or b or c)*
4 months	Diphtheria, tetanus and pertussis	DTP - Triple antigen
	Poliomyelitis	OPV - Sabin vaccine
	Hib (Schedule 1 or 2)**	Hib vaccine (a or b or c)*
6 months	Diphtheria, tetanus and pertussis	DTP - Triple antigen
	Poliomyelitis	OPV - Sabin vaccine
	Hib (Schedule 1 only)**	Hib vaccine (a or b)*
12 months	Measles, mumps and rubella	MMR
	Hib (Schedule 2 only)**	Hib vaccine (c)*
18 months	Diphtheria, tetanus and pertussis	DTP - Triple antigen
	Hib (Schedule 1 only)**	Hib vaccine (a or b)*
Prior to school entry (4-5 years)	Diphtheria, tetanus and pertussis	DTP - Triple antigen
	Poliomyelitis	OPV - Sabin vaccine
10-16 years	Measles, mumps and rubella	MMR
Prior to leaving school (15-19 years)	Diphtheria and tetanus	ADT - Adult diphtheria and tetanus
	Poliomyelitis	OPV - Sabin vaccine

*   Abbreviations for Hib vaccines - (a) is HbOC ['HibTITER']; (b) is PRP-T ['Act-HIB']; (c) is PRP-OMP ['PedvaxHIB'].

** There are two different schedules for Hib vaccines. Schedule 1 Hib vaccination applies to the use of HbOC and PRP-T. The selected vaccine is given at 2, 4, 6, and 18 months. Schedule 2 Hib vaccination refers to the use of PRP-OMP. This vaccine is given at 2, 4, and 12 months.

Note that a 4th Hib vaccine (PRP-D; 'ProHIBit') is approved for use as single injection for children over 18 months of age.

All of the vaccines in the standard schedule, except OPV, are given by deep subcutaneous or intramuscular injection. OPV is given orally. OPV should never be injected.

NHMRC   National Health and Medical Research Council

NH&MRC, The Australian immunisation procedures handbook 5th ed. The Council Canbera 1995. Commonwealth of Australia copyright, reproduced with permission.

Index

All index entries numbering from **page 695** *onwards occur in* **Volume 2**